CONTENTS

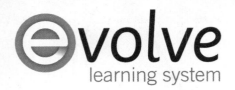
evolve
learning system

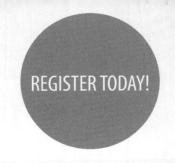
REGISTER TODAY!

To access your Student Resources, visit the web address below:

http://evolve.elsevier.com/Sorrentino/essentials/

Register today and gain access to:

- **Video Clips**
  Demonstrate important steps in procedures included in this textbook

- **Audio Glossary**
  Provides definitions of all key terms in addition to audio pronunciations for selected key terms

- **Useful Spanish Vocabulary and Phrases**
  Includes helpful translations of common healthcare terms and phrases

- **Skills Evaluation**
  Reviews procedures that may be covered on competency evaluations

- **Checklists**
  Allow for instructor use and student self-evaluation

- **Body Spectrum**
  Provides interactive review of Anatomy and Physiology content

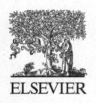
ELSEVIER

4ᵀᴴedition

MOSBY'S
Essentials
for NURSING
ASSISTANTS

SHEILA A. SORRENTINO, PhD, RN
Curriculum and Health Care Consultant
Anthem, Arizona

LEIGHANN N. REMMERT, BSN, RN
Clinical Instructor, Capital Area School of Practical Nursing
Springfield, Illinois

Retired Author
BERNIE GOREK, BS, MA
Gerontology Consultant
New England, North Dakota

MOSBY

ELSEVIER

3251 Riverport Lane
St. Louis, Missouri 63043
800-545-2522

MOSBY'S ESSENTIALS FOR NURSING ASSISTANTS   ISBN: 978-0-323-06621-1

NOTICE

The content and procedures in this book are based on information currently available. They were reviewed by instructors and practicing professionals in various regions of the United States. However, agency policies and procedures may vary from the information and procedures in this book. In addition, research and new information may require changes in standards and practices.

Standards and guidelines from the Centers for Disease Control and Prevention (CDC) and the Occupational Safety and Health Administration (OSHA) may change as new information becomes available. Other federal and state agencies also may issue new standards and guidelines. So may accrediting agencies and national organizations.

You are responsible for following the policies and procedures of your employer and the most current standards, practices, and guidelines as they relate to the safety of your work.

To the fullest extent of the law, neither the Publisher nor the authors or editors assume any liability for any injury and/or damage to persons or property as a matter of products liability, negligence or otherwise, or from any use or operation of any methods, products, instructions, or ideas contained in the material herein.

Library of Congress Cataloging-in-Publication Data

Sorrentino, Sheila A.
 Mosby's essentials for nursing assistants / Sheila A. Sorrentino, Leighann N. Remmert, Bernie Gorek. -- 4th ed.
  p. ; cm.
 Includes bibliographical references and index.
 ISBN 978-0-323-06621-1 (pbk.)
 1. Nurses' aides--Handbooks, manuals, etc. 2. Care of the sick--Handbooks, manuals, etc.
 I. Remmert, Leighann N. II. Gorek, Bernie. III. Title. IV. Title: Essentials for nursing assistants.
 [DNLM: 1. Nurses' Aides. 2. Nursing Care--methods. WY 193 S714m 2010]
 RT84.S666 2010
 610.7306'98--dc22

            2009042169

Executive Editor: Susan R. Epstein
Senior Developmental Editor: Maria Broeker
Publishing Services Manager: Jeff Patterson
Designer: Jessica Williams

Printed in the United States of America

Last digit is the print number: 9 8 7 6 5 4

DEDICATION

To my cousins, Pat and Buck (Everett),
for the caring and kindnesses
shown to my parents and me over the years.
Love,
Sheila

To Colin and Gracie,
for the joy, laughter, and love
you have brought into my life.
Love,
Aunt Leighann

To Kip and Luckie Greig, my loyal, forever friends.
Bernie

ABOUT THE AUTHORS

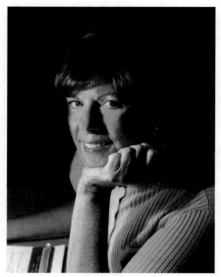

http://www.spindelvisions.com

Sheila A. Sorrentino is currently a curriculum and health care consultant focusing on effective delegation and partnering with assistive personnel in hospitals, long-term care centers, and home care agencies.

Dr. Sorrentino was instrumental in the development and approval of CNA-PN-ADN programs in the Illinois Community College System and has taught in nursing assistant, practical nursing, associate degree, and baccalaureate and higher degree programs. Her career includes experiences as a nursing assistant, staff nurse, charge nurse, head nurse, nursing educator, assistant dean, dean, and consultant.

A Mosby author since 1982, Dr. Sorrentino is the author of *Mosby's Textbook for Nursing Assistants* and several other textbooks for nursing assistive personnel. She was also involved in the development of *Mosby's Nursing Assistant Video Skills* and *Mosby's Nursing Video Skills,* winner of the 2003 AJN Book of the Year Award (electronic media). An earlier version of nursing assistant video skills won the 1992 International Medical Films Award on caregiving.

Dr. Sorrentino has a bachelor of science degree in nursing, a master of arts degree in education, a master of science degree in community nursing, and a PhD in higher education administration. She is a member of Sigma Theta Tau International, the Honor Society of Nursing, the Rotary Club of Anthem (Anthem, Arizona), the Provena Senior Services Board of Directors (Mokena, Illinois), and former member and chair of the Central Illinois Higher Education Health Care Task Force. She also served on the Iowa-Illinois Safety Council Board of Directors and the Board of Directors of Our Lady of Victory Nursing Center in Bourbonnais, Illinois.

In 1998 she received an alumni achievement award from Lewis University for outstanding leadership and dedication in nursing education. In 2005 she was inducted into the Illinois State University College of Education Hall of Fame. Her presentations at national and state conferences focus on delegation and other issues relating to nursing assistive personnel.

Dr. Sorrentino sponsors two nursing scholarships. One is for a senior high school student from her high school alma mater intending to major in nursing, and another is for a nursing assistant working at one of the three agencies in which she worked during and after college (Heritage Manor, Peru, Illinois; Illinois Valley Community Hospital, Peru, Illinois; and St. Margaret's Hospital, Spring Valley, Illinois).

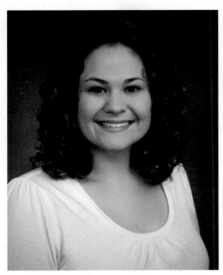

Terry Farmer Photography

Leighann N. Remmert is currently a clinical nursing instructor at the Capital Area School of Practical Nursing in Springfield, Illinois. She supervises, instructs, and evaluates student learning in various long-term care and acute care settings.

Graduating summa cum laude, with highest honors, Leighann received her bachelor of science degree in nursing from Bradley University in Peoria, Illinois. She was selected as the student representative to address the faculty, families, and classmates in attendance at the nursing department's pinning ceremony for her graduating class. Leighann is pursuing a master's degree in nursing education at Southern Illinois University Edwardsville. She is a member of Sigma Theta Tau International, the Honor Society of Nursing.

Leighann's background includes the roles of nursing assistant/tech, nurse extern, staff nurse, charge nurse, nurse preceptor, and trauma nurse. As a nursing assistant/tech and extern, Leighann acquired diverse clinical experience in the areas of general-medical, intermediate care, pediatric, cardiac, oncology, emergency, and post-surgical nursing at St. John's Hospital in Springfield, Illinois. As a registered nurse, Leighann concentrated in the area of emergency nursing at Memorial Medical Center in Springfield, Illinois. She is certified as a Trauma Nurse Specialist and a basic life support instructor. Leighann is licensed as an Emergency Communication Registered Nurse (ECRN) and is certified in Pediatric Advanced Life Support (PALS) and Advanced Cardiac Life Support (ACLS).

Leighann and her husband, Shane, volunteer as senior high youth sponsors at Elkhart Christian Church in Elkhart, Illinois. Leighann regularly participates in community blood drives and instructs CPR and First Aid training courses for the church and community.

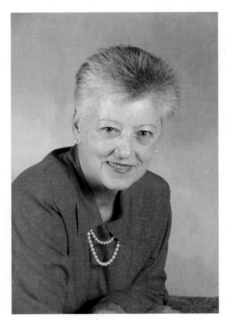

Photos by Jonathan

Retired author **Bernie Gorek** is a gerontology consultant. She received her nursing diploma from St. Mary's School of Nursing in Rochester, Minnesota, and a bachelor's degree in Health Arts from the College of St. Francis in Joliet, Illinois. Bernie also received certification as a gerontological nurse practitioner from the University of Colorado in Denver and a master's degree in gerontology from the University of Northern Colorado in Greeley, Colorado, where she received the Dean's Citation for Excellence.

Bernie has had 26 years of experience in gerontological nursing—in a clinical role as a nurse practitioner and in administrative roles as Director of Community Health Services, Director of Nursing, and Director of Resident Care and Services at Bonell Good Samaritan Center in Greeley, Colorado. She has also had experience as a licensed nursing home administrator in Colorado and Wyoming.

Bernie has been a leader in developing and implementing innovative programs for residents in independent living and long-term health care settings. She was instrumental in the development and implementation of a community nursing assistant training program. She received a credential for Career and Technical Education from the Colorado State Board of Community Colleges and Occupational Education. She has consulted for the School of Nursing at the University of Northern Colorado in various grant-writing projects. Bernie served two terms as president of the National Conference of Gerontological Nurse Practitioners. She served on the editorial board for *Geriatric Nursing* for 3 years.

REVIEWERS

Jane Bruker, MSEd, MSN, RN
Consultant
Navajo Technical College
Crownpoint, New Mexico

Nancy E. Redente, BSN, RN
Manager: Nursing Home Education
A.O. Fox Nursing Home
Oneonta, New York

Beth Skeen, MSN, RN
Education Facilitator
Memorial Hospital
Gulfport, Mississippi

ACKNOWLEDGMENTS

Many individuals and agencies have contributed to this new, fourth edition of *Mosby's Essentials for Nursing Assistants* by providing information, insights, and resources. We are especially grateful and appreciative of the efforts by:

- Connie March (President and CEO) and Kathy Dennis (Vice President, Clinical Support) of Provena Senior Services in Mokena, Illinois, for being valuable resources for information and insights.
- Pamela Randolph, MSN, RN—Associate Director of Education and Evidence Based Regulation at the Arizona State Board of Nursing (Phoenix, Arizona)—for providing Board information.
- Mary Beth Sorrentino Herron for promptly accommodating countless requests for documents, deliveries, research, and many favors.
- The artists at Graphic World in St. Louis, Missouri, for their talented work.
- Photographer Mike DeFilipo of St. Louis, Missouri, for his great photos. He is very patient, cooperative, and flexible during photo shoots.
- Jane Bruker, MSEd, MSN, RN; Nancy E. Redente, BSN, RN; and Elizabeth Skeen, MSN, RN for reviewing the manuscript and for their candor and suggestions. They have contributed to the thoroughness and accuracy of this book.
- Beth Welch (Columbus, Ohio) for serving as copy editor. It was a pleasure talking to her.

- And finally, to the talented and dedicated Elsevier/Mosby staff, especially:
  - Suzi Epstein (Executive Editor)—Suzi once again gave guidance and support and kept the project on track. She also stressed the importance of taking care of self and family. Suzi believes in and supports her authors. Her vision, creativity, and resourcefulness are amazing. She is dedicated to her authors and titles and is a master at what she does.
  - Maria Broeker (Senior Developmental Editor)—Maria handled numerous details, manuscript needs, tasks, and issues. She always has an empathetic ear and time to listen to author wants, needs, and frustrations. What would we do without Maria?
  - Sarah Graddy (Editorial Assistant)—Sarah provided prompt clerical and secretarial assistance. She is simply pleasant and a delight to work with.
  - Jeff Patterson (Publishing Services Manager)—With all the design elements and layout considerations inherent in this book, Jeff produced a user friendly and attractive book.
  - Jessica Williams (Book Designer)—Jessica took all of our ideas, some rather abstract, and created a unique and colorful book and cover design. As always, the book is distinctive from the rest.

And to all those who contributed to this effort in any way, we are sincerely grateful.

Sheila A. Sorrentino

Leighann N. Remmert

Bernie Gorek

INSTRUCTOR PREFACE

As with previous editions of *Mosby's Essentials for Nursing Assistants,* the fourth edition serves to prepare students to function as nursing assistants in nursing centers and hospitals. This textbook serves the needs of students and instructors in community colleges, technical schools, high schools, nursing centers, hospitals, and other agencies. As students complete their education, the book is a valuable resource for the competency test review. As part of one's personal library, the book is a reference for the nursing assistant who seeks to review or learn additional information for safe care.

Patients and residents are presented as *persons* with dignity and value who have a past, a present, and a future. Caring, understanding, and protecting and respecting the person's rights, and respecting patients and residents as persons with dignity and value, are attitudes conveyed throughout the book.

Nursing assistants of today and tomorrow must have a firm understanding of the legal principles affecting their role. Both federal and state laws directly and indirectly define their roles, range of functions, and limitations. Nursing assistant roles and functions also vary among states and agencies. Therefore emphasis is given to nursing assistant responsibilities, limitations, and professional boundaries (Chapter 2), which focus on the legal and ethical aspects of the role. This includes reporting abuse.

Nursing assistant functions and role limits also depend on effective delegation. Building on the delegation principles presented in Chapter 2, *Delegation Guidelines* are presented as they relate to procedures. They empower the student to seek information from the nurse and the care plan about critical aspects of the procedure and the observations to report and record. Step 1 of most procedures refers the student to the appropriate *Delegation Guidelines* boxes.

Since the first edition, safety and comfort have been core values of *Mosby's Essentials for Nursing Assistants. Promoting Safety and Comfort* boxes focus the student's attention on the need to be safe and cautious and to promote comfort when giving care. Step 1 of most procedures refers the student to the appropriate *Promoting Safety and Comfort* boxes.

Besides legal aspects, delegation, and safety and comfort, work ethics also affect how nursing assistants function. To foster a positive work ethic, Chapter 3 focuses on workplace behaviors and practices. The goal is for the nursing assistant to be a proud, professional member of the nursing and health teams.

Being a productive and efficient member of the nursing team requires good communication, and good communication skills are needed when interacting with patients and residents. A new feature, *Focus on Communication* boxes suggest what to say and questions to ask when interacting with patients, residents, and the nursing team.

Mosby's Essentials for Nursing Assistants, third edition, featured a chapter ending summary called *Focus on the PERSON,* with PERSON spelled out in the first letter of each bullet: *P*roviding Comfort, *E*thical Behavior, *R*emaining independent, *S*peaking Up, *O*BRA and other laws, and *N*ursing teamwork. To expand the feature and promote pride in the person, family, and one's self, this new edition features *Focus on PRIDE—The Person, Family, and Yourself:*

- **Personal and Professional Responsibility**—focuses on how the nursing assistant can have pride in himself or herself through personal and professional behaviors and development.
- **Rights and Respect**— focuses on how the nursing assistant can promote the person's rights and respect him or her as a person with inherent dignity.
- **Independence and Social Interaction**—presents ways the nursing assistant can help the person remain or attain independence and interact socially with others.
- **Delegation and Teamwork**— focuses on how the nursing assistant can work efficiently with and help other nursing team members.
- **Ethics and Laws**— focuses on the laws affecting nursing care and doing the right thing when dealing with patients, residents, and co-workers.

Because some chapters in the third edition were long and were going to be longer because of new guidelines and content, some lengthy chapters are divided into shorter ones to facilitate the teaching/learning process:

- Fall prevention content was moved from the Safety chapter to Chapter 9: Preventing Falls.
- Body mechanics, moving the person in bed, turning, and transferring content and procedures are in two chapters—Chapter 12: Body Mechanics and Chapter 13: Safely Handling, Moving, and Transferring the Person.
- Mental health problems were moved from the common health problems chapter to Chapter 27: Caring for Persons With Mental Health Problems.

An exciting feature is the CD-ROM in this book. Using video clips and animations, key procedures are presented along with interactive exercises. The CD also includes an audio glossary and the *Body Spectrum* program.

ORGANIZATIONAL STRATEGIES

These concepts and principles—that the patient or resident is a person, ethical and legal aspects, delegation, safety and comfort, and work ethics—serve as the guiding framework for this book. Other organizational strategies and values include:

- Understanding the work setting and the individuals in that setting
- Respecting patients and residents as physical, social, psychological, and spiritual beings with basic needs and protected rights
- Respecting personal choice and the person's dignity
- Appreciating the role of cultural heritage and religion in health and illness practices
- Understanding that knowledge about body structure and function is needed to give safe care and to safely perform nursing skills
- Following the principle that learning proceeds from the simple to the complex
- Recognizing that certain concepts and functions are foundational—safety, body mechanics, and preventing infection are central to other procedures
- Embracing the nursing process as the basis for planning and delivering nursing care and the role that nursing assistants play in assisting with the process

CONTENT ISSUES

With every edition, revision and content decisions are made. When changes are made in laws or in guidelines and standards issued by government or accrediting agencies, the decisions are easy. Content decisions also are based on state curricula and competency testing services. Every attempt is made to make the book as up-to-date as possible with changes sometimes made right before publication.

Other content issues are more difficult. Student learning needs and abilities, instructor desires, work-related issues, and course/program and book length are among the factors considered. With such issues in mind, new and expanded content includes:

New Chapters

- Chapter 9: Preventing Falls
- Chapter 13: Safely Handling, Moving, and Transferring the Person
- Chapter 27: Caring for Persons With Mental Health Problems

New Content

- Meeting Standards
- Boundaries
- Vulnerable Adults
- Managing Stress
- Drug Testing
- End-of-Shift Report
- Addressing the Person
- Protecting the Person
- Color-Coded Wristbands
- Healthcare-Associated Infection
- Preventing Work-Related Injuries
- Bed Safety
- Assisting With Pain Relief
- Providing Drinking Water
- PROCEDURE: Providing Drinking Water
- Using Reagent Strips
- Measures to Prevent Skin Tears
- Loss of Limb
- Amyotrophic Lateral Sclerosis
- Traumatic Head Injury
- Age-Related Macular Degeneration
- Diabetic Retinopathy
- Prostate Enlargement
- PROCEDURE: Adult CPR With AED—Two Rescuers

New Boxes

- Box 2-1: Reasons for Losing Certification, Licensure, or Registration
- Box 2-4: Nursing Assistant Standards
- Box 4-2: Observations to Report at Once
- Box 11-1: Signs and Symptoms of Infection
- Box 13-1: Preventing Work-Related Injuries
- Box 13-2: Levels of Dependence
- Box 19-2: High-Sodium Foods
- Box 23-5: Rules for Applying Binders
- Box 26-2: Care of the Person After Total Joint Replacement Surgery—Hip and Knee
- Box 28-3: Causes of Permanent Dementia

New Delegation Guidelines

- Positioning the Person
- Preventing Work-Related Injuries
- Using Mechanical Lifts
- Changing Hospital Gowns
- Providing Drinking Water
- Corrective Lenses

New Promoting Safety and Comfort

- Paying for Health Care
- End-of-Shift Report
- Preventing Falls
- Disinfection
- Goggles and Face Shields

New Promoting Safety and Comfort—cont'd

- Positioning the Person
- Safely Handling, Moving, and Transferring the Person
- Preventing Work-Related Injuries
- Moving the Person Up in Bed With an Assist Device
- Transferring the Person to and From the Toilet
- Closet and Drawer Space
- Changing Hospital Gowns
- Diarrhea
- The Oil-Retention Enema
- Providing Drinking Water
- Flow Rate
- Body Temperature
- Using Reagent Strips
- Deep Breathing and Coughing
- Pulse Oximetry
- Corrective Lenses

New Persons With Dementia

- Vulnerable Adults
- Communicating With the Person
- The Falling Person
- Applying Restraints
- Meeting Basic Needs
- Preventing Work-Related Injuries
- Factors Affecting Pain
- Dressing and Undressing
- Vital Signs
- Electronic Thermometers
- Assisting With Exercise and Activity
- Skin Tears

New Feature: Focus on Communication

- The Health Team
- Refusing a Task
- Informed Consent
- Confidentiality
- Harassment
- Dealing With Conflict
- Behavior Issues
- Communication Barriers
- The Sexually Aggressive Person
- Fire and the Use of Oxygen
- Preventing Falls
- Legal Aspects
- Safety Guidelines
- Isolation Precautions
- Positioning the Person

- Safely, Handling, Moving, and Transferring the Person
- The Occupied Bed
- Bathing
- Perineal Care
- Skin and Scalp Conditions
- Dressing and Undressing
- Normal Urination
- Urinals
- Observations
- Meeting Food and Fluid Needs
- Vital Signs
- Taking Temperatures
- Using a Stethoscope
- Signs and Symptoms
- The Midstream Specimen
- Stool Specimens
- Complications of Bedrest
- Range-of-Motion Exercises
- Ambulation
- Pressure Ulcer Stages
- Elastic Bandages
- Tape
- Applying Dressings
- Binders
- Applying Heat and Cold
- Deep Breathing and Coughing
- Communication
- Psychological and Social Aspects
- Your Role
- Hearing Loss
- Care of Persons With AD and Other Dementias
- Chain of Survival for Adults
- Psychological and Spiritual Needs

FEATURES AND DESIGN

Besides content issues, attention also is given to improving the book's features and designs. To make the book readable and user friendly, new features and design elements are added while others are retained. See "Student Preface," p. xiii.

May this book serve you and your students well. Our intent is to provide you and your students with the current information needed to teach and learn safe and effective care during this time of dynamic change in health care.

Sheila A. Sorrentino, BSN, MA, MSN, PhD, RN
Leighann N. Remmert, BSN, RN
Bernie Gorek, GNP, MA, RNC

STUDENT PREFACE

This book was designed for you. It was designed to help you learn. The book is a useful resource as you gain experience and expand your knowledge.

This preface gives some study guidelines and helps you use the book. When given a reading assignment, do you read from the first page to the last page without stopping? How much do you remember? You will learn more if you use a study system. A useful study system has these steps:

- Survey or preview
- Question
- Read and record
- Recite and review

PREVIEW

Before you start a reading assignment, preview or survey the assignment. This gives you an idea of what the assignment covers. It also helps you recall what you already know about the subject. Carefully look over the assignment. Preview the chapter title, headings, subheadings, and terms or ideas in bold print or italics. Also survey the objectives, key terms, boxes, and review questions at the end of the chapter. Previewing only takes a few minutes. Remember, previewing helps you become familiar with the material.

QUESTION

After previewing, you need to form questions to answer while you read. Questions should relate to what might be asked on a test or how the information applies to giving care. Use the title, headings, and subheadings to form questions. Avoid questions that have one word answers. Questions that begin with what, how, or why are helpful. While reading, you may find that a question does not help you study. If so, just change the question. Remember, questioning sets a purpose for reading. So changing a question only makes this step more useful.

READ AND RECORD

Reading is the next step. Reading is more productive after determining what you already know and what you need to learn. Read to find answers to your questions. The purpose of reading is to:

- Gain new information
- Connect new information to what you know already

Break the assignment into smaller parts. Then answer your questions as you read each part. Also, mark important information—underline, highlight, or make notes. Underlining and highlighting remind you of what you need to learn. Go back and review the marked parts later. Making notes results in more immediate learning. To make notes, write down important information in the margins or in a notebook. Use words and statements to jog your memory about the material.

You need to remember what you read. To do so, work with the information. Organize information into a study guide. Study guides have many forms. Diagrams or charts show relationships or steps in a process. Note taking in outline format is also very useful. The following is a sample outline:

1. Main heading
   a. Second level
   b. Second level
      i. Third level
      ii. Third level
2. Main heading

RECITE AND REVIEW

Finally, recite and review. Use your notes and study guides. Answer the questions you formed earlier. Also answer other questions that came up when reading and answering the Review Questions at the end of a chapter. Answer all questions out loud (recite).

Reviewing is more about when to study rather than what to study. You already determined what to study during the preview, question, and reading steps. The best times to review are right after the first study session, one week later, and before a quiz or test.

This book was also designed to help you study. Special design features are described on the next pages.

We hope you enjoy learning and your work. You and your work are important. You and the care you give make a difference in the person's life!

Sheila A. Sorrentino
Leighann N. Remmert
Bernie Gorek

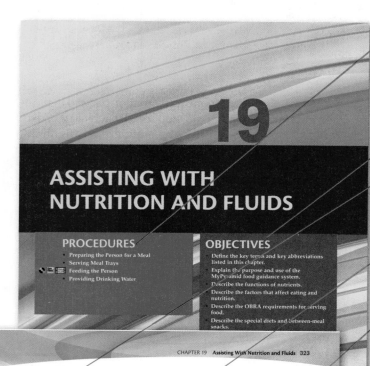

Procedures list identifies the procedures presented in the chapter. A CD icon follows those procedures that are also on the CD-ROM in this book. A video icon follows those procedures for which there is a related clip on the EVOLVE website.

Objectives tell what is presented in the chapter.

Key Terms are the important words and phrases in the chapter. Definitions are given for each term. The key terms introduce you to the chapter content. They are also a useful study guide.

Bolded type is used to highlight the key terms in the text. You again see the key term and read its definition. This helps reinforce your learning.

Key Abbreviations are a quick reference of the main abbreviations used in the chapter. They are listed after the "Key Terms."

Persons With Dementia boxes focus on information and insights about caring for persons with dementia.

Caring About Culture boxes contain information to help you learn about the various practices of other cultures.

CHAPTER 19 Assisting With Nutrition and Fluids 323

KEY TERMS

anorexia The loss of appetite
aspiration Breathing fluid, food, vomitus, or an object into the lungs
calorie The amount of energy produced when the body burns food
dehydration A decrease in the amount of water in body tissues
dysphagia Difficulty (*dys*) swallowing (*phagia*)
edema The swelling of body tissues with water
enteral nutrition Giving nutrients into the gastro-intestinal (GI) tract (*enteral*) through a feeding tube
flow rate The number of drops per minute
gavage The process of giving a tube feeding
intravenous (IV) therapy Giving fluids through a needle or catheter inserted into a vein; IV and IV infusion
nutrition The processes involved in the ingestion, digestion, absorption, and use of foods and fluids by the body
regurgitation The backward flow of stomach contents into the mouth

KEY ABBREVIATIONS

GI Gastro-intestinal
ID Identification
IV Intravenous
mg Milligram
mL Milliliter
NG Nasogastric
NPO Non per os; nothing by mouth
OBRA Omnibus Budget Reconciliation Act of 1987
oz Ounce

Food and water are physical needs. They are necessary for life. The person's diet affects physical and mental well-being. A poor diet and poor eating habits:
* Increase the risk for diseases and infection
* Cause healing problems
* Affect physical and mental function, increasing the risk for accidents and injuries

BASIC NUTRITION

Nutrition is the processes involved in the ingestion, digestion, absorption, and use of foods and fluids by the body. Good nutrition is needed for growth, healing, and body functions. A *nutrient* is a substance that is ingested, digested, absorbed, and used by the body. Nutrients are grouped into fats, proteins, carbohydrates, vitamins, minerals, and water.

Fats, proteins, and carbohydrates give the body fuel for energy. A **calorie** is the amount of energy produced when the body burns food:
* 1 gram of fat—9 calories
* 1 gram of protein—4 calories
* 1 gram of carbohydrate—4 calories

MyPyramid

The MyPyramid food guidance ... p. 324) encourages smart and ... and daily activity. The MyPyr... "Steps To a Healthier You." ...
* *The kind and amounts of fo...* pends on the person's ag... male), and activity level...gov website.)
* *Gradual improvement.* Peop... each day to improve diet a...
* *Physical activity.* This is sho... person climbing them. The ... importance of physical acti... 30 minutes of physical activ... days of the week. It is best ... tivity should be moderate c... 325). Activity can be done ... riod. Or it can be done in 2 ... total time is at least 30 min...
* *Variety.* The 6 color band... groups and oils. Food fr... needed each day for good ...
* *Moderation.* This means t... bands narrow as they go ... top of the pyramid. Foo... the most nutritional value ... They have little or no solic... caloric sweeteners. Choos... band more often than thos...
* *The right amount from each...* widths suggest how muc... each group. The wider the ... the person should choose f...

Factors Affecting Pain

Many factors affect pain.
* *Past experience.* The severity of pain, its cause, how long it lasted, and if relief occurred all affect the person's response to pain. Knowing what to expect can help or hinder how the person handles pain. Some people have not had pain. When it occurs, pain can cause fear and anxiety. They can make pain worse.
* *Anxiety.* Anxiety relates to feelings of fear, dread, worry, and concern. The person is uneasy and tense. Pain and anxiety are related. Pain can cause anxiety. Anxiety increases how much pain the person feels. Reducing anxiety helps lessen pain.
* *Rest and sleep.* Pain seems worse when tired or restless. Also, the person tends to focus on pain when tired and unable to rest or sleep.
* *Personal and family duties.* Often pain is ignored when there are children to care for. Some people go to work with pain. Others deny pain if a serious illness is feared. The illness can interfere with a job, going to school, or caring for children, a partner, or ill parents.
* *The value or meaning of pain.* To some people, pain is a sign of weakness. It may mean a serious illness and the need for painful tests and treatments. Sometimes pain gives pleasure. The pain of childbirth is one example. For some persons, pain is used to avoid certain people or things. Some people like doting and pampering by others. The person values and wants such attention.
* *Support from others.* Dealing with pain is often easier when family and friends offer comfort and support. The use of touch by a valued person is very comforting. Just being nearby also helps. Some people do not have caring family or friends. Dealing with pain alone can increase anxiety.
* *Culture.* Culture affects pain responses. Non-English speaking persons may have problems describing pain. The agency uses interpreters to communicate with the person. See *Caring About Culture: Pain Reactions.*
* *Illness.* Some diseases cause decreased pain sensations. Central nervous system disorders are examples. The person may not feel pain. Or it may not feel severe.
* *Age.* Older persons may have decreased pain sensations. They may not feel pain or it may not feel severe. See *Persons With Dementia: Factors Affecting Pain.*

PERSONS WITH DEMENTIA

Factors Affecting Pain

Persons with dementia may not be able to complain of pain. Changes in usual behavior may signal pain. A person who moans and groans may become quiet and withdrawn. A person who is friendly and outgoing may become agitated and aggressive. One who is nonverbal and quiet may become restless and cry easily. Loss of appetite also signals pain.

Report any changes in a person's usual behavior to the nurse. All persons have the right to correct pain management. The nurse needs to do a pain assessment when the person's behavior changes.

PROMOTING SLEEP

Sleep is a basic need. The mind and body rest. The body saves energy. Body functions slow. Vital signs (temperature, pulse, respirations, and blood pressure) are lower than when awake. Tissue healing and repair occur. Sleep lowers stress, tension, and anxiety. It refreshes and renews the person. The person regains energy and mental alertness. The person thinks and functions better after sleep.

The nurse uses the nursing process to promote sleep. Report your observations about how the person slept. The person's care plan may include the measures in Box 14-4.

See *Persons With Dementia: Promoting Sleep.*

Heading icons alert you to associated procedures. Procedure boxes contain the same icon.

Delegation Guidelines boxes describe what information you need from the nurse and care plan before performing a procedure. They also tell you what information to report and record.

Focus on Communication boxes suggest what to say and questions to ask when interacting with patients, residents, and the nursing team.

Promoting Safety and Comfort boxes focus your attention on the need to be safe and cautious and promote comfort when giving care. "Safety" and "Comfort" subtitles are used.

Procedure icons in the title bar alert you to associated content areas. Heading icons and procedure icons are the same.

CD icons appear in the chapter procedures lists and the procedure box title bar for the skills included on the CD-ROM in the book.

View Video Icons indicate procedures included on *Mosby's Nursing Assistant Video Skills 3.0.*

Video Clip Icons indicate related video clips available online on EVOLVE Student Learning Resources.

NNAAP™ in the procedure title bar alerts you to those skills that are part of the National Nurse Aide Assessment Program (NNAAP™). Note: All states do not participate in NNAAP™. Ask your instructor for a list of the skills tested in your state.

The Quality of Life section in the Procedure boxes lists six simple courtesies that show respect for the patient or resident as a person.

Procedure boxes are written in a step-by-step format. They are divided into Quality of Life, Pre-Procedure, Procedure, and Post-Procedure sections for easy studying.

Color illustrations and photographs visually present key ideas, concepts, or procedure steps. They help you apply and remember the written material.

---

398 MOSBY'S ESSENTIALS FOR NURSING ASSISTANTS

AMBULATION

Ambulation is the act of walking. After bedrest, activity increases slowly and in steps. First the person dangles (sits on the side of the bed). Sitting in a bedside chair follows. Next the person walks in the room and then in the hallway.

Some people are weak and unsteady from bedrest, illness, surgery, or injury. Follow the care plan when helping a person walk. Use a gait (transfer) belt if the person is weak or unsteady. The person also uses hand rails along the wall. Always check the person for orthostatic hypotension (p. 390).

See *Focus on Communication: Ambulation.*
See *Delegation Guidelines: Ambulation.*
See *Promoting Safety and Comfort: Ambulation.*

FOCUS ON COMMUNICATION
Ambulation

Before ambulating, talk with the person about the activity. Doing so promotes comfort and reduces fear. Explain to the person:
* The distance to walk
* What assistive devices will be used
* How you will assist
* What the person is to report to you
* How you will help if the person begins to fall

For example, you can say:
"Mr. Owens, I am going to help you walk from your bed to the doorway and back. This belt is to help support you while you walk. I will stay by your side and keep hold of the belt at all times. Let me know right away if you feel unsteady, dizzy, or weak. Also tell me if you feel any pain or discomfort. If you do begin to fall, I will use the belt to pull you close to me and gently lower you to the ground. Do you have any questions?"

DELEGATION GUIDELINES
Ambulation

Before helping with ambulation, you need this information from the nurse and the care plan:
* How much help the person needs
* If the person uses a cane, walker, crutches, or a brace
* Areas of weakness—right arm or leg, left arm or leg
* How far to walk the person
* What observations to report and record:
  * How well the person tolerated the activity
  * Shuffling, sliding, limping, or walking on tip-toes
  * Complaints of pain or discomfort
  * Complaints of orthostatic hypotension—weakness, dizziness, spots before the eyes, feeling faint
  * The distance walked
* When to report observations
* What specific patient or resident concerns to report at once

PROMOTING SAFETY AND COMFORT
Ambulation

Safety
Practice the safety measures to prevent falls (Chapter 9). Use a gait belt to help the person stand. Also use it during ambulation.

Comfort
The fear of falling affects the person's mental comfort. Explain the purpose of the gait belt. Also explain how you will help the person if he or she starts to fall (Chapter 9).

HELPING THE PERSON WALK   NNAAP

QUALITY OF LIFE

Remember to:
* Knock before entering the person's room.
* Address the person by name.
* Introduce yourself by name and title.

* Explain the procedure to the person before beginning and during the procedure.
* Protect the person's rights during the procedure.
* Handle the person gently during the procedure.

PRE-PROCEDURE

1 Follow *Delegation Guidelines: Ambulation.* See *Promoting Safety and Comfort: Ambulation.*
2 Practice hand hygiene.
3 Collect the following:
   * Robe and non-skid shoes
   * Paper or sheet to protect bottom linens
   * Gait (transfer) belt
4 Identify the person. Check the ID bracelet against the assignment sheet. Also call the person by name.
5 Provide for privacy.

CHAPTER 22 Assisting With Exercise and Activity 399

PROCEDURE

6 Lower the bed to its lowest position. Lock the bed wheels. Lower the bed rail if up.
7 Fan-fold top linens to the foot of the bed.
8 Place the paper or sheet under the person's feet. Put the shoes on the person. Fasten the shoes.
9 Help the person sit on the side of the bed. (See procedure: *Sitting on the Side of the Bed [Dangling],* Chapter 13.)
10 Help the person put on the robe.
11 Make sure the person's feet are flat on the floor.
12 Apply the gait belt. (See procedure: *Applying a Transfer/Gait Belt,* Chapter 9.)
13 Help the person stand. (See procedure: *Transferring the Person to a Chair or Wheelchair,* Chapter 13.) Grasp the gait belt at each side. If not using a gait belt, place your arms under the person's arms around to the shoulder blades.
14 Stand at the person's weak side while he or she gains balance. Hold the belt at the side and back. If not using a gait belt, have one arm around the back and the other at the elbow to support the person.

15 Encourage the person to stand erect with the head up and back straight.
16 Help the person walk. Walk to the side and slightly behind the person on the person's weak side. Provide support with the gait belt (Fig. 22-23). If not using a gait belt, have one arm around the back and the other at the elbow to support the person. Encourage the person to use the hand rail on his or her strong side.
17 Encourage the person to walk normally. The heel strikes the floor first. Discourage shuffling, sliding, or walking on tip-toes.
18 Walk the required distance if the person tolerates the activity. Do not rush the person.
19 Help the person return to bed. Remove the gait belt. (See procedure: *Transferring the Person From a Chair or Wheelchair to a Bed,* Chapter 13.)
20 Lower the head of the bed. Help the person to the center of the bed.
21 Remove the shoes. Remove and discard the paper or sheet over the bottom sheet.

POST-PROCEDURE

22 Provide for comfort. (See the inside of the front book cover.)
23 Place the signal light within reach.
24 Raise or lower bed rails. Follow the care plan.
25 Return the robe and shoes to their proper place.
26 Unscreen the person.

27 Complete a safety check of the room. (See the inside of the front book cover.)
28 Decontaminate your hands.
29 Report and record your observations.

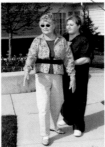

FIGURE 22-23 The nursing assistant walks at the person's side and slightly behind her.

Boxes and tables contain important rules, principles, guidelines, signs and symptoms, nursing measures, and other information in a list format. They identify important information and are useful study guides.

Focus on PRIDE: The Person, Family, and Yourself build on the concepts and principles presented in the chapter to help you promote pride in the person, family, and yourself. PRIDE is spelled out in the first letter of each bullet.

- *Personal and Professional Responsibility*—the focus is on how the you can have pride in yourself through personal and professional behaviors and development.
- *Rights and Respect*—the focus is on how you can promote the person's rights and respect him or her as a person with dignity.
- *Independence and Social Interaction*—presents ways you can help the person remain or attain independence and interact socially with others.
- *Delegation and Teamwork*—focuses on how you can work efficiently with and help other nursing team members.
- *Ethics and Laws*—the focus is on the laws affecting nursing care and doing the right thing when dealing with patients, residents, and co-workers.

Review Questions are useful study guides. They help you review what you have learned. They can also be used when studying for a test or the competency evaluation. Answers are given at the back of the book beginning on p. 527.

Inset page 1:

CHAPTER 19   Assisting With Nutrition and Fluids   345

BOX 19-7   Signs and Symptoms of IV Therapy Complications

Local—At the IV Site
- Bleeding
- Puffiness, swelling, or leaking fluid
- Pale or reddened skin
- Complaints of pain at or above the IV site
- Hot or cold skin near the site

Systemic—Involving the Whole Body
- Fever
- Itching
- Drop in blood pressure
- Pulse rate greater than 100 beats per minute
- Irregular pulse
- Cyanosis (bluish color)
- Confusion or changes in mental function
- Loss of consciousness
- Difficulty breathing
- Shortness of breath
- Decreasing or no urine output
- Chest pain
- Nausea

Focus on PRIDE
The Person, Family, and Yourself

Personal and Professional Responsibility—Many hospitals are serving food in new ways. The purpose is to allow freedom and personal choice. For example, some hospitals offer:
- *24-hour catering.* Meals and snacks are provided 24 hours a day. This is for persons who cannot or do not want to eat at the usual mealtimes. The person can order food directly from the food service department. The person orders the foods he or she wants within the person's ordered diet.
- *Mobile food carts.* Food service staff bring a food cart to the nursing unit. The patient selects food and a tray is prepared.

With such systems, you may have new responsibilities. For example, you may need to watch for the arrival of food trays more often. Or you may need to assist persons with reading or filling out menus. Know your agency's food ordering and delivery system and your role in that system. Take pride in helping others meet their nutritional needs.

Rights and Respect—Persons have different food preferences. Cultural, social, religious, medical, and personal factors affect a person's food choices. Persons commonly express their food likes and dislikes. You may hear a person say the food is too cold. Or it is too bland. Or the food tastes bad.

Persons have the right to express their preferences. Do not become angry or upset. The person should not feel as if he or she is complaining or being picky. Learning the person's likes and dislikes can improve nutrition. It also shows interest and concern for the person. Respect the person's right to express personal food choices.

Independence and Social Interaction—Meals can provide a time for social contact with others. A friendly, social setting is important. Some nursing centers have areas where residents can dine with a partner, family, or friends. They can enjoy holidays, birthdays, anniversaries, and other special events together. The dietary department provides the meal. Or the meal is brought by the family.

Delegation and Teamwork—In some agencies, meal trays arrive on the nursing unit in a meal cart. Each tray is in a slot. Trays are served in the order that they appear in the cart. The entire nursing team serves trays. You may serve trays to patients or residents of other staff members. They do the same for you. The team works together to serve food promptly and at the correct temperature.

Ethics and Laws—OBRA requires that patients and residents receive proper nutrition. Survey teams make sure that:
- Needed help is provided
- Assistive devices are provided
- Medical asepsis is practiced when serving food and fluids
- Meals and snacks are served promptly
- Other food is offered if the person refuses the food served

---

Inset page 2:

428 MOSBY'S ESSENTIALS FOR NURSING ASSISTANTS

REVIEW QUESTIONS

Circle the BEST answer.

1 Which can cause skin tears?
   a Keeping your nails trim and smooth
   b Dressing the person in soft clothing
   c Wearing rings
   d Padding wheelchair footplates

2 The first sign of a pressure ulcer is
   a a blister   c Drainage
   b A reddened area   d Gangrene

3 Which can cause pressure ulcers?
   a Repositioning the person every 2 hours
   b Scrubbing and rubbing the skin
   c Applying lotion to dry areas
   d Keeping linens clean, dry, and wrinkle-free

4 Pressure ulcers usually occur
   a On the feet
   b Over a bony area
   c On the buttocks
   d Where skin has contact with skin

5 What is the preferred position for preventing pressure ulcers?
   a 30-degree lateral position   c Prone position
   b Semi-Fowler's position   d Supine position

6 A person is at risk for pressure ulcers. Which measure should you question?
   a Apply lotion to the hands, elbows, legs, ankles, and heels.
   b Massage bony areas.
   c Give a back massage when repositioning the person.
   d Apply powder under the breasts.

7 A person has a circulatory ulcer. Which measure should you question?
   a Hold socks in place with elastic garters.
   b Do not cut or trim toenails.
   c Apply elastic stockings.
   d Reposition the person every hour.

8 Persons with diabetes are at risk for diabetic foot ulcers because of
   a Gangrene   d Nerve and blood
   b Amputation   vessel damage
   c Infection

9 A person has diabetes. You should check the person's feet every
   a 2 hours   c Week
   b Day   d Month

10 Elastic stockings are applied
    a Before the person gets out of bed
    b When the person is standing
    c After the person's shower or bath
    d For 30 minutes and then removed

11 When applying an elastic bandage
    a Position the part in good alignment
    b Cover the fingers or toes if possible
    c Apply it from the largest to smallest part of the extremity
    d Apply it from the upper to lower part of the extremity

12 To secure a dressing, apply tape
    a Around the entire part
    b Along the sides of the dressing
    c To the top, middle, and bottom of the dressing
    d As the person prefers

13 To remove tape
    a Pull it toward the wound
    b Pull it away from the wound
    c Use an adhesive remover
    d Use a saline solution

14 An abdominal binder is used to
    a Prevent blood clots
    b Prevent wound infection
    c Provide support and hold dressings in place
    d Decrease swelling and circulation

15 The *greatest* threat from heat applications is
    a Infection   c Chilling
    b Burns   d Pressure ulcers

16 A person uses an aquathermia pad. Which is *false*?
    a It is a dry heat application.
    b A flannel cover is used.
    c Electrical safety precautions are practiced.
    d Pins secure the pad in place.

17 Before applying an ice bag
    a Place the bag in the freezer
    b Measure the temperature of the bag
    c Place the bag in a cover
    d Provide perineal care

18 Moist cold compresses are left in place no longer than
    a 20 minutes   c 45 minutes
    b 30 minutes   d 60 minutes

Answers to these questions are on p. 528.

CONTENTS

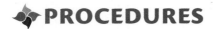

PROCEDURES

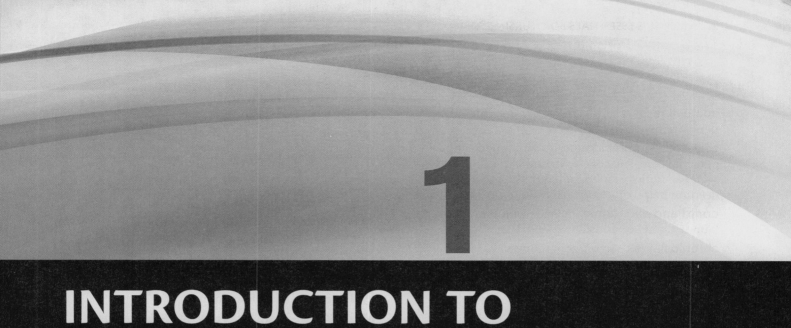

1

INTRODUCTION TO HOSPITALS AND NURSING CENTERS

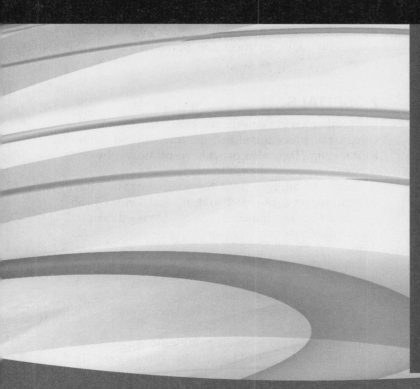

OBJECTIVES

- Define the key terms and key abbreviations listed in this chapter.
- Describe hospitals and long-term care centers.
- Describe the persons cared for in long-term care centers.
- Identify members of the health team and nursing team.
- Describe the nursing care patterns.
- Describe the programs that pay for health care.
- Describe the Omnibus Budget Reconciliation Act of 1987.
- Explain the rights of patients and residents.
- Explain how to promote PRIDE in the person, the family, and yourself.

KEY TERMS

acute illness A sudden illness from which the person is expected to recover

assisted living residence (ALR) Provides housing, personal care, support services, health care, and social activities in a home-like setting to persons needing help with daily activities

board and care home Provides a room, meals, laundry, and supervision

chronic illness An on-going illness that is slow or gradual in onset; it has no known cure; it can be controlled and complications prevented with proper treatment

health team The many health care workers whose skills and knowledge focus on the person's total care; interdisciplinary health care team

hospice An agency or program for persons who are dying

licensed practical nurse (LPN) A nurse who has completed a 1-year nursing program and has passed a licensing test; called *licensed vocational nurse (LVN)* in some states

licensed vocational nurse (LVN) See "licensed practical nurse"

nursing assistant A person who has passed a nursing assistant training and competency evaluation program; performs delegated nursing tasks under the supervision of a licensed nurse

nursing center A long-term care center that provides health care services to persons who need regular or continuous care; nursing facility or nursing home

nursing facility See "nursing center"

nursing home See "nursing center"

nursing team Those who provide nursing care— RNs, LPNs/LVNs, and nursing assistants

ombudsman Someone who supports or promotes the needs and interests of another person

Omnibus Budget Reconciliation Act of 1987 (OBRA) A federal law requiring that nursing centers provide care in a manner and in a setting that maintains or improves each person's quality of life, health, and safety

registered nurse (RN) A nurse who has completed a 2-, 3-, or 4-year nursing program and has passed a licensing test

skilled nursing facility (SNF) A long-term care center that provides complex care for severe health problems

subacute care Complex medical care or rehabilitation when hospital care is no longer needed

terminal illness An illness or injury from which the person will not likely recover

KEY ABBREVIATIONS

ALR Assisted living residence

DON Director of nursing

HMO Health maintenance organization

LPN Licensed practical nurse

LVN Licensed vocational nurse

MS-DRG Medicare Severity-adjusted Diagnosis Related Group

OBRA Omnibus Budget Reconciliation Act of 1987

PPO Preferred provider organization

RN Registered nurse

RUG Resource utilization group

Hospitals and long-term care centers provide health care services. Staff members use their talents, knowledge, and skills to meet the person's needs. The *person* is the focus of care.

HOSPITALS

Hospitals provide emergency care, surgery, nursing care, x-ray procedures and treatments, and laboratory testing. They also provide respiratory, physical, occupational, and speech therapies.

People of all ages need hospital care. They have babies, surgery, physical and mental health problems, and broken bones. Some people need hospital care to diagnose and treat medical problems or when dying.

Hospital patients have acute, chronic, or terminal illnesses:

- **Acute illness** is a sudden illness from which the person is expected to recover. Heart attack is an example.
- **Chronic illness** is an on-going illness that is slow or gradual in onset. There is no known cure. The illness can be controlled and complications prevented with proper treatment. Diabetes is an example.
- **Terminal illness** is an illness or injury from which the person will not likely recover. The person will die (Chapter 30). Cancers that do not respond to treatment are examples.

Some surgeries, diagnostic tests, and therapies do not require 24-hour stays. Other hospital stays can last days, weeks, or months.

Patient Rights

In April 2003, the American Hospital Association adopted *The Patient Care Partnership: Understanding Expectations, Rights, and Responsibilities.* The document explains the person's rights and expectations during hospital stays. They include:

- High quality care
- A clean and safe setting
- Being involved in care
- Having privacy protected
- Being prepared to leave the hospital
- Help understanding the hospital bill and filing insurance claims

LONG-TERM CARE CENTERS

Some persons cannot care for themselves. Hospital care is not needed. Long-term care centers are designed to meet their needs. Care needs range from simple to complex. Medical, nursing, dietary, recreational, rehabilitative, and social services are provided.

Persons in long-term care centers are *residents.* They are not *patients.* The center is their temporary or permanent home.

Most residents are older. They have chronic diseases, poor nutrition, or poor health. Not all residents are old. Some are disabled from birth defects, accidents, or diseases. People are often discharged from hospitals while still recovering from illness, surgery, or an injury. Some residents recover and return home. Others need nursing care until death.

Long-term care centers meet the needs of:

- *Alert, oriented persons.* They know who they are, where they are, the year, and the time of day. They have physical problems. Disability level affects the amount of care required. Some require complete care. Others need help with daily activities.
- *Confused and disoriented persons.* They are mildly to severely confused and disoriented. Some cannot remember names or dates. Others are more confused and disoriented—they do not know who or where they are. They cannot remember how to dress or feed themselves. Sometimes the problem is temporary. Some persons have Alzheimer's disease and other dementias (Chapter 28). Confusion and disorientation are permanent and become worse.

- *Persons needing complete care.* They are very disabled, confused, or disoriented. They cannot meet any of their own needs. Some cannot say what they need or want.
- *Short-term residents.* These persons need to recover from acute illness, surgery, fractures, and other injuries. Often they are younger than most residents. They usually recover and return home.
- *Persons needing respite care.* Some people cared for at home go to nursing centers for short stays. This is *respite care.* Respite means rest or relief. The caregiver can go on a trip, tend to business, or simply rest. Respite care may be for a few days or several weeks.
- *Life-long residents.* Some disabilities occur before 22 years of age. Called *developmental disabilities,* they are caused by birth defects and childhood diseases and injuries. Impairments may be physical, intellectual, or both. The person has limited function in at least three areas: self-care, understanding or expressing language, learning, mobility, self-direction, independent living, financial support of oneself. The person needs life-long assistance, support, and special devices. Some nursing centers admit developmentally disabled children and adults.
- *Mentally ill persons.* Behavior and function are affected. In severe cases, self-care and independent living are impaired. Some persons have physical and mental illnesses.
- *Terminally ill persons.* Some are alert and oriented; others are comatose. Comatose persons cannot respond to what people say to them. But they may still feel pain. Some have severe pain. Terminally ill persons may need hospice care. The goal is a peaceful, dignified death.

Board and Care Homes

Board and care homes provide a room, meals, laundry, and supervision. Residents—4 to 30 or more—share common living areas and eat together.

A safe setting is provided but not 24-hour nursing care. Residents can usually dress themselves and meet grooming and elimination needs with little help.

Some homes are for older persons. Others are for people with certain problems. Dementia, mental health problems, and developmental disabilities are examples.

Assisted Living Residences

An **assisted living residence (ALR)** provides housing, personal care, support services, health care, and social activities in a home-like setting. ALR residents need help with some daily activities—taking drugs and with bathing, dressing, elimination, and eating. Many have problems with thinking, reasoning, and judgment.

Mobility is often required. The person walks or uses a wheelchair or motor scooter. The person can leave the building in an emergency. Stable health also is required. The person needs limited health care or treatment.

A home-like, secure setting is provided. Residents have 24-hour supervision and three meals a day. They have laundry, housekeeping, transportation, social, recreational, and some health services. Services are added or reduced as the person's needs change.

Some ALRs are part of nursing centers or retirement communities. Others are separate facilities. ALRs must follow state laws and rules.

Nursing Centers

A **nursing center (nursing facility, nursing home)** provides health care services to persons who need regular or continuous care. Licensed nurses are required. Medical, nursing, dietary, recreation, rehabilitation, and social services are provided.

Skilled nursing facilities (SNFs) provide complex care for severe health problems. They are part of nursing centers. Some hospitals have skilled nursing units. Many people are admitted to SNFs from hospitals. They stay for a short time to recover or for rehabilitation. Others never go home.

Some nursing centers and hospitals provide subacute care. **Subacute care** is complex medical care or rehabilitation when hospital care is no longer needed. Often called *patients*, they may have nervous system injuries, bone or joint injuries or surgeries, or wounds that are not healing. Short stays are common.

See "The Omnibus Budget Reconciliation Act of 1987" and "Resident Rights" on p. 8.

Hospices

A **hospice** is an agency or program for persons who are dying. Such persons no longer respond to treatments aimed at cures. Usually they have less than 6 months to live.

The physical, emotional, social, and spiritual needs of the person and family are met. The focus is on comfort, not cure. Hospice care is provided by hospitals, nursing centers, and home care agencies.

Alzheimer's Units (Dementia Care Units)

An Alzheimer's unit is designed for persons with Alzheimer's disease and other dementias (Chapter 28). Such persons suffer increasing memory loss and confusion. Over time, they cannot tend to simple personal needs. They often wander about and may become agitated and combative. The unit is usually closed off from other parts of the center. The closed unit provides a safe setting where residents can wander freely.

HOSPITAL AND NURSING CENTER ORGANIZATION

A hospital has a governing body called the *board of trustees* or *board of directors.* The board makes policies. It makes sure that safe care is given at the lowest possible cost.

An administrator manages the agency. He or she reports directly to the board. Directors or department heads manage certain areas.

Nursing centers are usually owned by an individual or a corporation. Some are owned by county health departments.

Each center has an administrator. Department directors report to the administrator. Most nursing centers have nursing, therapy, and food service departments (Fig. 1-1). They also have social service and activity departments.

Hospitals and nursing centers must follow local, state, and federal laws and rules. This is to ensure safe care.

The Health Team

The **health team** involves the many health care workers whose skills and knowledge focus on the person's

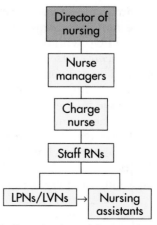

FIGURE 1-1 Organization of the nursing department.

TABLE 1-1 Health Team Members

Activities director	Assesses, plans, and implements recreational needs
Audiologist	Tests hearing; prescribes hearing aids; works with persons who are hard-of-hearing
Cleric (clergyman; clergywoman)	Assists with spiritual needs
Clinical nurse specialist	Provides nursing care and consults in a nursing speciality—geriatrics, critical care, diabetes, rehabilitation, wound care, and so on
Dietitian	Assesses and plans for nutritional needs; teaches good nutrition, food selection, and preparation
Licensed practical/vocational nurse (LPN/LVN)	Provides direct nursing care, including giving drugs, under the direction of an RN
Medical records and health information technician	Maintains medical records; transcribes medical reports; files records; completes required reports
Medical technologist (MT)	Performs complicated laboratory tests on blood, urine, and other body fluids, secretions, and excretions; organizes, supervises, and performs diagnostic analyses; supervises medical laboratory technicians (MLTs)
Medication assistant-certified (MA-C)	Gives medications as allowed by state law under the supervision of a licensed nurse
Nurse practitioner	Works with the health team to plan and provide care; does physical exams, health assessments, and health education
Nursing assistive personnel	Assists nurses and gives nursing care; supervised by a licensed nurse; nursing assistant
Occupational therapist (OT)	Assists persons to learn or retain skills needed to perform activities of daily living; designs adaptive equipment for activities of daily living
Pharmacist	Fills drug orders written by doctors; monitors and evaluates drug interactions; consults with doctors and nurses about drug actions and interactions
Physical therapist (PT)	Assists persons with musculoskeletal problems; focuses on restoring function and preventing disability
Physician (doctor)	Diagnoses and treats diseases and injuries
Podiatrist	Prevents, diagnoses, and treats foot disorders
Radiographer/radiologic technologist	Takes x-rays and processes film for viewing
Registered nurse (RN)	Assesses, makes nursing diagnoses, plans, implements, and evaluates nursing care; supervises LPNs/LVNs and nursing assistants
Respiratory therapist (RT)	Assists in the treatment of lung and heart disorders; gives respiratory treatments and therapies
Social worker	Deals with social, emotional, and environmental issues affecting illness and recovery; coordinates community agencies to assist patients, residents, and families
Speech-language pathologist	Evaluates speech and language and treats persons with speech, voice, hearing, communication, and swallowing disorders

total care (Table 1-1). In nursing centers, it is called the *interdisciplinary health care team*. The goal is to provide quality care. The person is the focus of care.

Many staff members are involved in the care of each person. Coordinated care is needed. An RN leads this team.

See *Focus on Communication: The Health Team*, p. 6.

FOCUS ON COMMUNICATION
The Health Team

Many staff members work together to provide a person's care. Each member has a different role. Health team members must communicate often. You may have questions or concerns about a person and his or her care. Tell the team leader. The leader will communicate with other health team members.

Nursing Service

Nursing service is a large department. The director of nursing (DON) is a registered nurse (RN). The DON is responsible for the entire nursing staff and the care given.

Nurse managers oversee a work shift, a nursing area, or a certain function. Functions include staff development, restorative nursing, infection control, and continuous quality care. Nurse managers are responsible for all nursing care and the actions of nursing staff in their areas.

Nursing areas may have charge nurses for each shift. Usually RNs, some states allow LPNs/LVNs to serve as charge nurses. A charge nurse reports to the nurse manager. The charge nurse is responsible for all patient or resident care and for the actions of nursing staff during that shift. Staff RNs report to the charge nurse. LPNs/LVNs report to staff RNs or to the charge nurse. You report to the nurse supervising your work.

Nursing education is part of nursing service. Nursing education staff:
- Plan and present educational programs (in-service programs) that meet federal and state requirements
- Provide new and changing information
- Instruct on the use of new equipment
- Review key policies and procedures on a regular basis
- Teach and train nursing assistants
- Conduct new employee orientation programs

THE NURSING TEAM

The **nursing team** involves those who provide nursing care—RNs, LPNs/LVNs, and nursing assistants. All focus on the physical, social, emotional, and spiritual needs of the person and family.

Registered Nurses

A **registered nurse (RN)** has completed a 2-, 3-, or 4-year nursing program and has passed a licensing test:
- Community college programs—2 years
- Hospital-based diploma programs—2 or 3 years
- College or university programs—4 years

The graduate nurse takes a licensing test offered by a state board of nursing. The nurse receives a license and becomes *registered* when the test is passed. RNs must have a license recognized by the state in which they work.

RNs assess, make nursing diagnoses, plan, implement, and evaluate nursing care (Chapter 4). They develop care plans, provide care, and delegate nursing care and tasks to the nursing team. They evaluate how the care plans and nursing care affect each person. RNs teach persons how to improve health and independence. They also teach the family.

RNs carry out the doctor's orders. They may delegate them to other nursing team members. RNs do not diagnose or prescribe treatments or drugs. However, some RNs become *clinical nurse specialists* or *nurse practitioners.* They have limited diagnosing and prescribing functions.

Licensed Practical Nurses and Licensed Vocational Nurses

A **licensed practical nurse (LPN)** has completed a 1-year nursing program and has passed a licensing test. Hospitals, community colleges, vocational schools, and technical schools offer programs. Some programs are 18 months long. Some high schools offer 2-year programs.

Graduates take a licensing test for practical nursing. After passing the test, the person receives a license and the title of *licensed practical nurse.* **Licensed vocational nurse (LVN)** is used in some states. LPNs/LVNs must have a license required by the state in which they work.

LPNs/LVNs are supervised by RNs, licensed doctors, and licensed dentists. They have fewer responsibilities and functions than RNs do. They need little supervision when the person's condition is stable and care is simple. They assist RNs in caring for acutely ill persons and with complex procedures.

Nursing Assistants

A **nursing assistant** has passed a nursing assistant training and competency evaluation program. Nursing assistants perform delegated nursing tasks under the supervision of a licensed nurse. Nursing assistants are discussed in Chapter 2.

NURSING CARE PATTERNS

Nursing care is given in many ways. The pattern used depends on how many persons need care, the staff, and the cost.

- *Functional nursing* focuses on tasks and jobs. Each nursing team member has certain tasks and jobs to do. For example, one nurse gives all drugs. Another gives all treatments. Nursing assistants give baths, make beds, and serve meals.
- *Team nursing* involves a team of nursing staff led by an RN. Called the "team leader," he or she delegates care to other nurses. Some nursing tasks and procedures are delegated to nursing assistants. Delegation (Chapter 2) is based on the person's needs and team member abilities. Team members report to the team leader about observations made and the care given.
- *Primary nursing* involves total care. An RN is responsible for the person's total care. The nursing team assists as needed. The RN ("primary nurse") gives nursing care and makes discharge plans. The RN teaches and counsels the person and family.
- *Case management* is like primary nursing. A case manager (an RN) coordinates a person's care from admission through discharge and into the home setting. He or she communicates with the doctor and health team. There also is communication with community agencies as needed. Some case managers work with certain doctors. Others deal with certain health problems. Heart diseases and cancer are examples.
- *Patient-focused care* is when services are moved from departments to the bedside. The nursing team performs basic skills usually done by other health team members. The number of people caring for each person is reduced. This reduces care costs.

PAYING FOR HEALTH CARE

Health care is costly. Most people cannot afford these costs. Some avoid health care because they cannot pay. Others pay doctor bills before buying food or drugs. If the person has insurance, some care costs are covered. Rarely is the total cost of care covered.

These programs help pay for health care:

- *Private insurance* is bought by individuals and families. The insurance company pays for some or all health care costs.
- *Group insurance* is bought by groups or organizations for individuals. This is often an employee benefit.

PROMOTING SAFETY AND COMFORT
Paying for Health Care Safety

Safety

Some conditions can be prevented with proper care. Medicare will pay a lower rate for such conditions if they are acquired during a hospital stay. Pressure ulcers (Chapter 23) and certain types of falls, trauma, and infections are examples. You must assist the nursing and health teams in preventing such conditions.

- *Medicare* is a federal health insurance program for persons 65 years of age or older. Some younger people with certain disabilities are covered. Part A pays for some hospital, SNF, hospice, and home care costs. Part B helps pay for doctors' services, out-patient hospital care, physical and occupational therapists, some home care, and many other services. Part B is voluntary. The person pays a monthly premium.
- *Medicaid* is a health care payment program. Sponsored by the federal government, it is operated by the states. People with low incomes usually qualify. So do some older, blind, and disabled persons. There is no insurance premium. The amount paid for covered services is limited.

See *Promoting Safety and Comfort: Paying for Health Care.*

Prospective Payment Systems

Prospective payment systems limit the amount paid by insurers, Medicare, and Medicaid. Prospective means *before* care. The amount paid for services is determined before giving care.

- Medicare Severity-adjusted Diagnosis Related Groups (MS-DRGs) are for hospital costs.
- Resource utilization groups (RUGs) are for SNF payments.
- Case mix groups (CMGs) are used for rehabilitation centers.

Length of stay and treatment costs are determined for each group. If the treatment costs are less than the amount paid, the agency keeps the extra money. If costs are greater, the agency takes the loss.

Managed Care

Managed care deals with health care delivery and payment (Box 1-1, p. 8). Insurers contract with doctors and hospitals for reduced rates or discounts. The insured person uses doctors and agencies providing the lower rates. The person pays for costs not covered by insurance.

BOX 1-1   Types of Managed Care
■ **Health Maintenance Organization (HMO)** For a pre-paid fee, persons receive needed services offered by the HMO. Some have an annual physical exam. Others need hospital care. HMOs stress preventing disease and maintaining health. Keeping someone healthy costs far less than treating illness.
■ **Preferred Provider Organization (PPO)** A group of doctors and hospitals provide health care at reduced rates. Usually the agreement is between the PPO and an employer or an insurance company. Employees or those insured receive reduced rates for the services used. The person can choose any doctor or hospital in the PPO.

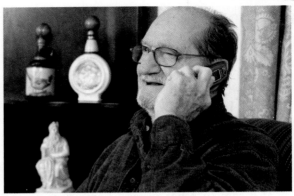

FIGURE 1-2 A resident talks privately on the phone.

Managed care limits the choice of where to go for health care. It also limits the care that doctors provide. Many states require managed care for Medicaid and Medicare coverage.

THE OMNIBUS BUDGET RECONCILIATION ACT OF 1987

The **Omnibus Budget Reconciliation Act of 1987 (OBRA)** is a federal law. It applies to all 50 states. Nursing centers must provide care in a manner and in a setting that maintains or improves each person's quality of life, health, and safety. Nursing assistant training and competency evaluation are part of OBRA. Resident rights are a major part of OBRA.

Resident Rights

Residents have rights as United States citizens. They also have rights relating to their everyday lives and care in a nursing center. Nursing centers must protect and promote such rights. The center cannot interfere with a resident's rights. Some residents are incompetent (not able). They cannot exercise their rights. A responsible party (partner, adult child) or legal representative does so for them.

Nursing centers must inform residents of their rights. This is done orally and in writing before or during admission to the center. It is given in the language the person uses and understands. Interpreters are used as needed. Resident rights also are posted throughout the center.

Information The person has the right to all of his or her records. They include the medical record, contracts, incident reports, and financial records. The request can be oral or written.

The person has the right to be fully informed of his or her health condition. The person must also have information about his or her doctor. This includes the doctor's name and contact information.

You do not give information to the person or family (Chapter 2). Report the request to the nurse.

Refusing Treatment The person has the right to refuse treatment or to take part in research. Treatment means the care provided to relieve symptoms, improve function, or maintain or restore health. If a person does not give consent or refuses treatment, it cannot be given. The center must find out what the person is refusing and why. Report any treatment refusal to the nurse. The nurse may need to change the person's care plan.

Privacy and Confidentiality Residents have the right to personal privacy. Body areas are exposed only as needed. Only staff directly involved in care and treatments are present. Consent is needed for others to be present.

A person has the right to use the bathroom in private. Privacy is maintained for all personal care measures. Bathing and dressing are examples.

Residents have the right to visit where others cannot see or hear them. This includes phone calls (Fig. 1-2). If requested, the center must provide private space. Offices, chapels, dining rooms, and meeting rooms are used as needed.

The right to privacy also involves mail. No one can interfere with the person sending or getting mail. Consent is needed to open any of the person's mail.

Information about the person's care, treatment, and condition is kept confidential. So are medical and financial records.

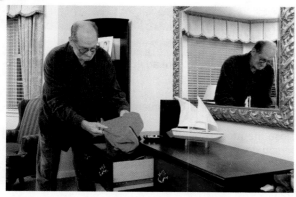

FIGURE 1-3 Resident chooses what clothing to wear.

Personal Choice Residents can choose their doctors. They also help plan and decide about their care and treatment. They can choose activities, schedules, and care. They can choose when to get up and go to bed, what to wear, how to spend time, and what to eat (Fig. 1-3). They can choose friends and visitors inside and outside the center. Allow personal choice whenever possible.

Disputes and Grievances Residents have the right to voice concerns, questions, and complaints about care. The problem may involve another person. It may be about how care was given or not given. The center must promptly try to correct the matter. No one can punish the person in any way for voicing the dispute or grievance.

Work The person does not work for care, care items, or other things or privileges. The person is not required to perform services for the center.

However, the person *can* work or perform services if he or she wants to. Some people like to garden, repair or build things, sew, or cook. Other persons need work for rehabilitation or activity reasons. The desire or need for work is part of the person's care plan.

Taking Part in Resident and Family Groups The person has the right to form and take part in resident and family groups. Families have the right to meet with other families. These groups can discuss concerns, suggest center improvements, and plan activities. They can provide support and comfort to group members.

Residents have the right to take part in social, cultural, religious, and community events. They have the right to help in getting to and from events of their choice.

Care and Security of Personal Items Residents have the right to keep and use personal items. Treat the person's property with care and respect. The items may not have value to you but have meaning to the person. They also relate to personal choice, dignity, and quality of life.

The person's property is protected. Items are labeled with the person's name. The center must investigate reports of lost, stolen, or damaged items. Police help is sometimes needed.

Protect yourself and the center from being accused of stealing a person's property. Do not go through a person's closet, drawers, purse, or other space without the person's consent. A nurse may ask you to inspect closets and drawers. If so, have a co-worker and the person or legal representative with you. They witness your actions.

Freedom From Abuse, Mistreatment, and Neglect Residents have the right to be free from all abuse—verbal, sexual, physical, mental, and so on (Chapter 2). They also have the right to be free from *involuntary seclusion:*
- Separating a person from others against his or her will
- Confining the person to a certain area
- Keeping the person away from his or her room without consent

No one can abuse, neglect, or mistreat a resident. This includes staff, volunteers, other residents, family members, visitors, and legal representatives. Centers must investigate suspected or reported cases of abuse. They cannot employ persons who were convicted of abusing, neglecting, or mistreating others.

Freedom From Restraint Residents have the right not to have body movements restricted. Restraints and certain drugs can restrict body movements (Chapter 10). Some drugs are restraints because they affect mood, behavior, and mental function. Sometimes residents are restrained to protect them from harming themselves or others. A doctor's order is needed for restraint use. Restraints are not used for staff convenience or to discipline a person.

BOX 1-2   OBRA-Required Actions to Promote Dignity and Privacy

Courteous and Dignified Interactions

- Use the right tone of voice.
- Use good eye contact.
- Stand or sit close enough as needed.
- Use the person's proper name and title. For example: "Mrs. Crane."
- Gain the person's attention before interacting with him or her.
- Use touch if the person approves.
- Respect the person's social status.
- Listen with interest to what the person is saying.
- Do not yell at, scold, or embarrass the person.

Courteous and Dignified Care

- Groom hair, beards, and nails as the person wishes.
- Assist with dressing in the right clothing for time of day and personal choice.
- Promote independence and dignity in dining.
- Respect private space and property.
- Assist with walking and transfers. Do not interfere with independence.
- Assist with bathing and hygiene preferences. Do not interfere with independence.
  - Appearance is neat and clean.
  - Person is clean shaven or has a groomed beard and mustache.
  - Nails are trimmed and clean.
  - Dentures, hearing aids, eyeglasses, and other devices are used correctly.
  - Clothing is clean.
  - Clothing is properly fitted and fastened.
  - Shoes, hose, and socks are properly fitted and fastened.
  - Extra clothing is available for warmth (sweaters and lap blanket are examples).

Privacy and Self-Determination

- Drape properly during care and procedures to avoid exposure and embarrassment.
- Drape properly in chair.
- Use privacy curtains or screens during care and procedures.
- Close the room door during care and procedures as the person desires. Also close window coverings.
- Knock on the door before entering. Wait to be asked in.
- Close the bathroom door when the person uses the bathroom.

Maintain Personal Choice and Independence

- Person smokes in allowed areas.
- Person takes part in activities according to his or her interests.
- Person takes part in scheduling activities and care.
- Person gives input into the care plan about preferences and independence.
- Person is involved in room or roommate change.

Quality of Life Residents must be cared for in a manner that promotes dignity and self-esteem. Care must also promote physical, psychological, and mental well-being. Protecting resident rights promotes quality of life. It shows respect for the person.

Speak to the person in a polite and courteous manner (Chapter 5). Good, honest, and thoughtful care enhances the person's quality of life. Box 1-2 lists OBRA-required actions that promote dignity and privacy.

Activities Nursing centers must provide activity programs that promote physical, intellectual, social, spiritual, and emotional well-being. Religious services promote spiritual health. Assist residents to and from activity programs. You may need to help them with activities.

Environment The center's environment must promote quality of life. It must be clean, safe, comfortable, and as home-like as possible. Personal items enhance quality of life. They allow personal choice and promote a home-like setting.

MEETING STANDARDS

Health care agencies must meet certain standards. Standards are set by the federal and state governments and accrediting agencies. Standards relate to agency policies and procedures, budget and finances, and quality of care.

Surveys are done to see if the agency meets set standards. A survey team will:

- Review policies, procedures, and medical records
- Interview staff, patients and residents, and families
- Observe how care is given
- Observe if dignity and privacy are promoted
- Check for cleanliness and safety
- Make sure the staff meets state requirements (Are doctors and nurses licensed? Are nursing assistants on the state registry?)

The survey team decides if the agency meets the standards. Sometimes problems are found. A problem is called a *deficiency*. The agency usually has 60 days to correct the problem. Sometimes less time is given. The agency can be fined for uncorrected or serious deficiencies. Or it can lose its license, certification, or accreditation.

Your Role

You have an important role in meeting standards and in the survey process. You must:

- Provide quality care.
- Protect the person's rights.
- Provide for the person's and your own safety.
- Help keep the agency clean and safe.
- Conduct yourself in a professional manner.
- Have good work ethics.
- Follow agency policies and procedures.
- Answer questions honestly and completely.

Focus on PRIDE
The Person, Family, and Yourself

Personal and Professional Responsibility—Health care is a rewarding profession. The health team works hard to provide quality care to patients and residents. You are an important part of that team. You spend most of your shift giving care to patients and residents. Remember to show them patience, compassion, dignity, and respect. You have a great impact on the quality of care each person receives.

Rights and Respect—Every person has the right to refuse treatment. This does not mean that the health team stops helping that person. The team offers other treatment options. For example, the doctor suggests the need for short-term placement in a nursing center. The person refuses. A family member agrees to help the person at home. A social worker helps the person and family arrange for home health care and respite care.

Independence and Social Interaction—Many patients and residents feel a loss of independence. Help promote independence by having them choose food, clothing, visitors, activities, and schedules. For example, a person needs help with bathing. He or she likes to bathe at night. However, the day shift gives baths. Share the person's preference with the nurse. The daytime and evening staffs must work together so the person can bathe when he or she chooses.

Delegation and Teamwork—The health team has many different members. Each has a certain role. Everyone must work together to reach the goal of quality care. Offer to help other team members when you are able to. Helping others shows you are dependable and value teamwork.

Ethics and Laws—The Older Americans Act is a federal law. The act addresses nutrition services, health promotion, disease prevention, family caregiver support, and other support services for older persons.

The act also serves to prevent elder abuse and protect the elder's rights. The act requires a long-term care ombudsman program in every state. An **ombudsman** is someone who supports or promotes the needs and interests of another person. Ombudsmen protect the health, safety, welfare, and rights of residents in long-term care centers. Centers must post contact information for local and state ombudsmen. If a person or family has a concern, know where to get this information.

REVIEW QUESTIONS

Circle the BEST answer.

1 An on-going illness that is slow or gradual in onset is called
   a An acute illness
   b A chronic illness
   c A terminal illness
   d A major illness

2 Persons in nursing centers are called
   a Patients
   b Residents
   c Clients
   d Patrons

3 A health care program for dying persons is a
   a Hospice
   b Board and care home
   c Skilled nursing facility
   d Dementia care unit

4 Who controls policy in a health care agency?
   a The survey team
   b The board of directors
   c The health team
   d Medicare and Medicaid

5 In nursing centers, the health team is called
   a The interdisciplinary health care team
   b The nursing team
   c A diagnosis-related group
   d A resident group

6 Who is responsible for the entire nursing staff and safe nursing care?
   a The case manager
   b The director of nursing
   c The charge nurse
   d The RN

7 You are supervised by
   a Licensed nurses
   b Nursing assistive personnel
   c The health team
   d The administrator

8 Nursing tasks are delegated according to a person's needs and staff member abilities. This nursing care pattern is called
   a Team nursing
   b Functional nursing
   c Case management
   d Primary nursing

9 Medicare is for persons who
   a Are 65 years of age and older
   b Receive MS-DRGs and RUGs
   c Have group insurance
   d Have low incomes

10 A survey team is at your agency. A team member asks you some questions. You should
   a Refer all questions to the nurse
   b Answer as the DON tells you to
   c Give as little information as possible
   d Give honest and complete answers

Circle T if the statement is *true*. Circle F if the statement is *false*.

11 T F   A person has the right to refuse treatment.
12 T F   A person has the right to use the bathroom in private.
13 T F   You can expose part of a person's body for care measures.
14 T F   You can open a person's mail.
15 T F   You can listen to a person's phone calls.
16 T F   A person can decide when he or she will bathe.
17 T F   You can punish a person for complaining about a nursing center.
18 T F   A person has the right to attend religious services.
19 T F   The person's items are treated with care and respect.
20 T F   The person's items are labeled with his or her name.
21 T F   You can decide when to search a person's closet and drawers.
22 T F   The person must be free from abuse, mistreatment, and neglect.
23 T F   You can decide when to restrain a person.
24 T F   The person can take part in activities of his or her choice.
25 T F   Nursing centers must be as home-like as possible.

Answers to these questions are on p. 527.

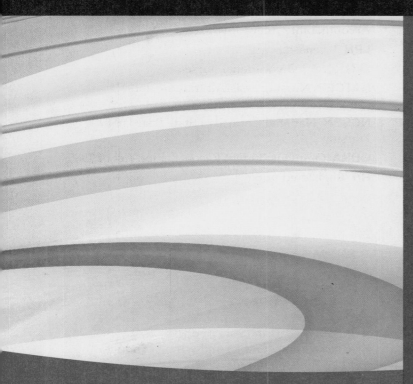

2

THE NURSING ASSISTANT

OBJECTIVES

- Define the key terms and key abbreviations listed in this chapter.
- List the reasons for denying, suspending, or revoking a nursing assistant's certification, license, or registration.
- Describe what nursing assistants can do and their role limits.
- Describe the standards for nursing assistants developed by the National Council of State Boards of Nursing.
- Explain why a job description is important.
- Describe the delegation process.
- Explain your role in the delegation process.
- Explain how to accept or refuse a delegated task.
- Give examples of intentional and unintentional torts.
- Explain how to protect the right to privacy.
- Explain the importance of informed consent.
- Describe elder abuse.
- Explain how to promote PRIDE in the person, the family, and yourself.

KEY TERMS

abuse The intentional mistreatment or harm of another person

assault Intentionally attempting or threatening to touch a person's body without the person's consent

battery Touching a person's body without his or her consent

boundary crossing A brief act or behavior outside of the helpful zone

boundary sign An act, behavior, or thought that warns of a boundary crossing or boundary violation

boundary violation An act or behavior that meets your needs, not the person's needs

civil law Laws dealing with relationships between people

crime An act that violates a criminal law

criminal law Laws concerned with offenses against the public and society in general

defamation Injuring a person's name and reputation by making false statements to a third person

delegate To authorize another person to perform a nursing task in a certain situation

elder abuse Any knowing, intentional, or negligent act by a caregiver or any other person to an older adult

ethics Knowledge of what is right conduct and wrong conduct

false imprisonment Unlawful restraint or restriction of a person's freedom of movement

fraud Saying or doing something to trick, fool, or deceive a person

invasion of privacy Violating a person's right not to have his or her name, photo, or private affairs exposed or made public without giving consent

job description A document that describes what the agency expects you to do

law A rule of conduct made by a government body

libel Making false statements in print, writing, or through pictures or drawings

malpractice Negligence by a professional person

neglect Failure to provide the person with the goods or services needed to avoid physical harm, mental anguish, or mental illness

negligence An unintentional wrong in which a person did not act in a reasonable and careful manner and a person or the person's property was harmed

nursing task Nursing care or a nursing function, procedure, activity, or work that can be delegated to nursing assistants when it does not require an RN's professional knowledge or judgment

professional boundary That which separates helpful behaviors from those that are not helpful

professional sexual misconduct An act, behavior, or comment that is sexual in nature

protected health information Identifying information about the person's health care that is maintained or sent in any form (paper, electronic, oral)

self-neglect A person's behaviors that threaten his or her health and safety

slander Making false statements orally

vulnerable adult A person 18 years old or older who has a disability or condition that makes him or her at risk to be wounded, attacked, or damaged

KEY ABBREVIATIONS

CNA Certified nursing assistant; certified nurse aide

HIPAA Health Insurance Portability and Accountability Act of 1996

LPN Licensed practical nurse

LVN Licensed vocational nurse

NATCEP Nursing assistant training and competency evaluation program

NCSBN National Council of State Boards of Nursing

OBRA Omnibus Budget Reconciliation Act of 1987

RN Registered nurse

You must protect patients and residents from harm. To do so, you need to know:
- What you can and cannot do
- What is right conduct and wrong conduct
- Rules and standards of conduct affecting your work
- Your legal limits

Laws, job descriptions, and the person's condition shape your work. So does the amount of supervision you need.

OBRA REQUIREMENTS

The Omnibus Budget Reconciliation Act of 1987 (OBRA) is a federal law. It applies to all 50 states. Each state must have a nursing assistant training and competency evaluation program (NATCEP). It must be successfully completed by nursing assistants working in nursing centers, hospital long-term care units, and home care agencies receiving Medicare funds.

The Training Program

OBRA requires at least 75 hours of instruction provided by a nurse. Some states require more hours. The training program includes the knowledge and skills needed to give basic nursing care. Sixteen hours are supervised practical training. It occurs in a laboratory or clinical setting. Students perform nursing care and procedures on other persons.

Competency Evaluation

The competency evaluation has a written test and a skills test (Appendix A, p. 529). The written test has multiple-choice questions. For the skills test, you perform certain skills learned in your training program.

You take the competency evaluation after your training program. Your instructor tells you when and where the tests are given. He or she helps you complete the application. There is a fee for the evaluation. If you work in a nursing center, the employer pays this fee.

If you listen, study hard, and practice safe care, you should do well. If your first attempt was not successful, you can retest. OBRA allows at least 3 attempts to successfully complete the evaluation.

After successfully completing your state's NATCEP, you have the title used in your state:
- Certified nursing assistant (CNA) or certified nurse aide (CNA). CNA is used in most states.
- Licensed nursing assistant (LNA).
- Registered nurse aide (RNA).

Nursing assistants can have their certification, license, or registration denied, revoked, or suspended. See Box 2-1 for the reasons listed by the National Council of State Boards of Nursing (NCSBN).

Nursing Assistant Registry

Each state must have a nursing assistant registry. It is an official listing of persons who have successfully completed a NATCEP. The registry has information about each nursing assistant:
- Full name, including maiden name and any married names.

BOX 2-1 Reasons for Losing Certification, a License, or Registration

- Substance abuse or dependency.
- Abandoning a patient or resident.
- Abusing a patient or resident.
- Fraud or deceit. Examples include:
  - Filing false personal information
  - Providing false information when applying for initial certification
  - Providing false information when applying to have certification re-instated
  - Providing false information when applying for certification renewal
- Neglecting a patient or resident.
- Violating professional boundaries (p. 24).
- Giving unsafe care.
- Performing acts beyond the nursing assistant role.
- Misappropriation (stealing, theft) or mis-using property.
- Obtaining money or property from a patient or resident. Fraud, falsely representing oneself, and force are examples.
- Having been convicted of a crime. Examples include murder, assault, kidnapping, rape or sexual assault, robbery, sexual crimes involving children, criminal mistreatment of children or a vulnerable adult (p. 27), drug trafficking, embezzlement (to take a person's property for one's own use), theft, and arson (starting fires).
- Failing to conform to the standards of nursing assistants (p. 17).
- Putting patients and residents at risk for harm.
- Violating the privacy of a patient or resident.
- Failing to maintain the confidentiality of patient or resident information.

- Last known home address.
- Registration number and the date it expires.
- Date of birth.
- Last known employer, date hired, and date employment ended.
- Date the competency evaluation was passed.
- Information about findings of abuse, neglect, or dishonest use of property. It includes the nature of the offense and supporting evidence. If a hearing was held, the date and its outcome are included. The person has the right to include a statement disputing the finding. All information stays in the registry for at least 5 years.

Any agency can access registry information. You also receive a copy of your registry information. The copy is provided when the first entry is made and when information is changed or added. You can correct wrong information.

Other OBRA Requirements

Retraining and a new competency evaluation program are required for nursing assistants who have not worked for 24 months. It does not matter how long you worked as a nursing assistant. What matters is how long you did *not* work. States can require:

- A new competency evaluation
- Both retraining and a new competency evaluation

Agencies must provide 12 hours of educational programs to nursing assistants every year. Performance reviews also are required. That is, your work is evaluated. These requirements help ensure that you have the current knowledge and skills to give safe, effective care.

ROLES, RESPONSIBILITIES, AND STANDARDS

OBRA, state laws, and legal and advisory opinions direct what you can do. To protect persons from harm, you must understand what you can do, what you cannot do, and the legal limits of your role.

Licensed nurses supervise your work. You perform nursing tasks related to the person's care. A **nursing task** is the nursing care or a nursing function, procedure, activity, or work that can be delegated to nursing assistants when it does not require an RN's professional knowledge or judgment. Often you function without a nurse in the room. At other times you help nurses give care. The rules in Box 2-2 will help you understand your role.

What you are allowed to do varies among states and agencies. Before you perform a nursing task make sure that:

- Your state allows nursing assistants to do so
- It is in your job description
- You have the necessary education and training
- A nurse is available to answer questions and to supervise you

You perform nursing tasks to meet hygiene, safety, comfort, nutrition, exercise, and elimination needs. You also handle and move persons and make observations. You also measure temperatures, pulses, respirations, and blood pressures. And you have a role in the person's mental comfort.

Box 2-3 describes what you should never do. State laws differ. You must know what you can do in the state in which you are working. State laws and rules limit nursing assistant functions. Your job description

---

BOX 2-2   Rules for Nursing Assistants

- You are an assistant to the nurse.
- A nurse assigns and supervises your work.
- You report observations about the person's physical and mental status to the nurse. Report changes in the person's condition or behavior at once.
- The nurse decides what should be done for a person. The nurse decides what should not be done for a person. You do not make these decisions.
- Review directions and the care plan with the nurse before going to the person.
- Perform only those nursing tasks for which you are trained.
- Ask a nurse to supervise you if you are not comfortable performing a nursing task.
- Perform only the nursing tasks that your state and job description allow.

BOX 2-3   Role Limits for Nursing Assistants

- **Never give drugs.** Nurses give drugs. Many states allow nursing assistants to give drugs after completing a state-approved medication assistant training program.
- **Never insert tubes or objects into body openings. Do not remove them from the body.** Exceptions to this rule are the procedures you will study during your training. Giving enemas is an example.
- **Never take oral or phone orders from doctors.** Politely give your name and title, and ask the doctor to wait for a nurse. Promptly find a nurse to speak with the doctor.
- **Never perform procedures that require sterile technique.** With sterile technique, all objects in contact with the person are free of microorganisms (Chapter 11). You can assist a nurse with a sterile procedure. However, you will not perform the procedure yourself.
- **Never tell the person or family the person's diagnosis or medical or surgical treatment plans.** This is the doctor's responsibility. Nurses may clarify what the doctor has said.
- **Never diagnose or prescribe treatments or drugs for anyone.** Doctors diagnose and prescribe.
- **Never supervise others including other nursing assistants.** This is a nurse's responsibility. You will not be trained to supervise others. Supervising others can have serious legal problems.
- **Never ignore an order or request to do something.** This includes nursing tasks that you can do, those you cannot do, and those beyond your legal limits. Promptly and politely explain to the nurse why you cannot carry out the order or request. The nurse assumes you are doing what you were told to do unless you explain otherwise. You cannot neglect the person's care.

reflects those laws and rules. An agency can further limit what you can do. So can a nurse based on the person's needs. However, no agency or nurse can expand your range of functions beyond what is allowed by your state's laws and rules.

OBRA defines the basic range of functions for nursing assistants. All NATCEPs include those functions (p. 15). Some states allow other functions. NATCEPs also prepare nursing assistants to meet the standards listed in Box 2-4.

JOB DESCRIPTION

The **job description** is a document that describes what the agency expects you to do (Fig. 2-1). It also states educational requirements.

Always obtain a written job description when you apply for a job. Ask questions about it during your job interview. Before accepting a job, tell the employer about functions you did not learn. Also advise the employer of functions you cannot do for moral or

Text continued on p. 20

BOX 2-4 **Nursing Assistant Standards**

The nursing assistant:
- Performs nursing tasks within the range of functions allowed by his or her state.
- Is honest and shows integrity in performing nursing tasks. (*Integrity* involves following a code of ethics [p. 24].)
- Bases nursing tasks on his or her education and training. Also bases them on the nurse's directions.
- Is accountable for his or her behavior and actions while assisting the nurse and helping patients and residents.
- Performs delegated aspects of the person's nursing care.
- Assists the nurse in observing patients and residents. Also assists in identifying their needs.

- Communicates:
  - Progress toward completing delegated nursing tasks
  - Problems in completing delegated nursing tasks
  - Changes in the person's status
- Asks the nurse to clarify what is expected when unsure.
- Uses educational and training opportunities as available.
- Practices safety measures to protect the person, others, and self.
- Respects the person's rights, concerns, decisions, and dignity.
- Functions as a member of the health team. Helps implement the care plan (Chapter 4).
- Respects the person's property and the property of others.
- Protects confidential information unless required by law to share the information.

Modified from National Council of State Boards of Nursing, Inc.: *Model Nursing Practice Act and Model Nursing Administrative Rules,* Chicago, Ill, 2006, Author.

JOB DESCRIPTION

Illinois Valley Community Hospital
925 West Street, Peru, Illinois 61354
815-223-3300

Caring Professionals

CRITERIA: NURSE ASSISTANT   NAME: _____   UNIT: _____

The following criteria are to be considered as an integral part of this job description and are used in the evaluation process.

ASSISTING WITH NURSING CARE	Met	Not Met
ASSISTS WITH ASSESSING Recognizes abnormal vital signs and reports them to the nurse in charge immediately.		
Observes patients and reports problems (e.g., bleeding, drainage, voiding, machine functions, IV drip, safety situations) immediately and/or current status to the nurse in charge.		
Checks on patients regularly, making frequent rounds.		

FIGURE 2-1 Nursing assistant job description. Note that the job description is also a performance evaluation tool. (*Modified from Illinois Valley Community Hospital, Peru, Ill.*)

Continued

ASSISTING WITH NURSING CARE (cont'd)	Met	Not Met
ASSISTS WITH PLANNING/ORGANIZING Consistently organizes and appropriately executes personal work assignments in an effort to achieve maximum productivity and efficiency during the assigned shift.		
Demonstrates a time-conscious awareness and consistently strives to use time effectively, completing assigned procedures during scheduled shift.		
Responds to changes in the unit workload, patient census, and staffing levels; plans patient care accordingly.		
Demonstrates an ability to recognize and deal with priorities promptly.		
ASSISTS WITH IMPLEMENTING Administers patient care based on the plan of care.		
Effectively implements nursing orders after consulting appropriate sources regarding unfamiliar or questionable orders.		
Responds to patient's condition/needs and acts in a timely and appropriate manner.		
Demonstrates a reliable and dependable ability to follow through with designated responsibilities in collecting, labeling, and transporting specimens to the proper area at the appropriate time: always correctly labels type of specimen collected, including patient's name and room number.		
Assists the nurse with complicated treatment procedures.		
Completes work left from previous shifts and reports all incomplete assignments to ensure continuity of care.		
As required, provides for patient comfort (by positioning, extra bathing, straightening linens, putting personal articles within reach) with courtesy and responsiveness.		
Routinely assists patients with elimination (bedpan, bathroom) as required.		
Regularly ambulates patients as assigned; demonstrates proper techniques.		
Consistently demonstrates competence in providing morning, evening, and general care routines in accordance with established nursing care procedures to ensure patients' comfort and safety.		
Regularly prepares patients for meals, sets up each patient and patient's tray, assists in feeding patients (if necessary), positions patients to avoid choking and for ease in eating, and distributes water and other nourishments according to patients' needs; regularly provides patients with fresh water.		
Always follows the nursing care plan; observes established policies and procedures for proper patient treatment and care.		
Promptly answers patient signal lights, whether that of assigned patient or not.		
ASSISTS WITH EVALUATING Checks physical environment of unit to determine what needs to be done in terms of smooth operation.		
Evaluates need for linen changes.		
Reviews basic care provided to patients and reports if changes are needed.		
ASSISTS WITH TEACHING/LEARNING Regularly provides patient information on admission in regard to: correct storage of patients' valuables, eyeglasses, and dentures; use of equipment, bed controls, nurse/patient communication system; location of bathroom and emergency call signals; and specimen collection.		
Serves as a resource person for new employees during orientation.		
Demonstrates the knowledge of the principles of growth and development over the life span. (Completes two age-related modules.)		
Recognizes own inadequacies, and seeks assistance appropriately.		

FIGURE 2-1, cont'd Nursing assistant job description. Note that the job description is also a performance evaluation tool.

	Met	Not Met
COMMUNICATING		
Communicates to appropriate members of the health care team specific observations or changes in patient's condition.		
Explains information to patients, visitors, and co-workers in a clear and thorough manner; leaves no questions unanswered and follows up on information not readily available.		
Consistently communicates appropriately with patients: speaks respectfully, addresses patients by name, responds to patients' needs or requests for assistance.		
JUDGMENT/LEADERSHIP		
Promotes teamwork among staff.		
Reports all patient care or management problems as appropriate, using chain of command.		
Functions in a calm manner during emergency and crisis situations.		
MAINTAINING SAFETY/INFECTION CONTROL/PATIENT RIGHTS		
Always demonstrates knowledge of and rationale for safe use of equipment; reports any equipment malfunctions and orders service, as necessary.		
Ensures patient safety by maintaining bed in a low position and signal light within reach at all times. Identifies patients before performing procedures. Follows the care plan for bed rail use.		
Uses proper techniques of body mechanics.		
Assists in maintaining a clean, safe, and attractive environment in all areas of the patient unit.		
Practices hand hygiene before and after each patient contact; uses aseptic technique during procedures and treatments.		
Uses principles of Standard and Transmission-Based Precautions. Follows the Bloodborne Pathogen Standard.		
Adheres to *The Patient Care Partnership: Understanding Expectations, Rights, and Responsibilities,* and respects the patient's right to privacy, dignity, and confidentiality.		
Handles all patients' clothing, dentures, eyeglasses, and other valuables with care.		
RELATIONSHIP WITH OTHERS		
Demonstrates a high level of mental and emotional tolerance and even temperament when dealing with ill people; uses tact, sensitivity, sound judgment, and a professional attitude when relating with patients, families, co-workers, and physicians.		
Greets all patients in a courteous manner by introducing self and calling the patient by name.		
Displays an unhurried, caring manner in all personal contact; demonstrates the ability to remain friendly and cooperative during all work situations.		
Consistently responds to others in a helpful manner, especially in times of increased patient activities or short staffing situations.		
Promotes an atmosphere of acceptance for new staff members on the unit.		

FIGURE 2-1, cont'd Nursing assistant job description. Note that the job description is also a performance evaluation tool.

Continued

	Met	Not Met
ATTENDANCE AND RELIABILITY		
Consistently is on time and ready to work at the start of the shift; requires no start-up time.		
Willingly accepts re-assignments to other units when necessary.		
Consistently returns promptly from errands, coffee breaks, and meals.		
Complies with Absenteeism Policy.		
COOPERATION/SUPPORT		
Attends and actively participates in unit meetings (75% of the time).		
Accepts additional assignments willingly.		
Consistently promotes good public relations for the unit, nursing department, and hospital.		
Supports hospital philosophy, policies and procedures, and management decisions.		
WORKS EXTRA WEEKENDS/HOLIDAYS AND/OR ROTATES SHIFTS TO ASSIST IN PROVIDING ADEQUATE STAFFING. **BONUS**		
INITIATIVE		
Takes initiative in recognition and resolution of problems.		
Reports to the nurse manager or appropriate supervisor any suggestions or recommendations for positive changes within the departmental policies and procedures.		
Ensures that supplies are maintained according to established guidelines, and notifies appropriate person to restock.		
PROFESSIONAL GROWTH/APPEARANCE		
Always appears well-groomed and observes the hospital dress code; wears identification badge while on duty; maintains a professional appearance at all times; is clean and well-groomed.		
Maintains professional code of ethics.		
Completes all mandatory programs including those on safety, infection control, and CPR.		
Identifies own self-development needs, and writes goals for same. Strives to achieve those goals.		
Demonstrates ability to perform unit-specific competencies.		

FIGURE 2-1, cont'd Nursing assistant job description. Note that the job description is also a performance evaluation tool.

religious reasons. Clearly understand what is expected before taking a job. Do not take a job that requires you to:

- Act beyond the legal limits of your role
- Function beyond your training limits
- Perform acts that are against your morals or religion

No one can force you to do something beyond the legal limits of your role. Sometimes jobs are threatened for refusing to follow a nurse's orders. Often staff obey out of fear. That is why you must understand nursing assistant roles, responsibilities, and standards. You also need to know what you can safely do, the things you should never do, and your job description.

DELEGATION

Delegate means to authorize another person to perform a nursing task in a certain situation. The person must be competent to perform a task in a given situation. For example, you know how to give a bed bath. However, the RN wants to spend time with a new resident and assess nursing needs. You do not assess. Therefore the RN gives the bath.

Who Can Delegate

RNs can delegate nursing tasks to LPNs/LVNs and nursing assistants. In some states, LPNs/LVNs can delegate tasks to nursing assistants. Delegation decisions must protect the person's health and safety.

The delegating nurse must make sure that the task was completed safely and correctly. If the RN delegates, the RN is responsible for the delegated task. If the LPN/LVN delegates, the LPN/LVN is responsible for the delegated task. The RN also supervises LPNs/LVNs. Therefore the RN also is responsible for the tasks that LPNs/LVNs delegate to nursing assistants. The RN is accountable for all nursing care.

Nursing assistants cannot delegate. You cannot delegate any task to other nursing assistants or to any other worker. You can ask someone to help you. But you cannot ask or tell someone to do your work.

Delegation Process

To make delegation decisions, the nurse follows a process. The person's needs, the nursing task, and the staff member doing the task must fit. The nurse may or may not decide to delegate the task to you. The person's needs and the task may require a nurse's knowledge, judgment, and skill. You may be asked to assist.

Delegation decisions must result in the best care for the person. Poor delegation decisions affect the person's health and safety. The NCSBN describes the delegation process in four steps.

Step 1—Assess and Plan
The nurse needs to understand the person's needs. And the nurse needs to know your knowledge, skills, and job description.

When assessing the person's needs, the nurse answers these questions:

- What is the nature of the person's needs? How complex are the needs? How can they vary? How urgent are the care needs?
- What are the most important long-term needs? What are the most important short-term needs?
- How much judgment is needed to meet the person's needs and give care?
- How predictable is the person's health status? How does the person respond to health care?
- What problems might arise from the nursing task? How severe might the problems be?
- What actions are needed if a problem arises? How complex are those actions?
- What emergencies or incidents might arise? How likely might they occur?
- How involved is the person in health care decisions? How involved is the family?
- How will delegating the nursing task help the person? What are the risks to the person?

To assess your knowledge and skills, the nurse answers these questions:

- What knowledge and skills are needed to safely perform the nursing task?
- What is your role in the agency? What is in your job description?
- What are the conditions under which the nursing task will be performed?
- What is expected after the nursing task is performed?
- What problems can arise from the nursing task? What problems might the person develop during the nursing task?

The nurse then decides if delegating the task is safe for the person and safe for you. If unsafe, the nurse stops the delegation process. If it is safe for the person and you, the nurse moves to step two.

Step 2—Communication
This step involves the nurse and you. The nurse must provide clear and complete directions about:

- How to perform and complete the task
- What observations to report and record
- When to report observations
- What specific patient and resident concerns to report at once
- Priorities for nursing tasks
- What to do if the person's needs change or condition changes

The nurse must be sure that you understand the directions. The nurse asks you questions to make sure you understand. He or she may ask you to explain what you are going to do. Do not be insulted by the nurse's questions. The nurse must make sure that safe care is given. This protects the person and you.

Before performing a delegated task, you must have the opportunity to discuss the task with the nurse. Make sure that you:

- Ask questions about the delegated task.
- Ask questions about what you are expected to do.
- Tell the nurse if you have not done the task before or if you have not done it often.
- Ask for needed training or supervision.
- Re-state what is expected of you.
- Re-state what specific patient or resident concerns to report to the nurse.
- Explain how and when you will report your progress in completing the task.
- Know how to contact the nurse for an emergency.
- Know what the nurse wants you to do during an emergency.

After completing a delegated task, you must report and record the care given. You also report and record your observations. See "Reporting and Recording" in Chapter 4.

Step 3—Surveillance and Supervision Surveillance means to keep a close watch over someone or something. Supervise means to oversee, direct, or manage. In this step, the nurse observes the care you give. The nurse makes sure that you complete the task correctly. The nurse also observes the person's condition and response to your care. How often the nurse makes observations depends on:

- The person's health status and needs
- If the person's condition is stable or unstable
- If the nurse can predict the person's responses and risks to care
- The setting where the nursing task occurs
- The resources and support available
- If the nursing task is simple or complex

The nurse must follow-up on any problems or concerns. For example, the nurse must take action if you did not complete the task in a timely manner. The nurse also must take action if the task did not meet expectations. An unexpected change in the person's condition is also cause for the nurse to act.

The nurse must be alert for signs and symptoms that signal a possible change in the person's condition. This way the nurse, with your help, can take action before the person's condition changes in a major way.

Sometimes problems arise in completing a task. By supervising you, the nurse can detect and solve problems early. This helps you complete the task safely and on time.

After you complete the task, the nurse may review and discuss what happened with you. This helps you learn. If a similar situation happens in the future, you have ideas about how to adjust.

Step 4—Evaluation and Feedback This step is done by the nurse. Evaluate means to judge. The nurse decides if the delegation was successful. The nurse answers these questions:

- Was the task done correctly?
- Did the person respond to the task as expected?
- Was the outcome (the result) as desired? Was it satisfactory or not satisfactory?
- Was communication between you and the nurse timely and effective?
- What went well? What were the problems?
- Does the care plan need to change (Chapter 4)? Or can the plan stay the same?
- Did the task present ways for the nurse or you to learn?
- Did the nurse give you the right feedback? Feedback means to respond. The nurse tells you what you did correctly. If you did something wrong, the nurse tells you that too. Feedback is another way in which you can learn and improve the care you give.
- Did the nurse thank you for completing the task?

The Five Rights of Delegation

The NCSBN's Five Rights of Delegation is another way to view the delegation process. The nurse answers the questions listed in the four steps described above. The Five Rights of Delegation are:

- The right task. Can the task be delegated? Is the nurse allowed to delegate the task? Is the task in your job description?
- The right circumstances. What are the person's physical, mental, emotional, and spiritual needs at this time?
- The right person. Do you have the training and experience to safely perform the task for this person?
- The right directions and communication. The nurse must give clear directions. The nurse tells you what to do and when to do it. The nurse tells you what observations to make and when to report back. The nurse allows questions and helps you set priorities.

- *The right supervision.* The nurse guides, directs, and evaluates the care you give. The nurse demonstrates tasks as necessary and is available to answer questions. The less experience you have with a task, the more supervision you need. Complex tasks require more supervision than do basic tasks. Also, the person's circumstances affect how much supervision you need. The nurse assesses how the task affected the person and how well you performed the task. The nurse tells you what you did well and how to improve your work. This helps you learn and give better care.

Your Role in Delegation

You perform delegated nursing tasks for or on *a person.* You must protect the person from harm. You have two choices when a task is delegated to you. You either *agree* or *refuse* to do the task. Use the *Five Rights of Delegation* in Box 2-5.

Accepting a Task When you agree to perform a task, you are responsible for your own actions. What you do or fail to do can harm the person. *You must complete the task safely.* Ask for help when you are unsure or have questions about a task. Report to the nurse what you did and the observations you made.

Refusing a Task You have the right to say "no." Sometimes refusing to follow the nurse's directions is your right and duty. You should refuse to perform a task when:

- The task is beyond the legal limits of your role.
- The task is not in your job description.
- You were not prepared to perform the task.
- The task could harm the person.
- The person's condition has changed.
- You do not know how to use the supplies or equipment.
- Directions are not ethical or legal.
- Directions are against agency policies or procedures.
- Directions are not clear or not complete.
- A nurse is not available for supervision.

Use common sense. This protects you and the person. Ask yourself if what you are doing is safe for the person.

Never ignore an order or a request to do something. Tell the nurse about your concerns. If the task is within the legal limits of your role and in your job

---

BOX 2-5 The Five Rights of Delegation for Nursing Assistants

The Right Task
- Does your state allow you to perform the task?
- Were you trained to do the task?
- Do you have experience performing the task?
- Is the task in your job description?

The Right Circumstances
- Do you have experience performing the task given the person's condition and needs?
- Do you understand the purposes of the task for the person?
- Can you perform the task safely under the current circumstances?
- Do you have the equipment and supplies to safely complete the task?
- Do you know how to use the equipment and supplies?

The Right Person
- Are you comfortable performing the task?
- Do you have concerns about performing the task?

The Right Directions and Communication
- Did the nurse give clear directions and instructions?
- Did you review the task with the nurse?
- Do you understand what the nurse expects?

The Right Supervision
- Is a nurse available to answer questions?
- Is a nurse available if the person's condition changes or if problems occur?

Modified from the National Council of State Boards of Nursing, Inc.: *The Five Rights of Delegation,* Chicago, Ill, 1997, Author.

---

description, the nurse can help increase your comfort with the task. The nurse can:

- Answer your questions
- Demonstrate the task
- Show you how to use supplies and equipment
- Help you as needed
- Observe you performing the task
- Check on you often
- Arrange for needed training

Do not refuse a task because you do not like it or do not want to do it. You must have sound reasons. Otherwise, you place the person at risk for harm. You also could lose your job.

See *Focus on Communication: Refusing a Task, p. 24.*

FOCUS ON COMMUNICATION
Refusing a Task

A nurse may delegate a task that you did not learn in your training program. The task is in your job description. You can say: "I know this task is in my job description, but I did not learn it in school. Can you show me what to do and then observe me doing it? That would really help me."

A nurse may ask you to do something that is not in your job description. With respect, you must firmly refuse the nurse's request. You can say: "I'm sorry. I am not trained to do that. That task is not in my job description. Can I help you with something else?"

ETHICAL ASPECTS

Ethics is knowledge of what is right conduct and wrong conduct. Morals are involved. It also deals with choices or judgments about what should or should not be done. An ethical person behaves and acts in the right way. He or she does not cause a person harm.

Ethical behavior also involves not being *prejudiced* or *biased.* To be prejudiced or biased means to make judgments and have views before knowing the facts. Judgments and views usually are based on one's values and standards. They are based in the person's culture, religion, education, and experiences. For example, children want their mother to have nursing home care. In your culture, children care for older parents at home.

Do not judge the person by your values and standards. Do not avoid persons whose standards and values differ from your own.

Ethical problems involve making choices. You must decide what is the right thing to do.

Codes of ethics are rules or standards of conduct. Nursing organizations have codes of ethics for RNs and LPNs/LVNs. The rules of conduct in Box 2-6 can guide your thinking and behavior. See Chapter 3 for ethics in the workplace.

BOX 2-6   Code of Conduct for Nursing Assistants

- Respect each person as an individual.
- Know the limits of your role and knowledge.
- Perform only those tasks that are within the legal limits of your role.
- Perform only those tasks that you have been prepared to do.
- Perform no act that will cause the person harm.
- Take drugs only if prescribed and supervised by a doctor.
- Carry out the directions and instructions of the nurse to your best possible ability.
- Follow the agency's policies and procedures.
- Complete each task safely.
- Be loyal to your employer and co-workers.
- Act as a responsible citizen at all times.
- Keep the person's information confidential.
- Protect the person's privacy.
- Protect the person's property.
- Consider the person's needs to be more important than your own.
- Report errors and incidents at once.
- Be accountable for your actions.

Boundaries

A *boundary* limits or separates something. A fence forms a boundary. It tells you to stay within or on the side of the fenced area. Nursing assistants help patients, residents, and families. Therefore you enter into a helping relationship with them. The helping relationship has professional boundaries.

Professional boundaries separate helpful behaviors from those that are not helpful (Fig. 2-2). The boundaries create a helpful zone. If your behaviors are outside of the helpful zone, you are over-involved with the person or under-involved. The following can occur:

- A **boundary crossing** is a brief act or behavior outside of the helpful zone. The act or behavior may be thoughtless or something you did not mean to do. Or it could be on purpose if it meets the person's needs. For example, giving a crying person a hug meets the person's needs at that time. If giving a hug meets your needs, the act is wrong. Also, it is wrong to hug the person every time you see him or her.

PROFESSIONAL BOUNDARIES

Under-involved	Helpful zone	Over-involved

FIGURE 2-2 Professional boundaries. *(Modified from the National Council of State Boards of Nursing, Inc.:* Professional boundaries: a nurse's guide to the importance of appropriate professional boundaries, *Chicago, Ill, 1996, Author.)*

- A **boundary violation** is an act or behavior that meets your needs, not the person's. The act or behavior is unethical. It violates the code of conduct in Box 2-6. The person could be harmed. Boundary violations include:
  - Abuse (p. 27).
  - Giving a lot of personal information about yourself. You tell a person about your personal relationships or problems.
  - Keeping secrets with the person.
- **Professional sexual misconduct** is an act, behavior, or comment that is sexual in nature. It is sexual misconduct even if the person consents or makes the first move.

Some boundary violations and some types of professional sexual misconduct also are crimes (p. 26). To maintain professional boundaries, follow the rules in Box 2-7. Be alert to boundary signs. **Boundary signs** are acts, behaviors, or thoughts that warn of a boundary crossing or boundary violation. Examples include:

- You spend free time with the person.
- You give more attention to the person at the expense of other patients and residents.
- The person gives you gifts or money. Or you give the person gifts or money.
- You flirt with the person.
- You make comments that have a sexual message.
- You notice more touch between you and the person.

BOX 2-7 Rules for Maintaining Professional Boundaries

- Follow the code of conduct listed in Box 2-6.
- Talk to the nurse if you sense a boundary sign, crossing, or violation.
- Avoid caring for family, friends, and people with whom you do business. This may be hard to do in a small community. Always tell the nurse if you know the person. The nurse may need to change your assignment.
- Do not date, flirt with, kiss, or have a sexual relationship with current patients or residents. The same applies to family members of current patients or residents.
- Do not make sexual comments or jokes.
- Do not use offensive language.
- Do not discuss your sexual relationships with patients, residents, or their families.
- Do not say or write things that could suggest a romantic or sexual relationship with a patient, resident, or family member.
- Use touch correctly (Chapter 5). Do not touch or handle sexual and genital areas except when necessary to give care. Such areas include the breasts, nipples, perineum, buttocks, and anus.
- Do not accept gifts, loans, money, credit cards, or other valuables from a patient, resident, or family member.
- Do not give gifts, loans, money, credit cards, or other valuables to a patient, resident, or family member.
- Do not borrow from a patient, resident, or family member. This includes money, personal items, and transportation.
- Maintain a professional relationship at all times. Do not develop any personal relationship or friendship with the person or family member.
- Do not visit or spend extra time with a person that is not part of your assignment.
- Do not share personal or financial information with a person or family member.
- Do not help a person or family member with his or her finances.
- Do not take a person home with you. This includes for holidays or other events.
- Ask these questions before you date or marry a person whom you cared for. Be aware of the risk for sexual misconduct.
  - How long ago did you assist with the person's care?
  - Was the person's care short-term or long-term?
  - What kind and how much information do you have about the person? How will that information affect your relationship with the person?
  - Will the person need more care in the future?
  - Does dating or marrying the person place the person at risk for harm?

LEGAL ASPECTS

A **law** is a rule of conduct made by a government body. The U.S. Congress and state legislatures make laws. Enforced by the government, laws protect the public welfare.

Criminal laws are concerned with offenses against the public and society in general. An act that violates a criminal law is called a **crime**—murder, rape, theft, abuse. A person found guilty of a crime is fined or sent to prison.

Civil laws deal with relationships between people. Examples include contracts and nursing practice. A person found guilty of breaking a civil law usually has to pay a sum of money to the injured person.

Tort comes from the French word meaning wrong. Torts are part of civil law. A tort is a wrong committed against a person or the person's property. Some torts are unintentional—harm was not intended. Other torts are intentional—harm was intended.

Unintentional Torts

Negligence is an unintentional wrong. The negligent person did not act in a reasonable and careful manner. As a result, a person or the person's property was harmed. The person causing the harm did not intend or mean to cause harm. The person failed to do what a reasonable and careful person would have done. Or he or she did what a reasonable and careful person would not have done.

Malpractice is negligence by a professional person. A person has professional status because of training and the services provided. Nurses, doctors, dentists, and pharmacists are examples.

What you do or do not do can lead to a lawsuit if a person or property is harmed. You are legally responsible (*liable*) for your own actions. The nurse is liable as your supervisor. However, you are not relieved of personal liability. Sometimes refusing to follow the nurse's directions is your right and duty.

Intentional Torts

Intentional torts are acts meant to be harmful.
- **Defamation** is injuring a person's name and reputation by making false statements to a third person. **Libel** is making false statements in print, writing, or through pictures or drawings. **Slander** is making false statements orally.
- **False imprisonment** is the unlawful restraint or restriction of a person's freedom of movement. It involves:
  - Threatening to restrain a person
  - Restraining a person
  - Preventing a person from leaving the agency

BOX 2-8	Protecting the Right to Privacy

- Keep all information about the person confidential.
- Cover the person when he or she is being moved in hallways.
- Screen the person. Close the privacy curtain as in Figure 2-3. Close the door when giving care. Also close window coverings.
- Expose only the body part involved in care or a procedure.
- Do not discuss the person or the person's treatment with anyone except the nurse supervising your work.
- Ask visitors to leave the room when care is given.
- Do not open the person's mail.
- Allow the person to visit with others in private.
- Allow the person to use the phone in private.
- Follow agency policies and procedures required to protect privacy.

- **Invasion of privacy** is violating a person's right not to have his or her name, photo, or private affairs exposed or made public without giving consent. You must treat the person with respect and ensure privacy. Only staff involved in the person's care should see, handle, or examine his or her body. See Box 2-8 for measures to protect privacy. The Health Insurance Portability and Accountability Act of 1996 (HIPAA) protects the privacy and security of a person's health information. **Protected health information** refers to identifying information and information about the person's health care that is maintained or sent in any form (paper, electronic, oral). Failure to comply with HIPAA rules can result in fines, penalties, and criminal action including jail time. You must follow agency policies and procedures. Direct any questions about the person or the person's care to the nurse. Also follow the rules for using computers and other electronic devices (Chapter 4).
- **Fraud** is saying or doing something to trick, fool, or deceive a person. The act is fraud if it does or could cause harm to a person or the person's property. Telling a person that you are a nurse is fraud. So is giving wrong or incomplete information on a job application.
- **Assault** is intentionally attempting or threatening to touch a person's body without the person's consent. The person fears bodily harm.
- **Battery** is touching a person's body without his or her consent. The person must consent to any procedure, treatment, or other act that involves touching the body. The person has the right to withdraw consent at any time.

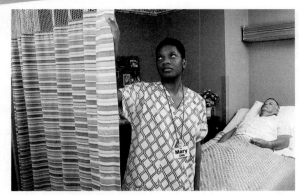

FIGURE 2-3 Pulling the privacy curtain around the bed helps protect the person's privacy.

Informed Consent

A person has the right to decide what will be done to his or her body and who can touch his or her body. The doctor is responsible for informing the person about all aspects of treatment. Consent is informed when the person clearly understands all aspects of treatment.

Persons under legal age (usually 18 years of age) cannot give consent. Nor can mentally incompetent persons. Such persons are unconscious, sedated, or confused. Or they have certain mental health problems. Informed consent is given by a responsible party—a wife, husband, adult child, or a legal representative.

You are never responsible for obtaining written consent. In some agencies, you can witness the signing of a consent. To be a witness, you must be present when the person signs the consent.

See *Focus on Communication: Informed Consent.*

REPORTING ABUSE

Abuse is the intentional mistreatment or harm of another person. Abuse is a crime. It can occur at home or in a health care agency. Abuse has one or more of these elements:

* Willful causing of injury
* Unreasonable confinement
* Intimidation (to make afraid with threats of force or violence)
* Punishment
* Depriving the person of the goods or services needed for physical, mental, or psychosocial well-being

Abuse causes physical harm, pain, or mental anguish. Protection against abuse extends to persons in a coma. The abuser is usually a family member or

---

FOCUS ON COMMUNICATION
Informed Consent

There are different ways to give consent:
* *Written consent.* The person signs a form agreeing to a treatment or procedure. You are not responsible for obtaining written consent.
* *Verbal consent.* The person says aloud that he or she consents. "Yes" and "okay" are examples.
* *Implied consent.* For example, you ask Mr. Jones if you can check his blood pressure. He extends his arm. His movement implies consent.

Before any procedure, explain the steps to the person. This is how you obtain verbal or implied consent. Also explain each step during a procedure. This allows the person the chance to refuse at any time.

PERSONS WITH DEMENTIA
Vulnerable Adults

Some persons have behaviors that threaten their health and safety. This is called **self-neglect.** Causes include declining health and chronic disease. Other causes are disorders that impair judgment or memory. Alzheimer's disease and dementia are examples.

The warning signs of self-neglect are:
* Hoarding. The person saves, hides, or stores things. Newspapers, magazines, food containers, and shopping bags are examples.
* No food, water, heat, and other necessities.
* Not taking needed drugs.
* Refusing medical treatment for serious illnesses.
* Dehydration—poor urinary output, dry skin, dry mouth, confusion.
* Poor hygiene.
* Wearing the wrong clothing for the weather.
* Confusion.

---

caregiver. The abuser can be a friend, neighbor, landlord, or other person. Both men and women are abusers. Both men and women are abused.

Vulnerable Adults

Vulnerable comes from the Latin word *vulnerare* which means *to wound.* **Vulnerable adults** are persons 18 years old or older who have disabilities or conditions that make them at risk to be wounded, attacked, or damaged. They have problems caring for or protecting themselves due to:

* A mental, emotional, physical, or developmental disability
* Brain damage
* Changes from aging

Patients and residents, regardless of age, are considered vulnerable.

See *Persons With Dementia: Vulnerable Adults.*

Elder Abuse

Elder abuse is any knowing, intentional, or negligent act by a caregiver or any other person to an older adult. The act causes harm or serious risk of harm. Elder abuse can take these forms:

- *Physical abuse.* This involves inflicting, or threatening to inflict, physical pain or injury. Grabbing, hitting, slapping, kicking, pinching, hair-pulling, or beating are examples. It also includes *corporal punishment*—punishment inflicted directly on the body. Beatings, lashings, and whippings are examples. Depriving the person of a basic need also is physical abuse.
- *Neglect.* Failure to provide the person with the goods or services needed to avoid physical harm, mental anguish, or mental illness is called **neglect.** This includes failure to provide health care or treatment, food, clothing, hygiene, shelter, or other needs. In health care, neglect includes but is not limited to:
  - Leaving persons lying or sitting in urine or feces
  - Keeping persons alone in their rooms or other areas
  - Failing to answer signal lights
- *Verbal abuse.* Using oral or written words or statements that speak badly of, sneer at, criticize, or condemn the person. It includes unkind gestures.
- *Involuntary seclusion.* Confining the person to a certain area. People have been locked in closets, basements, attics, bathrooms, and other spaces.
- *Financial exploitation or misappropriation.* To *exploit* means to use unjustly. *Misappropriate* means to dishonestly, unfairly, or wrongly take for one's own use. The older person's resources (money, property, assets) are mis-used by another person. Or the resources are used for the other person's profit or benefit. The person's money is stolen or used by another person. It is also mis-using a person's property. For example, an adult child sells his or her parent's house without the parent's consent.
- *Emotional abuse.* This involves inflicting mental pain, anguish, or distress through verbal or non-verbal acts. Humiliation, harassment, ridicule, and threats of punishment are examples. It includes being deprived of needs such as food, clothing, care, a home, or a place to sleep.
- *Sexual abuse.* The person is harassed about sex or is attacked sexually. The person may be forced to perform sexual acts out of fear of punishment or physical harm.

| BOX 2-9 | Signs of Elder Abuse |

- Living conditions are unsafe, unclean, or inadequate.
- Personal hygiene is lacking. The person is not clean. Clothes are dirty.
- Weight loss—there are signs of poor nutrition and inadequate fluid intake.
- Assistive devices are missing or broken—eyeglasses, hearing aids, dentures, cane, walker, and so on.
- Medical needs are not met.
- Frequent injuries—conditions behind the injuries are strange or seem impossible.
- Old and new injuries—bruises, pressure marks, welts, scars, fractures, punctures, and so on.
- Complaints of pain or itching in the genital area.
- Bleeding and bruising around the breasts or in the genital area.
- Burns on the feet, hands, buttocks, or other parts of the body. Cigarettes and cigars cause small circle-like burns.
- Pressure ulcers (Chapter 23) or contractures (Chapter 22).
- The person seems very quiet or withdrawn.
- Unexplained withdrawal from normal activities.
- The person seems fearful, anxious, or agitated.
- Sudden change in alertness.
- Depression.
- Sudden changes in finances.
- The person does not seem to want to talk or answer questions.
- The person is restrained. Or the person is locked in a certain area for long periods.
- The person cannot reach toilet facilities, food, water, and other needed items.
- Private conversations are not allowed. The caregiver is present during all conversations.
- Strained or tense relationships with a caregiver.
- Frequent arguments with a caregiver.
- The person seems anxious to please the caregiver.
- Drugs are not taken properly. Drugs are not bought. Or too much or too little of the drug is taken.
- Visits to the emergency room may be frequent.
- The person may change doctors often. Some people do not have a doctor.

- *Abandonment. Abandon* means to leave or desert someone. The person is deserted by someone who is responsible for his or her care.

The abused person may show only some of the signs in Box 2-9. Federal and state laws require the reporting of elder abuse or suspected abuse. If you suspect abuse, share your concerns and observations with the nurse. Give as many details as possible. The nurse contacts health team members as needed. The nurse also contacts community agencies that investigate elder abuse. Sometimes the police or the courts need to help.

OBRA Requirements

Agencies cannot employ persons who were convicted of abuse, neglect, or mistreatment. Before hiring, the agency must thoroughly check the applicant's work history. All references are checked. Efforts must be made to find out about any criminal records.

The agency also checks the nursing assistant registry for findings of abuse, neglect, or mistreatment. It also is checked for mis-using or stealing a person's property.

OBRA requires these actions if abuse is suspected within the center:

- The incident is reported at once to:
  - The administrator
  - Other officials as required by federal and state laws
- All claims of abuse are thoroughly investigated.
- The center must prevent further potential for abuse while the investigation is in progress.
- Investigation results are reported to the center administrator within 5 days of the incident. They also are reported to other officials as required by federal and state laws.
- Corrective actions are taken if the claim is found to be true.

Other Laws

See "Ethics and Laws" in the *Focus on PRIDE: The Person, Family, and Yourself* boxes at the end of each chapter. They describe other laws affecting your work as a nursing assistant.

Focus on P R I D E
The Person, Family, and Yourself

Personal and Professional Responsibility—The work you do has value. Continued education increases your skills and knowledge. It adds to your value. It offers you more opportunities. Your current training is just the start of a life-time of learning and possibilities.

Agencies have educational programs, commonly called in-services, for staff. Some in-services are required. Others are optional. In-service announcements and schedules are posted on bulletin boards, in staff lounges, by the time clock, and in other areas. Or they are e-mailed. Know where to find in-service information. Check those areas often.

Some states have higher levels of nursing assistants. Medication Assistant-Certified (MA-C) is an example. MA-Cs are nursing assistants with extra training. Supervised by a licensed nurse, they give drugs as allowed by state law.

You will have many opportunities to continue learning. Find out the options available in your state and agency. Take advantage of them. Be proud of your training. And never stop learning!

Rights and Respect—Every person has the right to privacy. HIPAA protects a person's health information. You must follow HIPAA rules. Only discuss a person's health information with the nurse. Visitors may ask questions about a person's care. Respect the person's privacy. You can say: "I'm sorry. I'm not allowed to give any information." Direct the visitor to the nurse.

Independence and Social Interaction—You will interact with many persons daily. Some are family and friends. Work relationships differ from social ones. Make sure your actions and conversations are appropriate. Patients, residents, and families notice what you do and say. Always show good judgment.

Delegation and Teamwork—Delegation of tasks may change. Do not get offended if you cannot perform a task usually delegated to you. The nurse decides what is best for the person at the time. That decision is also best for you. For example, you always care for Mrs. Mills. Now she is weak and not eating well. The nurse wants to observe and evaluate the changes in her condition. The nurse decides to give her care. This does not mean the nurse is worried about your quality of care. At this time, Mrs. Mills needs the nurse's assessment and judgment.

Ethics and Laws—Some nursing assistants work in more than one setting. Some work in a nursing center and a hospital. Others are also emergency medical technicians (EMTs). EMTs provide emergency care outside health care settings. State laws and rules for EMTs and nursing assistants differ. For example, you work as an EMT and a nursing assistant. Your state allows EMTs to start intravenous (IV) lines. Nursing assistants do not start IVs. The ability to do something does not give the right to do so in all settings. There are legal limits to your role. Be proud of your advanced skills and training. But when working as a nursing assistant, follow your state's laws and rules for nursing assistants.

REVIEW QUESTIONS

Circle the BEST answer.

1 Which requires a training and competency evaluation program for nursing assistants?
   a Medicare
   b Medicaid
   c NCSBN
   d OBRA

2 Your nursing assistant certification can be revoked for
   a Refusing a nursing task
   b Asking the nurse questions
   c Performing acts beyond your role
   d Keeping the person's information confidential

3 As a nursing assistant, you
   a Must perform all nursing tasks as directed by the nurse
   b Make decisions about a person's care
   c Should have a written job description before employment
   d Should give a drug when a nurse tells you to

4 As a nursing assistant, you
   a Can take verbal or phone orders from doctors
   b Are responsible for your own actions
   c Can remove tubes from the person's body
   d Should ignore a nursing task if it is not in your job description

5 Who assigns and supervises your work?
   a Other nursing assistants
   b The health team
   c Nurses
   d Doctors

6 You are responsible for
   a Supervising other nursing assistants
   b Delegation decisions
   c Completing delegated tasks safely
   d Obtaining written consent

7 These statements are about delegation. Which is *false*?
   a Nurses can delegate their responsibilities to you.
   b A delegated task must be safe for the person.
   c The delegated task must be in your job description.
   d The delegating nurse is responsible for the safe completion of the task.

8 A task is in your job description. Which is *false*?
   a The nurse must delegate the task to you.
   b The nurse can delegate the task if the person's circumstances are right.
   c You must have the necessary education and training to complete the task.
   d You must have clear directions before you perform the task.

9 A nurse delegates a task to you. You must
   a Complete the task
   b Decide to accept or refuse the task
   c Delegate the task if you are busy
   d Ignore the request if you do not know what to do

10 You can refuse to perform a task for these reasons *except*
   a The task is beyond the legal limits of your role
   b The task is not in your job description
   c You do not like the task
   d A nurse is not available to supervise you

11 You decide to refuse a task. What should you do?
   a Delegate the task to a nursing assistant.
   b Communicate your concerns to the nurse.
   c Ignore the request.
   d Talk to the director of nursing.

12 Ethics is
   a Making judgments before you have the facts
   b Knowledge of what is right and wrong conduct
   c A behavior that meets your needs, not the person's
   d Skills, care, and judgments required of a health team member

13 Which of the following is ethical behavior?
   a Sharing information about a patient with your family
   b Accepting gifts from a resident's family
   c Reporting errors
   d Calling your family before answering a signal light

14 To maintain professional boundaries, your behaviors must
   a Help the person
   b Meet your needs
   c Be biased
   d Show that you care

15 A patient asks you out to dinner. You accept. This is a
   a Professional boundary
   b Boundary crossing
   c Boundary violation
   d Professional sexual misconduct

16 Which is *not* a crime?
   a Abuse
   b Murder
   c Negligence
   d Robbery

17 These statements are about negligence. Which is *false*?
   a It is an unintentional tort.
   b The negligent person did not act in a reasonable manner.
   c Harm was caused to a person or a person's property.
   d A prison term is likely.

18 Threatening to touch the person's body without the person's consent is
   a Assault
   b Battery
   c Defamation
   d False imprisonment

19 Restraining a person's freedom of movement is
   a Assault
   b Battery
   c Defamation
   d False imprisonment

20 You show photos of a resident without that person's consent. This is
   a Battery
   b Fraud
   c Invasion of privacy
   d Malpractice

21 A person asks if you are a nurse. You answer "yes." This is
   a Negligence
   b Fraud
   c Libel
   d Slander

22 Informed consent is when the person
   a Fully understands all aspects of his or her treatment
   b Signs a consent form
   c Is admitted to the agency
   d Decides how to distribute property after his or her death

23 Who is at risk for being wounded, attacked, or damaged?
   a Children
   b Older adults
   c Persons with disabilities
   d All patients and residents

24 Self-neglect is when
   a A caregiver harms a person
   b The person's behaviors put him or her at risk for harm
   c A person is deprived of food, clothing, hygiene, and shelter
   d The person does not receive attention or affection

25 Which is *not* a sign of elder abuse?
   a Stiff joints and joint pain
   b Old and new bruises
   c Poor personal hygiene
   d Frequent injuries

26 You suspect a person was abused. What should you do?
   a Tell the family.
   b Call the police.
   c Tell the nurse.
   d Ask the person about the abuse.

Answers to these questions are on p. 527.

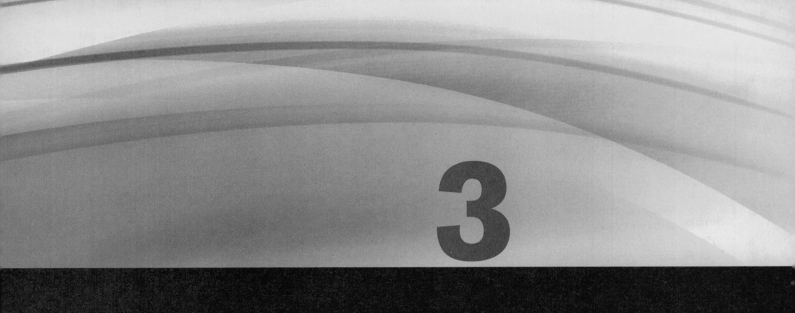

3

WORK ETHICS

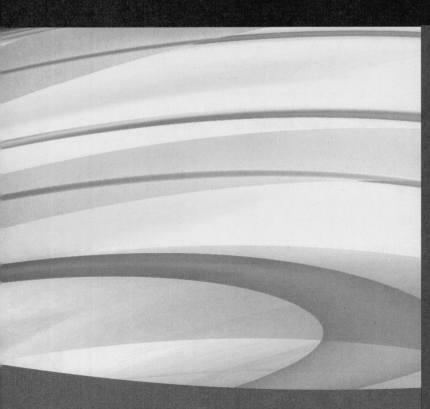

OBJECTIVES

- Define the key terms listed in this chapter.
- Describe the practices for good health, hygiene, and professional appearance.
- Describe the qualities and traits of a successful nursing assistant.
- Explain how to get a job.
- Explain how to plan for childcare and transportation.
- Describe ethical behavior on the job.
- Explain how to manage stress.
- Explain the aspects of harassment.
- Explain how to resign from a job.
- Identify the common reasons for losing a job.
- Explain the reasons for drug testing.
- Explain how to promote PRIDE in the person, the family, and yourself.

KEY TERMS

confidentiality Trusting others with personal and private information

gossip To spread rumors or talk about the private matters of others

harassment To trouble, torment, offend, or worry a person by one's behavior or comments

priority The most important thing at the time

professionalism Following laws, being ethical, having good work ethics, and having the skills to do your work

stress The response or change in the body caused by any emotional, physical, social, or economic factor

teamwork Staff members work together as a group; each person does his or her part to provide safe and effective care

work ethics Behavior in the workplace

You must act and function in a professional manner. **Professionalism** involves following laws, being ethical, having good work ethics, and having the skills to do your work. In the workplace, certain behaviors (conduct), choices, and judgments are expected. **Work ethics** deals with behavior in the workplace. Your conduct reflects your choices and judgments. Work ethics involves:

* How you look
* What you say
* How you behave
* How you treat and work with others

HEALTH, HYGIENE, AND APPEARANCE

Patients, residents, families, and visitors expect the health team to look and act healthy. Your health, appearance, and hygiene need careful attention.

Your Health

To function at your best, you need good physical and mental health.

* *Diet.* You need a balanced diet for good nutrition (Chapter 19).
* *Sleep and rest.* Most adults need about 7 hours of sleep daily.
* *Body mechanics.* You will bend, carry heavy objects, and handle, move, and turn persons. Use your muscles correctly (Chapter 12).
* *Exercise.* Regular exercise is needed for muscle tone, circulation, and weight loss.
* *Your eyes.* You will read instructions and take measurements. Wrong readings can harm the person. Have your eyes checked. Wear needed eyeglasses or contact lenses. Provide enough light for reading and fine work.
* *Smoking.* Smoking causes lung, heart, and circulatory disorders. Smoke odors stay on your breath, hands, clothing, and hair. Practice hand washing and good personal hygiene.
* *Drugs.* Some drugs affect thinking, feeling, behavior, and function. Working under the influence of drugs affects the person's safety. Take drugs only if prescribed by a doctor.
* *Alcohol.* Alcohol is a drug that affects thinking, balance, coordination, and alertness. Never report to work under the influence of alcohol. Do not drink alcohol while working.

Your Hygiene

Your hygiene needs careful attention. Bathe daily. Use a deodorant or antiperspirant to prevent body odors. Brush your teeth upon awakening, before and after meals, and at bedtime. Use a mouthwash to prevent breath odors. Shampoo often. Style hair in a simple, attractive way.

Foot care prevents odors and infection. Wash your feet daily. Dry thoroughly between the toes. Cut toenails straight across after bathing or soaking them.

Practice menstrual hygiene. Change tampons or sanitary pads often, especially for heavy flow. Wash your genital area with soap and water at least twice a day. And practice good hand washing.

Your Appearance

Good health and hygiene practices help you look and feel well. Follow the practices in Box 3-1, p. 34 to look clean, neat, and professional (Fig. 3-1, p. 34).

GETTING A JOB

There are easy ways to find out about agencies and jobs:

* Newspaper ads
* Local state employment services
* Agencies you would like to work at
* Phone book yellow pages
* People you know—your instructor, family, and friends
* The Internet
* Your school's or college's job placement counselors
* Your clinical experience site

BOX 3-1 Practices for a Professional Appearance

- Practice good hygiene.
- Wear uniforms that fit well. They are modest in length and style. Follow the agency's dress code.
- Keep uniforms clean, pressed, and mended. Sew on buttons. Repair zippers, tears, and hems.
- Wear a clean uniform daily.
- Wear your name badge or photo ID (identification) at all times when on duty. Make sure it is visible. Follow agency policy.
- Wear undergarments that are clean and fit properly. Change them daily.
- Wear undergarments in the correct color for your skin tone. Do not wear colored (red, pink, blue, and so on) ones. They can be seen through white and light-colored uniforms.
- Cover tattoos (body art). They may offend others.
- Follow the agency's dress code for jewelry. Wedding and engagement rings may be allowed. Rings and bracelets can scratch a person. Confused or combative persons can easily pull on jewelry (necklaces, dangling earrings). So can young children.
- Do not wear jewelry in pierced eyebrows, nose, lips, or tongue while on duty.

- Follow the agency's dress code for earrings. Usually small, simple earrings are allowed. For multiple ear piercings, usually only one set of earrings is allowed.
- Wear a wristwatch with a second hand.
- Wear clean stockings and socks that fit well. Change them daily.
- Wear shoes that fit properly, are comfortable, give needed support, and have non-skid soles. Do not wear sandals or open-toed shoes.
- Clean and polish shoes often. Wash and replace laces as needed.
- Keep fingernails clean, short, and neatly shaped. Long nails can scratch a person. Nails must be natural.
- Do not wear nail polish. Chipped nail polish may provide a place for microbes to grow.
- Have a simple, attractive hairstyle. Hair is off your collar and away from your face. Use simple pins, combs, barrettes, and bands to keep long hair up and in place.
- Keep beards and mustaches clean and trimmed.
- Use makeup that is modest in amount and moderate in color. Avoid a painted and severe look.
- Do not wear perfume, cologne, or after-shave lotion. The scents may offend, nauseate, or cause breathing problems in patients and residents.

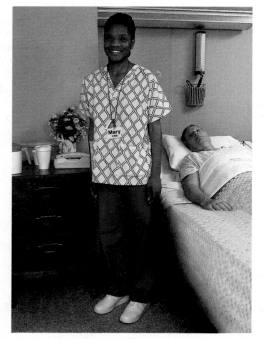

FIGURE 3-1 This nursing assistant is well-groomed. Her uniform and shoes are clean. Her hair has a simple style. It is away from her face and off of her collar. She does not wear jewelry.

What Employers Look For

If you owned a business, who would you want to hire? Your answer helps you understand the employer's point of view. Employers want to hire people who:

- Are dependable
- Are well-groomed
- Have needed job skills and training
- Have values and attitudes that fit with the agency
- Have the qualities and traits described in Box 3-2

You must be at work on time and when scheduled. Undependable people cause everyone problems. Other staff have extra work. Fewer people give care. Quality of care suffers. You want co-workers to work when scheduled. Otherwise, you have extra work. You have less time to spend with patients and residents. Likewise, co-workers also expect you to work when scheduled.

Job Skills and Training The employer checks the nursing assistant registry and requests proof of training:

- A certificate of course completion
- A high school, college, or technical school transcript
- An official grade report (report card)

Give the employer only a *copy* of the document you present. Never give the original to the employer.

BOX 3-2 Qualities and Traits for Good Work Ethics

- **Caring.** Have concern for the person. Help make the person's life happier, easier, or less painful.
- **Dependable.** Report to work on time and when scheduled. Perform delegated tasks. Keep obligations and promises.
- **Considerate.** Respect the person's physical and emotional feelings. Be gentle and kind toward patients, residents, families, and co-workers.
- **Cheerful.** Greet and talk to people in a pleasant manner. Do not be moody, bad-tempered, or unhappy while at work.
- **Empathetic.** Empathy is seeing things from the person's point of view—putting yourself in the person's place. How would you feel if you had the person's problems?
- **Trustworthy.** Patients, residents, and staff have confidence in you. They believe you will keep information confidential. They trust you not to gossip about patients, residents, or the health team.
- **Respectful.** Patients and residents have rights, values, beliefs, and feelings. They may differ from yours. Do not judge or condemn the person. Treat the person with respect and dignity at all times. Also show respect for the health team.
- **Courteous.** Be polite and courteous to patients, residents, families, visitors, and co-workers. See p. 39 for common courtesies in the workplace.
- **Conscientious.** Be careful, alert, and exact in following instructions. Give thorough care. Do not lose or damage the person's property.
- **Honest.** Accurately report the care given, your observations, and any errors.
- **Cooperative.** Willingly help and work with others. Also take that "extra step" during busy and stressful times.
- **Enthusiastic.** Be eager, interested, and excited about your work. Your work is important.
- **Self-aware.** Know your feelings, strengths, and weaknesses. You need to understand yourself before you can understand patients and residents.

Box 3-3 Guidelines for Completing a Job Application

- Read and follow the directions. They may ask you to print using black ink. Following directions is needed on the job. Employers look at job applications to see if you can follow directions.
- Write neatly. Writing must be readable. A messy application gives a bad image. Readable writing gives the correct information. The agency cannot contact you if unable to read your phone number. You may miss getting the job.
- Complete the entire form. Something may not apply to you. If so, write "N/A" for non-applicable. Or draw a line through the space. This tells the employer that you read the section. It also shows that you did not skip the item on purpose.
- Report any felony convictions as directed. Write "no" or "none" as appropriate. Criminal background and fingerprint checks are common requirements.
- Give information about employment gaps. If you did not work for a time, the employer wonders why. Provide this information to give a good impression about your honesty. Some reasons are an illness, going to school, raising your children, or caring for an ill or older family member.
- Tell why you left a job, if asked. Be brief, but honest. People leave jobs for one that pays better. Some leave for career advancement. Other reasons include those given for employment gaps. If you were fired from a job, give an honest but positive response. Do not talk badly about a former employer.
- Provide references. Be prepared to give names, titles, addresses, and phone numbers of at least four references who are not relatives. Have this information written down before completing an application. (Always ask references if an employer can contact them.) You may get the job faster or over another applicant if the employer can quickly check references. If they are missing or not complete, the employer waits for all of the information. This wastes your time and the employer's time. Also, the employer wonders if you are hiding something with incomplete reference information.
- Be prepared to provide the following:
  - Social security number
  - Proof of citizenship or legal residency
  - Proof of required training and competency evaluation
  - Identification—driver's license or government-issued ID card
- Give honest responses. Lying on an application is fraud. It is grounds for being fired.
- Keep a file of your education and work history.

Keep it for future use. The employer may want a transcript sent directly from the school or college. A criminal background check and drug testing are common requirements.

Job Applications

You get a job application from the *personnel office* or *human resources* office. You can complete the application there. Or take it home, and return it by mail or in person. Be well-groomed and behave pleasantly when seeking or returning a job application. It often is your first chance to make a good impression.

To complete a job application, see Box 3-3. A neat, readable, and complete application gives a good image. A sloppy or incomplete one does not.

Many agencies provide applications on-line. Follow the agency's instructions for completing and sending one on-line.

BOX 3-4 Common Interview Questions

What the Interviewer May Ask You

- Tell me about yourself.
- Tell me about your career goals.
- What are you doing to reach these goals?
- Describe your idea of *professional* behavior.
- Tell me about your last job. Why did you leave?
- What did you like the most about your last job? What did you like the least?
- What would your supervisor and co-workers tell me about you? Your dependability? Your skills? Your flexibility?
- Which functions are the hardest for you? How do you handle this difficulty?
- How do you set your priorities?
- How have your experiences prepared you for this job?
- What would you like to change about your last job?
- How do you handle problems with patients, residents, and co-workers?
- Why do you want to work here?
- Why should this agency hire you?

What You May Ask the Interviewer

- Which job functions do you think are the most important?
- What employee qualities and traits are the most important to you?
- What nursing care pattern is used here (Chapter 1)?
- Who will I work with?
- When are performance evaluations done? Who does them? How are they done?
- What performance factors are evaluated?
- How does the supervisor handle problems?
- What are the most common reasons that nursing assistants lose their jobs here?
- What are the most common reasons that nursing assistants resign from their jobs here?
- How do you see this job in the next year? In the next 5 years?
- What is the greatest reward from this job?
- What is the greatest challenge from this job?
- What do you like the most about nursing assistants who work here? What do you like the least?
- Why should I work here rather than in another agency?
- Why are you interested in hiring me?
- How much will I make an hour?
- What hours will I work?
- What uniforms are required?
- What benefits do you offer:
  - Health and disability insurance?
  - Continuing education?
  - Vacation time?
- Does the agency have a new employee orientation program?
- May I have a tour of the agency and the unit I will work on? Will you introduce me to the nurse manager and unit staff?
- Can I have a few minutes to talk to the nurse manager?

The Job Interview

An employer gets to know and evaluate you during a job interview. You also learn about the agency. Box 3-4 lists common interview questions. Prepare your answers before the interview. Also prepare a list of your skills for the interviewer.

You must appear neat, clean, well-groomed, and neatly dressed (Fig. 3-2). Follow the guidelines in Box 3-5. You must present a good image.

Be on time. It shows you are dependable. Go to the agency some day before your interview. Note how long it takes and where to park. Also find the personnel office. A *dry run* (practice run) shows how long it takes to get from your home to the personnel office.

When you arrive for the interview, turn off your wireless phone or pager. Tell the receptionist your name and why you are there. Give the interviewer's name. Then sit quietly in the waiting area. Do not smoke or chew gum. Review your answers to the common interview questions. Waiting may be part of the interview. The interviewer may ask the receptionist about how you acted while waiting. Smile, and be polite and friendly.

Politely greet the interviewer. A firm hand-shake is correct for men and women. Address him or her as Miss, Mrs., Ms., Mr., or Doctor. Stand until asked to take a seat. Sit with good posture and in a professional way. If offered a beverage, you can accept. Be sure to say "thank you."

Look at the interviewer when answering or asking questions. Poor eye contact sends negative information—shy, insecure, dishonest, or lacking interest.

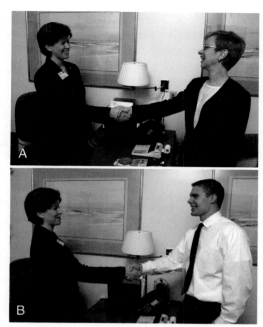

FIGURE 3-2 **A,** A simple suit is worn for a job interview. **B,** This man wears slacks and a shirt and tie for his interview.

Watch your body language (Chapter 5). What you say is important. However, how you use and move your body tells a great deal. Avoid distracting habits—biting nails; playing with jewelry, clothing, or your hair; crossing your arms; and swinging legs back and forth.

Give complete and honest answers. Speak clearly and with confidence. Avoid short and long answers. "Yes" and "no" answers give little information. Briefly explain "yes" and "no" responses.

You will be asked about your skills. Share your skills list. He or she may ask about skills not on your list. Explain that you are willing to learn the skill if your state allows nursing assistants to perform the tasks.

You can ask questions at the end of the interview (see Box 3-4). Review the job description with the interviewer. If you have questions about it, ask them at this time. Advise the interviewer of functions you cannot perform because of training, legal, ethical, or religious reasons.

You may be offered a job when the interview ends. Or you are told when to expect a call or letter. Follow-up is acceptable. Ask when you can check on your application. Before leaving, thank the interviewer and shake hands. Say that you look forward to hearing from him or her.

Write a thank-you letter within 24 hours of the interview. Use a computer or typewriter or write the letter by hand. Include:

- The date
- The interviewer's formal name using Miss, Mrs., Ms., Mr., or Dr.
- A statement thanking the person for the interview
- Comments about the interview, the agency, and your eagerness to hear about the job
- Your signature using your first and last names

Accepting a Job

When accepting a job, agree on a starting date, pay rate, and work hours. Find out where to report on your first day. Ask for such information in writing. Use the written offer later if questions arise. Also ask for the employee handbook and other agency information. Read everything before you start working.

New Employee Orientation

Agencies have orientation programs for new employees. The policy and procedure manual is reviewed. Your skills are checked for safety and correctness. Also, you learn how to use the agency's supplies and equipment.

Preceptor programs are common. A *preceptor* is a

staff member who guides another staff member. A nurse or nursing assistant:

- Helps you learn the agency's layout and where to find things
- Introduces you to patients, residents, and staff
- Helps you organize your work
- Helps you feel part of the nursing team
- Answers questions about the policy and procedure manual

A nursing assistant preceptor is not your supervisor. Only nurses can supervise. A preceptor program usually lasts 2 to 4 weeks. When the program ends, you should feel comfortable with the setting and your role. If not, ask for more orientation time.

PREPARING FOR WORK

A job is a privilege. You must work when scheduled, be on time, and stay the entire shift. Absences and tardiness (being late) are common reasons for losing a job. Childcare and transportation issues often interfere with getting to work.

Childcare

Someone needs to care for your children when you leave for work, while you are at work, and before you get home from work. Also plan for emergencies:

- Your childcare provider is ill or cannot care for your children that day.
- A child becomes ill while you are at work.
- You will be late getting home from work.

Transportation

Plan for getting to and from work. If you drive, keep your car in good working order. Keep plenty of gas in the car. Or leave early to get enough gas.

Carpooling is an option. Carpool members depend on each other. If the driver is late leaving, everyone is late for work. If one person is not ready when the driver arrives, everyone is late for work. Carpool with persons who are always ready and on time. Be on time as a driver or a passenger.

Know bus or train schedules. Know what bus or train to take if delays occur. Carry enough money for fares to and from work.

Always have a back-up plan for getting to work. Your car may not start, the carpool driver may not go to work, or public transportation may not operate.

TEAMWORK

You are an important member of the health team. Teamwork is important for safe and effective care. **Teamwork** means that staff members work together as a group. Each person does his or her part to provide safe and effective care. Teamwork involves:

- Working when scheduled
- Being cheerful and friendly
- Performing delegated tasks
- Being available to help others
- Helping others willingly
- Being kind to others

Attendance

Report to work when scheduled and on time. The entire unit is affected when just one person is late. Call the agency if you will be late or cannot go to work. Follow the attendance policy in your employee handbook.

Be *ready to work* when your shift starts. Store your belongings. Use the restroom before your shift starts. Arrive on your nursing unit a few minutes early. This gives you time to greet others and settle yourself.

You must stay the entire shift. Prepare to stay longer to work over-time. When it is time to leave, report off-duty to the nurse.

Your Attitude

You need a good attitude. Show that you enjoy your work. Listen to others. Be willing to learn. Stay busy, and use your time well.

Always think before you speak. These statements signal a bad attitude:

- "That's not my resident (patient)."
- "I can't. I'm too busy."
- "I didn't do it."
- "I don't feel like it."
- "It's not my fault."
- "Don't blame me."
- "It's not my turn. I did it yesterday."
- "Nobody told me."
- "That's not my job."
- "You didn't say that you needed it right away."
- "I work harder than anyone else."
- "No one appreciates what I do."
- "I'm tired of this place."
- "Is it time to leave yet?"

Gossip

To **gossip** means to spread rumors or talk about the private matters of others. Gossiping is unprofessional and hurtful. To avoid being a part of gossip:

- Remove yourself from a group or situation where others are gossiping.
- Do not make or repeat any comment that can hurt a person, family member, visitor, co-worker, or the agency.

- Do not make or repeat any comment that you do not know to be true. This includes written comments and e-mail and other electronic messages.
- Do not talk about patients, residents, families, visitors, co-workers, or the agency at home or in social settings.

Confidentiality

The person's information is private and personal. **Confidentiality** means trusting others with personal and private information. The person's information is shared only among staff involved in his or her care. Agency and co-worker information also is confidential.

Avoid talking about patients, residents, the agency, or co-workers when others are present. Do not talk about them in hallways, elevators, dining areas, or outside the agency. Others may overhear you. Share information only with the nurse.

Do not eavesdrop. To eavesdrop means to listen in or overhear what others are saying. It invades a person's privacy.

Many agencies have intercom systems. They allow for communication between the bedside and the nurses' station. Be careful what you say over the intercom. It is like a loud speaker. Others nearby can hear what you are saying.

See *Focus on Communication: Confidentiality.*

Hygiene and Appearance

Home and social attire is not proper at work. You cannot wear jeans, halter tops, tank tops, or short skirts. Clothing must not be tight, revealing, or sexual. Females cannot show cleavage, the tops of breasts, or upper thighs. Males must avoid tight pants and exposing their chests. Only the top shirt button is open. Follow the practices in Box 3-1.

Speech and Language

Some speech and language used in home and social settings is not proper at work. Words used with family and friends may offend the person, family, visitors, and co-workers. Remember the following:
- Do not swear or use foul, vulgar, slang, or abusive language.
- Speak softly and gently.
- Speak clearly. The person may have a hearing problem.
- Do not shout or yell.
- Do not fight or argue with a person, family member, visitor, or co-worker.

FOCUS ON COMMUNICATION
Confidentiality

Your family members and friends may ask you about people they know in the agency. They may ask about patients, residents, or employees. For example, your mother says: "Mrs. Drew goes to our church. I heard that she's in your nursing home. What's wrong with her?"

You must not share information with your family and friends. To do so violates the person's right to privacy. You can say: "I'm sorry, but I can't tell you about any person in the center. It's unprofessional and against center policies. And it violates the person's right to privacy. Please don't ask me about anyone in the center."

Courtesies

Courtesies are polite, considerate, or helpful comments or acts. They take little time or energy. And they mean so much to people.
- Address others by Miss, Mrs., Ms., Mr., or Doctor.
- Begin or end each request with "please."
- Say "thank you" whenever someone does something for you.
- Apologize. Say "I'm sorry" when you make a mistake or hurt someone.
- Hold doors open for others. If you are at the door first, open the door and let others pass through.
- Hold elevator doors open for others coming down the hallway.
- Let patients, residents, families, and visitors enter elevators first.

Personal Matters

Personal matters cannot interfere with the job. Otherwise care is neglected. This is a reason for losing your job. To keep personal matters out of the workplace:
- Make phone calls during meals and breaks. Use a pay phone or your wireless phone.
- Do not let family and friends visit you on the unit. If they must see you, have them meet you during a meal or break.
- Make appointments (doctor, dentist, lawyer, beauty, and others) for your days off.
- Do not use the agency's computers, printers, fax machines, copiers, or other equipment for your personal use.
- Do not take agency supplies (pens, paper, and others) for your personal use.
- Do not discuss personal problems.
- Do not borrow money from or lend it to co-workers.
- Do not sell things or engage in fund-raising.
- Turn off personal pagers and wireless phones.
- Do not send or check text messages.

Meals and Breaks

Meal breaks are usually 30 minutes. Other breaks are usually 15 minutes. Meals and breaks are scheduled so that some staff are always on the unit. Staff remaining on the unit cover for the staff on break.

Staff members depend on each other. Leave for and return from breaks on time. That way other staff can have their turn. Do not take longer than allowed. Tell the nurse when you leave and return to the unit.

Planning Your Work

You will give care and perform routine tasks on the nursing unit. Some tasks are done at certain times. Others are done by the end of the shift.

The nurse, the Kardex, care plan, and your assignment sheet help you decide what to do and when (Chapter 4). This is called *priority setting*. A **priority** is the most important thing at the time. Setting priorities involves deciding:

- Which person has the greatest or most life-threatening needs
- What tasks the nurse or person needs done first
- What tasks need to be done at a set time
- What tasks need to be done when your shift starts
- What tasks need to be done at the end of your shift
- How much time it takes to complete a task
- How much help you need to complete a task
- Who can help you and when

Priorities change as the person's needs change. A person's condition can improve or worsen. New patients or residents are admitted. Others are transferred to other nursing units or discharged. These and many other factors can cause priorities to change.

Setting priorities is hard at first. It becomes easier as you gain experience. You can ask the nurse to help you set priorities. Plan your work to give safe, thorough care and to make good use of your time (Box 3-6).

MANAGING STRESS

Stress is the response or change in the body caused by any emotional, physical, social, or economic factor. Stress is normal. It occurs every minute of every day and in everything you do. No matter the cause—pleasant or unpleasant—stress affects the whole person:

- *Physically*—sweating, increased heart rate, faster and deeper breathing, increased blood pressure, dry mouth, and so on.

BOX 3-6   Planning Your Work

- Discuss priorities with the nurse.
- Know the routine of your shift and nursing unit.
- Follow unit policies for shift reports.
- List tasks that are on a schedule. For example, some persons are turned or offered the bedpan every 2 hours.
- Judge how much time you need for each person and task.
- Identify the tasks to do while patients or residents are eating, visiting, or involved with activities or therapies.
- Plan care around meal times, visiting hours, and therapies. In a nursing center, also consider recreation and social activities.
- Identify when you will need a co-worker's help. Ask a co-worker to help you. Give the time when you will need help and for how long.
- Schedule equipment or rooms for the person's use. The shower room is an example.
- Review delegated tasks. Gather needed supplies beforehand.
- Do not waste time. Stay focused on your work.
- Leave a clean work area. Make sure rooms are neat and orderly. Also clean utility areas.
- Be a self-starter. Ask others if they need help. Follow unit routines, stock supply areas, and clean utility rooms. Stay busy.

- *Mentally*—anxiety, fear, anger, dread, depression, and using defense mechanisms (Chapter 27).
- *Socially*—changes in relationships, avoiding others, needing others, blaming others, and so on.
- *Spiritually*—changes in beliefs and values and strengthening or questioning one's belief in God or a higher power.

Prolonged or frequent stress threatens physical and mental health. Some problems are minor—headaches, sleep problems, muscle tension, and so on. Others are life-threatening—high blood pressure, heart attack, stroke, ulcers, and so on.

Job stresses affect your family and friends. Stress in your personal life affects your work. Stress affects you, the care you give, the person's quality of life, and relating to co-workers. To reduce or cope with stress:

- Exercise regularly.
- Get enough rest and sleep.
- Eat healthy.
- Plan personal and quiet time for you.
- Use common sense about what you can do. Do not try to do everything that family and friends ask you to do.
- Do one thing at a time. Set priorities.

- Do not judge yourself harshly. Do not try to be perfect or expect too much from yourself.
- Give yourself praise. You do good and wonderful things every day.
- Have a sense of humor. Laugh at yourself. Laugh with others. Spend time with those who make you laugh.
- Talk to the nurse if your work or a person is causing too much stress. The nurse can help you deal with the matter.

HARASSMENT

Harassment means to trouble, torment, offend, or worry a person by one's behavior or comments. Harassment can be sexual. Or it can involve age, race, ethnic background, religion, or disability. You must respect others. Do not offend others by your gestures, remarks, or use of touch. Do not offend others with jokes, photos, or other pictures (drawings, cartoons, and so on). Harassment is not legal in the workplace.

See *Focus on Communication: Harassment.*

Sexual Harassment

Sexual harassment involves unwanted sexual behaviors by another. It may be a sexual advance or a request for a sexual favor. Some comments and touch are sexual. The behavior affects the person's work and comfort. In extreme cases, jobs are threatened if sexual favors are not granted.

Victims of sexual harassment may be men or women. Men harass women or men. Women harass men or women. You might feel that you are being harassed. If so, tell your supervisor and the human resource officer.

Even innocent remarks and behaviors can be viewed as harassment. Employee orientation programs address harassment. You might not be sure about your own or another person's remarks or behaviors. If so, talk to the nurse. You cannot be too careful.

RESIGNING FROM A JOB

Whatever your reason for resigning, you need to tell your employer. Give a written notice. Write a resignation letter. Or complete a form in the human resource office. Giving a 2-week notice is a good practice. Include the following in your notice:

- Reason for leaving
- The last date you will work
- Comments thanking the employer for the opportunity to work in the agency

---

FOCUS ON COMMUNICATION
Harassment

You have the right to feel safe and unthreatened. If someone's comments make you uncomfortable, you can say: "Please don't say things like that. It's unprofessional." If someone's actions make you uneasy, you can say: "Please don't do that. It's unprofessional." Leave the area. Report the person's statements or actions to the nurse.

BOX 3-7 Common Reasons for Losing a Job

- Poor attendance—not going to work or excessive tardiness (being late).
- Abandonment—leaving the job during your shift.
- Falsifying a record—job application or a person's medical record.
- Violent behavior in the workplace.
- Weapons in the work setting—guns, knives, explosives, or other dangerous items.
- Having, using, or distributing alcohol or drugs in the work setting. This excludes taking drugs ordered by a doctor.
- Taking a person's drugs for your own use or giving it to others.
- Harassment.
- Using offensive speech and language.
- Stealing or destroying the agency's or a person's property.
- Showing disrespect to patients, residents, families, visitors, co-workers, or supervisors.
- Abusing or neglecting a person.
- Invading a person's privacy.
- Failing to maintain patient, resident, agency, or co-worker confidentiality. This includes access to computer and other electronic information.
- Using the agency's supplies and equipment for your own use.
- Defamation—see Chapter 2 and "Gossip," p. 38.
- Abusing meal breaks and break periods.
- Sleeping on the job.
- Violating the agency's dress code.
- Violating any agency policy.
- Failing to follow agency care procedures.
- Tending to personal matters while on duty.

LOSING A JOB

You must perform your job well and protect patients and residents from harm. Otherwise you could lose your job. Failure to follow agency policy is often grounds for termination. So is failure to get along with others. Box 3-7 lists the many reasons why you can lose your job.

DRUG TESTING

Drug and alcohol use affects patient, resident, and staff safety. Quality of care suffers. Those who use drugs or alcohol are late to work or absent more often than staff members who do not use such substances. Therefore drug testing policies are common. Review your agency's policy for when and how you might be tested.

Focus on P R I D E
The Person, Family, and Yourself

Personal and Professional Responsibility—How you look affects the way people think about you and the agency. If staff members are clean and neat, people think the agency is clean and neat. They think the agency is unclean if staff members are messy and unkept. People also wonder about the quality of care given. You are responsible for dressing in a professional manner. Follow your agency's dress code.

Rights and Respect—Your attitude affects your feelings and behaviors. So do the attitudes of others. Quality care is affected by how you work with others and how you feel about your job. You will work with many different personalities. You may be more comfortable with some than with others. Show respect to all persons.

Sometimes you may work without enough staff. It may be hard to keep a good attitude. Do not complain about not having enough help. Do not put down another staff member. For example, do not say: "She calls in sick all the time. You know she's not sick." Every team member has value. Treat everyone with respect.

Independence and Social Interaction—Social interaction is a vital part of your job. Employers look for good social skills. During an interview, smile, give a firm hand-shake, make eye contact, and answer questions confidently. At work, smile and greet patients and residents by name. Politely introduce yourself. Do not appear hurried. Display a caring and friendly manner all the time. Remain calm and helpful in stressful situations. These actions promote good relationships and reflect positively on you.

Delegation and Teamwork—Your work ethics impact the team. Greet co-workers pleasantly. Help others willingly when asked. Offer to help others if you are able. After completing your tasks, ask the nurse if you can help with anything else. Be available. Stay in an area where you can be easily found. If you will be in one area for a while, tell the nurse. When you would like a break, ask the nurse. Return from breaks on time. Help others so they may take a break. Set a positive example with your behavior. Your actions help build a strong team.

Ethics and Laws—To be professional, you must be safe. You must follow federal, state, and agency laws and rules. Many agencies require a background check and drug testing before hiring.

Show good judgment with your actions inside and outside the workplace. Be honest and give accurate information to employers. Giving wrong or incomplete information to an employer is fraud (Chapter 2).

REVIEW QUESTIONS

Circle T if the statement is *true*. Circle F if the statement is *false*.

1. **T** F You wear needed eyeglasses. This helps protect the person's safety.
2. **T** F Childcare requires planning before you go to work.
3. T **F** Being on time for work means arriving at the agency when your shift begins.
4. **T** F You share information about a person with a friend. You could lose your job.
5. **T** F You wear jeans to work. You could lose your job.
6. T **F** You can use the agency's computer for your homework.
7. T **F** You can keep your wireless phone turned on while at work.
8. T **F** Harassment is legal in the workplace.
9. T **F** In a resignation letter, you should include any work problems.

Circle the BEST answer.

10 Which will *not* help you do your job well?
  a Enough rest and sleep
  b Regular exercise
  c Using drugs and alcohol
  d Good nutrition
11 Which is *not* a good hygiene practice?
  a Bathing daily
  b Using a deodorant
  c Brushing teeth after meals
  d Having long and polished fingernails
12 When do you ask questions about your job description?
  a After completing the job application
  b Before completing the job application
  c When your interview is scheduled
  d During the interview
13 To complete a job application, do the following *except*
  a Write neatly and clearly
  b Provide references
  c Give information about employment gaps
  d Leave spaces blank that do not apply to you
14 Which of the following do employers look for the *most?*
  a Cooperation
  b Courtesy
  c Dependability
  d Empathy
15 What is proper to wear to a job interview?
  a A uniform
  b Party clothes
  c A simple dress or suit
  d What is most comfortable
16 Which is a poor behavior during a job interview?
  a Good eye contact with the interviewer
  b Shaking hands with the interviewer
  c Asking the interviewer questions
  d Crossing your arms and legs
17 Which is the best response to an interview question?
  a "Yes" or "no"
  b Long answers
  c Brief explanations
  d A written response

18 A co-worker says that a doctor and nurse are dating. This is
  a Gossip
  b Eavesdropping
  c Confidential information
  d Sexual harassment
19 Which is professional speech and language?
  a Speaking clearly
  b Using vulgar words
  c Shouting
  d Arguing
20 You are on a meal break. Which is *false?*
  a You can make personal phone calls.
  b Family members can meet you.
  c You can take a few extra minutes if needed.
  d The nurse needs to know that you are off the unit.
21 To plan your work, do the following *except*
  a Discuss priorities with the nurse
  b Ask others if they need help
  c Stay busy
  d Plan care so that you can watch the person's TV
22 Which does *not* help reduce stress?
  a Exercise, rest, and sleep
  b Blaming yourself for things you did not do
  c Planning quiet time
  d Having a sense of humor
23 Which is *not* harassment?
  a Using touch to comfort a person
  b Joking about a person's religion
  c Asking for a sexual favor
  d Acting like a disabled person
24 Which is *not* a reason for losing your job?
  a Leaving the job during your shift
  b Using alcohol in the work setting
  c Sleeping on the job
  d Taking a meal break

Answers to these questions are on p. 527.

4

COMMUNICATING WITH THE HEALTH TEAM

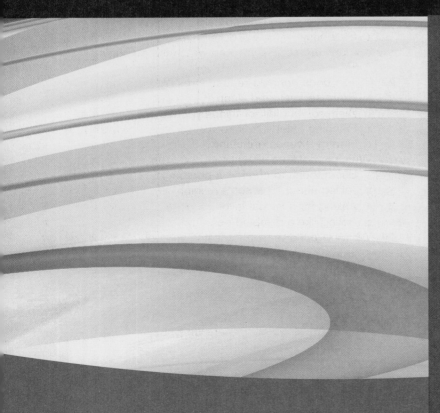

OBJECTIVES

- Define the key terms and key abbreviations listed in this chapter.
- Describe the rules for good communication.
- Explain the purpose, parts, and information found in the medical record.
- Describe the legal and ethical aspects of medical records.
- Describe the purpose of the Kardex.
- Explain your role in the nursing process.
- List the information you need to report to the nurse.
- List the rules for recording.
- Use the 24-hour clock, medical terminology, and medical abbreviations.
- Explain how computers and other electronic devices are used in health care.
- Explain how to protect the right to privacy when using computers and other electronic devices.
- Describe the rules for answering phones.
- Explain how to problem solve and deal with conflict.
- Explain how to promote PRIDE in the person, the family, and yourself.

KEY TERMS

chart See "medical record"

communication The exchange of information—a message sent is received and correctly interpreted by the intended person

comprehensive care plan A written guide giving direction for the resident's care; required by OBRA

medical record A written or electronic account of a person's condition and response to treatment and care; chart

nursing care plan A written guide about the person's care; care plan

nursing process The method nurses use to plan and deliver nursing care; its five steps are assessment, nursing diagnosis, planning, implementation, and evaluation

objective data Information that is seen, heard, felt, or smelled by an observer; signs

observation Using the senses of sight, hearing, touch, and smell to collect information

recording The written account of care and observations; charting

reporting The oral account of care and observations

signs See "objective data"

subjective data Things a person tells you about that you cannot observe through your senses; symptoms

symptoms See "subjective data"

KEY ABBREVIATIONS

MDS Minimum Data Set

NANDA-I North American Nursing Diagnosis Association International

OBRA Omnibus Budget Reconciliation Act of 1987

PDA Personal digital assistant

PHI Protected health information

RAPs Resident Assessment Protocols

RN Registered nurse

Health team members communicate with each other to give coordinated and effective care. They share information about:
- What was done for the person
- What needs to be done for the person
- The person's response to treatment

COMMUNICATION

Communication is the exchange of information—a message sent is received and correctly interpreted by the intended person. For good communication:
- Use words that mean the same thing to you and the receiver of the message. Avoid words with more than one meaning.
- Use familiar words. Avoid terms that the person and family do not understand.
- Be brief and concise. Do not add unrelated or unnecessary information. Stay on the subject. Avoid wandering in thought. Do not get wordy.
- Give information in a logical and orderly manner. Organize your thoughts. Present them step-by-step.
- Give facts and be specific. You report a pulse rate of 110. It is more specific and factual than the "pulse is fast."

THE MEDICAL RECORD

The **medical record (chart)** is a written or electronic account of a person's condition and response to treatment and care. It is used by the health team to share information about the person. The record is permanent. It can be used in court as legal evidence of the person's problems, treatment, and care.

The record has many forms. Each page has the person's name, room and bed number, and other identifying information. This helps prevent errors and the improper placement of records.

Agencies have policies about medical records and who can see them. Policies address who records, when to record, abbreviations, correcting errors, ink color, and signing entries.

Some agencies allow nursing assistants to record observations and care. Others do not. You must know your agency's policies.

Professional staff involved in a person's care can read and use charts. If you have access to charts, you must keep information confidential. This is your ethical and legal duty. If you are not involved in a person's care, you have no right to see the person's chart. To do so is an invasion of privacy.

Med-Forms, Inc.
FORM #MF37079 (Rev 9/95)

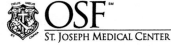

OSF ℠
ST. JOSEPH MEDICAL CENTER
Bloomington, Illinois 61701

DAILY SUMMARY AND GRAPHIC

TEMPERATURE
Write in 105° or over

	2400	0400	0800	1200	1600	2000	2400	0400	0800	1200	1600	2000	2400	0400	0800	1200	1600	2000	2400	0400	0800	1200	1600	2000
DATE	5-7						5-8																	
HOSPITAL DAY	4						5																	
POST OP DAY																								
HOUR	2400	0400	0800	1200	1600	2000	2400	0400	0800	1200	1600	2000	2400	0400	0800	1200	1600	2000	2400	0400	0800	1200	1600	2000
B/P			130/80	120/76	130/76	130/80			120/72	120/80	130/80	130/82												

TEMPERATURE (°F / °C):
- 104 40
- 102.2 39
- 100.4 38
- 98.6 37
- 96.6 36

PULSE			74	80	76	74			74	74	76	72												
RESPIRATION			18	18	16	16			18	20	18	16												
WEIGHT																								
DR. VISIT	@ 0900																							

INTAKE	2300-0700	0700-1500	1500-2300	TOTAL	2300-0700	0700-1500	1500-2300	TOTAL	2300-0700	0700-1500	1500-2300	TOTAL	2300-0700	0700-1500	1500-2300	TOTAL
Oral	100	1200	800	2100	100	1050	820	1970								
IV																
Tube Feedings																
PPN/TPN/Lipids																
Blood/Blood Products																
IV Meds																
Chemotherapy																
Unreturned irr. sol.																
TOTAL INTAKE	100	1200	800	2100	100	1050	820	1970								

OUTPUT	2300-0700	0700-1500	1500-2300	TOTAL	2300-0700	0700-1500	1500-2300	TOTAL	2300-0700	0700-1500	1500-2300	TOTAL	2300-0700	0700-1500	1500-2300	TOTAL
Urine	0	1050	800	1850	200	850	750	1800								
GI																
Emesis	100			100												
Drains																
TOTAL OUTPUT	100	1050	800	1950	200	850	750	1800								
Feces		✓				✓										

FIGURE 4-1 Graphic sheet. *(Modified from OSF St. Joseph Medical Center, Bloomington, Ill.)*

Date	Time	Nursing Margin	Other Depts Margin
3-19	1700	Out with family for dinner. Jane Doe, LPN	
	1930	Returned from outing accompanied by her son. States she had a pleasant time Mary Smith, CNA	
3-20	0900	IN BED. COMPLAINS OF HEADACHE. T 98.4 ORALLY, RADIAL PULSE 72 AND REGULAR, RESPIRATIONS 18 AND UNLABORED. BP 134/84 LEFT ARM LYING DOWN. ALICE JONES, RN NOTIFIED OF RESIDENT COMPLAINT AND VITAL SIGNS. ANN ADAMS, CNA	
	0910	In bed resting. States she has had a headache for about 1/2 hour. Denies nausea and dizziness. No other complaints. PRN Tylenol given. Instructed resident to use signal light if headache worsens or other symptoms occur. Alice Jones, RN	
	0945	Resting quietly. Denies headache at this time. T 98.4 orally, radial pulse 70 and regular, respirations 18 and unlabored. BP 132/84 left arm lying down. Alice Jones, RN	

FIGURE 4-2 Progress notes. Note that other members of the health team also can record on this form.

THE NURSING PROCESS

The **nursing process** is the method nurses use to plan and deliver nursing care. It has five steps: assessment, nursing diagnosis, planning, implementation, and evaluation.

The nursing process deals with the person's nursing needs. All nursing team members do the same things for the person. They have the same goals.

The nursing process is on-going. New information is gathered and the person's needs may change. However, the steps remain the same. You will see the continuous nature of the nursing process as each step is explained.

You have a key role in the nursing process. The nurse uses your observations for nursing diagnoses and planning. You may help develop the care plan. In the implementation step, you perform nursing actions and measures in the care plan. Your assignment sheet tells you what to do. Your observations are used for the evaluation step.

Text continued on p. 50

The following medical record forms relate to your work:

- *Admission sheet*—is completed when the person is admitted to the agency. It has the person's identifying information. Use it to complete forms that require the same information.
- *Health history*—is completed by the nurse. The nurse asks about current and past illnesses, signs and symptoms, allergies, and drugs.
- *Graphic sheet*—is used to record measurements and observations made daily, every shift, or 3 to 4 times a day (Fig. 4-1). Information includes temperature, pulse, respirations, blood pressure, weight, intake and output, bowel movements (feces), and doctor's visits.
- *Progress notes*—are used to describe observations, the care given, the person's response and progress (Fig. 4-2). They are used to record information about treatments, some drugs, and procedures performed by the doctor. In long-term care, summaries of care describe the person's progress toward goals and response to care.
- *Flow sheets*—are used to record frequent measurements or observations (Fig. 4-3, p. 48). The activities of daily living flow sheet is used to record the person's every day activities.

THE KARDEX

The *Kardex* is a type of card file. It summarizes the person's drugs, treatments, diagnoses, care measures, equipment, and special needs. The Kardex is a quick, easy source of information about the person (Fig. 4-4, p. 49).

Activities of Daily Living Flow Sheet

JAN FEB (MAR) APR MAY JUN JUL AUG SEP OCT NOV DEC

ORDER/INSTRUCTION	TIME	1	2	3	4	5	6	7	8	9	10	11	12	13	14	15	16	17	18	19	20	21	22	23	24	25	26	27	28	29	30	31
Bowel Movements L = Large M = Medium S = Small IC = Incontinent	11-7	M																														
	7-3			L																												
	3-11																															
Bladder Elimination I = Independent IC = Incontinent FC = Foley catheter	11-7	I	I	I	I																											
	7-3	I	I	I	I																											
	3-11	I	IC	I	I																											
Weight Bearing Status TT = Toe touch AT = As tol. P = Partial F = Full NWB = No weight bearing	11-7	AT	AT	AT	AT																											
	7-3	AT	AT	AT	AT																											
	3-11	AT	AT	AT	AT																											
Transfer Status ML = Mech lift SBA = Stand by assist; Assist of 1 or 2	11-7	SBA	SBA	SBA	SBA																											
	7-3	SBA	SBA	SBA	SBA																											
	3-11	SBA	SBA	SBA	A-1																											
Activity A = Ambulate GC = Gerichair T = Turn every 2 hrs. W/C = Wheelchair	11-7	T	T	T	T																											
	7-3	A	A	A	A																											
	3-11	A	A	A	A																											
Safety LT = Lap tray BR = Bed rails BA = Bed alarm SB = Seat belt	11-7																															
	7-3																															
	3-11																															
Feeding Status I = Independent S = Set up F = Staff feed SP = Swallow precautions TL = Thickened liquids	Breakfast	S	S	S	S																											
	Lunch	S	S	S	S																											
	Supper	S	S	S	S																											
Amount of food taken in %	Breakfast	75	100	100	75																											
	Lunch	75	75	100	75																											
	Supper	50	50	50	75																											
Bath and Shampoo every *Monday* & *Thursday* on *7-3* shift T = Tub S = Shower B = Bed bath	11-7																															
	7-3		T																													
	3-11																															
Oral Care Own/(Dentures)/No teeth I = Independent S = Set up A = Assist	11-7	S	S	S	S																											
	7-3	S	S	S	S																											
	3-11	S	S	S	S																											
Dressing I = Independent S = Set up A = Assist T = Total care	11-7	A	A	S	S																											
	7-3																															
	3-11	A	A	A	A																											
Grooming: Washing Face and Hands Combing Hair I = Independent S = Set up A = Assist T = Total care	11-7	A	A	A	A																											
	7-3	A	A	A	A																											
	3-11	A	A	A	A																											
Trim Fingernails weekly *Thursday*	11-7																															
	7-3		✓																													
	3-11																															
Lotion Arms and Legs twice daily	11-7																															
	7-3	✓	✓	✓	✓																											
	3-11	✓	✓	✓	✓																											
Shave Men daily Shave (Women) every *Monday* & *Thursday* on *7-3* shift	11-7																															
	7-3		✓																													
	3-11																															
Amount Between-Meal Snack taken in %	AM	100	75	100	50																											
	PM	100	100	75	75																											
	HS	50	75	75	75																											
Intake and Output	11-7																															
	7-3																															
	3-11																															
Vital Signs Every *Thursday*	11-7																															
	7-3		✓																													
	3-11																															
Weight Every *Thursday*	11-7		✓																													
	7-3																															
	3-11																															

FIGURE 4-3 Some items on an Activities of Daily Living Flow Sheet.

DIET	NOURISHMENT/SPECIAL FEEDING	INTAKE/OUTPUT
Regular	*Health shake at Bedtime*	Encourage/(Restrict) Fluids ___*2000*___ mL/24 Hr.
Hold:		7-3 ___*1000*___ 3-11 ___*800*___ 11-7 ___*200*___

FUNCTIONAL STATUS

	SELF	ASSIST	TOTAL	OTHER	SPECIFY
Feeding	☐	☒	☐	☐	
Bathing	☐	☒	☐	☐	
Toileting	☐	☒	☐	☐	
Oral Care	☐	☒	☐	☐	
Positioning	☒	☐	☐	☐	
Transferring	☒	☐	☐	☐	
Wheeling	☐	☐	☐	☐	
Walking	☒	☐	☐	☐	
	☐	☐	☐	☐	

ACTIVITIES

- Bedrest & BRP _____
- Bedside Commode _____
- Up ad Lib ___*X*___
- Chair _____
- Ambulatory ___*X*___
- Ambulate & Assist _____
- Turn _____
- Dangle _____
- Mode of Travel _____

ELIMINATION

- Bladder - Cont. (Incont)
- Catheter _____
- Date Changed _____
- Irrigations _____
- Bowel - (Cont.) / Incont.
- Ostomy _____
- Irrigations _____

VITALS

Temp.	*qid*
Pulse	*qid*
Resp.	*qid*
BP	*qid*
Weight	*daily*
Other:	*Pulse OX daily*

COMMUNICATION DEFICITS ☐ None

- Hearing *Hard-of-hearing*
- Vision *Impaired*
- Speech _____
- Language *Impaired*

PROSTHESIS ☐ None

- Glasses ___*X*___   Dentures ___*X*___
- Contacts _____   Limb _____
- Hearing Aid ___*L ear*___

SPECIAL CONDITIONS (Paralysis, Pressure Ulcers, Etc.)

SAFETY/SUPPORTIVE MEASURES

- Bed rails: ☐ Nights Only ☐ Constant ☐ No Need
- Restraints: ☐ PRN ☐ Constant
- Support Devices: ☐ PRN ☐ Constant

RESPIRATORY THERAPY

- Aerosol
- IPPB
- Ultrasonic
- Rx Med _____

OXYGEN

- ___*2*___ Liter/Minute
- ☒ PRN ☐ Constant
- ___ Tent ___ Catheter
- ___ Mask ___*X*___ Cannula

SPECIAL EQUIPMENT/PROCEDURES/ANCILLARY SERVICES/ETC.

Speech therapy 3 times/wk.

ORDERED	SCHEDULED	COMPLETED	X-RAY AND SPECIAL DIAGNOSTIC EXAMS
10-20	*10-20*	*10-20*	*Chest x-ray*

DATE	TREATMENTS/MISCELLANEOUS

START DATE	SCHEDULED MEDICATIONS	STOP DATE	RENEW	START DATE	STOP OR RENEW	SITE	IV FLUID & RATE	TUBING	DRESS.	SITE
10-19	*Lasix 40 mg PO daily*									
10-19	*Lanoxin 0.25 mg PO daily*									

DATE	ONE TIME ORDERS

DATE	DAILY/REPEATING ORDERS
10-20	*Serum potassium daily*

DATE	TIME	PRN MEDICATIONS
10-19	*2100*	*Ativan 0.25 mg PO q4h PRN anxiety*

MISCELLANEOUS

ALLERGIES:	NURSING ALERTS:	EMERGENCY CONTACT:	
☒ None Known		Name: *Parker, Marie*	Telephone No. Home: *555-1212*
		Relationship: *Wife*	Bus:

ROOM	NAME	PHYSICIAN	ADMITTING DIAGNOSIS/PROBLEM	HOSP. NO.
310	*Parker, Edwin*	*Dr. S Epstein*	1. *CHF* 2. *Dementia*	*1035B*

FIGURE 4-4 A sample Kardex. (*Modified from Briggs Corporation, Des Moines, Iowa.*)

Assessment

Assessment involves collecting information about the person. A health history is taken about current and past health problems. It includes the family's history. Information from the doctor is reviewed. So are test results and past medical records.

An RN assesses the person's body systems and mental status. You assist with assessment. You make many observations as you give care and talk to the person.

Observation is using the senses of sight, hearing, touch, and smell to collect information:

- You *see* how the person lies, sits, or walks. You see flushed or pale skin. You see red and swollen body areas.
- You *listen* to the person breathe, talk, and cough.
- Through *touch,* you feel if the skin is hot or cold, or moist or dry.
- *Smell* is used to detect body, wound, and breath odors. You also smell odors from urine and bowel movements.

Objective data (signs) are seen, heard, felt, or smelled by an observer. You can feel a pulse. You can see the color of urine. **Subjective data (symptoms)** are things a person tells you about that you cannot observe through your senses. You cannot feel or see the person's pain, fear, or nausea.

Box 4-1 lists the basic observations you need to make and report to the nurse. Box 4-2, p. 52 lists the observations that you must report at once. Make notes of your observations. Use them when reporting and recording observations. Carry a note pad and pen in your pocket. That way you can note observations as you make them.

The Omnibus Budget Reconciliation Act of 1987 (OBRA) requires the *Minimum Data Set* (MDS) for nursing center residents. It provides extensive information about the person. Examples include memory, communication, hearing and vision, physical function, and activities. The MDS is updated before each care conference (p. 53). A new MDS is completed once a year and whenever a change occurs in the person's health status.

Nursing Diagnosis

The RN uses assessment information to make a nursing diagnosis. A *nursing diagnosis* describes a health problem that can be treated by nursing measures. It is different from a medical diagnosis. A *medical diagnosis* is the identification of a disease or condition by a doctor. Cancer, stroke, heart attack, and diabetes are examples.

A person can have many nursing diagnoses. They may change as assessment information changes. Or new nursing diagnoses are added. For example, "Acute pain" is added after surgery. Box 4-3, p. 52 lists some common nursing diagnoses.

Planning

Planning involves setting priorities and goals. Priorities are what is most important for the person. Goals are aimed at the person's highest level of well-being and function—physical, emotional, social, spiritual. Goals promote health and prevent health problems.

A *nursing intervention* is an action or measure taken by the nursing team to help the person reach a goal. *Nursing intervention, nursing action,* and *nursing measure* mean the same thing. A nursing intervention does not need a doctor's order.

The **nursing care plan** (care plan) is a written guide about the person's care. It has the person's nursing diagnoses, goals, and measures for each goal. The care plan is a communication tool. Nursing staff use it to see what care to give. The care plan helps ensure that the nursing team members give the same care.

Each agency has a care plan form. It is found in the medical record, on the Kardex, or on a computer.

The RN may conduct a care conference to share information and ideas about the person's care. The purpose is to develop or revise the person's nursing care plan. Effective care is the goal. Nursing assistants usually take part in the conference.

The plan is carried out. It may change as the person's nursing diagnoses change.

The Comprehensive Care Plan

OBRA requires a **comprehensive care plan.** It is a written guide giving direction for the resident's care. The plan identifies person's problems, goals for care, and actions to take.

Problems identified on the MDS give *triggers* (clues) for the Resident Assessment Protocols (RAPs). RAPs are guidelines used to develop the person's care plan. For example, the MDS shows that Mr. Smith has problems walking. This triggers the RAPs. They provide guidelines to solve the problem. The goal is for Mr. Smith to walk without help. Actions to help him reach the goal are:

- Physical therapy to work with Mr. Smith on exercises daily
- Nursing staff member to walk Mr. Smith 20 yards twice daily

The comprehensive care plan also states the person's strengths. For example, Mr. Smith can feed himself. This strength increases his independence. The health team helps Mr. Smith continue to feed himself.

BOX 4-1   Basic Observations

Ability to Respond

- Is the person easy or hard to wake up?
- Can the person give his or her name, the time, and location when asked?
- Does the person identify others correctly?
- Does the person answer questions correctly?
- Does the person speak clearly?
- Are instructions followed correctly?
- Is the person calm, restless, or excited?
- Is the person conversing, quiet, or talking a lot?

Movement

- Can the person squeeze your fingers with each hand?
- Can the person move arms and legs?
- Are the person's movements shaky or jerky?
- Does the person complain of stiff or painful joints?

Pain or Discomfort

- Where is the pain located? (Ask the person to point to the pain.)
- Does the pain go anywhere else?
- How does the person rate the severity of the pain—mild, moderate, severe?
- How does the person rate the pain on a scale of 0 to 10 (Chapter 20)?
- When did the pain begin?
- What was the person doing when the pain began?
- How long does the pain last?
- How does the person describe the pain?
  - Sharp
  - Severe
  - Knife-like
  - Dull
  - Burning
  - Aching
  - Comes and goes
  - Depends on position
- Was a pain-relief drug given?
- Did the pain-relief drug relieve the pain? Is the pain still present?
- Is the person able to sleep and rest?
- What is the position of comfort?

Skin

- Is the skin pale or flushed?
- Is the skin cool, warm, or hot?
- Is the skin moist or dry?
- What color are the lips and nail beds?
- Is the skin intact? Are there broken areas? If so, where?
- Are sores or reddened areas present?
- Are bruises present? Where are they located?
- Does the person complain of itching? If yes, where?

Eyes, Ears, Nose, and Mouth

- Is there drainage from the eyes? What color is the drainage?
- Are the eyelids closed? Do they stay open?
- Are the eyes reddened?
- Does the person complain of spots, flashes, or blurring?
- Is the person sensitive to bright lights?
- Is there drainage from the ears? What color is the drainage?
- Can the person hear? Is repeating necessary? Are questions answered appropriately?
- Is there drainage from the nose? What color is the drainage?
- Can the person breathe through the nose?
- Is there breath odor?
- Does the person complain of a bad taste in the mouth?
- Does the person complain of painful gums or teeth?

Respirations

- Do both sides of the person's chest rise and fall with respirations?
- Is breathing noisy?
- Does the person complain of pain or difficulty breathing?
- What is the amount and color of sputum?
- What is the frequency of the person's cough? Is it dry or productive?

Bowels and Bladder

- Is the abdomen firm or soft?
- Does the person complain of gas?
- What are the amount, color, and consistency of bowel movements?
- What is the frequency of bowel movements?
- Can the person control bowel movements?
- Does the person have pain or difficulty urinating?
- What is the amount of urine?
- What is the color of urine?
- Is the urine clear? Are there particles in the urine?
- Does the urine have a foul smell?
- Can the person control the passage of urine?
- What is the frequency of urination?

Appetite

- Does the person like the food served?
- How much of the meal is eaten?
- What foods does the person like?
- Can the person chew food?
- What is the amount of fluid taken?
- What fluids does the person like?
- How often does the person drink fluids?
- Can the person swallow food and fluids?
- Does the person complain of nausea?
- What is the amount and color of material vomited?
- Does the person have hiccups?
- Is the person belching?
- Does the person cough when swallowing?

Continued

BOX 4-1   Basic Observations—cont'd

Activities of Daily Living

- Can the person perform personal care without help?
  - Bathing?
  - Brushing teeth?
  - Combing and brushing hair?
  - Shaving?
- Which does the person use: toilet, commode, bedpan, or urinal?
- Does the person feed himself or herself?
- Can the person walk?
- What amount and kind of help is needed?

Other

- Is the person bleeding from any body part? If yes, where and how much?

BOX 4-2   Observations to Report at Once

- A change in the person's ability to respond
  - A responsive person is no longer responding.
  - A non-responsive person is now responding.
- A change in the person's mobility
  - The person cannot move a body part.
  - The person is now able to move a body part.
- Complaints of sudden, severe pain
- A sore or reddened area on the person's skin
- Complaints of a sudden change in vision
- Complaints of pain or difficulty breathing
- Abnormal respirations
- Complaints of or signs of difficulty swallowing
- Vomiting
- Bleeding
- Vital signs outside their normal ranges

BOX 4-3   Common Nursing Diagnoses Approved by the North American Nursing Diagnosis Association International

- Activity Intolerance
- Activity Intolerance, Risk for
- Airway Clearance, Ineffective
- Anxiety
- Aspiration, Risk for
- Bathing Self-Care Deficit
- Body Image, Disturbed
- Body Temperature, Risk for Imbalanced
- Breathing Pattern, Ineffective
- Communication, Impaired Verbal
- Confusion, Acute
- Confusion, Chronic
- Confusion, Risk for Acute
- Constipation
- Contamination
- Death Anxiety
- Denial, Ineffective
- Dentition, Impaired

- Diarrhea
- Disuse Syndrome, Risk for
- Diversional Activity, Deficient
- Dressing Self-Care Deficit
- Failure to Thrive, Adult
- Falls, Risk for
- Family Processes, Interrupted
- Fatigue
- Fear
- Feeding Self-Care Deficit
- Fluid Balance, Readiness for Enhanced
- Fluid Volume, Deficient
- Fluid Volume, Excess
- Glucose Level, Blood, Risk for Unstable
- Grieving
- Grieving, Complicated
- Health Behavior, Risk-Prone
- Health Maintenance, Ineffective

BOX 4-3	Common Nursing Diagnoses Approved by the North American Nursing Diagnosis Association International—cont'd

- Hopelessness
- Incontinence, Bowel
- Incontinence, Urinary, Functional
- Incontinence, Urinary, Overflow
- Incontinence, Urinary, Reflex
- Incontinence, Urinary, Stress
- Incontinence, Urinary, Total
- Incontinence, Urinary, Urge
- Incontinence, Urinary, Urge, Risk for
- Infection, Risk for
- Injury, Risk for
- Insomnia
- Latex Allergy Response
- Loneliness, Risk for
- Memory, Impaired
- Mobility, Impaired Bed
- Mobility, Impaired Physical
- Mobility, Impaired Wheelchair
- Nausea
- Nutrition, Imbalanced: Less Than Body Requirements
- Nutrition, Imbalanced: More Than Body Requirements
- Nutrition, Imbalanced: More Than Body Requirements, Risk for
- Nutrition, Readiness for Enhanced
- Oral Mucous Membrane, Impaired
- Pain, Acute
- Pain, Chronic
- Post-Trauma Syndrome

- Powerlessness
- Relocation Stress Syndrome
- Self-Esteem, Chronic Low
- Sensory Perception, Disturbed (Specify: visual, auditory, kinesthetic, gustatory, tactile, olfactory)
- Sexuality, Ineffective Pattern
- Skin Integrity, Impaired
- Sleep Deprivation
- Social Interaction, Impaired
- Social Isolation
- Sorrow, Chronic
- Spiritual Distress
- Spiritual Distress, Risk for
- Suffocation, Risk for
- Suicide, Risk for
- Surgical Recovery, Delayed
- Swallowing, Impaired
- Therapeutic Regimen Management, Effective
- Thought Processes, Disturbed
- Tissue Integrity, Impaired
- Toileting Self-Care Deficit
- Transfer Ability, Impaired
- Trauma, Risk for
- Urinary Elimination, Impaired
- Urinary Elimination, Readiness for Enhanced
- Urinary Retention
- Walking, Impaired
- Wandering

Implementation

To *implement* means to perform or carry out. The *implementation* step is performing the nursing measures in the care plan. Care is given in this step. The nurse delegates nursing tasks that are within your legal limits and job description.

Assignment Sheets The nurse uses an assignment sheet to communicate delegated measures and tasks to you (Fig. 4-5, p. 54). Talk to the nurse about unclear assignments. You can also check the care plan and Kardex if you need more information.

Evaluation

Evaluate means to measure. The *evaluation* step involves measuring if the goals in the planning step were met. Progress is evaluated. Changes in nursing diagnoses, goals, and the care plan may result.

RESIDENT CARE CONFERENCES

OBRA requires two types of resident care conferences:
- *Interdisciplinary care planning (IDCP) conference.* This is held regularly to review and update care plans. It also is held to develop care plans for new residents. The RN, doctor, and other health team members attend.
- *Problem-focused conference.* This is held when one problem affects a person's care. Only staff directly involved with the problem attend.

The person has the right to take part in these planning conferences. Sometimes the family is involved. The person may refuse actions suggested by the health team.

Assignment Sheet

Date: 9–10
Shift: Day
Nursing assistant: John Reed
Supervisor: Mary Adams, RN

Breaks: 1000   1400
Lunch: 1230
Unit Tasks: Pass ice water at 0900
Clean utility room at 1430

*Check the care plan for other care measures and information

Room # 501A Name: Mrs. Ann Lopez	Functional status/other care measures and procedures
ID Number: S1514491530 Date of birth: 11/04/1925	Total assist with ADL
VS: Daily at 0700	Stand-pivot transfers
T _____ P _____ R _____ BP _____	Uses w/c
Wt: Weekly (Monday at 0700) _____	Incontinent of bowel and bladder – uses briefs
Intake _____ BM _____	Bilateral passive ROM exercises to extremities twice daily
Bath: Portable tub	Turn and reposition q2h when in bed
Shampoo Bed rails	Wears eyeglasses and dentures
	Diet: High fiber (Total Assist)
Room # 510B Name: Mr. Mark Monroe	Functional status/other care measures and procedures
ID Number: D4468947762 Date of birth: 12/29/1926	Independent with ADL
VS: 2 times daily, at 0700 and 1500	Independent with ambulation
0700: T _____ P _____ R _____ BP _____	Attends exercise group every morning
1500: T _____ P _____ R _____ BP _____	Continent of bowel and bladder – q4h bathroom schedule
Wt: Daily at 0700 _____	to maintain continence
Intake _____ Output _____ BM _____	Wears eyeglasses
Bath: Shower	Coughing and deep breathing exercises q4h
	Diet: Sodium-controlled (Independent)

FIGURE 4-5 Sample Assignment Sheet. Note: this Assignment Sheet is a computer printout.

REPORTING AND RECORDING

Reporting and recording are accounts of what was done and observed about the person. **Reporting** is the oral account of care and observations. **Recording** (*charting*) is the written account of care and observations.

Reporting

You report care and observations to the nurse. Report to the nurse:
- Whenever there is a change from normal or a change in the person's condition. Report these changes at once (see Box 4-2).
- When the nurse asks you to do so.
- When you leave the unit for meals, breaks, or for other reasons.
- Before the end-of-shift report.

Follow these rules:
- Be prompt, thorough, and accurate.
- Give the person's name and room and bed number.
- Give the time your observations were made or the care was given.
- Report only what you observed or did yourself.
- Report care measures that you expect the person to need. For example, you expect that the person will need the bedpan during your meal break.
- Report expected changes in the person's condition. For example, you expect that the person may be tired after physical therapy.
- Use your written notes to give a specific, concise, and clear report.

End-of-Shift Report The nurse gives a report at the end of the shift. This is called the *end-of-shift report* or the *change-of-shift report*. It is given to the nursing team of the on-coming shift. The nurse reports about:
- The care given
- The care that must be given during other shifts
- The person's current condition
- Likely changes in the person's condition

In some agencies, the entire nursing team hears the end-of-shift report as they come on duty. In other agencies, only nurses hear the report. After the report, the nurses share important information with nursing assistants.

See *Promoting Safety and Comfort: End-of-Shift Report.*

Recording

When recording on the person's chart, communicate clearly and thoroughly. Follow the rules in Box 4-4. Anyone who reads your charting should know:
- What you observed
- What you did
- The person's response

See *Focus on Communication: Reporting and Recording,* p. 56.

PROMOTING SAFETY AND COMFORT
End-of-Shift Report

Safety

You may not hear the end-of-shift report as you come on duty. Yet you need to answer signal lights and give care before the nurse shares new information with you. To give safe care:
- Check the care plan and Kardex before granting a request. The person's condition or care plan may have changed since you last worked. Or there may be new orders.
- Ask a nurse about the care needs of new patients or residents. If necessary, politely interrupt the end-of-shift report to ask your questions.
- Do not take directions or orders from another nursing assistant. Remember, nursing assistants cannot supervise or delegate to other nursing assistants.

BOX 4-4   Rules for Recording

General Rules

- Follow your agency's policies and procedures for recording. Ask for training as needed.
- Include the date and time for every recording. Use conventional time (AM or PM) or 24-hour clock time according to agency policy (p. 56).
- Use only agency-approved medical abbreviations (p. 59).
- Use correct spelling, grammar, and punctuation.
- Sign all entries with your name and title as required by agency policy.
- Make sure each form has the person's name and other identifying information.
- Record only what you observed and did yourself. Do not record for another person.
- Never chart a procedure, treatment, measurement, or care measure until after it is completed.
- Chart a procedure, treatment, measurement, or care measure after it is done. If not recorded, the action is considered not done.
- Be accurate, concise, and factual. Do not record judgments or interpretations.
- Record in a logical and sequential manner.
- Be descriptive. Avoid terms with more than one meaning.
- Use the person's exact words whenever possible. Use quotation marks to show that the statement is a direct quote.
- Do not use ditto marks.
- Chart any changes from normal or changes in the person's condition. Also chart that you informed the nurse (include the nurse's name), what you told the nurse, and the time you made the report.

- Do not omit information.
- Record safety measures. Examples include placing the signal light within reach, assisting a person when up, or reminding a person not to get out of bed.

Paper Charting

- Always use ink. Use the ink color required by the agency.
- Make sure writing is readable and neat.
- Never erase or use correction fluid. Draw a line through the incorrect part. Date and initial the line. Write "mistaken entry" over it if this is agency policy. Then rewrite the part. Follow agency policy for correcting errors.
- Do not skip lines. Draw a line through the blank space of a partially completed line or to the end of the page. This prevents others from recording in a space with your signature.

Electronic Charting

- Log in using your "unique user identification" (username) and password. Do not chart using another person's username.
- Check the time your entry is made. Make sure it is the intended time.
- Check for accuracy. Review your entry before saving.
- Save your entries. Unsaved data will be lost.
- Follow the manufacturer's instructions for changing or uncharting a mistaken entry. Most electronic charting systems keep a record of what was entered before a change was made. This works in the same manner as drawing a line through a mistaken entry in paper charting. The first entry is still visible.
- Log off after you are done charting. This prevents others from charting under your username.

"Small," "moderate," and "large" mean different things to different people. Is small the size of a dime? Or is it the size of a quarter? In health care, different meanings can cause serious problems. Give accurate descriptions and measurements. If you have a question, ask the nurse to look at what you are trying to describe.

MEDICAL TERMINOLOGY AND ABBREVIATIONS

Medical terminology and abbreviations are used in health care. Like all words, medical terms are made up of parts or *word elements*—prefixes, roots, and suffixes (Box 4-5). Most are from Greek or Latin. They are combined to form medical terms. A term is translated by separating the word into its elements.

Recording Time The 24-hour clock (military time or international time) has four digits (Fig. 4-6). The first two digits are for the hours: 0100 = 1:00 AM; 1300 = 1:00 PM. The last two digits are for minutes: 0110 = 1:10 AM. The AM and PM abbreviations are not used.

As Figure 4-6 shows, the hour is the same for morning times, but AM is not used. For PM times add 12 to the clock time. If it is 2:00 PM, add 12 and 2 for 1400. For 8:35 PM, add 12 and 835 for 2035.

Some agencies use 0000 for midnight. Others use 2400. Follow agency policy.

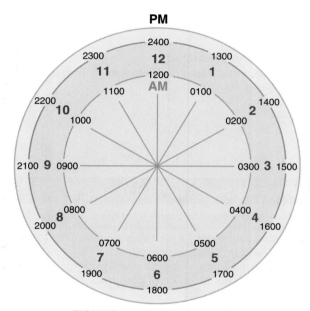

FIGURE 4-6 The 24-hour clock.

BOX 4-5	Medical Terminology		
PREFIX	**MEANING**	**PREFIX**	**MEANING**
a-, an-	without, not, lack of	ex-	out, out of, from, away from
ab-	away from	hemi-	half
ad-	to, toward, near	hyper-	excessive, too much, high
ante-	before, forward, in front of	hypo-	under, decreased, less than normal
anti-	against	in-	in, into, within, not
auto-	self	inter-	between
bi-	double, two, twice	intra-	within
brady-	slow	intro-	into, within
circum-	around	leuk-	white
contra-	against, opposite	macro-	large
de-	down, from	mal-	bad, illness, disease
dia-	across, through, apart	meg-	large
dis-	apart, free from	micro-	small
dys-	bad, difficult, abnormal	mono-	one, single
ecto-	outer, outside	neo-	new
en-	in, into, within	non-	not
endo-	inner, inside	olig-	small, scant
epi-	over, on, upon	para-	beside, beyond, after
eryth-	red	per-	by, through
eu-	normal, good, well, healthy	peri-	around

BOX 4-5 Medical Terminology—cont'd

PREFIX	MEANING
poly-	many, much
post-	after, behind
pre-	before, in front of, prior to
pro-	before, in front of
re-	again, backward
retro-	backward, behind
semi-	half
sub-	under, beneath
super-	above, over, excess
supra-	above, over
tachy-	fast, rapid
trans-	across
uni-	one

ROOT (combining vowel)	MEANING
abdomin (o)	abdomen
aden (o)	gland
adren (o)	adrenal gland
angi (o)	vessel
arterio	artery
athr (o)	joint
broncho	bronchus, bronchi
card, cardi (o)	heart
cephal (o)	head
chole, chol (o)	bile
chondr (o)	cartilage
colo	colon, large intestine
cost (o)	rib
crani (o)	skull
cyan (o)	blue
cyst (o)	bladder, cyst
cyt (o)	cell
dent (o)	tooth
derma	skin
duoden (o)	duodenum
encephal (o)	brain
enter (o)	intestines
fibr (o)	fiber, fibrous
gastr (o)	stomach
gloss (o)	tongue
gluc (o)	sweetness, glucose
glyc (o)	sugar
gyn, gyne, gyneco	woman
hem, hema, hemo, hemat (o)	blood
hepat (o)	liver
hydr (o)	water
hyster (o)	uterus
ile (o), ili (o)	ileum
laparo	abdomen, loin, flank
laryng (o)	larynx
lith (o)	stone
mamm (o)	breast, mammary gland
mast (o)	mammary gland, breast

ROOT (combining vowel)	MEANING
meno	menstruation
my (o)	muscle
myel (o)	spinal cord, bone marrow
necro	death
nephr (o)	kidney
neur (o)	nerve
ocul (o)	eye
oophor (o)	ovary
ophthalm (o)	eye
orth (o)	straight, normal, correct
oste (o)	bone
ot (o)	ear
ped (o)	child, foot
pharyng (o)	pharynx
phleb (o)	vein
pnea	breathing, respiration
pneum (o)	lung, air, gas
proct (o)	rectum
psych (o)	mind
pulmo	lung
py (o)	pus
rect (o)	rectum
rhin (o)	nose
salping (o)	eustachian tube, uterine tube
splen (o)	spleen
sten (o)	narrow, constriction
stern (o)	sternum
stomat (o)	mouth
therm (o)	heat
thoraco	chest
thromb (o)	clot, thrombus
thyr (o)	thyroid
toxic (o)	poison, poisonous
toxo	poison
trache (o)	trachea
urethr (o)	urethra
urin (o)	urine
uro	urine, urinary tract, urination
uter (o)	uterus
vas (o)	blood vessel, vas deferens
ven (o)	vein
vertebr (o)	spine, vertebrae

SUFFIX	MEANING
-algia	pain
-asis	condition, usually abnormal
-cele	hernia, herniation, pouching
-centesis	puncture and aspiration of
-cyte	cell
-ectasis	dilation, stretching
-ectomy	excision, removal of
-emia	blood condition
-genesis	development, production, creation
-genic	producing, causing
-gram	record
-graph	a diagram, a recording instrument

Continued

BOX 4-5	Medical Terminology—cont'd		
SUFFIX	**MEANING**	**SUFFIX**	**MEANING**
-graphy	making a recording	-phobia	an exaggerated fear
-iasis	condition of	-plasty	surgical repair or reshaping
-ism	a condition	-plegia	paralysis
-itis	inflammation	-ptosis	falling, sagging, dropping down
-logy	the study of	-rrhage, -rrhagia	excessive flow
-lysis	destruction of, decomposition	-rrhaphy	stitching, suturing
-megaly	enlargement	-rrhea	profuse flow, discharge
-meter	measuring instrument	-scope	examination instrument
-oma	tumor	-scopy	examination using a scope
-osis	condition	-stasis	maintenance, maintaining a constant level
-pathy	disease		
-penia	lack, deficiency	-stomy, -ostomy	creation of an opening
-phagia	to eat or consume, swallowing	-tomy, -otomy	incision, cutting into
-phasia	speaking	-uria	condition of the urine

Prefixes, Roots, and Suffixes

A *prefix* is a word element placed before a root. It changes the meaning of the word. The prefix *olig* (scant, small amount) is placed before the root *uria* (urine) to make *oliguria*. It means a scant amount of urine. Prefixes are always combined with other word elements. They are never used alone.

The *root* contains the basic meaning of the word. It is combined with another root, with prefixes, and with suffixes. A vowel (an *o* or an *i*) is added when two roots are combined or when a suffix is added to a root. The vowel makes the word easier to pronounce.

A *suffix* is placed after a root. It changes the meaning of the word. Suffixes are not used alone. When translating medical terms, begin with the suffix. For example, *nephritis* means inflammation of the kidney. It was formed by combining *nephro* (kidney) and *itis* (inflammation).

Medical terms are formed by combining word elements. Prefixes always come before roots. Suffixes always come after roots. Roots are combined with prefixes, roots, and suffixes. Combining a prefix, root, and suffix is another way to form medical terms. *Endocarditis* has the prefix *endo* (inner), the root *card* (heart), and the suffix *itis* (inflammation). *Endocarditis* means inflammation of the inner part of the heart.

Directional Terms

Certain terms describe the position of one body part in relation to another. These terms give the direction

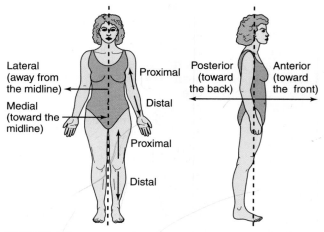

FIGURE 4-7 Directional terms describe the position of one body part in relation to another.

of the body part when a person is standing and facing forward (Fig. 4-7):

- *Anterior (ventral)*—at or toward the front of the body or body part
- *Distal*—the part farthest from the center or from the point of attachment
- *Lateral*—away from the midline; at the side of the body or body part
- *Medial*—at or near the middle or midline of the body or body part
- *Posterior (dorsal)*—at or toward the back of the body or body part
- *Proximal*—the part nearest to the center or to the point of origin

Medical Abbreviations

Abbreviations are shortened forms of words or phrases. They save time and space when recording. Each agency has a list of accepted medical abbreviations. Obtain the list when you are hired. Use only those accepted by the agency. If not sure that an abbreviation is acceptable, write the term out in full. This promotes accurate communication.

Common abbreviations are on the inside of the back book cover for easy use.

COMPUTERS AND OTHER ELECTRONIC DEVICES

Computer systems collect, record, send, receive, and store information. So do some personal digital assistants (PDAs). Many agencies store charts and care plans on computers. Entering data on a computer or PDA is easier and faster than writing care and observations.

The health team uses computers, PDAs, and faxes to send messages and reports to the nursing unit. This reduces clerical work and phone calls. And information is sent with greater speed and accuracy.

Computers and other electronic devices save time. Quality care and safety are increased. Fewer errors are made in recording. Records are more complete. Staff is more efficient.

Computers store vast amounts of information. Therefore the right to privacy must be protected.

Each staff member using computers and other electronic devices is issued a "unique user identification" (username) and a password. They are used to access, send, receive, or store protected health information (PHI).

You must follow the agency's policies when using computers and other electronic devices. You must maintain the confidentiality of PHI and electronic protected health information (ePHI; EPHI). To do so, follow the rules in Box 4-6 and the ethical and legal rules about privacy, confidentiality, and defamation.

BOX 4-6   Using the Agency's Computer and Other Electronic Devices

Computers and PDAs

- Do not tell anyone your "unique user identification" (username) or password. If someone has your information, he or she can access, record, send, receive, or store PHI under your name. It will be hard to prove that someone else did so and not you.
- Do not write down, post, or expose your "unique user identification" or password in a manner that is not secure. For example, do not write them on a notepad or post them at your work station.
- Change your password often. Follow agency policy.
- Do not use another person's "unique user identification" or password.
- Follow the rules for recording (see Box 4-4).
- Enter data carefully. Double-check your entries.
- Prevent others from seeing what is on the screen:
  - Position the monitor or PDA so the screen cannot be seen in the hallway or by others.
  - Be aware of anyone standing behind you.
  - Stand or sit with your back to the wall if recording on a mobile computer unit.
  - Do not leave the computer unattended.
- Log off after making an entry.
- Do not leave printouts where others can read them or pick them up.
- Shred or destroy computer-printed documents or worksheets. Follow agency policy.
- Send e-mail and messages only to those needing the information.

- Do not use e-mail for information or messages that require immediate reporting. Give the report in person. (The person may not read the e-mail in a timely manner.)
- Do not use e-mail or messages to report confidential information. This includes addresses, phone numbers, and Social Security numbers. The computer system may not be secure.
- Do not use the agency's computer or PDA to:
  - Send personal e-mail messages
  - Send or receive e-mail or messages that are offensive, not legal, or sexual
  - Send or receive e-mail or messages for illegal activities, jokes, politics, gambling (including football and other pools), chain letters, or other non-work activities
  - Post information, opinions, or comments on Internet message boards
  - Take part in Internet discussion groups
  - Upload, download, or send materials containing a copyright, trademark, or patent
- Remember that any communication can be read or heard by someone other than the intended person.
- Remember that deleted communications can be retrieved by authorized staff.
- Remember that the agency has the right to monitor your use of computers, PDAs, or other electronic devices. This includes Internet use.
- Do not open another person's e-mail or messages.
- Follow agency policy for misdirected e-mails.

Continued

BOX 4-6 Using the Agency's Computer and Other Electronic Devices—cont'd

Faxes

- Use the agency's approved "cover sheet." The sheet has instructions about:
  - The confidentiality of PHI
  - The receiver's responsibilities concerning PHI
  - The receiver's responsibilities if the fax is received in error (misdirected fax)

- Complete the "cover sheet" according to agency policy. Usually the following information is required:
  - Name of the person to receive the PHI
  - Receiver's fax number
  - Date
  - Name of person sending the fax
  - Number of pages being faxed
  - Department name
  - Name and phone number of the employee sending the fax
- Follow agency policy for a misdirected fax.
- Do not leave sent or received faxes unattended in the fax machine or lying around.

BOX 4-7 Guidelines for Answering Phones

- Answer the call after the first ring if possible. Be sure to answer by the fourth ring.
- Do not answer the phone in a rushed or hasty manner.
- Give a courteous greeting. Identify the nursing unit, and give your name and title. For example: "Good morning. Three center. Mark Wills, nursing assistant."
- Write the following information when taking a message:
  - The caller's name and phone number (include area code and extension number)
  - The date and time
  - The message
- Repeat the message and phone number back to the caller.
- Ask the caller to "Please hold" if necessary. First find out who is calling. Then ask if the caller can hold. Do not put callers with an emergency on hold.
- Do not lay the phone down or cover the receiver with your hand when not speaking to the caller. The caller may overhear confidential conversations.
- Return to a caller on hold within 30 seconds. Ask if the caller can wait longer or if the call can be returned.
- Do not give confidential information to any caller. Patient, resident, and employee information is confidential. Refer such calls to a nurse.
- Transfer the call if appropriate:
  - Tell the caller that you are going to transfer the call.
  - Give the name of the department if appropriate.
  - Give the caller the phone number in case the call gets disconnected or the line is busy.
- End the conversation politely. Thank the person for calling, and say good-bye.
- Give the message to the appropriate person.

PHONE COMMUNICATIONS

You will answer phones at the nurse's station or in the person's room. You need good communication skills. The caller cannot see you. But you give much information by your tone of voice, how clearly you speak, and your attitude. Be professional and courteous. Also practice good work ethics. Follow the agency's policy and the guidelines in Box 4-7.

DEALING WITH CONFLICT

People bring their values, attitudes, opinions, experiences, and expectations to the work setting. Differences often lead to *conflict*—a clash between opposing interests or ideas. People disagree and argue. There are misunderstandings and unrest.

Conflicts arise over issues or events. Work schedules, absences, and the amount and quality of work performed are examples. The problems must be worked out. Otherwise, unkind words or actions may occur. The work setting becomes unpleasant. Care is affected.

To resolve conflict, know the real problem. This is part of *problem solving*. The problem solving process involves these steps:

- Step 1: Define the problem. *A nurse ignores me.*
- Step 2: Collect information about the problem. *The nurse does not look at me. The nurse does not talk to me. The nurse does not respond when I ask for help. The nurse does not ask me to help with tasks that require two people. The nurse talks to other staff members.*
- Step 3: Identify possible solutions. *Ignore the nurse. Talk to my supervisor. Talk to co-workers about the problem. Change jobs.*

- Step 4: Select the best solution. *Talk to my supervisor.*
- Step 5: Carry out the solution. *See below.*
- Step 6: Evaluate the results. *See below.*

Communication and good work ethics help prevent and resolve conflicts. Identify and solve problems before they become major issues. To deal with conflict:

- Ask your supervisor for some time to talk privately. Explain the problem. Give facts and specific examples. Ask for advice in solving the problem.
- Approach the person with whom you have the conflict. Ask to talk privately. Be polite and professional.
- Agree on a time and place to talk.
- Talk in a private setting. No one should hear you or the other person.
- Explain the problem and what is bothering you. Give facts and specific behaviors. Focus on the problem. Do not focus on the person.
- Listen to the person. Do not interrupt.
- Identify ways to solve the problem. Offer your thoughts. Ask for the co-worker's ideas.
- Set a date and time to review the matter.
- Thank the person for meeting with you.
- Carry out the solution.
- Review the matter as scheduled.

    See *Focus on Communication: Dealing With Conflict.*

FOCUS ON COMMUNICATION
Dealing With Conflict

You may find it hard to talk to someone with whom you have a conflict. This is hard for many people. However, letting the problem or issue continue only makes the matter worse. The following may help you start talking to the person:

- "You say 'no' when I ask you to help me. I help you when you ask me to. This really bothers me. Can we talk privately for a few minutes?"
- "I heard you tell John that you saw me sitting in Mr. Gordon's room. You seemed angry when you said it. Can we talk privately? I want to explain why I was sitting and find out why that bothers you."
- "The new schedule shows me working every weekend this month. Please tell me why. The employee handbook says that we work every other weekend."

Focus on P R I D E
The Person, Family, and Yourself

Personal and Professional Responsibility—You are responsible for your speech, actions, and charting. This is called being accountable. For example, you are delegated a task. You are responsible for completing the task and reporting or recording its completion. If you do not complete it, you are still held accountable. You must tell the nurse why it was not done. Or you must complete the task.

Do not be offended when asked if you completed a task or charted. This is part of accountability. The delegating nurse must know what was done and what was not done. Show you are accountable by completing tasks in a timely manner. Record accurately. Tell the nurse when you are done with a task. Also tell the nurse if a task was not done and why.

Rights and Respect—Conflict among co-workers will arise. Dealing with conflict can be hard. But, it must be addressed. Deal with conflict in a respectful and mature way. Do not gossip, put down others, or talk about people behind their backs. These are not professional behaviors.

Everyone, including you, deserves to be treated with respect. If you feel someone has wronged you, address the issue. Politely ask to talk to the person in private. Speak calmly and respectfully. Focus on the problem and the solution. Do not attack the person's character. For example, do not say: "You are always so mean. I can't believe you were talking about me behind my back." Instead, you can say: "It bothers me that you didn't come to me about this. Next time could you talk to me first?" For good working relationships, identify and resolve conflict in a respectful and professional manner.

Independence and Social Interaction—You spend a lot of time with patients and residents. You see how they interact with others, what they like and do not like, and what they can and cannot do. Patients and residents talk to you. They tell you about their families and interests. You make observations every time you are with them. Share this information during care conferences. Also share your ideas about the person's care. For example, you can say:

- "Mr. Antonio never eats his squash. He says that he misses the fresh green beans and broccoli from his garden. Can he have those more often?"
- "Mrs. Clark said she used to love sitting on the patio in the evening. Can I take her outside after lunch?"
- "Miss Walsh never talks when her family visits. She just sits there. Yet she talks to her roommate all the time."

Your sharing can improve the person's independence and quality of life.

Delegation and Teamwork—Two staffs are present at the end of a shift—the staff going off duty and the staff coming on duty. The entire on-coming shift may attend the end-of-shift report. If so, staff members going off duty answer all signal lights, provide care, and tend to routine tasks. If only nurses attend the end-of-shift report, nursing assistants of the on-coming shift also answer signal lights, provide care, and tend to routine tasks.

The end-of-shift is a time for good teamwork. Continue to do your job. Your attitude is important. If going off duty, avoid saying or thinking the following:
- "I'm ready to go home. Let them do it."
- "It's their turn. I've been here all day (evening or night)."
- "No one helped us when we came on duty."

Use this time to work as a team. For example, those going off duty can answer signal lights. They know about changes in the person's condition and care plan and about new orders. They also know about the care needs of new patients or residents. The on-coming shift has yet to learn this information. The on-coming shift uses this time to perform routine tasks for the shift and to collect needed supplies and equipment.

Talk to the on-coming shift about what routine tasks were completed and what still needs to be done. This saves time and promotes accountability. All shifts are part of the team. Show you respect the on-coming shift during change-of-shift interactions. Say "please" and "thank you" as appropriate.

Ethics and Laws—A person's chart is a legal, permanent, and private record. The information you record in a person's chart is important. It must be accurate. Chart what you do. If not charted, there is no legal proof that you completed a task. And it is wrong to chart something that you did not do. Only chart after completing a delegated task. If events change, your charting is wrong. You are accountable for the information you record.

REVIEW QUESTIONS

Circle the BEST answer.

1 To communicate, you should do the following *except*
   a Use terms with many meanings
   b Be brief and concise
   c Present information logically and in sequence
   d Give facts and be specific

2 These statements are about medical records. Which is *false?*
   a They are used to communicate information about patients and residents.
   b They are a written or electronic account of illness and response to treatment.
   c They can be used as legal evidence of the care given.
   d Anyone working in the agency can read them.

3 A person is weighed daily. The measurement is recorded on the
   a Admission sheet
   b Graphic sheet
   c Flow sheet
   d Progress notes

4 Where does the nurse describe the nursing care given?
   a Admission sheet
   b Health history
   c Progress notes
   d Graphic sheet

5 What happens during assessment?
   a Goals are set.
   b Information is collected.
   c Nursing measures are carried out.
   d Progress is evaluated.

6 Which is a symptom?
   a Redness
   b Vomiting
   c Pain
   d Pulse rate of 78
7 Which is a sign?
   a Nausea
   b Headache
   c Dizziness
   d Dry skin
8 Which should you report at once?
   a The person had a bowel movement.
   b The person complains of sudden, severe pain.
   c The person does not like the food served for lunch.
   d The person complains of stiff, painful joints.
9 The nursing care plan is
   a Written by the doctor
   b The measures to help the person
   c The same for all persons
   d Also called the Kardex
10 What is used to communicate the nursing tasks delegated to you?
   a The care plan
   b The Kardex
   c An assignment sheet
   d Care conferences
11 When recording, you do the following *except*
   a Use ink
   b Include the date and time
   c Erase errors
   d Sign all entries with your name and title
12 These statements are about recording. Which is *false*?
   a Use the person's exact words when possible.
   b Record only what you did and observed.
   c Sign your initials to a mistaken entry.
   d Chart a procedure before completing it.
13 In the evening the clock shows 9:26. In 24-hour clock time this is
   a 9:26 PM
   b 926
   c 0926
   d 2126

14 A suffix is
   a Placed at the beginning of a word
   b Placed after a root
   c A shortened form of a word or phrase
   d The main meaning of the word
15 You have access to the agency's computer. Which is *true?*
   a E-mail and messages are sent only to those needing the information.
   b E-mail is used for reports the nurse needs at once.
   c You can open another person's e-mail.
   d You can use the computer for your personal needs.
16 You answer a person's phone. How should you answer?
   a "Good morning. Mrs. Park's room."
   b "Good morning. Third floor."
   c "Hello."
   d "Good morning. Tammy Brown, nursing assistant, speaking."
17 Which term relates to the side of the body?
   a Anterior
   b Lateral
   c Posterior
   d Proximal
18 A co-worker is often late for work. This means extra work for you. To resolve the conflict you should do the following *except*
   a Explain the problem to your supervisor
   b Discuss the matter during the end-of-shift report
   c Give facts and specific behaviors
   d Suggest ways to solve the problem

Answers to these questions are on p. 527.

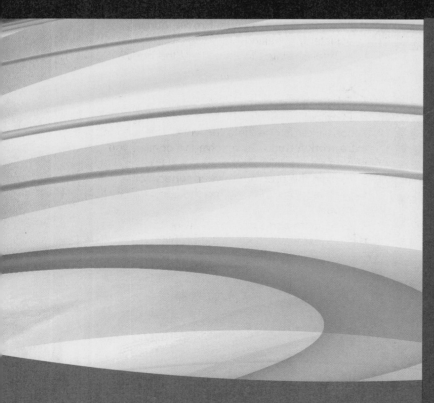

5

UNDERSTANDING THE PERSON

OBJECTIVES

- Define the key terms listed in this chapter.
- Identify the parts that make up the whole person.
- Explain how to properly address the person.
- Explain Abraham Maslow's theory of basic needs.
- Explain how culture and religion influence health and illness.
- Explain how to deal with behavior issues.
- Identify the elements needed for good communication.
- Explain the methods and barriers to good communication.
- Explain why family and visitors are important to the person.
- Identify the courtesies given to the person, family, and friends.
- Explain how to promote PRIDE in the person, the family, and yourself.

KEY TERMS

body language Messages sent through facial expressions, gestures, posture, hand and body movements, gait, eye contact, and appearance

comatose Being unable to respond to verbal stimuli

culture The characteristics of a group of people—language, values, beliefs, habits, likes, dislikes, customs—passed from one generation to the next

disability Any lost, absent, or impaired physical or mental function

holism A concept that considers the whole person; the whole person has physical, social, psychological, and spiritual parts that are woven together and cannot be separated

need Something necessary or desired for maintaining life and mental well-being

nonverbal communication Communication that does not use words

religion Spiritual beliefs, needs, and practices

verbal communication Communication that uses written or spoken words

The patient or resident is the most important person in the agency. Each person has value. Each has needs, fears, and rights. Each has suffered losses—loss of home, family, friends, and body functions.

CARING FOR THE PERSON

Holism is a concept that considers the whole person. Holism means *whole*. The whole person has physical, social, psychological, and spiritual parts. These parts are woven together and cannot be separated (Fig. 5-1).

Each part relates to and depends on the others. As a social being, a person speaks and communicates with others. Physically, the brain, mouth, tongue, lips, and throat structures must function for speech. Communication is also psychological. It involves thinking and reasoning.

To consider only the physical part is to ignore the person's ability to think, make decisions, and interact with others. It also ignores the person's experiences, life-style, culture, religion, joys, sorrows, and needs.

Addressing the Person

You must know and respect the whole person to provide effective, quality care. Too often a person is referred to as a room number. For example: "12A needs the bedpan," rather than "Mrs. Brown in 12A needs the bedpan."

Follow these rules to address patients and residents with dignity and respect:

- Use the person's title—Mrs. Dennison, Mr. Smith, Miss Turner, or Dr. Gonzalez.
- Do not use a first name unless the person asks you to do so.
- Do not use any other name unless the person asks you to do so.
- Do not call the person Grandma, Papa, Sweetheart, Honey, or other name.

BASIC NEEDS

A **need** is something necessary or desired for maintaining life and mental well-being. According to psychologist Abraham Maslow, basic needs must be met for a person to survive and function. These needs are arranged in order of importance (Fig. 5-2).

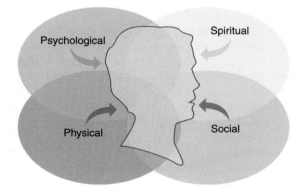

FIGURE 5-1 A person is a physical, psychological, social, and spiritual being. The parts overlap and cannot be separated.

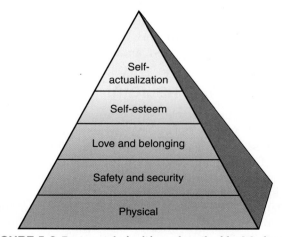

FIGURE 5-2 Basic needs for life as described by Maslow. *(From Maslow AH:* Motivation and personality; *Copyright 1987. Reprinted with permission of Pearson Education, Upper Saddle River, NJ.)*

Lower-level needs must be met before the higher-level needs. Basic needs, from the lowest level to the highest level, are:

- *Physical needs*—oxygen, food, water, elimination, rest, and shelter are needed for life. A person dies within minutes without oxygen. Without food or water, a person feels weak and ill within a few hours. The kidneys and intestines must function. Otherwise wastes build up in the blood. This can cause death. Without enough rest and sleep, a person becomes very tired. Without shelter, the person is exposed to extremes of heat and cold.
- *Safety and security needs*—relate to feeling safe from harm, danger, and fear. Health care agencies are strange places with strange routines and equipment. Strangers provide care. Fear of pain or discomfort is common. People feel safer and more secure if they know what will happen. For every task, the person should know:
  - Why it is needed
  - Who will do it
  - How it will be done
  - What sensations or feelings to expect
- *Love and belonging needs*—relate to love, closeness, affection, and meaningful relationships with others. Some people become weaker or die from the lack of love and belonging. This is seen in older persons who have outlived family and friends.
- *Self-esteem needs*—self-esteem means to think well of oneself and to see oneself as useful and having value. It also relates to being thought well of by others. People often lack self-esteem when ill, injured, older, or disabled.
- *The need for self-actualization*—self-actualization means experiencing one's potential. It involves learning, understanding, and creating to the limit of a person's capacity. This is the highest need. Rarely, if ever, is it totally met. Most people constantly try to learn and understand more. This need can be postponed, and life will continue.

CULTURE AND RELIGION

Culture is the characteristics of a group of people—language, values, beliefs, habits, likes, dislikes, and customs. They are passed from one generation to the next. The person's culture influences health beliefs and practices. Culture also affects thinking and behavior during illness.

People come from many cultures, races, and nationalities. Their family practices and food choices may differ from yours. So might their hygiene habits and clothing styles. Some speak a foreign language. Some cultures have beliefs about what causes and cures illness. (See *Caring About Culture: Health Care*

 CARING ABOUT CULTURE
Health Care Beliefs

Some *Mexican Americans* believe that illness is caused by prolonged exposure to hot or cold. If hot causes illness, cold is used for the cure. Likewise, hot is used to cure illnesses caused by cold. Hot and cold are found in body organs, medicines (drugs), the air, and food. For example, an earache may occur from cold air entering the body. Hot remedies are used to cure the earache.

The hot-cold balance is also a belief of some *Vietnamese Americans*. Illnesses, food, drugs, and herbs are hot or cold. Hot is given to balance cold illnesses. Cold is given for hot illnesses.

(Modified from Giger JN, Davidhizar RE: *Transcultural nursing: assessment and intervention*, ed 5, St Louis, 2008, Mosby.)

 CARING ABOUT CULTURE
Sick Care Practices

Folk practices are common among some *Vietnamese Americans*. They include *cao gio* ("rub wind")—rubbing the skin with a coin to treat the common cold. Skin pinching *(batgio*—"catch wind")* is used for headaches and sore throats. Herbs, oils, and soups are used for many signs and symptoms.

Some *Russian Americans* practice folk medicine. Herbs are taken through drinks or enemas. For headaches, an ointment is placed behind the ears and temples and at the back of the neck. A backache treatment involves placing a dough of dark rye flour and honey on the spine.

Folk healers are used by some *Mexican Americans*. Folk healers may be family members or from outside the family. A *yerbero* uses herbs and spices to prevent or cure disease. A *curandero* (*curandera* if female) deals with serious physical and mental illnesses. Witches use magic. A *brujos* is a male witch. A *brujas* is a female witch.

(Modified from Giger JN, Davidhizar RE: *Transcultural nursing: assessment and intervention*, ed 5, St Louis, 2008, Mosby.)

Beliefs.) They may perform rituals to rid the body of disease. (See *Caring About Culture: Sick Care Practices.*) Many have beliefs and rituals about dying and death (Chapter 30). Culture also is a factor in communication.

Religion relates to spiritual beliefs, needs, and practices. Religions may have beliefs and practices about daily living, behaviors, relationships with others, diet, healing, days of worship, birth and birth control, drugs, and death.

Many people find comfort and strength from religion during illness. They may want to pray and observe religious practices. Assist the person to attend services as needed.

The care plan includes the person's cultural and religious practices. You must respect and accept the person's culture and religion.

A person may not follow all beliefs and practices of his or her culture or religion. Some people do not practice a religion. Each person is unique. Do not judge the person by your standards. Do not force your ideas on the person.

BEHAVIOR ISSUES

People do not choose illness, injury, or disability. A **disability** is any lost, absent, or impaired physical or mental function. It may be temporary or permanent.

Many patients, residents, and families accept illness, injury, and disability. Others do not adjust well. They have some of the following behaviors. These behaviors are new for some people. For others, they are a life-long part of one's personality.

- *Anger.* Anger is a common emotion. Causes include fear, pain, and dying and death. Loss of function and loss of control over health and life are causes. So are long waits for care. Anger is a symptom of some diseases that affect thinking and behavior. Some people are generally angry. Anger is shown verbally and nonverbally (p. 68). Verbal outbursts, shouting, raised voices, and rapid speech are common. Some people are silent. Others are uncooperative. They may refuse to answer questions. Nonverbal signs include rapid movements, pacing, clenched fists, and a red face. Glaring and getting close to you when speaking are other signs. Violent behaviors can occur.
- *Demanding behavior.* Nothing seems to please the person. The person is critical of others. He or she wants care given at a certain time and in a certain way. Loss of independence, loss of health, loss of control, and unmet needs are causes.
- *Self-centered behavior.* The person cares only about his or her own needs. The needs of others are ignored. The person demands the time and attention of others. The person becomes impatient if needs are not met.
- *Aggressive behavior.* The person may swear, bite, hit, pinch, scratch, or kick. Fear, anger, pain, and dementia (Chapter 28) are causes. Protect the person, others, and yourself from harm (Chapter 8).
- *Withdrawal.* The person has little or no contact with others. He or she spends time alone and does not take part in social or group events. This may signal physical illness or depression. Some people are not social and like being alone.

BOX 5-1 **Dealing With Behavior Issues**

- Recognize frustrating and frightening situations. How would you feel in the person's situation? How do you want to be treated?
- Treat the person with dignity and respect.
- Answer questions clearly and thoroughly. Refer questions you cannot answer to the nurse.
- Keep the person informed. Tell the person what you are going to do and when.
- Do not keep the person waiting. Answer signal lights promptly. If you tell the person that you will do something, do it promptly.
- Explain the reason for long waits. Ask how you can increase the person's comfort.
- Stay calm and professional, especially if the person is angry or hostile. Often the person is not angry at you. He or she is angry at another person or situation.
- Do not argue with the person.
- Listen and use silence. The person may feel better if able to express feelings.
- Protect yourself from violent behaviors (Chapter 8).
- Report the person's behavior to the nurse. Discuss how to deal with the person.

FOCUS ON COMMUNICATION
Behavior Issues

Anger is a common response to illness and disability. Patients or residents may be angry with their situation. A person may direct anger at you. You might have difficulty dealing with the person's anger. You must continue to act in a professional manner. Remain calm. Do not yell at or insult the person. Listen to his or her concerns. Provide needed care. Try not to take his or her statements personally. If a patient or resident says hurtful things, you can kindly say: "Please don't say those things, I'm trying to help you." Tell the nurse about the person's behavior.

Caring for demanding or angry persons can be hard. Ask the nurse or co-workers to help if needed.

- *Inappropriate sexual behavior.* Some people make inappropriate sexual remarks. Or they touch others. Some disrobe or masturbate in public. These behaviors may be on purpose. Or they are due to disease, confusion, dementia, or drug side effects.

Some behaviors are not pleasant. You cannot avoid the person or lose control. Good communication is needed. Behaviors are addressed in the care plan. Follow the care plan and the guidelines in Box 5-1.

See *Focus on Communication: Behavior Issues.*

COMMUNICATING WITH THE PERSON

You communicate with the person every time you give care. For effective communication between you and the person, you must:

- Follow the rules of communication (Chapter 4):
  - Use words that have the same meaning for you and the person.
  - Avoid medical terms and words not familiar to the person.
  - Communicate in a logical and orderly manner. Do not wander in thought.
  - Give facts and be specific.
  - Be brief and concise.
- Understand and respect the patient or resident as a person.
- View the person as a physical, psychological, social, and spiritual human being.
- Appreciate the person's problems and frustrations.
- Respect the person's rights.
- Respect the person's religion and culture.
- Give the person time to process (understand) the information that you give.
- Repeat information as often as needed. Repeat exactly what you said. Use the exact same words. Do not give the person a new message to process.
- Ask questions to see if the person understood you.
- Be patient. People with memory problems may ask the same question many times. Do not say that you are repeating information.
- Include the person in conversations when others are present. This includes when a co-worker is assisting you with care.

See *Persons With Dementia: Communicating With the Person.*

Verbal Communication

Words are used in **verbal communication.** Words are spoken or written. Most verbal communication involves the spoken word. Follow these rules:

- Face the person. Look directly at the person.
- Position yourself at the person's eye level. Stand, sit, or squat by the person.
- Control the loudness and tone of your voice.
- Speak clearly, slowly, and distinctly.
- Do not use slang or vulgar words.
- Repeat information as needed.
- Ask one question at a time. Wait for an answer.
- Do not shout, whisper, or mumble.
- Be kind, courteous, and friendly.

Use the written word if the person cannot speak or hear but can read. The nurse and care plan tell you how to communicate with the person. The devices in

---

PERSONS WITH DEMENTIA
Communicating With the Person

Communicating with persons who have dementia is often difficult. The Alzheimer's Disease Education and Referral Center (ADEAR) recommends the following:

- Gain the person's attention before speaking. Call the person by name.
- Choose simple words and short sentences.
- Use a gentle, calm voice.
- Do not talk to the person as you would a baby.
- Do not talk about the person as if he or she is not there.
- Keep distractions and noise to a minimum.
- Help the person focus on what you are saying.
- Allow the person time to respond. Do not interrupt him or her.
- Try to provide the word the person is struggling to find.
- State questions and instructions in a positive way.

Figure 5-3 are often used. The person also may have poor vision. When writing messages:

- Be brief and concise.
- Use a black felt pen on white paper.
- Print in large letters.

Some persons cannot speak or read. Ask questions that have "yes" or "no" answers. The person can nod, blink, or use other gestures for "yes" and "no." Follow the care plan. Persons who are deaf may use sign language. See Chapter 26.

Nonverbal Communication

Nonverbal communication does not use words. Gestures, facial expressions, posture, body movements, touch, and smell send messages. Nonverbal messages more truly reflect a person's feelings than words do. They are usually involuntary and hard to control. A person may say one thing but act another way. Watch the person's eyes, hand movements, gestures, posture, and other actions.

Touch Touch is a very important form of nonverbal communication. It conveys comfort, caring, love, affection, interest, trust, concern, and reassurance. Touch means different things to different people. The meaning depends on age, gender (male or female), experiences, and culture. (See *Caring About Culture: Touch Practices*, p. 70.)

Some people do not like to be touched. However, stroking or holding a hand can comfort a person. Touch should be gentle—not hurried, rough, or sexual. To use touch, follow the person's care plan. Remember to maintain professional boundaries.

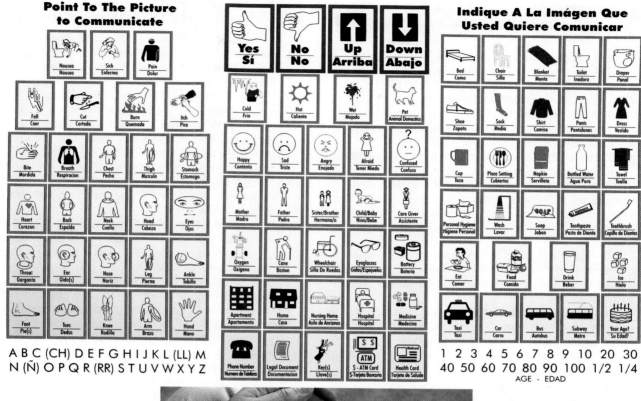

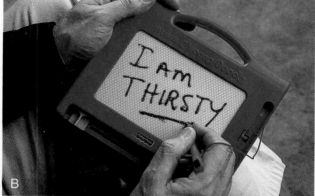

FIGURE 5-3 Communication aids. **A,** Picture board in English and Spanish. **B,** Magic Slate.

Body Language People send messages through their **body language:**

- Facial expressions (See *Caring About Culture: Facial Expressions,* p. 70.)
- Gestures
- Posture
- Hand and body movements
- Gait
- Eye contact
- Appearance (dress, hygiene, jewelry, perfume, cosmetics, tattoos, piercings, and so on)

Many messages are sent through body language. Slumped posture may mean the person is not happy or not feeling well. A person may deny pain. Yet a body part is protected by standing, lying, or sitting in a certain way.

Your actions, movements, and facial expressions send messages. So does how you stand, sit, walk, and look at the person. Your body language needs to show interest, enthusiasm, caring, and respect for the person.

Control your body language as needed. Control reactions to odors from body fluids, secretions, excretions, or the person's body. The person cannot control some odors. If you react to odors, you can embarrass the person and affect his or her pride.

CARING ABOUT CULTURE
Touch Practices

Touch practices vary among cultural groups. Touch is a friendly gesture in the *Philippine* culture. Touch is used often in *Mexico*. Some people believe that using touch while complimenting a person is important. It is thought to neutralize the power of the evil eye *(mal de ojo)*.

Persons from the *United Kingdom* tend to reserve touch for persons they know well. Within limits, touch is acceptable in *Poland*. Its use depends on age, gender, and the relationship.

In *India*, men shake hands with other men. Men do not shake hands with women. Instead, they place their palms together and bow slightly to women. As a sign of respect or to seek a blessing, people touch the feet of older adults.

In *Vietnam*, a person's head is not touched by others. It is considered the center of the soul. Men do not touch women who they do not know. Men commonly shake hands with men.

People from *China* do not like touching by strangers. A nod or slight bow is given during introductions. Patients prefer health care workers of the same gender.

In *Ireland*, a firm hand-shake is preferred. Only family and close friends are embraced.

(Modified from D'Avanzo CE, Geissler EM: *Pocket guide to cultural health assessment*, ed 4, St Louis, 2008, Mosby.)

CARING ABOUT CULTURE
Facial Expressions

Through facial expressions, *Americans* communicate:
- *Coldness*—there is a constant stare. Face muscles do not move.
- *Fear*—eyes are open wide. Eyebrows are raised. The mouth is tense with the lips drawn back.
- *Anger*—eyes are fixed in a hard stare. Upper lids are lowered. Eyebrows are drawn down. Lips are tightly compressed.
- *Tiredness*—eyes are rolled upward.
- *Disapproval*—eyes are rolled upward.
- *Disgust*—narrowed eyes. The upper lip is curled. There are nose movements.
- *Embarrassment*—eyes are turned away or down. The face is flushed. The person pretends to smile. He or she rubs the eyes, nose, or face. He or she twitches the hair, beard, or mustache.
- *Surprise*—direct gaze with raised eyebrows.

Italian, *Jewish*, *African-American*, and *Hispanic* persons smile readily. They use many facial expressions and gestures for happiness, pain, or displeasure. *Irish*, *English*, and *Northern European* persons tend to have less facial expression.

In some cultures, facial expressions mean the opposite of what the person is feeling. For example, *Asians* may conceal negative emotions with a smile.

(Modified from Giger JN, Davidhizar RE: *Transcultural nursing: assessment and intervention*, ed 5, St Louis, 2008, Mosby.)

Communication Methods

Certain methods help you communicate with others. They result in better relationships. More information is gained for the nursing process.

Listening Listening means to focus on verbal and nonverbal communication. You use sight, hearing, touch, and smell. You focus on what the person is saying. You observe nonverbal clues. They can support what the person says. Or they can show other feelings. For example, Mr. Hart says, "I want to stay here. That way my daughter won't have to care for me." You see tears, and he looks away from you. His verbal says *happy*. His nonverbal shows *sadness*.

Listening requires that you care and have interest. Follow these guidelines:
- Face the person.
- Have good eye contact with the person. See *Caring About Culture: Eye Contact Practices.*
- Lean toward the person (Fig. 5-4). Do not sit back with your arms crossed.

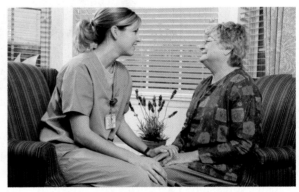

FIGURE 5-4 Listen by facing the person. Have good eye contact. Lean toward the person.

- Respond to the person. Nod your head. Say "uh huh," "mmm," and "I see." Repeat what the person says. Ask questions.
- Avoid the communication barriers (p. 72).

CARING ABOUT CULTURE

Eye Contact Practices

In the *American* culture, eye contact signals a good self-concept. It also shows openness, interest in others, attention, honesty, and warmth. Lack of eye contact can mean:
- Shyness
- Lack of interest
- Humility
- Guilt
- Embarrassment
- Low self-esteem
- Rudeness
- Dishonesty

For some *Asian* and *American Indian* cultures, eye contact is impolite. It is an invasion of privacy. In certain *Indian* cultures, eye contact is avoided with persons of higher or lower socio-economic class. It is also given a special sexual meaning.

In *Iraq*, men and women avoid direct eye contact. Long, direct eye contact is rude in *Mexico*. In rural parts of *Vietnam*, it is not respectful to look at another while talking. Blinking means that a message is received. In the *United Kingdom*, looking directly at a speaker means the listener is paying attention.

(Modified from Giger JN, Davidhizar RE: *Transcultural nursing: assessment and intervention*, ed 5, St Louis, 2008, Mosby. Modified from D'Avanzo CE, Geissler EM: *Pocket guide to cultural health assessment*, ed 4, St Louis, 2008, Mosby.)

Direct Questions Direct questions focus on certain information. You ask the person something you need to know. Some direct questions have "yes" or "no" answers. Others require more information. For example:

You: Mr. Hart, do you want to shave this morning?
Mr. Hart: Yes.
You: Mr. Hart, when would you like to do that?
Mr. Hart: Could we start in 15 minutes? I'd like to call my son first.
You: Yes, we can start in 15 minutes.

CARING ABOUT CULTURE

Silence

In the *English* and *Arabic* cultures, silence is used for privacy. Among *Russian, French,* and *Spanish* cultures, silence means agreement between parties. In some *Asian* cultures, silence is a sign of respect, particularly to an older person.

(Modified from Giger JN, Davidhizar RE: *Transcultural nursing: assessment and intervention*, ed 5, St Louis, 2008, Mosby.)

Open-Ended Questions Open-ended questions lead or invite the person to share thoughts, feelings, or ideas. The person chooses what to talk about. He or she controls the topic and the information given. Answers require a brief response. For example:
- "What do you like about living with your son?"
- "Tell me about your grandson."
- "What do you like about being retired?"

Clarifying You use clarifying to make sure that you understand the message. You can ask the person to repeat the message, say you do not understand, or restate the message. For example:
- "Could you say that again?"
- "I'm sorry, Mr. Hart. I don't understand what you mean."
- "Are you saying that you want to go home?"

Silence Silence is a very powerful way to communicate. Sometimes you do not need to say anything. This is true during sad times. Just being there shows you care. At other times, silence gives time to think, organize thoughts, or choose words. Silence is useful when the person is upset and needs to gain control. Silence on your part shows caring and respect for the person's situation and feelings.

Sometimes pauses or long silences are uncomfortable. You do not need to talk when the person is silent. The person may need silence. See *Caring About Culture: Silence.*

CARING ABOUT CULTURE

Communicating With Persons From Other Cultures

- Ask the nurse about the beliefs and values of the person's culture. Learn as much as you can about the person's culture.
- Do not judge the person by your own attitudes, values, beliefs, and ideas.
- Follow the person's care plan. It includes the person's cultural beliefs and customs.
- Do the following when communicating with foreign speaking persons:
  - Convey comfort by your tone of voice and body language.
  - Do not speak loudly or shout. It will not help the person understand English.
  - Speak slowly and distinctly.
  - Keep messages short and simple.
  - Be alert for words the person seems to understand.
  - Use gestures and pictures.
  - Repeat the message in other ways.
  - Avoid using medical terms and abbreviations.
  - Be alert for signs the person is pretending to understand. Nodding and answering "yes" to all questions are signs that the person does not understand what you are saying.

(Modified from Giger JN, Davidhizar RE: *Transcultural nursing: assessment and intervention,* ed 5, St Louis, 2008, Mosby.)

Communication Barriers

Communication barriers prevent the sending and receiving of messages. Communication fails.

- *Language.* You and the person must use and understand the same language. If not, messages are not accurately interpreted. See Appendix B, p. 530, for useful Spanish words and phrases.
- *Cultural differences.* The person may attach different meanings to verbal and nonverbal communication. See *Caring About Culture: Communicating With Persons From Other Cultures.*
- *Changing the subject.* Someone changes the subject when the topic is uncomfortable. Avoid changing the subject whenever possible.
- *Giving opinions.* Opinions involve judging values, behaviors, or feelings. Let others express feelings and concerns without adding your opinion. Do not make judgments or jump to conclusions.

FOCUS ON COMMUNICATION
Communication Barriers

Persons from different cultures may speak a language you do not understand. This presents a barrier to communication. Persons may normally use family or friends to translate. In the health care setting, the nurse may discourage this practice. The nurse contacts a translator from the agency.

Trained translators know medical terms. Family or friends may not know a term. They may state something different than what was meant. There is a risk of passing on incorrect information. Also, using family or friends as translators violates a person's right to privacy. The Health Insurance Portability and Accountability Act of 1996 (HIPAA) protects the privacy and security of a person's health information (Chapter 2). The person's privacy is protected when using a translator from the agency.

- *Talking a lot when others are silent.* Talking too much is usually because of nervousness and discomfort with silence.
- *Failure to listen.* Do not pretend to listen. It shows lack of interest and caring. You miss complaints or symptoms that you must report to the nurse.
- *Pat answers.* "Don't worry." "Everything will be okay." "Your doctor knows best." These make the person feel that you do not care about his or her concerns, feelings, and fears.
- *Illness and disability.* Speech, hearing, vision, cognitive function, and body movements are often affected.
- *Age.* Values and communication styles vary among age groups.
  See *Focus on Communication: Communication Barriers.*

PERSONS WITH SPECIAL NEEDS

A person may acquire a disability any time from birth through old age. Disease and injury are common causes. Common courtesies and manners *(etiquette)* apply to any person with a disability. See Box 5-2 for disability etiquette.

BOX 5-2　Disability Etiquette

- Extend the same courtesies to the person as you would to anyone else.
- Allow the person privacy.
- Do not hang on or lean on a person's wheelchair.
- Treat adults as adults. Do not use the person's first name unless he or she asks you to do so.
- Do not pat a person who is in a chair or wheelchair on the head.
- Speak directly to the person. Do not address questions intended for the person to his or her companion.
- Do not be embarrassed if you use words that relate to a disability. For example, you say "Did you see that?" to a person with a vision problem.
- Sit or squat to talk to a person in a wheelchair or chair. This puts you and the person at eye level.
- Ask the person if he or she needs help before acting. If the person says "no," respect the person's wishes. If the person wants help, ask the person what to do and how to do it.
- Think before giving directions to a person in a wheelchair. Think about distance, weather conditions, stairs, curbs, steep hills, and other obstacles.
- Allow the person extra time to say or do things. Let the person set the pace in walking, talking, or other activities.

Modified from *Disability Etiquette*, Easter Seals, 2009.

The Person Who Is Comatose

Comatose means being unable to respond to verbal stimuli. The person who is comatose is unconscious. The person cannot respond to others. Often the person can hear and can feel touch and pain. Often pain is shown by grimacing or groaning. Assume that the person hears and understands you. Use touch and give care gently. Practice these measures:

- Knock before entering the person's room.
- Tell the person your name, the time, and the place every time you enter the room.
- Give care on the same schedule every day.
- Explain what you are going to do. Explain care measures step by step as you do them.
- Tell the person when you are finishing care.
- Use touch to communicate care, concern, and comfort.
- Tell the person what time you will be back to check on him or her.
- Tell the person when you are leaving the room.

⬡CARING ABOUT CULTURE

Family Roles in Sick Care

In *Vietnam*, family members are involved in the person's hospital care. They stay at the bedside and sleep in the person's bed or on straw mats. In *Vietnam* and *China*, family members provide food, hygiene, and comfort.

In *Pakistan* hospitals, there are different sections for females and males. Adult family members of the opposite sex are not allowed to stay overnight.

(Modified from D'Avanzo CE, Geissler EM: *Pocket guide to cultural health assessment*, ed 4, St Louis, 2008, Mosby.)

FAMILY AND FRIENDS

Family and friends help meet basic needs. They offer support and comfort. They lessen loneliness. Some also help with the person's care. The presence or absence of family or friends affects the person's quality of life.

The person has the right to visit with family and friends in private and without unnecessary interruptions. You may need to give care when visitors are there. Protect the right to privacy. Do not expose the person's body in front of them. Politely ask them to leave the room. Show them where to wait. Promptly tell them when they can return. A partner or family member may want to help you. If the patient or resident consents, you may allow the person to stay.

Treat family and friends with courtesy and respect. They have concerns about the person's condition and care. They need support and understanding. However, do not discuss the person's condition with them. Refer their questions to the nurse.

Visiting rules depend on agency policy and the person's condition. Know your agency's visiting policies and what is allowed for the person.

Visitors may have questions about the chapel, gift shop, lounge, dining room, or business office. Know the location, special rules, and hours of these areas.

A visitor may upset or tire a person. Report your observations to the nurse. The nurse will speak with the visitor about the person's needs.

See *Caring About Culture: Family Roles in Sick Care.*

Focus on P R I D E
The Person, Family, and Yourself

Personal and Professional Responsibility— Improving communication is an on-going process. Do not feel bad if you are uncomfortable with patient or resident interactions at first. You will have many chances to develop better communication skills. You are responsible for taking advantage of these opportunities. To improve your communication skills:

- Learn from mistakes.
- Use methods such as listening and clarifying.
- Pay attention to the nonverbal messages you may be sending.
- Avoid communication barriers.
- Know where your agency keeps resources to aid with communication. These may include devices like those shown in Figure 5-3 or translation lists with useful words or phrases (Appendix B, p. 530).

With practice, you will communicate more effectively. This is a valuable skill.

Rights and Respect—Patients and residents have the right to quality of life. This includes promoting physical, mental, spiritual, and social well-being. Try not to focus on physical needs alone. Consider the person's thoughts and feelings. Small gestures make a difference. For example, give a person time to pray before eating if this is something he or she values. While giving care, ask about his or her friends and family. Or simply say: "How are you feeling today?" Respect all of the person's needs. All interact and affect the person's well-being. Provide care that focuses on the person as a whole.

Independence and Social Interaction—Fear and anxiety are common emotions for persons in a nursing center or hospital. Nursing center residents may feel lonely or abandoned by their families and friends. Patients may fear loss of function that will have social effects. For example, a stroke can cause a person to lose function on one side of the body. The person may lose the ability to work, live at home, perform daily activities, walk, drive a car, and so on. Feeling abandoned or worthless harms a person's self-esteem. Such feelings affect a person's overall health.

Your interactions can promote a sense of identity, worth, and belonging. The following actions ease a person's worries and help improve quality of life:

- Greet each person by name.
- Talk to the person while providing care.
- Take an extra minute to visit or just listen.
- Treat each person with respect and dignity.
- Encourage as much independence as possible.
- Focus on the person's abilities, not disabilities.
- Allow private time with visitors.

Delegation and Teamwork—Caring for persons with behavior issues requires great teamwork. Staff members may become frustrated. But the person's quality of care must not be lowered. The health team must work together to manage such persons. Care assignments may rotate to allow breaks. When not assigned to the person, you can assist your co-worker with the person or other tasks. When you interact with the person, be respectful. Treat the person as nicely as you treat other persons. Often when treated kindly, the person's behavior will improve. A supportive and encouraging team makes caring for difficult persons easier.

Ethics and Laws—You will care for persons with different ideas, values, and life-styles. These shape the person's character and identity. It is not ethical to:

- Force your views and beliefs on another person
- Make negative comments or insult the person's customs
- Argue with a person about health care or religious beliefs

Respect the person as a whole. This includes his or her cultural and religious practices.

REVIEW QUESTIONS

Circle the BEST answer.

1 You work in a health care agency. You focus on
   a The person's care plan
   b The person's physical, safety and security, and self-esteem needs
   c The person as a physical, psychological, social, and spiritual being — *Maslow*
   d The person's cultural and spiritual needs

2 Which basic need is the *most* essential?
   a Self-actualization
   b Self-esteem
   c Love and belonging
   d Safety and security

3 A person says "What are they doing to me?" Which basic needs are *not* being met?
   a Physical needs
   b Safety and security needs
   c Love and belonging needs
   d Self-esteem needs

4 A person wants care given at a certain time and in a certain way. Nothing seems to please the person. The person is most likely demonstrating
   a Angry behavior
   b Demanding behavior
   c Withdrawn behavior
   d Aggressive behavior

5 A person is demonstrating problem behavior. You should do the following *except*
   a Put yourself in the person's situation
   b Tell the person what you are going to do and when
   c Ask the person to be nicer
   d Listen and use silence

6 Which is *false?*
   a Verbal communication uses the written or spoken word.
   b Verbal communication is the truest reflection of a person's feelings.
   c Messages are sent by facial expressions, gestures, posture, and body movements.
   d Touch means different things to different people.

7 To communicate with a person you should
   a Use medical words and phrases
   b Change the subject often
   c Give your opinions
   d Be quiet when the person is silent

8 Which might mean that you are *not* listening?
   a You sit facing the person.
   b You have good eye contact with the person.
   c You sit with your arms crossed.
   d You ask questions.

9 Which is a direct question?
   a "Do you feel better now?"
   b "What are your plans for home?"
   c "What will you do at home?"
   d "You said that you can't sleep."

10 Which promotes communication?
   a "Don't worry."
   b "Everything will be just fine."
   c "This is a good nursing center."
   d "Why are you crying?"

11 Which is *not* a barrier to communication?
   a Using silence
   b Giving your opinions
   c Changing the subject
   d Illness

12 A person uses a wheelchair. For effective communication, you should
   a Lean on the wheelchair
   b Pat the person on the head
   c Direct questions to the companion
   d Sit or squat next to the person

13 A person is comatose. Which action is *not* correct?
   a Assume that the person can hear and can feel touch.
   b Explain what you are going to do.
   c Use listening and silence to communicate.
   d Tell the person when you are leaving the room.

14 A visitor seems to tire a person. What should you do?
   a Ask the person to leave.
   b Tell the nurse.
   c Stay in the room to observe the person and visitor.
   d Find out the visitor's relationship to the person.

Answers to these questions are on p. 527.

6

BODY STRUCTURE AND FUNCTION

OBJECTIVES

- Define the key terms and key abbreviations listed in this chapter.
- Identify the basic structures of the cell.
- Explain how cells divide.
- Describe four types of tissue.
- Identify the structures of each body system.
- Identify the functions of each body system.
- Explain how to promote PRIDE in the person, the family, and yourself.

KEY TERMS

artery A blood vessel that carries blood away from the heart

capillary A tiny blood vessel; food, oxygen, and other substances pass from the capillaries into the cells

cell The basic unit of body structure

digestion The process of physically and chemically breaking down food so that it can be absorbed for use by the cells

hemoglobin The substance in red blood cells that carries oxygen and gives blood its color

hormone A chemical substance secreted by the endocrine glands into the bloodstream

immunity Protection against a disease or condition; the person will not get or be affected by the disease

menstruation The process in which the lining of the uterus breaks up and is discharged from the body through the vagina

metabolism The burning of food for heat and energy by the cells

organ Groups of tissues with the same function

peristalsis Involuntary muscle contractions in the digestive system that move food down the esophagus through the alimentary canal

respiration The process of supplying the cells with oxygen and removing carbon dioxide from them

system Organs that work together to perform special functions

tissue A group of cells with similar functions

vein A blood vessel that returns blood to the heart

KEY ABBREVIATIONS

GI Gastro-intestinal
RBC Red blood cell
WBC White blood cell

You help patients and residents meet basic needs. Their bodies do not work at peak levels because of illness, disease, or injury. Your care promotes comfort, healing, and recovery. You need to know the body's normal structure and function. It will help you understand signs, symptoms, and the reasons for care and procedures. You will give safe and more efficient care.

See Chapter 7 for changes in body structure and function that occur with aging.

CELLS, TISSUES, AND ORGANS

The basic unit of body structure is the **cell.** Cells have the same basic structure. Function, size, and shape may differ. Cells are very small. You need a microscope to see them. Cells need food, water, and oxygen to live and function.

Figure 6-1, p. 78, shows the cell and its structures. The *cell membrane* is the outer covering. It encloses the cell and helps it hold its shape. The *nucleus* is the control center of the cell. It directs the cell's activities. The nucleus is in the center of the cell. The *cytoplasm* surrounds the nucleus. Cytoplasm contains smaller structures that perform cell functions. *Protoplasm* means "living substance." It refers to all structures, substances, and water within the cell. Protoplasm is a semi-liquid substance much like an egg white.

Chromosomes are thread-like structures in the nucleus. Each cell has 46 chromosomes. Chromosomes contain *genes*. Genes control the traits children inherit from their parents. Height, eye color, and skin color are examples.

The nucleus controls cell reproduction. Cells reproduce by dividing in half. The process of cell division is called *mitosis*. It is needed for tissue growth and repair. During mitosis, the 46 chromosomes arrange themselves in 23 pairs. As the cell divides, the 23 pairs are pulled in half. The two new cells are identical. Each has 46 chromosomes (Fig. 6-2, p. 78).

Cells are the body's building blocks. Groups of cells with similar functions combine to form **tissues:**

- *Epithelial tissue* covers internal and external body surfaces. Tissue lining the nose, mouth, respiratory tract, stomach, and intestines is epithelial tissue. So are the skin, hair, nails, and glands.
- *Connective tissue* anchors, connects, and supports other tissues. It is in every part of the body. Bones, tendons, ligaments, and cartilage are connective tissue. Blood is a form of connective tissue.
- *Muscle tissue* stretches and contracts to let the body move.
- *Nerve tissue* receives and carries impulses to the brain and back to body parts.

Groups of tissue with the same function form **organs.** An organ has one or more functions. Examples of organs are the heart, brain, liver, lungs, and kidneys. **Systems** are formed by organs that work together to perform special functions (Fig. 6-3, p. 78).

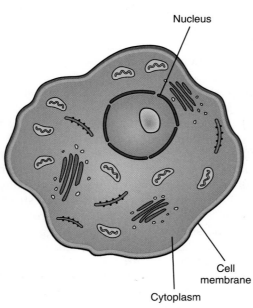

FIGURE 6-1 Parts of a cell.

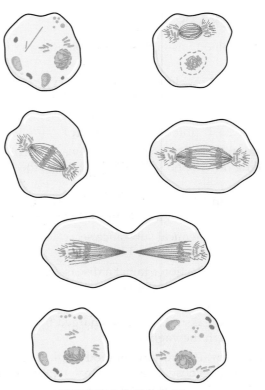

FIGURE 6-2 Cell division.

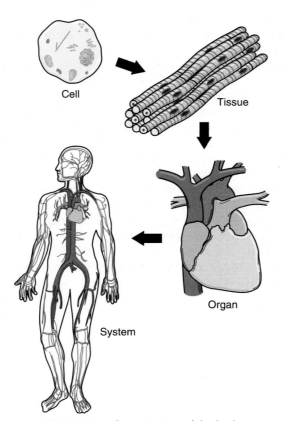

FIGURE 6-3 Organization of the body.

THE INTEGUMENTARY SYSTEM

The *integumentary system*, or *skin*, is the largest system. *Integument* means covering. The skin covers the body. It has epithelial, connective, and nerve tissue. It also has oil glands and sweat glands. There are two skin layers (Fig. 6-4):

- The *epidermis* is the outer layer. It has living cells and dead cells. The dead cells were once deeper in the epidermis. They were pushed upward as the cells divided. Dead cells constantly flake off. They are replaced by living cells. Living cells also die and flake off. Living cells of the epidermis contain *pigment*. Pigment gives skin its color. The epidermis has no blood vessels and few nerve endings.

- The *dermis* is the inner layer. It is made up of connective tissue. Blood vessels, nerves, sweat glands, and oil glands are found in the dermis. So are hair roots.

The epidermis and dermis are supported by *subcutaneous tissue*. The subcutaneous tissue is a thick layer of fat and connective tissue.

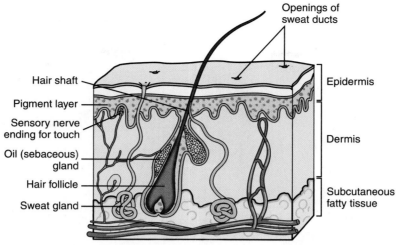

FIGURE 6-4 Layers of the skin.

Oil glands and *sweat glands, hair,* and *nails* are skin appendages:

- Hair—covers the entire body, except the palms of the hands and the soles of the feet. Hair in the nose and ears and around the eyes protects these organs from dust, insects, and other foreign objects.
- Nails—protect the tips of the fingers and toes. Nails help fingers pick up and handle small objects.
- Sweat glands—help the body regulate temperature. Sweat consists of water, salt, and a small amount of wastes. Sweat is secreted through pores in the skin. The body is cooled as sweat evaporates.
- Oil glands—lie near the hair shafts. They secrete an oily substance into the space near the hair shaft. Oil travels to the skin surface. This helps keep the hair and skin soft and shiny.

The skin has many functions:

- It is the body's protective covering.
- It prevents microorganisms and other substances from entering the body.
- It prevents excess amounts of water from leaving the body.
- It protects organs from injury.
- Nerve endings in the skin sense both pleasant and unpleasant stimulation. Nerve endings are over the entire body. They sense cold, pain, touch, and pressure to protect the body from injury.
- It helps regulate body temperature. Blood vessels dilate (widen) when temperature outside the body is high. More blood is brought to the body surface for cooling during evaporation. When blood vessels constrict (narrow), the body retains heat. This is because less blood reaches the skin.

THE MUSCULOSKELETAL SYSTEM

The musculoskeletal system provides the framework for the body. It lets the body move. This system also protects and gives the body shape.

Bones

The human body has 206 *bones* (Fig. 6-5, p. 80). There are four types of bones:

- *Long bones* bear the body's weight. Leg bones are long bones.
- *Short bones* allow skill and ease in movement. Bones in the wrists, fingers, ankles, and toes are short bones.
- *Flat bones* protect the organs. They include the ribs, skull, pelvic bones, and shoulder blades.
- *Irregular bones* are the vertebrae in the spinal column. They allow various degrees of movement and flexibility.

Bones are hard, rigid structures. They are made up of living cells. They are covered by a membrane called *periosteum*. Periosteum contains blood vessels that supply bone cells with oxygen and food. Inside the hollow centers of the bones is a substance called *bone marrow*. Blood cells are formed in the bone marrow.

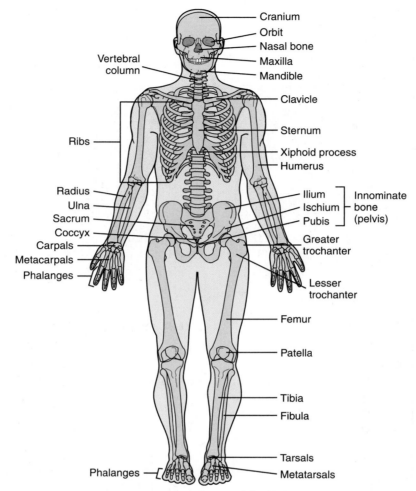

FIGURE 6-5 Bones of the body.

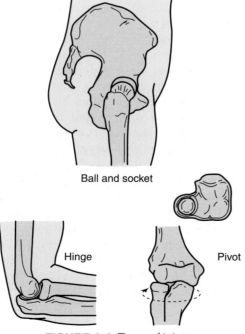

FIGURE 6-6 Types of joints.

Joints

A *joint* is the point at which two or more bones meet. Joints allow movement (Chapter 22). *Cartilage* is the connective tissue at the end of the long bones. It cushions the joint so that the bone ends do not rub together. The *synovial membrane* lines the joints. It secretes *synovial fluid*. Synovial fluid acts as a lubricant so the joint can move smoothly. Bones are held together at the joint by strong bands of connective tissue called *ligaments*.

There are three major types of joints (Fig. 6-6):

- *Ball-and-socket joint* allows movement in all directions. It is made up of the rounded end of one bone and the hollow end of another bone. The rounded end of one fits into the hollow end of the other. The joints of the hips and shoulders are ball-and-socket joints.
- *Hinge joint* allows movement in one direction. The elbow is a hinge joint.
- *Pivot joint* allows turning from side to side. A pivot joint connects the skull to the spine.

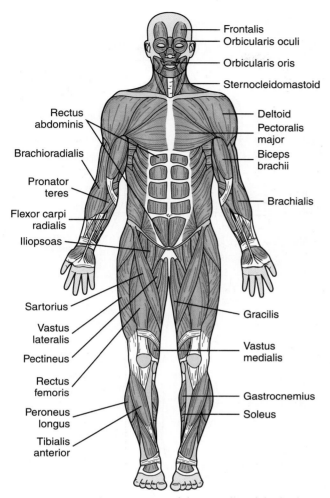

FIGURE 6-7 Anterior view of the muscles of the body.

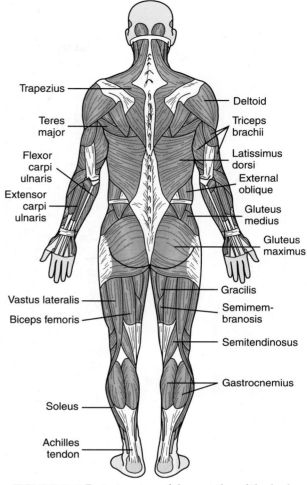

FIGURE 6-8 Posterior view of the muscles of the body.

Muscles

The human body has more than 500 *muscles* (Figs. 6-7 and 6-8). Some are voluntary. Others are involuntary.

- *Voluntary muscles* can be consciously controlled. Muscles attached to bones *(skeletal muscles)* are voluntary. Arm muscles do not work unless you move your arm; likewise for leg muscles. Skeletal muscles are *striated*. That is, they look striped or streaked.
- *Involuntary muscles* work automatically. You cannot control them. They control the action of the stomach, intestines, blood vessels, and other body organs. Involuntary muscles also are called *smooth muscles.* They look smooth, not streaked or striped.
- *Cardiac muscle* is in the heart. It is an involuntary muscle. However, it appears striated like skeletal muscle.

Muscles have three functions:

- Movement of body parts
- Maintenance of posture
- Production of body heat

Strong, tough connective tissues called *tendons* connect muscles to bones. When muscles contract (shorten), tendons at each end of the muscle cause the bone to move. The body has many tendons. See the Achilles tendon in Figure 6-8. Some muscles constantly contract to maintain the body's posture. When muscles contract, they burn food for energy. Heat is produced. The more muscle activity, the greater the amount of heat produced. Shivering is how the body produces heat when exposed to cold. Shivering is from rapid, general muscle contractions.

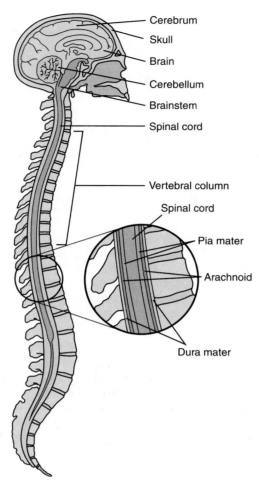

FIGURE 6-9 Central nervous system.

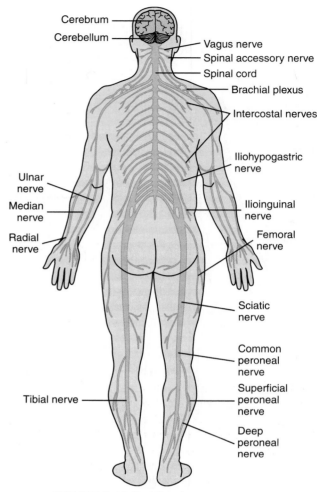

FIGURE 6-10 Peripheral nervous system.

THE NERVOUS SYSTEM

The nervous system controls, directs, and coordinates body functions. Its two main divisions are:

- The *central nervous system* (CNS). It consists of the brain and spinal cord (Fig. 6-9).
- The *peripheral nervous system*. It involves the *nerves* throughout the body (Fig. 6-10).

Nerves carry messages or impulses to and from the brain. Nerves connect to the spinal cord. They are easily damaged and take a long time to heal. Some nerve fibers have a protective covering called a *myelin sheath*. The myelin sheath also insulates the nerve fiber. Nerve fibers covered with myelin conduct impulses faster than those fibers without it.

The Central Nervous System

The *brain* and *spinal cord* make up the central nervous system. The brain is covered by the skull. The three

main parts of the brain are the *cerebrum*, the *cerebellum*, and the *brainstem* (Fig. 6-11).

The cerebrum is the largest part of the brain. It is the center of thought and intelligence. The cerebrum is divided into two halves called the *right* and *left hemispheres*. The right hemisphere controls movement and activities on the body's left side. The left hemisphere controls the right side.

The outside of the cerebrum is called the *cerebral cortex*. It controls the highest functions of the brain. These include reasoning, memory, consciousness, speech, voluntary muscle movement, vision, hearing, sensation, and other activities.

The cerebellum regulates and coordinates body movements. It controls balance and the smooth movements of voluntary muscles. Injury to the cerebellum results in jerky movements, loss of coordination, and muscle weakness.

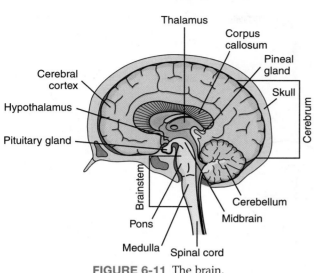

FIGURE 6-11 The brain.

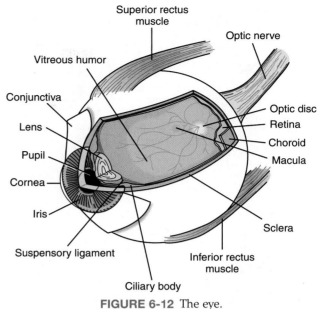

FIGURE 6-12 The eye.

The brainstem connects the cerebrum to the spinal cord. The brainstem contains the *midbrain, pons,* and *medulla.* The midbrain and pons relay messages between the medulla and the cerebrum. The medulla is below the pons. The medulla controls heart rate, breathing, blood vessel size, swallowing, coughing, and vomiting. The brain connects to the spinal cord at the lower end of the medulla.

The spinal cord lies within the spinal column. The cord is 17 to 18 inches long. It contains pathways that conduct messages to and from the brain.

The brain and spinal cord are covered and protected by three layers of connective tissue called *meninges:*

- The outer layer lies next to the skull. It is a tough covering call the *dura mater.*
- The middle layer is the *arachnoid.*
- The inner layer is the *pia mater.*

The space between the middle layer (arachnoid) and inner layer (pia mater) is the *arachnoid space.* The space is filled with *cerebrospinal fluid.* It circulates around the brain and spinal cord. Cerebrospinal fluid protects the central nervous system. It cushions shocks that could easily injure brain and spinal cord structures.

The Peripheral Nervous System

The peripheral nervous system has 12 pairs of *cranial nerves* and 31 pairs of *spinal nerves.* Cranial nerves conduct impulses between the brain and the head, neck, chest, and abdomen. They conduct impulses for smell, vision, hearing, pain, touch, temperature, and pressure. They also conduct impulses for voluntary and involuntary muscles. Spinal nerves carry impulses from the skin, extremities, and the internal structures not supplied by cranial nerves.

Some peripheral nerves form the *autonomic nervous system.* This system controls involuntary muscles and certain body functions. The functions include the heartbeat, blood pressure, intestinal contractions, and glandular secretions. These functions occur automatically.

The autonomic nervous system is divided into the *sympathetic nervous system* and the *parasympathetic nervous system.* They balance each other. The sympathetic nervous system speeds up functions. The parasympathetic nervous system slows functions. When you are angry, scared, excited, or exercising, the sympathetic nervous system is stimulated. The parasympathetic system is activated when you relax or when the sympathetic system is stimulated for too long.

The Sense Organs

The five senses are *sight, hearing, taste, smell,* and *touch.* Receptors for taste are in the tongue. They are called *taste buds.* Receptors for smell are in the nose. Touch receptors are in the dermis, especially in the toes and fingertips.

The Eye Receptors for vision are in the *eyes* (Fig. 6-12). The eye is easily injured. Bones of the skull, eyelids and eyelashes, and tears protect the eyes from

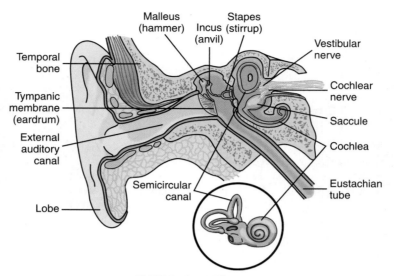

FIGURE 6-13 The ear.

injury. The eye has three layers:
- The *sclera*, the white of the eye, is the outer layer. It is made of tough connective tissue.
- The *choroid* is the second layer. Blood vessels, the *ciliary muscle*, and the *iris* make up the choroid. The iris gives the eye its color. The opening in the middle of the iris is the *pupil*. Pupil size varies with the amount of light entering the eye. The pupil constricts (narrows) in bright light. It dilates (widens) in dim or dark places.
- The *retina* is the inner layer. It has receptors for vision and the nerve fibers of the *optic nerve*.

Light enters the eye through the *cornea*. It is the transparent part of the outer layer that lies over the eye. Light rays pass to the *lens*, which lies behind the pupil. The light is then reflected to the retina. Light is carried to the brain by the optic nerve.

The *aqueous chamber* separates the cornea from the lens. The chamber is filled with a fluid called *aqueous humor*. The fluid helps the cornea keep its shape and position. The *vitreous humor* is behind the lens. It is a gelatin-like substance that supports the retina and maintains the eye's shape.

The Ear The *ear* is a sense organ (Fig. 6-13). It functions in hearing and balance. It has three parts: the *external ear, middle ear,* and *inner ear.*

The external ear (outer part) is called the *pinna* or *auricle.* Sound waves are guided through the external ear into the *auditory canal.* Glands in the auditory canal secrete a waxy substance called *cerumen.* The auditory canal extends about 1 inch to the *eardrum.* The eardrum *(tympanic membrane)* separates the external and middle ear.

The middle ear is a small space. It contains the

eustachian tube and three small bones called *ossicles.* The eustachian tube connects the middle ear and the throat. Air enters the eustachian tube so that there is equal pressure on both sides of the eardrum. The ossicles amplify sound received from the eardrum and transmit the sound to the inner ear. The three ossicles are:
- The *malleus.* It looks like a hammer.
- The *incus.* It looks like an anvil.
- The *stapes.* It is shaped like a stirrup.

The inner ear consists of *semicircular canals* and the *cochlea.* The cochlea looks like a snail shell. It contains fluid. The fluid carries sound waves from the middle ear to the *auditory nerve.* The auditory nerve then carries the message to the brain.

The three semicircular canals are involved with balance. They sense the head's position and changes in position. They send messages to the brain.

THE CIRCULATORY SYSTEM

The circulatory system is made up of the *blood, heart,* and *blood vessels.* The heart pumps blood through the blood vessels. The circulatory system has many functions:
- Blood carries food, oxygen, and other substances to the cells.
- Blood removes waste products from cells.
- Blood and blood vessels help regulate body temperature. The blood carries heat from muscle activity to other body parts. Blood vessels in the skin dilate to cool the body. They constrict to retain heat.
- The system produces and carries cells that defend the body from microbes that cause disease.

The Blood

The blood consists of blood cells and *plasma*. Plasma is mostly water. It carries blood cells to other body cells. Plasma also carries substances that cells need to function. This includes food (proteins, fats, and carbohydrates), hormones (p. 91), and chemicals.

Red blood cells (RBCs) are called *erythrocytes*. They give blood its red color because of a substance in the RBC called **hemoglobin.** As RBCs circulate through the lungs, hemoglobin picks up oxygen. Hemoglobin carries oxygen to the cells. When blood is bright red, hemoglobin in the RBCs is saturated (filled) with oxygen. As blood circulates through the body, oxygen is given to the cells. Cells release carbon dioxide (a waste product). It is picked up by the hemoglobin. RBCs saturated with carbon dioxide make the blood look dark red.

The body has about 25 trillion (25,000,000,000,000) RBCs. About 4.5 to 5 million cells are in a cubic millimeter of blood (the size of a tiny drop). RBCs live for 3 or 4 months. They are destroyed by the liver and spleen as they wear out. New RBCs are formed in the bone marrow. About 1 million RBCs are produced every second.

White blood cells (WBCs) are called *leukocytes*. They have no color. They protect the body against infection. There are about 5,000 to 10,000 WBCs in a cubic millimeter of blood. At the first sign of infection, WBCs rush to the infection site. There they multiply rapidly. The number of WBCs increases when there is an infection. WBCs are formed by the bone marrow. They live about 9 days.

Platelets (thrombocytes) are needed for blood clotting. They are formed by the bone marrow. There are about 200,000 to 400,000 platelets in a cubic millimeter of blood. A platelet lives about 4 days.

The Heart

The heart is a muscle. It pumps blood through the blood vessels to the tissues and cells. The heart lies in the middle to lower part of the chest cavity toward the left side (Fig. 6-14). The heart is hollow and has three layers (Fig. 6-15):

- The *pericardium* is the outer layer. It is a thin sac covering the heart.
- The *myocardium* is the second layer. It is the thick, muscular part of the heart.
- The *endocardium* is the inner layer. A membrane, it lines the inner surface of the heart.

The heart has four chambers (see Fig. 6-15). Upper chambers receive blood and are called *atria*. The *right atrium* receives blood from body tissues. The *left atrium* receives blood from the lungs. Lower chambers are called *ventricles*. Ventricles pump blood. The

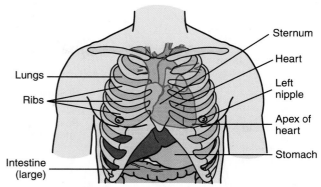

FIGURE 6-14 Location of the heart in the chest cavity.

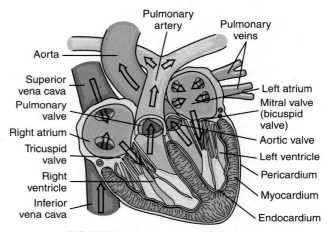

FIGURE 6-15 Structures of the heart.

right ventricle pumps blood to the lungs for oxygen. The *left ventricle* pumps blood to all parts of the body.

Valves are between the atria and ventricles. The valves allow blood flow in one direction. They prevent blood from flowing back into the atria from the ventricles. The *tricuspid valve* is between the right atrium and the right ventricle. The *mitral valve (bicuspid valve)* is between the left atrium and left ventricle.

Heart action has two phases:

- *Diastole.* It is the resting phase. Heart chambers fill with blood.
- *Systole.* It is the working phase. The heart contracts. Blood is pumped through the blood vessels when the heart contracts.

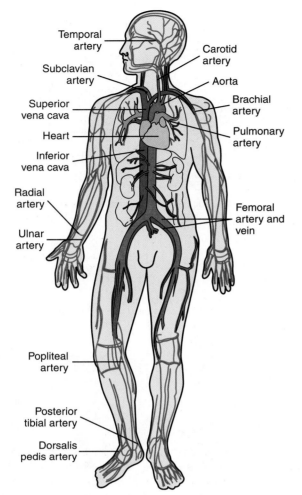

FIGURE 6-16 Arterial and venous systems. Arterial system is red. Venous system is blue.

The Blood Vessels

Blood flows to body tissues and cells through the blood vessels. There are three groups of blood vessels: arteries, capillaries, and veins.

Arteries carry blood away from the heart. Arterial blood is rich in oxygen. The *aorta* is the largest artery. It receives blood directly from the left ventricle. The aorta branches into other arteries that carry blood to all parts of the body (Fig. 6-16). These arteries branch into smaller parts within the tissues. The smallest branch of an artery is an *arteriole*.

Arterioles connect to **capillaries.** Capillaries are very tiny blood vessels. Food, oxygen, and other substances pass from capillaries into the cells. The capillaries pick up waste products (including carbon dioxide) from the cells. Veins carry waste products back to the heart.

Veins return blood to the heart. They connect to the capillaries by *venules.* Venules are small veins.

Venules branch together to form veins. The many veins also branch together as they near the heart to form two main veins (see Fig. 6-16). The two main veins are the *inferior vena cava* and the *superior vena cava.* Both empty into the right atrium. The inferior vena cava carries blood from the legs and trunk. The superior vena cava carries blood from the head and arms. Venous blood is dark red. It has little oxygen and a lot of carbon dioxide.

Blood flow through the circulatory system is shown in Figure 6-15. The path of blood flow is as follows:
- Venous blood, poor in oxygen, empties into the right atrium.
- Blood flows through the tricuspid valve into the right ventricle.
- The right ventricle pumps blood into the lungs to pick up oxygen.
- Oxygen-rich blood from the lungs enters the left atrium.
- Blood from the left atrium passes through the mitral valve into the left ventricle.
- The left ventricle pumps the blood to the aorta. It branches off to form other arteries.
- Arterial blood is carried to the tissues by arterioles and to the cells by capillaries.
- Cells and capillaries exchange oxygen and nutrients for carbon dioxide and waste products.
- Capillaries connect with venules.
- Venules carry blood that has carbon dioxide and waste products.
- Venules form veins.
- Veins return blood to the heart.

THE RESPIRATORY SYSTEM

Oxygen is needed to live. Every cell needs oxygen. Air contains about 21% oxygen. This meets the body's needs under normal conditions. The respiratory system (Fig. 6-17) brings oxygen into the lungs and removes carbon dioxide. **Respiration** is the process of supplying the cells with oxygen and removing carbon dioxide from them. Respiration involves *inhalation* (breathing in) and *exhalation* (breathing out). The terms *inspiration* (breathing in) and *expiration* (breathing out) also are used.

Air enters the body through the *nose.* The air then passes into the *pharynx* (throat). It is a tube-shaped passageway for air and food. Air passes from the pharynx into the *larynx* (voice box). A piece of cartilage, the *epiglottis,* acts like a lid over the larynx. The epiglottis prevents food from entering the airway during swallowing. During inhalation the epiglottis lifts up to let air pass over the larynx. Air passes from the larynx into the *trachea* (windpipe).

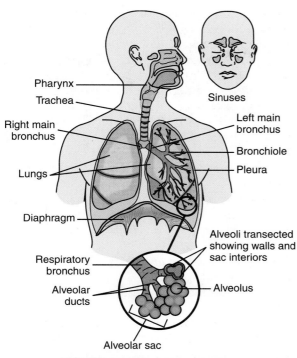

FIGURE 6-17 Respiratory system.

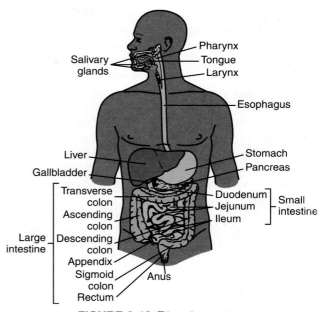

FIGURE 6-18 Digestive system.

The trachea divides at its lower end into the *right bronchus* and the *left bronchus.* Each bronchus enters a lung. Upon entering the lungs, the bronchi divide many times into smaller branches. The smaller branches are called *bronchioles.* Eventually the bronchioles subdivide. They end up in tiny one-celled air sacs called *alveoli.*

Alveoli look like small clusters of grapes. They are supplied by capillaries. Oxygen and carbon dioxide are exchanged between the alveoli and capillaries. Blood in the capillaries picks up oxygen from the alveoli. Then the blood is returned to the left side of the heart and pumped to the rest of the body. Alveoli pick up carbon dioxide from the capillaries for exhalation.

The lungs are spongy tissues. They are filled with alveoli, blood vessels, and nerves. Each lung is divided into lobes. The right lung has three lobes; the left lung has two. The lungs are separated from the abdominal cavity by a muscle called the *diaphragm.*

Each lung is covered by a two-layered sac called the *pleura.* One layer is attached to the lung and the other to the chest wall. The pleura secretes a very thin fluid that fills the space between the layers. The fluid prevents the layers from rubbing together during inhalation and exhalation. A bony framework made up of the ribs, sternum, and vertebrae protects the lungs.

THE DIGESTIVE SYSTEM

The digestive system breaks down food physically and chemically so it can be absorbed for use by the cells. This process is called **digestion.** The digestive system is also called the *gastro-intestinal (GI) system.* The system also removes solid wastes from the body.

The digestive system involves the *alimentary canal (GI tract)* and the accessory organs of digestion (Fig. 6-18). The alimentary canal is a long tube. It extends from the mouth to the anus. Its major parts are the mouth, pharynx, esophagus, stomach, small intestine, and large intestine. Accessory organs are the teeth, tongue, salivary glands, liver, gallbladder, and pancreas.

Digestion begins in the *mouth.* The mouth also is called the *oral cavity.* It receives food and prepares it for digestion. Using chewing motions, the *teeth* cut, chop, and grind food into small particles for digestion and swallowing. The *tongue* aids in chewing and swallowing. Taste buds on the tongue's surface contain nerve endings. Taste buds allow sweet, sour, bitter, and salty tastes to be sensed. *Salivary glands* in the mouth secrete *saliva.* Saliva moistens food particles to ease swallowing and begin digestion. During swallowing, the tongue pushes food into the *pharynx.*

The pharynx (throat) is a muscular tube. Swallowing continues as the pharynx contracts. Contraction of the pharynx pushes food into the *esophagus*. The esophagus is a muscular tube about 10 inches long. It extends from the pharynx to the *stomach*. Involuntary muscle contractions called **peristalsis** move food down the esophagus through the alimentary canal.

The stomach is a muscular, pouch-like sac. It is in the upper left part of the abdominal cavity. Strong stomach muscles stir and churn food to break it up into even smaller particles. A mucous membrane lines the stomach. It contains glands that secrete *gastric juices*. Food is mixed and churned with the gastric juices to form a semi-liquid substance called *chyme*. Through peristalsis, the chyme is pushed from the stomach into the small intestine.

The *small intestine* is about 20 feet long. It has three parts. The first part is the *duodenum*. There more digestive juices are added to the chyme. One is called *bile*. Bile is a greenish liquid made in the *liver*. Bile is stored in the *gallbladder*. Juices from the *pancreas* and small intestine are added to the chyme. Digestive juices chemically break down food so it can be absorbed.

Peristalsis moves the chyme through the two other parts of the small intestine: the *jejunum* and the *ileum*. Tiny projections called *villi* line the small intestine. Villi absorb the digested food into the capillaries. Most food absorption takes place in the jejunum and the ileum.

Some chyme is not digested. Undigested chyme passes from the small intestine into the *large intestine* (*large bowel* or *colon*). The colon absorbs most of the water from the chyme. The remaining semi-solid material is called *feces*. Feces contain a small amount of water, solid wastes, and some mucus and germs. These are the waste products of digestion. Feces pass through the colon into the *rectum* by peristalsis. Feces pass out of the body through the *anus*.

THE URINARY SYSTEM

The digestive system rids the body of solid wastes. The lungs rid the body of carbon dioxide. Water and other substances leave the body through sweat. There are other waste products in the blood from cells burning food for energy. The urinary system (Fig. 6-19):

- Removes waste products from the blood
- Maintains water balance within the body

The *kidneys* are two bean-shaped organs in the upper abdomen. They lie against the back muscles on each side of the spine. They are protected by the lower edge of the rib cage.

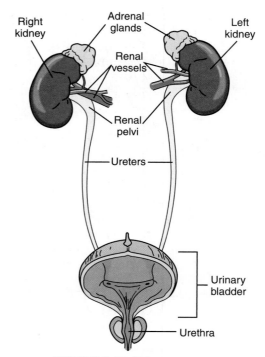

FIGURE 6-19 Urinary system.

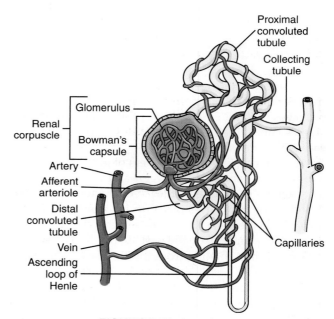

FIGURE 6-20 A nephron.

Each kidney has over a million tiny *nephrons* (Fig. 6-20). Each nephron is the basic working unit of the kidney. Each nephron has a *convoluted tubule*, which is a tiny coiled tubule. Each convoluted tubule has a *Bowman's capsule* at one end. The capsule partly surrounds a cluster of capillaries called a *glomerulus*. Blood passes through the glomerulus and is filtered by the capillaries. The fluid part of the blood is squeezed into the Bowman's capsule. The fluid then passes into the tubule. Most of the water and other needed substances are re-absorbed by the blood. The rest of the fluid and the waste products form *urine* in the tubule. Urine flows through the tubule to a *collecting tubule.* All collecting tubules drain into the *renal pelvis* in the kidney.

A tube, called the *ureter,* is attached to the renal pelvis of the kidney. Each ureter is about 10 to 12 inches long. The ureters carry urine from the kidneys to the *bladder.* The bladder is a hollow, muscular sac. It lies toward the front in the lower part of the abdominal cavity.

Urine is stored in the bladder until the need to urinate is felt. This usually occurs when there is about a half pint (250 milliliters [mL]) of urine in the bladder. Urine passes from the bladder through the *urethra.* The opening at the end of the urethra is the *meatus.* Urine passes from the body through the meatus. Urine is a clear, yellowish fluid.

THE REPRODUCTIVE SYSTEM

Human reproduction results from the union of a male sex cell and a female sex cell. The male and female reproductive systems are different. This allows for the process of reproduction.

The Male Reproductive System

The male reproductive system is shown in Figure 6-21. The *testes (testicles)* are the male sex glands. Sex glands also are called *gonads.* The two testes are oval or almond-shaped glands. Male sex cells are produced in the testes. Male sex cells are called *sperm* cells.

Testosterone, the male hormone, is produced in the testes. This hormone is needed for reproductive organ function. It also is needed for the development of the male secondary sex characteristics. There is facial hair; pubic and axillary (underarm) hair; and hair on the arms, chest, and legs. Neck and shoulder sizes increase.

The testes are suspended between the thighs in a sac called the *scrotum.* The scrotum is made of skin and muscle.

Sperm travel from a testis to the *epididymis.* The epididymis is a coiled tube on top and to the side of the testis. From the epididymis, sperm travel through a tube called the *vas deferens.* Each vas deferens joins a seminal vesicle. The two seminal vesicles store sperm and produce *semen.* Semen is a fluid that carries sperm from the male reproductive tract. The ducts of the seminal vesicles unite to form the *ejaculatory duct.* It passes through the *prostate gland.*

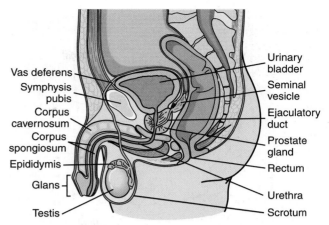

FIGURE 6-21 Male reproductive system.

The prostate gland lies just below the bladder. It is shaped like a donut. The gland secretes fluid into the semen. As the ejaculatory ducts leave the prostate, they join the *urethra.* The urethra runs through the prostate gland. The urethra is the outlet for urine and semen. The urethra is contained within the *penis.*

The penis is outside of the body and has *erectile* tissue. When a man is sexually excited, blood fills the erectile tissue. The penis enlarges and becomes hard and erect. The erect penis can enter a female's vagina. The semen, which contains sperm, is released into the vagina.

The Female Reproductive System

Figure 6-22, p. 90, shows the female reproductive system. The female gonads are two almond-shaped glands called *ovaries.* An ovary is on each side of the uterus in the abdominal cavity.

The ovaries contain *ova* or eggs. Ova are the female sex cells. One ovum (egg) is released monthly during the woman's reproductive years. Release of an ovum is called *ovulation.*

The ovaries secrete the female hormones *estrogen* and *progesterone.* These hormones are needed for reproductive system function. They also are needed for the development of secondary sex characteristics in the female. These include increased breast size, pubic and axillary (underarm) hair, slight deepening of the voice, and widening and rounding of the hips.

When an ovum is released from an ovary, it travels through a *fallopian tube.* There are two fallopian tubes, one on each side. The tubes are attached at one end to the uterus. The ovum travels through the fallopian tube to the *uterus.*

The *uterus* is a hollow, muscular organ shaped like a pear. It is in the center of the pelvic cavity behind the bladder and in front of the rectum. The main part

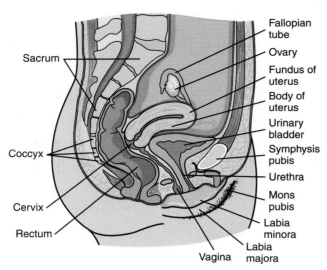

FIGURE 6-22 Female reproductive system.

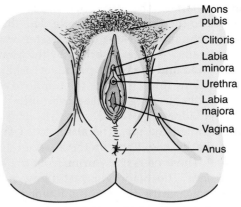

FIGURE 6-23 External female genitalia.

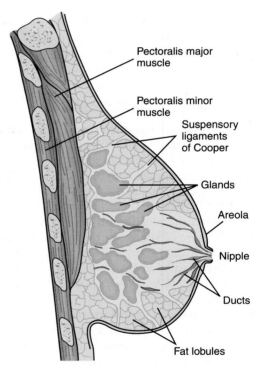

FIGURE 6-24 The female breast.

of the uterus is the *fundus.* The neck or narrow section of the uterus is the *cervix.* Tissue lining the uterus is called the *endometrium.* The endometrium has many blood vessels. If sex cells from the male and female unite into one cell, that cell implants into the endometrium. There the cell grows into a baby. The uterus serves as a place for the *fetus* (unborn baby) to grow and receive nourishment.

The cervix of the uterus projects into a muscular canal called the *vagina.* The vagina opens to the outside of the body. It is just behind the urethra. The vagina receives the penis during intercourse. It also is part of the birth canal. Glands in the vaginal wall keep it moistened with secretions. In young girls, the external vaginal opening is partially closed by a membrane called the *hymen.* The hymen ruptures when the female has intercourse for the first time.

The external female genitalia are called the *vulva* (Fig. 6-23):

- The *mons pubis* is a rounded, fatty pad over a bone called the *symphysis pubis.* The mons pubis is covered with hair in the adult female.
- The *labia majora* and *labia minora* are two folds of tissue on each side of the vaginal opening.
- The *clitoris* is a small organ composed of erectile tissue. It becomes hard when sexually stimulated.

The *mammary glands (breasts)* secrete milk after childbirth. The glands are on the outside of the chest. They are made up of glandular tissue and fat (Fig. 6-24). The milk drains into ducts that open onto the *nipple.*

Menstruation The endometrium is rich in blood to nourish the cell that grows into a fetus. If pregnancy does not occur, the endometrium breaks up. It is discharged from the body through the vagina. This process is called **menstruation.** Menstruation occurs about every 28 days. Therefore it is called the *menstrual cycle.*

The first day of the menstrual cycle begins with menstruation. Blood flows from the uterus through the vaginal opening. Menstrual flow usually lasts 3 to 7 days. Ovulation occurs during the next phase. An ovum matures in an ovary and is released. Ovulation usually occurs on or about day 14 of the cycle.

Meanwhile, estrogen and progesterone (the female hormones) are secreted by the ovaries. These hormones cause the endometrium to thicken for pregnancy. If pregnancy does not occur, the hormones decrease in amount. This causes the blood supply to the endometrium to decrease. The endometrium breaks up. It is discharged through the vagina. Another menstrual cycle begins.

Fertilization

To reproduce, a male sex cell (sperm) must unite with a female sex cell (ovum). The uniting of the sperm and ovum into one cell is called *fertilization*. A sperm has 23 chromosomes. An ovum has 23 chromosomes. When the two cells unite, the fertilized cell has 46 chromosomes.

During intercourse, millions of sperm are deposited into the vagina. Sperm travel up the cervix, through the uterus, and into the fallopian tubes. If a sperm and an ovum unite in a fallopian tube, fertilization results. Pregnancy occurs. The fertilized cell travels down the fallopian tube to the uterus. After a short time, the fertilized cell implants in the thick endometrium and grows during pregnancy.

THE ENDOCRINE SYSTEM

The endocrine system is made up of glands called the *endocrine glands* (Fig. 6-25). The endocrine glands secrete chemical substances called **hormones** into the bloodstream. Hormones regulate the activities of other organs and glands in the body.

The *pituitary gland* is called the *master gland*. About the size of a cherry, it is at the base of the brain behind the eyes. The pituitary gland is divided into the *anterior pituitary lobe* and the *posterior pituitary lobe*. The anterior pituitary lobe secretes:
- *Growth hormone (GH)*—needed for growth of muscles, bones, and other organs. It is needed throughout life to maintain normal-size bones and muscles. Growth is stunted if a baby is born with deficient amounts of growth hormone. Too much of the hormone causes excessive growth.
- *Thyroid-stimulating hormone (TSH)*—needed for thyroid gland function.
- *Adrenocorticotropic hormone (ACTH)*—stimulates the adrenal gland.

The anterior lobe also secretes hormones that regulate growth, development, and function of the male and female reproductive systems.

The posterior pituitary lobe secretes *antidiuretic hormone (ADH)* and *oxytocin*. ADH prevents the kidneys from excreting excessive amounts of water. Oxytocin causes uterine muscles to contract during childbirth.

The *thyroid gland,* shaped like a butterfly, is in the neck in front of the larynx. *Thyroid hormone (TH, thyroxine)* is secreted by the thyroid gland. It regulates

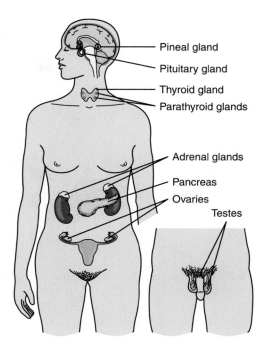

FIGURE 6-25 Endocrine system.

metabolism. Metabolism is the burning of food for heat and energy by the cells. Too little TH results in slowed body processes, slowed movements, and weight gain. Too much TH causes increased metabolism, excess energy, and weight loss. Some babies are born with deficient amounts of TH. Their physical growth and mental growth are stunted.

The four *parathyroid glands* secrete *parathormone.* Two lie on each side of the thyroid gland. Parathormone regulates calcium use. Calcium is needed for nerve and muscle function. Insufficient amounts of calcium cause *tetany.* Tetany is a state of severe muscle contraction and spasm. If untreated, tetany can cause death.

There are two *adrenal glands.* An adrenal gland is on the top of each kidney. The adrenal gland has two parts: the *adrenal medulla* and the *adrenal cortex.* The adrenal medulla secretes *epinephrine* and *norepinephrine.* These hormones stimulate the body to quickly produce energy during emergencies. Heart rate, blood pressure, muscle power, and energy all increase.

The adrenal cortex secretes three groups of hormones needed for life:
- *Glucocorticoids*—regulate the metabolism of carbohydrates. They also control the body's response to stress and inflammation.
- *Mineralocorticoids*—regulate the amount of salt and water that is absorbed and lost by the kidneys.
- Small amounts of male and female sex hormones— p. 89.

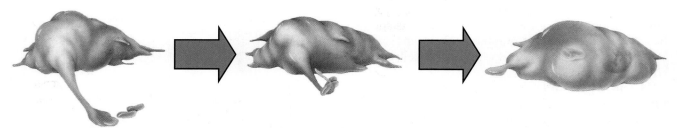

FIGURE 6-26 A phagocyte digests and destroys a microorganism. *(From Thibodeau GA, Patton KT:* Structure and function of the body, *ed 11, St Louis, 2000, Mosby.)*

The *pancreas* secretes *insulin*. Insulin regulates the amount of sugar in the blood available for use by the cells. Insulin is needed for sugar to enter the cells. If there is too little insulin, sugar cannot enter the cells. If sugar cannot enter the cells, excess amounts of sugar build up in the blood. This condition is called *diabetes*.

The *gonads* are the glands of human reproduction. Male sex glands (testes) secrete *testosterone*. Female sex glands (ovaries) secrete *estrogen* and *progesterone*.

THE IMMUNE SYSTEM

The immune system protects the body from disease and infection. Abnormal body cells can grow into tumors. Sometimes the body produces substances that cause the body to attack itself. Microorganisms (bacteria, viruses, and other germs) can cause an infection. The immune system defends against threats inside and outside the body.

The immune system gives the body **immunity.** Immunity means that a person has protection against a disease or condition. The person will not get or be affected by the disease:

- *Specific immunity* is the body's reaction to a certain threat.
- *Nonspecific immunity* is the body's reaction to anything it does not recognize as a normal body substance.

Special cells and substances function to produce immunity:

- *Antibodies*—normal body substances that recognize other substances. They are involved in destroying abnormal or unwanted substances.
- *Antigens*—substances that can cause an immune response. Antibodies recognize and bind with unwanted antigens. This leads to the destruction of unwanted substances and the production of more antibodies.
- *Phagocytes*—white blood cells that digest and destroy microorganisms and other unwanted substances (Fig. 6-26).
- *Lymphocytes*—white blood cells that produce antibodies. Lymphocyte production increases as the body responds to an infection.
- *B lymphocytes (B cells)*—cause the production of antibodies that circulate in the plasma. The antibodies react to specific antigens.
- *T lymphocytes (T cells)*—cells that destroy invading cells. *Killer T cells* produce poisons near the invading cells. Some T cells attract other cells. The other cells destroy the invaders.

When the body senses an antigen from an unwanted substance, the immune system acts. Phagocyte and lymphocyte production increases. Phagocytes destroy the invaders through digestion. The lymphocytes produce antibodies that identify and destroy the unwanted substances.

Focus on P R I D E
The Person, Family, and Yourself

Personal and Professional Responsibility—To function, you must care for your body. A healthy diet (Chapter 19), exercise, and rest are needed for over-all health. See your doctor for a check-up at least once a year. Or sooner if you have a concern. Take prescription or over the counter drugs as instructed. Keep your immunizations up to date. For example, get a tetanus booster every 10 years. Protect your bones and muscles from injury by using good body mechanics (Chapter 12). Follow Standard Precautions to protect yourself from infection (Chapter 11). Also practice good hand hygiene (Chapter 11). Taking care of yourself is a personal and professional responsibility. To care for others, you need a strong and healthy body.

Rights and Respect—Patients and residents have the right to make decisions about their bodies. You may not agree with those decisions. But you must respect the person's choice. If the decision will cause no harm, comply with the request. For example, Mr. Collins does not want to wear his hearing aid today. He says: "I don't need that thing." His request will not harm him. Respect his choice. Tell the nurse.

If the person's decision may cause harm, tell the nurse at once. For example, Ms. Lane's kidneys do not function. She goes to dialysis 3 times a week. (Dialysis is the process of artificially removing wastes from the blood when the kidneys do not function.) Ms. Lane tells you that she does not want to go today. She says: "I just can't sit there for that long." You know the importance of the urinary system. Without dialysis, she will become very sick. You tell the nurse. Ms. Lane cannot be forced to go to dialysis. But the nurse can talk with Ms. Lane about her decision, the consequences, and possible solutions.

Independence and Social Interaction—The body does not always work right. Persons become ill or injured. Some illnesses cannot be cured. Sometimes the health team cannot prevent loss of function. However, patients and residents are helped to maintain their optimal level of function. This is the person's highest potential for mental and physical performance.

You can help maintain optimal level of functioning. Do not treat the person as a sick, dependent person. This reduces quality of life. Encourage the person to be as independent as possible. Always focus on the person's abilities, not disabilities. Tell the person when you notice progress. Promote social interaction. This improves mental performance. Help each person regain or maintain the highest level of functioning possible.

Delegation and Teamwork—The body works like a team. Each system has independent functions. But all systems interact and depend on each other. They work together to keep the body functioning. When a person has a problem with one body system, other systems are affected. Understanding each system and how the systems interact helps you provide better care.

Ethics and Laws—Sometimes a person is not able to make decisions about his or her own body. For example, the person has dementia. Or the person is unconscious or under the influence of drugs or alcohol. Maybe the person is thinking of harming himself or herself. Or the person may be a child. Ethical issues may arise over who makes decisions for such persons.

Spouses, parents, family members, or legal guardians may make decisions. Some persons have a durable power of attorney (Chapter 30). This is someone assigned to make decisions for that person if he or she is unable to do so. Some fill out a legal document called an advance directive (Chapter 30). This document states a person's wishes about health care when that person is unable to make his or her own decisions. In cases such as drug and alcohol abuse or attempts to harm oneself, the person's safety is the priority. Sometimes the court appoints a guardian for a short time. Finally, the agency's ethics committee may address complex issues. In all cases, the person's safety and best interests guide the care given.

REVIEW QUESTIONS

Circle the BEST answer.

1 The basic unit of body structure is the
   a Cell
   b Neuron
   c Nephron
   d Ovum
2 The outer layer of the skin is called the
   a Dermis
   b Epidermis
   c Integument
   d Myelin
3 Which allows movement?
   a Bone marrow
   b Synovial membrane
   c Joints
   d Ligaments
4 Skeletal muscles
   a Are under involuntary control
   b Appear smooth
   c Are under voluntary control
   d Appear striped and smooth
5 The highest functions in the brain take place in the
   a Cerebral cortex
   b Medulla
   c Brainstem
   d Spinal nerves
6 The ear is involved with
   a Regulating body movements
   b Balance
   c Smoothness of body movements
   d Controlling involuntary muscles
7 The liquid part of the blood is the
   a Hemoglobin
   b Red blood cell
   c Plasma
   d White blood cell
8 Which part of the heart pumps blood to the body?
   a Right atrium
   b Left atrium
   c Right ventricle
   d Left ventricle
9 Which carry blood away from the heart?
   a Capillaries
   b Veins
   c Venules
   d Arteries

10 Oxygen and carbon dioxide are exchanged
    a In the bronchi
    b Between the alveoli and capillaries
    c Between the lungs and pleura
    d In the trachea
11 Digestion begins in the
    a Mouth
    b Stomach
    c Small intestine
    d Colon
12 Most food absorption takes place in the
    a Stomach
    b Small intestine
    c Colon
    d Large intestine
13 Urine is formed by the
    a Jejunum
    b Kidneys
    c Bladder
    d Liver
14 Urine passes from the body through the
    a Ureters
    b Urethra
    c Anus
    d Nephrons
15 The male sex gland is called the
    a Penis
    b Ovary
    c Testis
    d Vagina
16 The discharge of the lining of the uterus is called
    a The endometrium
    b Ovulation
    c Fertilization
    d Menstruation
17 The endocrine glands secrete
    a Hormones
    b Mucus
    c Semen
    d Insulin
18 The immune system protects the body from
    a Low blood sugar
    b Disease and infection
    c Loss of fluid
    d Stunted growth

Answers to these questions are on p. 527.

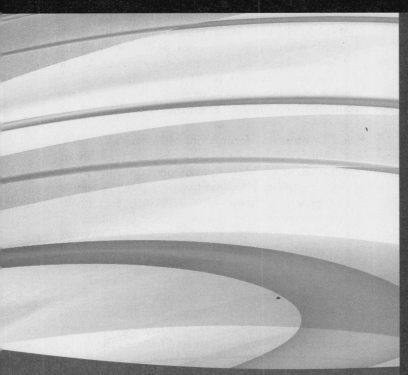

7

CARE OF THE OLDER PERSON

OBJECTIVES

- Define the key terms and key abbreviation listed in this chapter.
- Identify the developmental tasks of each age group.
- Identify the social changes common in older adulthood.
- Describe the physical changes from aging and the care required.
- Describe the gains and losses related to long-term care.
- Describe the sexual changes and needs of older persons.
- Explain how to deal with sexually aggressive persons.
- Explain how to promote PRIDE in the person, the family, and yourself.

KEY TERMS

development Changes in mental, emotional, and social function

developmental task A skill that must be completed during a stage of development

geriatrics The care of aging people

gerontology The study of the aging process

growth The physical changes that are measured and that occur in a steady, orderly manner

menopause The time when menstruation stops and menstrual cycles end

old Persons between 75 and 84 years of age

old-old Persons 85 years of age and older

sexuality The physical, emotional, social, cultural, and spiritual factors that affect a person's feelings and attitudes about his or her sex

young-old Persons between 65 and 74 years of age

KEY ABBREVIATION

OBRA Omnibus Budget Reconciliation Act of 1987

People live longer than ever before. They are healthier and more active. Most people in late adulthood live with a partner, children, or other family. Some live alone or with friends. Others live in nursing centers.

Late adulthood involves these age ranges:
- **Young-old**—between 65 and 74 years of age
- **Old**—between 75 and 84 years of age
- **Old-old**—85 years of age and older

Gerontology is the study of the aging process. **Geriatrics** is the care of aging people. Aging is normal. It is not a disease. Normal changes occur in body structure and function. They increase the risk for illness, injury, and disability. Psychological and social changes also occur. Often changes are slow. Most people adjust well to these changes. They lead happy, meaningful lives.

GROWTH AND DEVELOPMENT

People grow and develop throughout life. **Growth** is the physical changes that are measured and that occur in a steady and orderly manner. Growth is measured in weight and height. Changes in appearance and body functions also measure growth.

Development relates to changes in mental, emotional, and social function. A person behaves and thinks in certain ways in each stage of development. A 2-year-old thinks in simple terms. A 40-year-old thinks in complex ways. The entire person is affected.

Growth and development occur in a sequence, order, and pattern. Certain skills must be completed during each stage. A **developmental task** is a skill that must be completed during a stage of development. A stage cannot be skipped. Each stage is the basis for the next stage. Each stage has its own characteristics and developmental tasks (Box 7-1).

SOCIAL CHANGES

People cope with aging in their own way. The following social changes occur with aging.
- *Retirement*—Retirement is a reward for a life-time of work. The person can relax and enjoy life. Some people retire because of poor health or disability. Retired people may have part-time jobs or do volunteer work (Fig. 7-1, p. 98). Work helps meet love, belonging, and self-esteem needs. The person feels fulfilled and useful. Friendships form with co-workers.
- *Reduced income*—Retirement often means reduced income. Social Security may provide the only income. Rent or house payments continue. Food, clothing, utility bills, and taxes are other expenses. Car expenses, home repairs, drugs, and health care are other costs. Severe money problems can result. Some people have income from savings, investments, retirement plans, and insurance.
- *Social relationships*—Social relationships change throughout life. Children grow up, leave home, and have their own families. Some live far away. Older family members and friends die, move away, or are disabled. Yet most older people have regular contact with family and friends. Others are lonely. Separation from children is a common cause. So is lack of companionship with people their own age. Hobbies, religious and community events, and new friends help prevent loneliness. So does taking part in family activities (Fig. 7-2, p. 98).

BOX 7-1   Stages of Growth and Development

Infancy (birth to 1 year)

- Learning to walk
- Learning to eat solid foods
- Beginning to talk and communicate with others
- Learning to trust
- Beginning to have emotional relationships with parents, brothers, and sisters
- Developing stable sleep and feeding patterns

Toddlerhood (1 to 3 years)

- Tolerating separation from parents or primary caregivers
- Gaining control of bowel and bladder function
- Using words to communicate
- Becoming less dependent on parents or primary caregivers

Preschool (3 to 6 years)

- Increasing the ability to communicate and understand others
- Performing self-care
- Learning gender (male; female) differences and developing sexual modesty
- Learning right from wrong and good from bad
- Learning to play with others
- Developing family relationships

School Age (6 to 9 or 10 years)

- Developing social and physical skills needed for playing games
- Learning to get along with children of the same age and background (peers)
- Learning gender-appropriate behaviors and attitudes
- Learning basic reading, writing, and arithmetic skills
- Developing a conscience and morals
- Developing a good feeling and attitude about oneself

Late Childhood (9 or 10 to 12 years)

- Becoming independent of adults and learning to depend on oneself
- Developing and keeping friendships with peers
- Understanding the physical, psychological, and social roles of one's sex
- Developing moral and ethical behavior
- Developing greater muscular strength, coordination, and balance
- Learning how to study

Adolescence (12 to 18 years)

- Accepting changes in the body and appearance
- Developing appropriate relationships with males and females of the same age
- Accepting the male or female role appropriate for one's age
- Becoming independent from parents and adults
- Preparing for marriage and family life
- Preparing for a career
- Developing the morals, attitudes, and values needed to function in society

Young Adulthood (18 to 40 years)

- Choosing education and a career
- Selecting a partner
- Learning to live with a partner
- Becoming a parent and raising children
- Developing a satisfactory sex life

Middle Adulthood (40 to 65 years)

- Adjusting to physical changes
- Having grown children
- Developing leisure-time activities
- Adjusting to aging parents

Late Adulthood (65 years and older)

- Adjusting to decreased strength and loss of health
- Adjusting to retirement and reduced income
- Coping with a partner's death
- Developing new friends and relationships
- Preparing for one's own death

- *Children as caregivers*—Some children care for older parents. Parents and children change roles. The child cares for the parent. This helps some older persons feel more secure. Others feel unwanted, in the way, and useless. Some lose dignity and self-respect. Tensions may occur among the child, parent, and other household members. Lack of privacy is a cause. So are disagreements and criticisms about housekeeping, raising children, cooking, and friends.

- *Death of a partner*—A person may try to prepare for a partner's death. When death occurs, the loss is crushing. No amount of preparation is ever enough for the emptiness and changes that result. The person loses a lover, friend, companion, and confidant. Grief may be very great. The person's life will likely change. Serious physical and mental health problems may result. Some lose the will to live. Some attempt suicide.

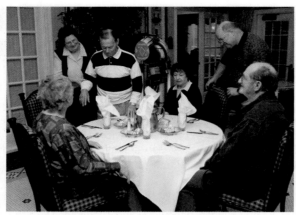

FIGURE 7-1 These older persons are nursing center volunteers.

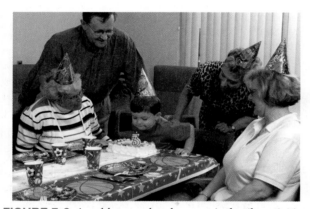

FIGURE 7-2 An older couple takes part in family activities.

PHYSICAL CHANGES

Physical changes occur with aging. Body processes slow down. Energy level and body efficiency decline. The changes occur over many years. Often they are not seen for a long time.

The Integumentary System

The skin loses its elasticity, strength, and fatty tissue layer. The skin thins and sags. Folds, lines, and wrinkles appear. Oil and sweat secretion decreases. Dry skin occurs. The skin is fragile and easily injured. Skin breakdown, skin tears, and pressure ulcers are risks (Chapter 23).

Brown spots—"age spots" or "liver spots"—appear on the skin. They are common on the wrists and hands.

The loss of the skin's fatty tissue layer makes the person more sensitive to cold. Protect the person from drafts and cold. Sweaters, lap blankets, socks, and extra blankets are helpful. So are higher thermostat settings.

The skin has fewer nerve endings. This affects the sensing of heat, cold, and pain. Burns are great risks. Fragile skin, poor circulation, and decreased sensing of heat and cold increase the risk of burns.

Dry skin causes itching. It is easily damaged. A shower or bath twice a week is enough for hygiene. Partial baths are taken at other times. Mild soaps or soap substitutes are used to clean the underarms, genitals, and under the breasts. Often soap is not used on the arms, legs, back, chest, and abdomen. Lotions, oils, and creams prevent drying and itching. Deodorants may not be needed. Sweat gland secretion is decreased.

Nails become thick and tough. Feet usually have poor circulation. A nick or cut can lead to a serious infection. Socks are helpful if the person complains of cold feet.

White or gray hair is common. Hair loss occurs in men. Hair thins on men and women. Thinning occurs on the head, in the pubic area, and under the arms. Facial hair (lip and chin) may occur in women.

Hair is drier from decreases in scalp oils. Brushing promotes circulation and oil production. Shampoo frequency depends on personal choice. It is done as needed for hygiene and comfort.

See Chapter 15 for hygiene. See Chapter 16 for grooming.

The Musculoskeletal System

Muscle cells decrease in number. Muscles atrophy (shrink). They decrease in strength. Bones lose strength, become brittle, and break easily. Joints become stiff and painful.

Vertebrae shorten. Hip and knee joints flex (bend) slightly. These changes cause gradual loss of height and strength. Mobility also decreases.

Activity, exercise, and diet help prevent bone loss and loss of muscle strength. Walking is good exercise. Exercise groups and range-of-motion exercises are helpful (Chapter 22). A diet high in protein, calcium, and vitamins is needed.

Bones can break easily. Protect the person from injury and prevent falls (Chapters 8 and 9). Turn and move the person gently and carefully (Chapter 13). Some persons need help and support getting out of bed. Some need help walking.

The Nervous System

Nerve cells are lost. Nerve conduction and reflexes slow. Responses are slower.

Blood flow to the brain is reduced. Dizziness may occur. It increases the risk for falls.

Changes occur in brain cells. This affects personality and mental function. So does reduced blood flow to the brain. Memory is shorter. Forgetfulness increases. Responses slow. Confusion, dizziness, and fatigue may occur. Long ago events are easier to re-call than recent ones. Many older people are mentally active and involved in current events. They show fewer personality and mental changes.

Less sleep is needed. Loss of energy and decreased blood flow may cause fatigue. They may rest or nap during the day. They may go to bed early and get up early. Sleep periods are shorter.

The Senses

Hearing and vision losses occur (Chapter 26). Taste and smell dull. Touch and sensitivity to pain and pressure are reduced. So is sensing heat and cold. These changes increase the risk for injury. The person may not notice painful injuries or diseases. Or the person feels minor pain. You need to:

- Protect older persons from injury (Chapters 8 and 9).
- Give good skin care (Chapter 15).
- Follow safety measures for heat and cold (Chapter 23).
- Check for signs of skin breakdown (Chapter 23).
- Prevent pressure ulcers (Chapter 23).

The Circulatory System

The heart muscle weakens. It pumps blood with less force. Activity, exercise, excitement, and illness increase the body's need for oxygen and nutrients. A damaged or weak heart cannot meet these needs.

Arteries narrow and are less elastic. Less blood flows through them. Poor circulation occurs in many body parts. A weak heart must work harder to pump blood through narrowed vessels.

Blood vessels decrease in number. Bruising and delayed healing are risks.

Sometimes circulatory changes are severe. Rest is needed during the day. The person should not walk far, climb many stairs, or carry heavy things. Personal care items, TV, phone, and other needed items are kept nearby. Doctors may order certain exercises and activity limits.

The Respiratory System

Respiratory muscles weaken. Lung tissue becomes less elastic. Difficult, labored, or painful breathing (*dyspnea*) may occur with activity. (*Dys* means difficult. *Pnea* means breathing.) The person may lack strength to cough and clear the airway of secretions. Respiratory infections and diseases may develop. These can threaten the older person's life.

Normal breathing is promoted. Avoid heavy bed linens over the chest. They prevent normal chest expansion. Turning, repositioning, and deep breathing are important. They help prevent respiratory complications from bedrest. Breathing usually is easier in semi-Fowler's position (Chapter 14). The person should be as active as possible.

The Digestive System

Salivary glands produce less saliva. This can cause difficulty swallowing (*dysphagia*). (*Dys* means difficult. *Phagia* means swallowing.) Dry foods may be hard to swallow. Taste and smell dull. This decreases appetite.

Secretion of digestive juices decreases. As a result, fried and fatty foods are hard to digest. They may cause indigestion.

Loss of teeth and ill-fitting dentures cause chewing problems. Hard-to-chew foods are avoided. Ground or chopped meat is easier to chew and swallow. Or food is pureed.

Peristalsis decreases. The stomach and colon empty slower. Flatulence and constipation can occur (Chapter 18).

Dry, fried, and fatty foods are avoided. This helps swallowing and digestion problems. Oral hygiene and denture care improve taste. Some people do not have teeth or dentures.

High-fiber foods are hard to chew and can irritate the intestines. They include apricots, celery, and fruits and vegetables with skins and seeds. Persons with chewing problems or constipation often need foods that provide soft bulk. They include whole-grain cereals and cooked fruits and vegetables.

The Urinary System

Kidney function decreases. The kidneys shrink (atrophy). Blood flow to the kidneys is reduced. Waste removal is less efficient. Urine is more concentrated.

The ureters, bladder, and urethra lose tone and elasticity. Bladder muscles weaken. Bladder size decreases. Therefore the bladder stores less urine. Urinary frequency or urgency may occur. Many older persons have to urinate during the night. Urinary incontinence (inability to control the passage of urine from the bladder) may occur (Chapter 17).

In men, the prostate gland enlarges. This puts pressure on the urethra. Difficulty urinating or frequent urination occurs.

Urinary tract infections are risks. Adequate fluids are needed. The person needs water, juices, milk, and gelatin. Provide fluids according to the care plan. Most fluids should be taken before 1700 (5:00 PM). This reduces the need to urinate during the night.

Persons with incontinence may need bladder training programs. Sometimes catheters are needed. See Chapter 17.

The Reproductive System

Reproductive organs change with aging.

- *Men.* The hormone *testosterone* decreases. It affects strength, sperm production, and reproductive tissues. These changes affect sexual activity. An erection takes longer. The phase between erection and orgasm also is longer. Orgasm is less forceful than when younger. Erections are lost quickly. The time between erections also is longer.
- *Women.* **Menopause** is when menstruation stops and menstrual cycles end. The woman can no longer have children. This occurs between 45 and 55 years of age. Female hormones (*estrogen* and *progesterone*) decrease. The uterus, vagina, and genitalia shrink (atrophy). Vaginal walls thin. There is vaginal dryness. These make intercourse uncomfortable or painful. Arousal takes longer. Orgasm is less intense.

NEEDING NURSING CENTER CARE

Some older persons cannot care for themselves. Nursing centers are options for them (Chapter 1). Some people stay in nursing centers until death. Others stay until they can return home. The nursing center is the person's temporary or permanent home. The setting is as home-like as possible.

The person needing nursing center care may suffer some or all of these losses:

- Loss of identity as a productive member of a family and community
- Loss of possessions—home, household items, car, and so on
- Loss of independence
- Loss of real-world experiences—shopping, traveling, cooking, driving, hobbies, and so on
- Loss of health and mobility

These losses may cause a person to feel useless, powerless, and hopeless. The health team helps the person cope with loss and improve quality of life. Treat the person with dignity and respect. Also practice good communication skills. Follow the care plan.

SEXUALITY

Sexuality is the physical, emotional, social, cultural, and spiritual factors that affect a person's feelings and attitudes about his or her sex. Part of the whole person, sexuality involves the personality and the body. It affects how a person behaves, thinks, dresses, and responds to others.

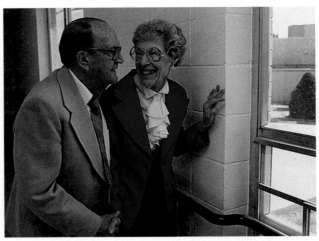

FIGURE 7-3 Relationships develop in nursing centers.

Love, affection, and intimacy are needed throughout life. Attitudes and sex needs change with aging. They are affected by life events. These include divorce, death of a partner, relationship break-ups, injury, illness, and surgery. However, sexual relationships remain important to older persons (Fig. 7-3). They love and fall in love, hold hands, embrace, and have sex.

Frequency of sex decreases for many older persons. Besides life events, reasons relate to weakness, fatigue, and pain. Reduced mobility, aging, and chronic illness are factors.

Some older people do not have intercourse. This does not mean loss of sexual needs or desires. Often needs are expressed in other ways. They hold hands, touch, caress, and embrace. These bring closeness and intimacy.

Meeting Sexual Needs

The nursing team promotes the meeting of sexual needs. The measures in Box 7-2 may be part of the person's care plan.

Married couples in nursing centers can share the same room. This is a requirement of the Omnibus Budget Reconciliation Act of 1987 (OBRA). They can share the same bed if their health permits. Single persons may develop relationships. They are allowed time together, not kept apart.

The Sexually Aggressive Person

Some patients and residents flirt or make sexual advances or comments. Some expose themselves, masturbate, or touch the staff. Often there are reasons for the person's behavior. Understanding this helps you deal with the matter.

BOX 7-2   Promoting Sexuality

- Let the person practice grooming routines. Assist as needed. For women, this includes applying makeup, nail polish, and cologne. Many women shave their legs and underarms and pluck eyebrows. Men may use after-shave lotion and cologne. Hair care is important to men and women.
- Let the person choose clothing. Street clothes are worn if the person's condition permits.
- Protect the right to privacy. Do not expose the person. Drape and screen the person.
- Accept the person's sexual relationships. The person may not share your sexual attitudes, values, or practices. The person may have a homosexual, premarital, or extramarital relationship. Do not judge or gossip about relationships.
- Allow privacy. You can usually tell when people want to be alone. If the person has a private room, close the door for privacy. Some agencies have Do Not Disturb signs for doors.
- Let the person and partner know how much time they have alone. For example, remind them about meal times, drugs, and treatments. Tell other staff members that the person wants time alone.
- Knock before you enter any room. This is a simple courtesy that shows respect for privacy.
- Consider the person's roommate. Privacy curtains provide little privacy. They do not block sound. Arrange for privacy when the roommate is out of the room. Sometimes roommates offer to leave for a while. If the roommate cannot leave, the nurse finds a private area.
- Allow privacy for masturbation. It is a normal form of sexual expression. Close the privacy curtain and the door. Knock before you enter any room. This saves you and the person embarrassment. Sometimes confused persons masturbate in public areas. Lead the person to a private area. Or distract him or her with an activity.

Sexually aggressive behaviors have many causes. They include:

- Nervous system disorders
- Confusion, disorientation, and dementia
- Drug side effects
- Fever
- Poor vision

The person may confuse someone with his or her partner. Or the person cannot control behavior. The cause is changes in mental function. The healthy person controls sexual urges. Changes in the brain make control difficult. Sexual behavior in these cases is usually innocent.

Sometimes touch serves to gain attention. For example, Mr. Green cannot speak. He cannot move his right side. Your buttocks are near him. To get your attention, he touches your buttocks. His behavior is not sexual.

Sometimes masturbation is a sexually aggressive behavior. Some persons touch and fondle the genitals for sexual pleasure. However, urinary or reproductive system disorders can cause genital soreness or itching. So can poor hygiene and being wet or soiled from urine or feces. Touching genitals could signal a health problem.

Sometimes touch is sexual. For example, a man wants to prove that he is attractive and can perform sexually. You must be professional about the matter.

- Ask the person not to touch you. State the places where you were touched.
- Tell the person that you will not do what he or she wants.
- Tell the person what behaviors make you uncomfortable. Politely ask the person not to act that way.
- Allow privacy if the person is becoming aroused. Provide for safety. Complete a safety check of the room (see the inside of the front book cover). Tell the person when you will return.
- Discuss the matter with the nurse. The nurse can help you understand the behavior.
- Follow the care plan. It has measures to deal with sexually aggressive behaviors. They are based on the cause of the behavior.

See *Focus on Communication: The Sexually Aggressive Person.*

FOCUS ON COMMUNICATION
The Sexually Aggressive Person

Confronting the sexually aggressive person is difficult. This is true for young and older staff and for new and experienced staff. Ask yourself these questions:

- Does the person have a health problem that affects impulse control? If yes, the behavior may not have a sexual purpose.
- Is the person's behavior on purpose? Is the intent sexual? If yes, you must confront the behavior. Be direct and matter-of-fact. For example, you can say:
  - "You brushed your hand across my breast (or other body part) two times this morning. Please don't do that again."
  - "No, I cannot kiss you. It would be unprofessional for me to do so."
  - "You exposed yourself to me again today. Please do not do that again."

The sexually aggressive person needs the nurse's attention. Discuss the matter with the nurse. Report what happened and when. Also report what you said and did. The nurse must deal with the problem. If other staff are reporting such behaviors, the nurse views the problem in a broader and different way.

Protecting the Person

The person must be protected from unwanted sexual comments and advances. This is sexual abuse (Chapter 2). Tell the nurse right away. No one should be allowed to sexually abuse another person. This includes staff members, patients, residents, family members or other visitors, and volunteers.

Focus on P R I D E
The Person, Family, and Yourself

Personal and Professional Responsibility—Most nursing centers receive Medicare or Medicaid funds. They must meet OBRA requirements. Surveys are conducted for center compliance. If requirements are not met, funding is lost. Surveys are not announced. A survey team will:

- Review policies, procedures, and medical records
- Interview staff, patients and residents, and families
- Check for cleanliness and safety
- Make sure staff meets state requirements
- Observe how care is given

You may be observed during a survey. Or you may be asked questions. You must provide safe, quality care and protect the person's rights. Also, you must help keep the agency clean and follow agency policies and procedures. Answer survey questions completely and honestly. Always act in a professional manner. And have good work ethics (Chapter 3).

You may be tempted to act differently when surveyors are present. This is wrong. Your conduct and care must reflect a normal day. It is your professional responsibility to provide the same quality care every day.

Rights and Respect—A person's home is more than a place to live. It brings pride and self-esteem. Aging can lead to changes in a person's home setting. A nursing center provides a temporary or permanent residence for some persons.

The person's setting must promote quality of life. It must be clean, safe, comfortable, and as home-like as possible. Give care that reflects these principles. To do so:

- Make sure the person, clothes, and linens are clean and dry.
- Keep the person's room clean and orderly. This includes measures to prevent or reduce noise and odors.
- Place soiled linens in designated containers. Empty the containers often. Do not let them overflow.
- Clean up after giving care.
- Help the person display personal items if asked. Do not touch the person's items without permission.
- Treat the person as if you were in his or her home.
- Respect the person and his or her environment.

Independence and Social Interaction—The social changes of aging can cause loneliness. If nursing center care is needed, the loneliness can seem even greater. The person may be in the same building with other people. However, those people do not replace relationships with family and friends. To help the person feel less lonely, you can:

- Suggest that the person call a family member or friend. Offer to assist with finding phone numbers and dialing.
- Keep the phone within the person's reach. This helps him or her place or answer calls with ease.
- Suggest that the person read cards and letters. Offer to assist.
- Visit with the person a few times during your shift.
- Introduce new residents to other residents and staff.

Delegation and Teamwork—Some persons will display sexually aggressive behavior. The health team must work together to deal with such persons. If someone makes you uncomfortable, tell the nurse. The nurse needs to talk to the person. Sometimes the person's behavior cannot be controlled. The nurse may need to change care assignments. Or certain tasks may be delegated to different staff. Bathing and hygiene measures are examples. The team must communicate professionally about the person and his or her conduct. The team must be flexible and willing to help each other in all situations.

Ethics and Laws—The Older Americans Act requires a long-term care ombudsman program in every state (Chapter 1). An ombudsman supports or promotes the needs and interests of another person. Long-term care ombudsmen are employed by a state agency. Some are volunteers. They are not nursing center employees. They act on behalf of nursing center and assisted-living residents. Their services are useful when:

- There is concern about a person's care or treatment.
- Someone interferes with a person's rights, health, safety, or welfare.

Ombudsmen:

- Investigate and resolve complaints
- Provide services to assist residents
- Provide information about long-term care services
- Monitor nursing center care and conditions
- Provide support to resident and family groups
- Represent residents' interests before local, state, and federal governments

Residents have the right to voice grievances and disputes. Nursing centers must post the names, addresses, and phone numbers of local and state ombudsmen. You must know state and center policies and procedures for contacting an ombudsman.

REVIEW QUESTIONS

Circle the BEST answer.

1   Which is a developmental task of late adulthood?
   a   Accepting changes in appearance
   b   Adjusting to decreased strength
   c   Developing a satisfactory sex life
   d   Performing self-care

2   Retirement usually means
   a   Lowered income
   b   Changes from aging
   c   Less free time
   d   Financial security

3   Which does *not* cause loneliness in older persons?
   a   Children moving away
   b   The death of family and friends
   c   Problems communicating with others
   d   Contact with other older persons

4   These statements are about a partner's death. Which is *false?*
   a   The person loses a lover, friend, companion, and confidant.
   b   Preparing for the event lessens grief.
   c   The survivor may develop health problems.
   d   The survivor's life will likely change.

5   Skin changes occur with aging. Care should include the following *except*
   a   Providing for warmth
   b   Applying lotion
   c   A daily bath with soap
   d   Providing good skin care

6   Aging causes changes in the musculoskeletal system. Which is *false?*
   a   Bones become brittle. They can break easily.
   b   Bedrest is needed for loss of strength.
   c   Joints become stiff and painful.
   d   Exercise slows musculoskeletal changes.

7   Changes occur in the nervous system. Which is *true?*
   a   Less sleep is needed than when younger.
   b   The person forgets events from long ago.
   c   Sensitivity to pain increases.
   d   Confusion occurs in all older persons.

8   An older person has cardiovascular changes. Care includes the following *except*
   a   Placing needed items nearby
   b   A moderate amount of daily exercise
   c   Avoiding exertion
   d   Long walks

9   Respiratory changes occur with aging. Which is *false?*
   a   Heavy bed linens are avoided.
   b   The person is turned often if on bedrest.
   c   The side-lying position is best for breathing.
   d   The person should be as active as possible.

10   Older persons should avoid dry foods because of
   a   Decreases in saliva
   b   Loss of teeth or ill-fitting dentures
   c   Decreased amounts of digestive juices
   d   Decreased peristalsis

11   The doctor orders increased fluid intake for an older person. You should give most of the fluid before
   a   1700 (5:00 PM)
   b   1900 (7:00 PM)
   c   2100 (9:00 PM)
   d   2300 (11:00 PM)

12   Changes occur in the reproductive system. Which is *true?*
   a   Hormones decrease.
   b   Orgasms do not occur.
   c   Men experience menopause.
   d   The prostate gland decreases in size.

13   A person is masturbating in the dining room. You should do the following *except*
   a   Cover the person and quietly take the person to his or her room
   b   Scold the person
   c   Provide privacy
   d   Tell the nurse

14   A person touches you sexually and asks for a kiss. You should do the following *except*
   a   Discuss the matter with the nurse
   b   Do what the person asks
   c   Explain that the behaviors make you uncomfortable
   d   Ask the person not to touch you

Answers to these questions are on p. 527.

8

PROMOTING SAFETY

PROCEDURES

- Relieving Choking—Adult or Child (Over 1 Year of Age)
- Using a Fire Extinguisher

OBJECTIVES

- Define the key terms and key abbreviations listed in this chapter.
- Describe accident risk factors.
- Explain why you identify a person before giving care.
- Explain how to correctly identify a person.
- Describe the safety measures to prevent burns, poisoning, and suffocation.
- Identify the signs and causes of choking.
- Explain how to prevent equipment accidents.
- Explain how to safely use wheelchairs and stretchers.
- Explain how to handle hazardous substances.
- Describe safety measures for fire prevention and oxygen use.
- Explain what to do during a fire.
- Give examples of natural and human-made disasters.
- Explain how to protect yourself from workplace violence.
- Describe your role in risk management.
- Explain how to use color-coded wristbands.
- Explain how to promote PRIDE in the person, the family, and yourself.
- Perform the procedures described in this chapter.

KEY TERMS

coma A state of being unaware of one's surroundings and being unable to react or respond to people, places, or things

dementia The loss of cognitive and social function caused by changes in the brain

disaster A sudden catastrophic event in which people are injured and killed and property is destroyed

hazardous substance Any chemical in the workplace that can cause harm

paralysis Loss of muscle function, loss of sensation, or loss of both muscle function and sensation

suffocation When breathing stops from the lack of oxygen

workplace violence Violent acts (including assault and threat of assault) directed toward persons at work or while on duty

KEY ABBREVIATIONS

AED Automated external defibrillator

CPR Cardiopulmonary resuscitation

EMS Emergency Medical Services

FBAO Foreign-body airway obstruction

ID Identification

MSDS Material safety data sheet

OSHA Occupational Safety and Health Administration

RRT Rapid Response Team

Safety is a basic need. You must protect patients and residents, visitors, yourself, and co-workers. The safety measures in this chapter apply to health care settings and everyday life. The care plan lists other safety measures needed by the person. The goal is to prevent accidents and injuries without limiting the person's mobility and independence.

ACCIDENT RISK FACTORS

Some people cannot protect themselves. They rely on others for safety. Certain factors increase the risk of accidents and injuries. Follow the person's care plan to provide for safety. Also see *Persons With Dementia: Accident Risk Factors.*

- *Age.* Body changes occur from aging. Older persons have decreased strength, move slowly, and are less steady. Often balance is affected. Older persons also are less sensitive to heat and cold. They have poor vision, hearing problems, and a dulled sense of smell. Confusion, poor judgment,

PERSONS WITH DEMENTIA
Accident Risk Factors

Dementia is the loss of cognitive and social function caused by changes in the brain (Chapter 28). *Cognitive* relates to knowledge. Cognitive function involves memory, thinking, reasoning, understanding, judgment, and behavior.

Persons with dementia are confused and disoriented. Their awareness of surroundings is reduced. They may not understand what is happening to and around them. Judgment is poor. They no longer know what is safe and what are dangers. They may access closets, cupboards, or other unsafe and unlocked areas. They may eat or drink cleaning products, drugs, or poisons. The health team must meet all safety needs.

memory problems, and disorientation may occur (Chapter 28).

- *Awareness of surroundings.* **Coma** is a state of being unaware of one's surroundings and being unable to react or respond to people, places, or things. The person relies on others for protection. Confused and disoriented persons may not understand what is happening to and around them.
- *Agitated and aggressive behaviors.* Pain can cause these behaviors. So can confusion, decreased awareness of surroundings, and fear of what may happen.
- *Impaired vision.* Persons with poor vision may not see toys, rugs, equipment, furniture, and cords. Some have problems reading labels on cleaners, drugs, and other containers. Poisoning can result.
- *Impaired hearing.* Persons with impaired hearing have problems hearing explanations and instructions. They may not hear warning signals or fire alarms. Some cannot hear approaching meal carts, drug carts, stretchers, or people in wheelchairs. They do not know to move to safety.
- *Impaired smell and touch.* Illness and aging affect smell and touch. The person may not detect smoke or gas odors. When touch is reduced, burns are a risk. The person has problems sensing heat and cold. Some people have a decreased pain sense. They may be unaware of injury.
- *Impaired mobility.* Some diseases and injuries affect mobility. A person may know there is danger but cannot move to safety. Some persons cannot walk or propel wheelchairs. Some persons are paralyzed. **Paralysis** means loss of muscle function, loss of sensation, or loss of both muscle function and sensation.
- *Drugs.* Drugs have side effects. They include loss of balance, drowsiness, and lack of coordination. Reduced awareness, confusion, and disorientation can occur.

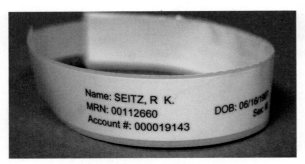

FIGURE 8-1 ID bracelet.

IDENTIFYING THE PERSON

Each person has different treatments, therapies, and activity limits. Life and health are threatened if the wrong care is given.

The person receives an identification (ID) bracelet when admitted to the agency (Fig. 8-1). The bracelet has the person's name, room and bed number, birth date, age, doctor, and other identifying information.

You use the bracelet to identify the person before giving care. The assignment sheet states what care to give. To identify the person:

- Compare identifying information on the assignment sheet with that on the ID bracelet (Fig. 8-2). Carefully check the information. Some people have the same first and last names. For example, John Smith is a very common name.
- Use at least two identifiers. An identifier cannot be the person's room or bed number. Some agencies require that the person state his or her name and birth date. Others require using the person's ID number. Always follow agency policy.
- Call the person by name when checking the ID bracelet. This is a courtesy given as you touch the person and before giving care. Just calling the person by name is not enough to identify him or her. Confused, disoriented, drowsy, hard-of-hearing, or distracted persons may answer to any name.

See *Promoting Safety and Comfort: Identifying the Person.*

Nursing Center Residents

Alert and oriented residents may choose not to wear ID bracelets. This is noted on the person's care plan. Follow center policy and the care plan to identify the person.

Some nursing centers have photo ID systems (Fig. 8-3). The person's photo is taken on admission. Then it is placed in the person's medical record. If your center uses such a system, learn to use it safely.

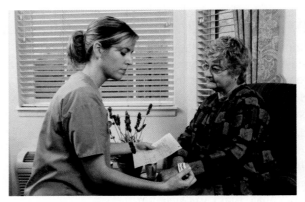

FIGURE 8-2 The ID bracelet is checked against the assignment sheet to accurately identify the person.

PROMOTING SAFETY AND COMFORT
Identifying the Person

Safety

Always identify the person right before you begin a task or procedure. Do not identify the person and then leave the room to collect supplies and equipment. You could go to the wrong room and give care to the wrong person. And the person for whom the care was intended would not receive it. This too could cause harm.

Sometimes ID bracelets become damaged from water, spilled food and fluids, and everyday wear and tear. Make sure you can read the information on the ID bracelet. If you cannot, tell the nurse. The nurse can have a new bracelet made for the person.

Comfort

Make sure the person's ID bracelet is not too tight. You should be able to slide 1 or 2 fingers under the bracelet. If it is too tight, tell the nurse.

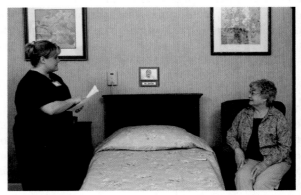

FIGURE 8-3 The person's photo is at the headboard. Her name is under the photo. The nursing assistant is using the photo to identify the person.

PREVENTING BURNS

Smoking, spilled hot liquids, very hot water, and electrical devices are common causes of burns. These safety measures can prevent burns:

- Be sure people smoke only in smoking areas.
- Check the person's care plan about leaving smoking materials at the bedside.
- Supervise the smoking of persons who cannot protect themselves.
- Do not allow smoking in bed.
- Do not allow smoking where oxygen is used or stored (Chapter 24).
- Be alert to ashes that may fall onto a person.
- Keep hot food and liquids away from counter and table edges.
- Do not pour hot liquids near a person.
- Turn on cold water first, then hot water. Turn off hot water first, then cold water.
- Measure bath or shower water temperature (Chapter 15). Check it before a person gets into the tub or shower.
- Check for "hot spots" in bath water. Move your hand back and forth.
- Do not let the person use a heating pad or an electric blanket.
- Follow safety guidelines when applying heat and cold (Chapter 23).

PREVENTING POISONING

Drugs and household products are common poisons. Poisoning in adults may be from carelessness, confusion, or poor vision when reading labels. To prevent poisoning:

- Make sure patients and residents cannot reach hazardous materials (p. 112).
- Follow agency policy for storing personal care items. Shampoo, mouthwash, lotion, perfume, and deodorant are examples. These products are harmful when swallowed.

PREVENTING SUFFOCATION

Suffocation is when breathing stops from the lack of oxygen. Death occurs if the person does not start breathing. Common causes include choking, drowning, inhaling gas or smoke, strangulation, and electrical shock. Entrapment in the hospital bed system is another cause (Chapter 14).

Measures to prevent suffocation are listed in Box 8-1. Clear the airway if the person is choking.

BOX 8-1	Safety Measures to Prevent Suffocation

- Cut food into small, bite-sized pieces for persons who cannot do so themselves.
- Make sure dentures fit properly and are in place.
- Make sure the person can chew and swallow the food served.
- Report loose teeth or dentures.
- Check the care plan for swallowing problems before serving snacks or fluids. The person may ask for something that he or she cannot swallow.
- Tell the nurse at once if the person has swallowing problems.
- Do not give oral food or fluids to persons with feeding tubes (Chapter 19).
- Follow aspiration precautions (Chapter 19).
- Do not leave a person unattended in a bathtub or shower.
- Move all persons from the area if you smell smoke.
- Position the person in bed properly (Chapter 12).
- Use bed rails correctly (Chapter 9).
- Use restraints correctly (Chapter 10).
- Prevent entrapment in the bed system (Chapter 14).
- See "Preventing Equipment Accidents" (p. 109).

Choking

Foreign bodies can obstruct the airway. This is called *choking* or *foreign-body airway obstruction (FBAO)*. Air cannot pass through the air passages to the lungs. The body does not get enough oxygen. It can lead to cardiac arrest. *Cardiac arrest* is when the heart stops suddenly and without warning (Chapter 29).

Choking often occurs during eating. A large, poorly chewed piece of meat is the most common cause. Laughing and talking while eating also are common causes. So is excessive alcohol intake.

Choking can occur in the unconscious person. Common causes are aspiration of vomitus and the tongue falling back into the airway. These occur during cardiac arrest.

Foreign bodies can cause mild or severe airway obstruction. With *mild airway obstruction,* some air moves in and out of the lungs. The person is conscious. Usually the person can speak. Often forceful coughing can remove the object. The person's

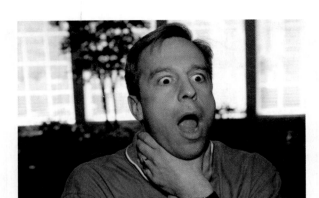

FIGURE 8-4 A choking person clutches at the throat.

breathing may sound like wheezing between coughs. To help a person with mild airway obstruction:

- Stay with the person.
- Encourage the person to keep coughing to expel the object.
- Do not interrupt the person's efforts to clear the airway. If the person is breathing and coughing, abdominal thrusts are not needed.
- If the obstruction persists, call for help.

A person with *severe airway obstruction* has difficulty breathing. Air does not move in and out of the lungs. The person may not be able to breathe, speak, or cough. If the person can cough, the cough is of poor quality. When the person tries to inhale, there is no noise or a high-pitched noise. The person may appear pale and cyanotic (bluish color).

The conscious person clutches at the throat (Fig. 8-4). Clutching at the throat is often called the "universal sign of choking." The conscious person is very frightened. If the obstruction is not removed, the person will die. Severe airway obstruction is an emergency.

Relieving Choking

Abdominal thrusts are used to relieve severe airway obstruction. Abdominal thrusts are quick, upward thrusts to the abdomen. They force air out of the lungs and create an artificial cough. They are done to try to expel the foreign body from the airway.

Abdominal thrusts are not used for very obese persons or pregnant women. Chest thrusts are used.

Relief of choking occurs when the foreign body is removed. Or it occurs when you feel air move and see the chest rise and fall when giving rescue breaths. The person may still be unresponsive.

Self-Administered Abdominal Thrusts You may choke when by yourself. You can perform abdominal thrusts to relieve the obstructed airway. To do so:

1. Make a fist with one hand.
2. Place the thumb side of the fist above your navel and below the lower end of the sternum.
3. Grasp your fist with your other hand.
4. Press inward and upward quickly.
5. Press the upper abdomen against a hard surface if the thrust did not relieve the obstruction. Use the back of a chair, a table, or railing.
6. Use as many thrusts as needed.

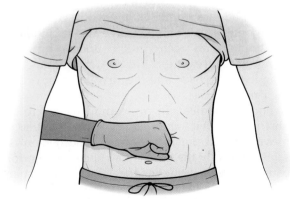

A

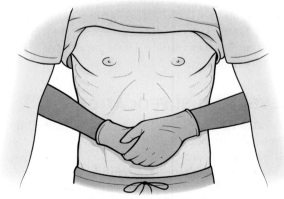

B

FIGURE 8-5 Hand positioning for abdominal thrusts. **A,** The fist is slightly above the navel in the midline of the abdomen. **B,** The other hand clasps the fist.

RELIEVING CHOKING—ADULT OR CHILD (Over 1 Year of Age)

PROCEDURE

1 Ask the person if he or she is choking. Help the person if he or she nods "yes" and cannot talk.
2 Have someone call for help:
   a *In a public area,* have someone activate the Emergency Medical Services (EMS) system by calling 911. Send someone to get an automated external defibrillator (AED). See Chapter 29.
   b *In an agency,* call the agency's Rapid Response Team (RRT). This is a team that quickly responds to provide care in life-threatening situations. Send someone to get the AED.
3 Give abdominal thrusts:
   a Stand or kneel behind the person.
   b Wrap your arms around the person's waist.
   c Make a fist with one hand.
   d Place the thumb side of the fist against the abdomen. The fist is slightly above the navel in the middle of the abdomen and well below the end of the sternum (breastbone). See Fig. 8-5, *A.*
   e Grasp the fist with your other hand (Fig. 8-5, *B*).
   f Press your fist into the person's abdomen with a quick, upward thrust.
   g Repeat thrusts until the object is expelled or the person becomes unresponsive.
4 *If the person is obese or pregnant,* give chest thrusts:
   a Stand behind the person.
   b Place your arms under the person's underarms. Wrap your arms around the person's chest.
   c Make a fist. Place the thumb side of the fist on the middle of the sternum (breastbone).
   d Grasp the fist with your other hand.
   e Give thrusts to the chest until the object is expelled or the person becomes unresponsive.
5 *If the object is dislodged,* encourage the person to go to the hospital. Injuries can occur from abdominal or chest thrusts.

6 *If the person becomes unresponsive,* lower the person to the floor or ground. Position the person supine (lying flat on the back). Make sure EMS or the RRT was called (step 2). If alone, provide 5 cycles (2 minutes) of CPR first. Then call EMS or the RRT.
7 Start CPR. See Chapter 29.
   a Do not check for a pulse. Begin with compressions. Give 30 compressions. Chest compressions help dislodge an obstruction.
   b Use the head tilt-chin lift method to open the airway (Fig. 8-6). Open the person's mouth. The mouth should be wide open. Look for an object. Remove the object if you see it and can remove it easily. Use your fingers.
   c Give 2 breaths.
   d Continue cycles of 30 compressions and 2 breaths. Look for an object every time you open the airway for rescue breaths.
8 *If you relieve choking in an unresponsive person:*
   a Check for a response, breathing, and a pulse.
      (1) *If no response, normal breathing, or pulse—* continue CPR. Attach an AED (Chapter 29).
      (2) *If no response and no normal breathing but there is a pulse—*give rescue breaths. For an adult, give 1 breath every 5 to 6 seconds (10 to 12 breaths per minute). For a child, give 1 breath every 3 to 5 seconds (12 to 20 breaths per minute). Check for a pulse every 2 minutes. If no pulse, begin CPR.
      (3) *If the person has normal breathing and a pulse—*place the person in the recovery position if there is no response (Chapter 29). Continue to check the person until help arrives. Encourage the person to go to the hospital if the person responds.

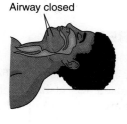 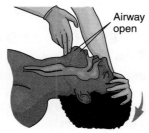

Airway closed

Airway open

FIGURE 8-6 The head tilt-chin lift method opens the airway. One hand is on the person's forehead. Pressure is applied to lift the head back. The chin is lifted with the fingers of the other hand.

PREVENTING EQUIPMENT ACCIDENTS

All equipment is unsafe if broken, not used correctly, or not working properly. This includes hospital beds (Chapter 14). Inspect all equipment before use. Check glass and plastic items for cracks, chips, and sharp or rough edges. They can cause cuts, stabs, or scratches. Follow the Bloodborne Pathogen Standard (Chapter 11). Also practice the safety measures in Box 8-2, p. 110.

BOX 8-2 Safety Measures to Prevent Equipment Accidents

General Safety

- Follow agency policies and procedures.
- Follow the manufacturer's instructions. Read all caution and warning labels.
- Do not use an unfamiliar item. Ask for needed training. Also ask a nurse to supervise you the first time you use an item.
- Use an item only for its intended purpose.
- Make sure the item works before you begin.
- Make sure you have all needed equipment. For example, you need to plug in an item. There must be an outlet.
- Do not use or give broken or damaged items to patients or residents.
- Show a broken or damaged item to the nurse. Follow the nurse's instructions and agency policies for discarding items or sending them for repair. Do not try to repair broken or damaged items.

Electrical Safety

- Inspect electrical cords and appliances for damage. Make sure they are in good repair.
- Use three-pronged plugs on all electrical devices (Fig. 8-7).
- Do not cover power cords with rugs, carpets, linens, or other materials. Do not run power cords under rugs.
- Connect a bed power cord directly to a wall outlet. Do not connect a bed power cord to an extension cord or outlet strip.
- Do not use electrical items owned by the person until they are safety checked. The maintenance staff does this.
- Keep electrical items away from water.
- Keep work areas clean and dry. Wipe up spills right away.
- Do not touch electrical items if you are wet, if your hands are wet, or if you are standing in water.
- Do not put a finger or any item into an outlet.
- Turn off equipment before unplugging it. Sparks occur when electrical items are unplugged while turned on.
- Hold onto the plug (not the cord) when removing it from an outlet.
- Do not give showers or tub baths during electrical storms. Lightning can travel through pipes.
- Do not use electrical items or phones during storms.
- Do not use water to put out an electrical fire. If possible turn off or unplug the item.
- Do not touch a person who is experiencing an electrical shock. If possible, turn off or unplug the item. Call for help at once.
- Keep electrical cords away from heating vents and other heat sources.
- Turn off the electrical device when done using the item.
- Unplug all electrical devices when not in use.

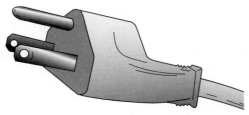

FIGURE 8-7 A three-pronged plug.

Electrical Equipment

Electrical items must work properly and be in good repair. Frayed cords and over-loaded electrical outlets can cause fires, burns, and electrical shocks (Fig. 8-8). *Electrical shock* is when electrical current passes through the body. It can burn the skin, muscles, nerves, and other tissues. It can affect the heart and cause death.

Warning signs of a faulty electrical item include:
- Shocks
- Loss of power or a power outage
- Dimming or flickering lights
- Sparks
- Sizzling or buzzing sounds
- Burning odor
- Loose plugs

WHEELCHAIR AND STRETCHER SAFETY

Some people use wheelchairs (Fig. 8-9). The handgrips/push handles are used to push wheelchairs. Stretchers are used to transport persons who cannot use wheelchairs.

Follow the safety measures in Box 8-3 when using wheelchairs and stretchers. The person can fall from the wheelchair or stretcher. Or the person can fall during transfers to and from the wheelchair or stretcher.

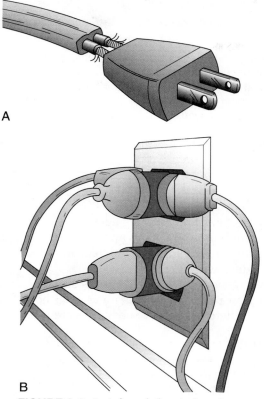

FIGURE 8-8 A, A frayed electrical cord. **B,** An over-loaded electrical outlet.

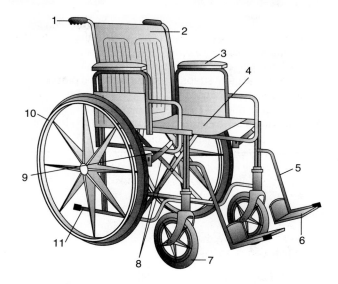

1. Handgrip/push handle	7. Caster
2. Back upholstery	8. Crossbrace
3. Armrest	9. Wheel lock/brake
4. Seat upholstery	10. Wheel and handrim
5. Front rigging	11. Tipping lever
6. Footplate	

FIGURE 8-9 Parts of a wheelchair.

BOX 8-3 Wheelchair and Stretcher Safety

Wheelchair Safety

- Check the wheel locks (brakes). Make sure you can lock and unlock them.
- Check for flat or loose tires. A wheel lock will not work on a flat or loose tire.
- Make sure the wheel spokes are intact. Damaged, broken, or loose spokes can interfere with moving the wheelchair or locking the wheels.
- Make sure the casters point forward. This keeps the wheelchair balanced and stable.
- Position the person's feet on the footplates.
- Make sure the person's feet are on the footplates before moving the chair. The person's feet must not touch or drag on the floor when the chair is moving.
- Push the chair forward when transporting the person. Do not pull the chair backward unless going through a doorway.
- Lock both wheels before you transfer a person to or from the wheelchair.
- Follow the care plan for keeping the wheels locked when not moving the wheelchair. Locking the wheels prevents the chair from moving if the person wants to move to or from the chair. (Locking the wheelchair may be considered a restraint. See Chapter 10.)
- Do not let the person stand on the footplates.
- Do not let the footplates fall back onto the person's legs.
- Make sure the person has needed wheelchair accessories—safety belt, pouch, tray, lapboard, cushion.
- Remove the armrests (if removable) when the person transfers to the bed, toilet, commode, tub, or car (Chapter 13).
- Swing front rigging out of the way for transfers to and from the wheelchair. Some front riggings detach for transfers.
- Clean the wheelchair according to agency policy.
- Ask a nurse or physical therapist to show you how to propel wheelchairs up steps and ramps and over curbs.
- Follow the safety measures to prevent equipment accidents.

Continued

BOX 8-3 | Wheelchair and Stretcher Safety—cont'd

Stretcher Safety

- Ask two co-workers to help you transfer the person to or from the stretcher (Chapter 13).
- Lock the stretcher wheels before the transfer.
- Fasten the safety straps when the person is properly positioned on the stretcher.
- Ask a co-worker to help with the transport.
- Raise the side rails. Keep them up during the transport.

- Make sure the person's arms, hands, legs, and feet do not dangle through the side rail bars.
- Stand at the head of the stretcher. Your co-worker stands at the foot of the stretcher.
- Move the stretcher feet first (Fig. 8-10).
- Do not leave the person alone.
- Follow the safety measures to prevent equipment accidents.

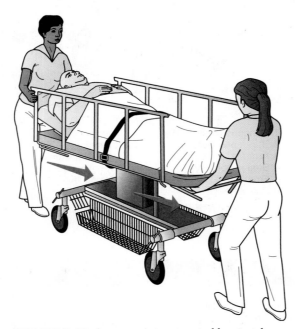

FIGURE 8-10 A person is transported by stretcher. The stretcher is moved feet first.

HANDLING HAZARDOUS SUBSTANCES

A **hazardous substance** is any chemical in the workplace that can cause harm. *Physical hazards* can cause fires or explosions. *Health hazards* are chemicals that can cause health problems. Hazardous substances include:

- Drugs used in cancer therapy (chemotherapy, anti-cancer drugs)
- Anesthesia gases
- Gases used to sterilize equipment
- Oxygen
- Disinfectants and cleaning agents
- Radiation used for x-rays and cancer treatments
- Mercury (found in thermometers and blood pressure devices)

Your agency provides hazardous substance training. It also provides eyewash and total body wash stations where hazardous substances are used.

Labeling

Hazardous substance containers need warning labels (Fig. 8-11). The manufacturer supplies all labels. Warning labels identify:

- Physical and health hazards
- Precaution measures (For example, "Do not use near open flame." Or "Avoid skin contact.")
- What personal protective equipment to wear—gown, mask, gloves, goggles, and so on
- How to use the substance safely
- Storage and disposal information

A container must have a label. If a warning label is removed or damaged, do not use the substance. Take the container to the nurse, and explain the problem. Do not leave the container unattended.

Material Safety Data Sheets

Every hazardous substance has a material safety data sheet (MSDS). It gives detailed information about the substance. Check the MSDS before using a hazardous substance, cleaning up a leak or spill, or disposing of the substance. Tell the nurse about a leak or spill right away. Do not leave a leak or spill unattended.

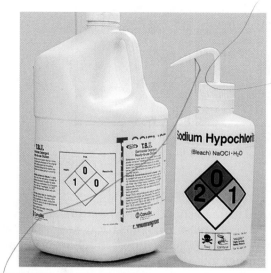

FIGURE 8-11 Warning labels on hazardous substances.

FIRE SAFETY

Faulty electrical equipment and wiring, over-loaded electrical circuits, and smoking are major causes of fires. The health team must prevent fires (Box 8-4) and act quickly during a fire.

Fire and the Use of Oxygen

Three things are needed for a fire:
- A spark or flame
- A material that will burn
- Oxygen

Air has some oxygen. However, doctors order oxygen therapy for some people (Chapter 24). Safety measures are needed where oxygen is used and stored:

- "No Smoking" signs are placed on the door and near the bed.
- The person and visitors are reminded not to smoke in the room.
- Smoking materials (cigarettes, cigars, and pipes), matches, and lighters are removed from the room.
- Safety measures to prevent equipment accidents are followed.
- Wool blankets and synthetic fabrics that cause static electricity are removed from the person's room.
- The person wears a cotton gown or pajamas.
- Materials that ignite easily are removed from the room. They include oil, grease, nail polish remover, and so on.

See *Focus on Communication: Fire and the Use of Oxygen.*

BOX 8-4 **Fire Prevention Measures**

- Practice safety measures to prevent burns.
- Practice safety measures to prevent equipment accidents.
- Follow the safety measures for oxygen use.
- Smoke only where allowed to do so.
- Be sure all ashes, cigars, cigarettes, and other smoking materials are out before emptying ashtrays.
- Empty ashtrays into a metal container partially filled with sand or water. Do not empty ashtrays into plastic containers or wastebaskets lined with paper or plastic bags.
- Provide ashtrays for persons who are allowed to smoke.
- Supervise persons who smoke. This is very important for persons who are confused, disoriented, or sedated.
- Keep matches, lighters, and flammable liquids and materials away from persons who are confused or disoriented.
- Do not leave cooking unattended on stoves, in ovens, or in microwave ovens.
- Store flammable liquids in their original containers. Follow the manufacturer's instructions.
- Do not light matches or lighters or smoke around flammable liquids or materials.

FOCUS ON COMMUNICATION
Fire and the Use of Oxygen

You may have to remind a patient, resident, or visitor not to smoke inside the agency. You can simply say:
- "Mrs. Murphy, this is a smoke-free area. Here is an ashtray to put out your cigarette. If you want to smoke, I'll be happy to show you the smoking area outside."
- "Mr. Garcia, please don't smoke inside the center. We have a smoking area outside the back entrance on hallway 2. I'll be happy to show you the way."

Tell the nurse what happened, what you said, and what you did. The nurse may need to speak with the person about not smoking.

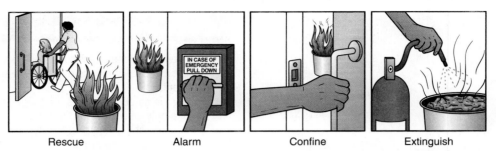

Rescue   Alarm   Confine   Extinguish

FIGURE 8-12 During a fire, RACE: **R**escue, **A**larm, **C**onfine, and **E**xtinguish.

What to Do During a Fire

Know your agency's policies and procedures for fire emergencies. Know where to find fire alarms, fire extinguishers, and emergency exits. Fire drills are held to practice emergency fire procedures. Remember the word RACE (Fig. 8-12):

- *R*—for *rescue.* Rescue persons in immediate danger. Move them to a safe place.
- *A*—for *alarm.* Sound the nearest fire alarm. Notify the switchboard operator.
- *C*—for *confine.* Close doors and windows to confine the fire. Turn off oxygen or electrical items used in the general area of the fire.
- *E*—for *extinguish.* Use a fire extinguisher on a small fire that has not spread to a larger area.

Clear equipment from all normal and emergency exits. *Do not use elevators if there is a fire.*

Using a Fire Extinguisher

Different extinguishers are used for different kinds of fires: oil and grease fires, electrical fires, and paper and wood fires. A general procedure for using a fire extinguisher follows.

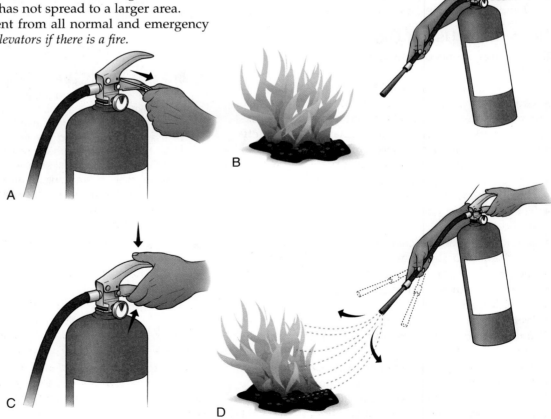

FIGURE 8-13 Using a fire extinguisher. **A,** *Pull* the safety pin. **B,** *Aim* the hose at the base of the fire. **C,** *Squeeze* the top handle down. **D,** *Sweep* back and forth.

USING A FIRE EXTINGUISHER

PROCEDURE

1 Pull the fire alarm
2 Get the nearest fire extinguisher.
3 Carry it upright.
4 Take it to the fire.
5 Follow the word *PASS:*
   a *P*—for *pull the safety pin* (Fig. 8-13, *A*). This unlocks the handle.
   b *A*—for *aim low* (Fig. 8-13, *B*). Direct the hose or nozzle at the base of the fire. Do not try to spray the tops of the flames.

c *S*—for *squeeze the lever* (Fig. 8-13, *C*). Squeeze or push down on the lever, handle, or button to start the stream. Release the lever, handle, or button to stop the stream.
d *S*—for *sweep back and forth* (Fig. 8-13, *D*). Sweep the stream back and forth (side to side) at the base of the fire.

DISASTERS

A **disaster** is a sudden catastrophic event. People are injured and killed. Property is destroyed. Natural disasters include tornadoes, hurricanes, blizzards, earthquakes, volcanic eruptions, floods, and some fires. Human-made disasters include auto, bus, train, and airplane accidents. They also include fires, bombings, nuclear power plant accidents, riots, gas or chemical leaks, explosions, and wars.

Communities, fire and police departments, and health care agencies have disaster plans. They include procedures to deal with the people needing treatment. A disaster may damage the agency. The disaster plan includes evacuation procedures.

Bomb Threats

Agencies have procedures for bomb threats. You must follow them if a caller makes a bomb threat or if you find an item that looks or sounds strange. Often bomb threats are sent by phone, mail, e-mail, messenger, or other means. Or the person can leave a bomb in the agency. If you see a stranger in the agency, tell the nurse at once. You cannot be too safe.

WORKPLACE VIOLENCE

Workplace violence is violent acts (including assault or threat of assault) directed toward persons at work or while on duty. It includes:
- Murders
- Beatings, stabbings, and shootings
- Rapes and sexual assaults
- Use of weapons—firearms, bombs, or knives
- Kidnapping
- Robbery
- Threats—obscene phone calls; threatening oral, written, or body language; and harassment of any nature (being followed, sworn at, or shouted at)

According to the Occupational Safety and Health Administration (OSHA), more assaults occur in health care settings than in other industries. Nurses and nursing assistants are at risk. They have the most contact with patients, residents, and visitors. Risk factors include:
- People with weapons
- Police holds—persons arrested or convicted of crimes
- Acutely disturbed and violent persons seeking health care
- Alcohol and drug abuse
- Mentally ill persons who do not take needed drugs, do not have follow-up care, and are not in hospitals unless they are an immediate threat to themselves or others
- Pharmacies have drugs and are a target for robberies
- Gang members and substance abusers are patients, residents, or visitors
- Upset, agitated, and disturbed family and visitors
- Long waits for emergency or other services
- Being alone with the person during care or transport to other areas
- Low staff levels during meals, emergencies, and at night
- Poor lighting in hallways, rooms, parking lots, and other areas
- Lack of training in recognizing and managing potentially violent situations

OSHA has guidelines for violence prevention programs. Work-site hazards are identified. Prevention measures are developed and followed. The staff receives safety and health training. Box 8-5, p. 116 lists measures to deal with agitated or aggressive persons.

BOX 8-5 Measures to Deal With Agitated or Aggressive Persons

- Stand away from the person. Judge the length of the person's arms and legs. Stand far enough away so that the person cannot hit or kick you.
- Stand close to the door. Do not become trapped in the room.
- Be aware of items in the room that can be used as weapons. Move away from such objects. Examples include vases, phones, radios, letter openers, paper weights, and belts.
- Know where to find panic buttons, signal lights, alarms, closed-circuit monitors, and other security devices.
- Keep your hands free.
- Stay calm. Talk to the person in a calm manner. Do not raise your voice or argue, scold, or interrupt the person.

- Be aware of your body language. Do not point a finger or glare at the person. Do not put your hands on your hips.
- Do not touch the person.
- Tell the person that you will get the nurse to speak to him or her.
- Leave the room as soon as you can. Make sure the person is safe.
- Tell the nurse about the matter. Report items in the room that can be used as weapons.
- Complete an incident report according to agency policy.

RISK MANAGEMENT

Risk management involves identifying and controlling risks and safety hazards affecting the agency. This includes accident and fire prevention, negligence and malpractice, abuse, workplace violence, and federal and state requirements. The intent is to:
- Protect everyone in the agency—patients, residents, visitors, and staff
- Protect agency property from harm or danger
- Protect the person's valuables
- Prevent accidents and injuries

Color-Coded Wristbands

Color-coded wristbands are used to promote the person's safety and prevent harm. They quickly communicate an alert or warning (Fig. 8-14). The type of alert is printed on the band. The printing is useful in dim lighting and for persons who are color blind. Many states use these three colors:
- Red—means an "allergy alert." Red is a warning to "stop." A red wristband is used to warn of allergies to food, drugs, treatment supplies such as tape or latex gloves, dust, plants, grass, and so on. Allergies are not listed on the wristband. Some persons have too many allergies to list on the wristband.
- Yellow—means a "fall risk." Yellow implies "caution." The person is at risk for falling. Yellow wristbands are used for persons with a history of falls. Or they are used for persons at risk for falls because of dizziness, balance problems, confusion, and so on. See Chapter 9.
- Purple—means the person has a "do not resuscitate" (DNR) order. See Chapter 30.

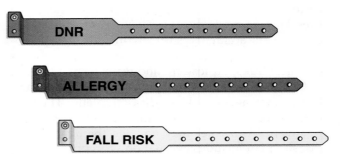

FIGURE 8-14 Color-coded wristbands. The alert is printed on the band.

Some agencies use other colors for other alerts. For example, pink is used for a "limb alert." This means that an arm or leg is not used for blood pressure measurements, blood draws, or intravenous infusions. To safely use color-coded wristbands:
- Know the wristband colors used in your agency. Colors may vary among agencies.
- Check the care plan and your assignment sheet when you see a color-coded wristband. You need to know the reason for the wristband and the care measures needed. Ask the nurse if you have questions.
- Do not confuse "social cause" bands with your agency's color-coded wristbands. "Live Strong" is an example.
- Check for wristbands on persons transferred from another agency. That agency may use different colored wristbands. Or the color meanings may differ from those in your agency. The nurse needs to remove wristbands from another agency.
- Tell the nurse if you think a person needs a color-coded wristband.

Personal Belongings

The person's belongings must be kept safe. Often they are sent home with the family. A personal belongings list is completed. Each item is listed and described. The staff member and person sign the completed list.

A valuables envelope is used for money and jewelry. Each jewelry item is listed and described on the envelope. Describe what you see. For example, describe a ring as having a white stone with four prongs in a yellow setting. Do not assume the stone is a diamond in a gold setting. For valuables:

- Count money with the person.
- Put money and each jewelry item in the envelope with the person watching. Seal the envelope. Sign the envelope like a personal belongings list.
- Give the envelope to the nurse. The nurse takes it to the safe or sends it home with the family.

Dentures, eyeglasses, hearing aids, watches, some jewelry, radios, music players, computers, and other electronic devices are kept at the bedside. Items kept at the bedside are listed in the person's record. Some people keep money for newspapers and personal items. The amount kept is noted in the person's record.

In nursing centers, clothing and shoes are labeled with the person's name. So are other items brought from home.

Reporting Incidents

An *incident* is any event that has harmed or could harm a patient, resident, visitor, or staff member. This includes:

- Accidents involving patients, residents, visitors, or staff.
- Errors in care. This includes giving the wrong care, giving care to the wrong person, or not giving care.
- Broken or lost items owned by the person. Dentures, hearing aids, and eyeglasses are examples.
- Lost money or clothing.
- Hazardous substance incidents.
- Workplace violence.

Report accidents and errors at once. Complete an incident report as soon as possible. Incident reports are reviewed by risk management and a committee of health care workers. They look for patterns and trends of accidents or errors. For example, are falls occurring on the same shift and on the same unit? Are lost or missing items being reported on the same shift or same unit? Are patients and residents being injured on the same shift or same unit? There may be new policies and procedures to prevent future incidents.

Focus on P R I D E
The Person, Family, and Yourself

Personal and Professional Responsibility—Accidents happen. Errors occur. No matter how much you try, mistakes are made. Do not lie or try to hide the incident. This is wrong. Be honest. Tell the nurse. Fill out an incident report. Incident reports are used to improve systems and promote safety, not to punish the person. Information gained signals areas for improvement. Processes may be changed to make mistakes more difficult. Or they are changed to make it easier to do the right thing.

Always do your best to give safe care. When errors or accidents happen, take responsibility. Be accountable. Take pride in doing the right thing by honest reporting.

Rights and Respect—Patients and residents have the right to the care and security of personal items. Treat the person's items with respect. The items may not have value to you but are important to the person. Label a person's belongings with his or her name. Put valuables in a secure place until a family member can take them home. Follow agency policies for charting and storing personal items.

Protect yourself and the agency from being accused of stealing. Do not go through a person's belongings without consent. Sometimes the nurse wants a person's items inspected for safety reasons. If so, make sure the nurse and the person or legal representative are present. Do not search on your own. Thorough documentation is important. The nurse charts the details of the search in the person's record.

Independence and Social Interaction—People want to be independent. They do not want to rely on others for simple, everyday things. Often accidents and injuries occur when the person tries to get needed items. The person has to reach too far and falls. Or he or she tries to get up without help. To promote independence and safety:

- Keep needed personal items within reach.
- Place assistive devices nearby. Walkers and canes are examples.
- Place the signal light within the person's reach. Answer signal lights and tend to the person's needs promptly.
- Let the person do as much as he or she safely can. Kindly communicate safety limits to the person. For example, you can say: "Mr. Dunn, you have been doing well using your walker. But I would like to be with you when you get up. Please call me if you need to get up. Here is your signal light."

Delegation and Teamwork—The entire health team must provide a safe setting. You may see something unsafe. Do what you can to correct the matter. For example:

- You see a water spill. Wipe up the spill right away. Do so even if you did not cause the spill.
- You see a person sliding out of a wheelchair. Position the person correctly in the chair. Do so even if a co-worker is responsible for the person's care.
- A person is having problems holding a cup of coffee. Offer to help the person.
- You notice a loose grab bar in the bathroom. Tell the nurse. Follow agency policy for reporting such problems.

Ethics and Laws—The Safe Medical Devices Act requires that agencies report equipment-related illnesses, injuries, and deaths. An incident report is completed if a patient, resident, visitor, or staff member has an equipment-related accident. Failing to report an incident can result in fines.

If you need to report an incident, tell the nurse. He or she will assist you with the form. Failing to report a problem is wrong. Tell the nurse any time there is an accident, error, or equipment-related incident.

Also follow agency policy for removing equipment from the area. This prevents others from being harmed.

REVIEW QUESTIONS

Circle the BEST answer.

1   Which is *not* a risk factor for accidents?
   a Needing eyeglasses
   b Hearing problems
   c Memory problems
   d Being able to respond to people, places, or things

2   A person in a coma
   a Has suffered an electrical shock
   b Has dementia
   c Is unaware of surroundings
   d Has stopped breathing

3   To identify a person, you
   a Call the person by name
   b Ask the person his or her name
   c Compare information on the ID bracelet against your assignment sheet
   d Ask both roommates their names

4   Burns are caused by the following *except*
   a Smoking
   b Spilled hot liquids
   c Very hot bath water
   d Oxygen

5   Which can cause suffocation?
   a Reporting loose teeth or dentures
   b Using electrical items that are in good repair
   c Cutting food into small, bite-size pieces
   d Over-loading an electrical outlet

6   The most common cause of choking in adults is
   a A loose denture
   b Meat
   c Marbles
   d Candy

7   If severe airway obstruction occurs, the person usually
   a Clutches at the throat
   b Can speak, cough, and breathe
   c Is calm
   d Has a seizure

8   These statements are about relieving FBAO. Which is *false?*
   a Abdominal thrusts can be self-administered.
   b A person is pregnant. Give abdominal thrusts.
   c Injuries can occur from abdominal or chest thrusts.
   d CPR is started if the responsive victim loses consciousness.

9   You need to shave a new resident. Before using the person's electric shaver
   a You need to inspect it
   b The maintenance staff must do a safety check
   c You need to check for a frayed cord
   d You need an electrical outlet

10 You are using electrical equipment. Which measure is *not* safe?
   a Following the manufacturer's instructions
   b Keeping electrical items away from water and spills
   c Pulling on the cord to remove a plug from an outlet
   d Turning off electrical items after using them

11 A person uses a wheelchair. Which measure is *not* safe?
   a The wheels are locked for transfers.
   b The chair is pulled backward to transport the person.
   c The feet are positioned on the footplates.
   d The casters point forward.

12 Stretcher safety involves the following *except*
   a Locking the wheels for transfers
   b Fastening the safety straps
   c Raising the side rails
   d Moving the stretcher head first

13 You spilled a hazardous substance. You should do the following *except*
   a Read the MSDS
   b Cover the spill and go tell the nurse
   c Wear personal protective equipment to clean up the spill
   d Complete an incident report

14 The fire alarm sounds. The following is done *except*
   a Turning off oxygen
   b Using elevators
   c Closing doors and windows
   d Moving patients and residents to a safe place

15 A severe weather alert was issued for your area. What should you do?
   a Take cover.
   b Follow the agency's disaster plan.
   c Make sure your family is safe.
   d Pull the fire alarm.

16 A person is agitated and aggressive. You should do the following *except*
   a Stand away from the person
   b Stand close to the door
   c Use touch to show you care
   d Talk to the person without raising your voice

17 A person has a red wristband. This means that the person
   a Is at risk for bleeding
   b Has an allergy
   c Is at risk for falling
   d Has an acute illness

18 You see a color-coded wristband. You should
   a Read the wristband for special instructions or care measures
   b Ask the person what it means
   c Check your assignment sheet and the person's care plan
   d Remove the wristband when the risk is no longer present

19 A resident brought a radio from home. Which helps prevent property loss?
   a Completing a personal belongings list
   b Labeling the item with the person's name
   c Putting the item in a safe
   d Using a wheelchair pouch for the item

20 You gave a person the wrong treatment. Which is *true*?
   a Report the error at the end of the shift.
   b Take action only if the person was injured.
   c You are guilty of negligence.
   d You must complete an incident report.

Answers to these questions are on p. 527.

9

PREVENTING FALLS

PROCEDURES

- Applying a Transfer/Gait Belt
- Helping the Falling Person

OBJECTIVES

- Define the key terms listed in this chapter.
- Identify the causes and risk factors for falls.
- Describe the safety measures that prevent falls.
- Explain how to use bed rails safely.
- Explain the purpose of hand rails and grab bars.
- Explain how to use wheel locks safely.
- Describe how to use transfer/gait belts.
- Explain how to help the person who is falling.
- Explain how to promote PRIDE in the person, the family, and yourself.
- Perform the procedures described in this chapter.

KEY TERMS

bed rail A device that serves as a guard or barrier along the side of the bed; side rail

gait belt See "transfer belt"

transfer belt A device used to support a person who is unsteady or disabled; gait belt

The risk of falling increases with age. Persons older than 65 years are at risk. Falls are a leading cause of injuries and deaths among older persons. A history of falls increases the risk of falling again. Most falls occur:

- In patient and resident rooms and in bathrooms.
- Between 1800 (6:00 PM) and 2100 (9:00 PM).
- During shift changes. Staff are busy going off and coming on duty. Confusion can occur about who gives care and answers signal lights.

The accident risk factors described in Chapter 8 can lead to falls. The problems listed in Box 9-1 increase a person's risk of falling.

Agencies have fall prevention programs. The measures listed in Box 9-2, p. 122 are part of such programs and care plans. The care plan also lists measures for the person's risk factors.

See *Promoting Safety and Comfort: Preventing Falls.*

See *Focus on Communication: Preventing Falls.*

Text continued on p. 124

PROMOTING SAFETY AND COMFORT
Preventing Falls

Safety

Some people are visually impaired or blind. Besides the measures in Box 9-1, other safety measures are needed to protect them from falling. See Chapter 26.

FOCUS ON COMMUNICATION
Preventing Falls

Often falls occur when the person tries to get needed items. The person has to reach too far and falls out of bed or from a chair. Or the person tries to get up without help. Prevent falls by asking the person these questions:

- "What things would you like near you?"
- "Can I move this closer to you?"
- "Can you reach the signal light?"
- "Can you reach your cane?" (Walker and wheelchair are other examples.)
- "Do you need to use the bathroom now?"
- "Is there anything else you need before I leave the room?"

BOX 9-1   Factors Increasing the Risk of Falls

Care Setting

- Bed: incorrent height
- Care equipment: IV poles, drainage tubes and bags, and others
- Cluttered floors
- Furniture out-of-place
- Lighting: poor
- Setting: strange and unfamiliar
- Throw rugs
- Wet and slippery floors, bathtubs, and showers

The Person

- Alcohol: over-use
- Balance problems
- Blood pressure: low or high
- Confusion
- Depression
- Disorientation
- Dizziness; dizziness on standing
- Drug side effects
  - Low blood pressure when standing or sitting
  - Drowsiness
  - Fainting
  - Dizziness
  - Coordination: poor
  - Unsteadiness
  - Urination: frequent
  - Diarrhea
  - Confusion and disorientation
- Elimination needs
- Falls: history of
- Foot problems
- Incontinence: urinary and fecal
- Joint pain and stiffness
- Judgment: poor
- Light-headedness
- Memory problems
- Mobility: decreased
- Muscle weakness
- Reaction time: slow
- Shoes that fit poorly
- Vision problems
- Weakness
- Wheelchairs, walkers, canes, and crutches: improper use

BOX 9-2   Safety Measures to Prevent Falls

Basic Needs

- Fluid needs are met.
- Eyeglasses and hearing aids are worn as needed. Reading glasses are not worn when up and about.
- Tasks are explained before and while performing them.
- Help is given with elimination needs. It is given at regular times and whenever requested. Assist the person to the bathroom. Or provide the bedpan, urinal, or commode.
- The bedpan, urinal, or commode is kept within easy reach if the person can use the device without help.
- A warm drink, soft lights, or a back massage is used to calm the person who is agitated.
- Barriers are used to prevent wandering (Fig. 9-1).
- The person is properly positioned when in bed, a chair, or a wheelchair. Use pillows, wedge pads, or seats as the nurse and care plan direct (Chapters 12 and 13).
- Correct procedures are used for transfers (Chapter 13).
- The person is involved in meaningful activities.

Bathrooms and Shower/Tub Rooms

- Tubs and showers have non-slip surfaces or non-slip bath mats.
- Grab bars (safety bars) are in showers. They also are by tubs and toilets.
- Bathrooms have grab bars.
- Shower chairs are used (Chapter 15).
- Safety measures for tub baths and showers are followed (Chapter 15).

Floors

- Scatter, area, and throw rugs are not used.
- Loose floor boards and tiles are reported. So are frayed rugs and carpets.
- Floors and stairs are free of clutter, cords, and other items that can cause tripping.
- Floors are free of spills. Wipe up spills at once. Put a "Wet Floor" sign by the wet area.
- Floors are free of excess furniture and equipment.
- Electrical and extension cords are out of the way.
- Equipment and supplies are kept on one side of the hallway.

Furniture

- Furniture is placed for easy movement.
- Furniture is kept in place. It is not re-arranged.
- Chairs have armrests. Armrests give support when standing or sitting.
- A phone, lamp, and personal belongings are within the person's reach.

Beds and Other Equipment

- The bed is in the lowest horizontal position, except when giving bedside care. The distance from the bed to the floor is reduced if the person falls or gets out of bed.
- Bed rails are used according to the care plan (p. 124).
- A mattress, special mat, or floor cushion is placed on the floor beside the bed (Fig. 9-2). This reduces the chance of injury if the person falls or gets out of bed.
- Wheelchairs, walkers, canes, and crutches fit properly.
- Crutches, canes, and walkers have non-skid tips.
- Correct equipment is used for transfers (Chapter 13). Follow the care plan.
- Wheelchair and stretcher safety is followed (Chapter 8).
- Wheel locks on beds (p. 124), wheelchairs, and stretchers are in working order.
- Bed and wheelchair or stretcher wheels are locked for transfers.
- Linens are checked for sharp objects and for the person's property (dentures, eyeglasses, hearing aids, and so on).

Lighting

- Rooms, hallways, and stairways have good lighting. So do bathrooms and shower/tub rooms.
- Light switches (including those in bathrooms) are within reach and easy to find.
- Night-lights are in bedrooms, hallways, and bathrooms.

Shoes and Clothing

- Non-skid footwear is worn. Socks, bedroom slippers, and long shoelaces are avoided.
- Clothing fits properly. Clothing is not loose. It does not drag on the floor. Belts are tied or secured in place.

Signal Lights and Alarms

- The person is taught how to use the signal light (Chapter 14).
- The signal light is always within the person's reach. This includes when in the bathroom and tub/shower room.
- The person is asked to call for assistance when help is needed:
  - When getting out of bed or a chair
  - With walking
  - With getting to or from the bathroom or commode
  - With getting on or off the bedpan
- Signal lights are answered promptly. The person may need help right away. He or she may not wait for help.
- Bed, chair, door, mat, and belt alarms are used. They sense when the person tries to get up, get out of bed, or open a door (Fig. 9-3).
- Alarms are responded to at once.

BOX 9-2 Safety Measures to Prevent Falls—cont'd

Other

- Color-coded alerts are used to warn of a fall risk. Yellow is the common color for a fall alert. Besides wristbands (Chapter 8), some agencies also use color-coded blankets, non-skid footwear, socks, and magnets or stickers to place on room doors.
- The person is checked often. This may be every 15 minutes or as required by the care plan. Careful and frequent observation is important.
- Frequent checks are made on persons with poor judgment or memory. This may be every 15 minutes or as required by the care plan.
- Hand rails are on both sides of stairs and hallways.

- Non-slip strips are on the floor next to the bed and in the bathroom. They are intact.
- Caution is used when turning corners, entering corridor intersections, and going through doors. You could injure a person coming from the other direction.
- Pull (do not push) wheelchairs, stretchers, carts, and other wheeled equipment through doorways. This allows you to lead the way and to see where you are going.
- A safety check is made of the room after visitors leave. (See the inside of the front book cover.) They may have lowered a bed rail, removed a signal light, or moved a walker out of reach. Or they may have brought an item that could harm the person.

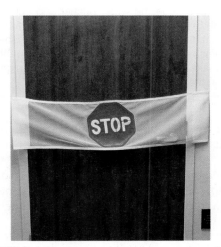

FIGURE 9-1 Barriers are used to prevent wandering.

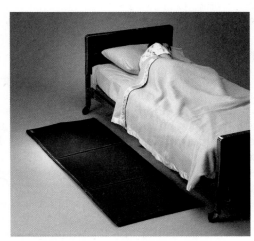

FIGURE 9-2 Floor cushion. (*Image courtesy J. T. Posey Co., Arcadia, Calif.*)

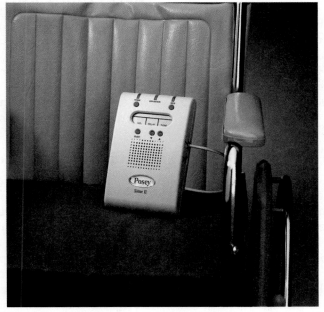

FIGURE 9-3 Chair alarm. (*Image courtesy J. T. Posey Co., Arcadia, Calif.*)

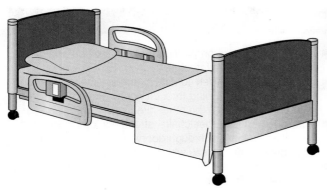

FIGURE 9-4 Bed rails. The far bed rail is raised. The near bed rail is lowered.

BED RAILS

A **bed rail** (*side rail*) is a device that serves as a guard or barrier along the side of the bed. Bed rails are raised and lowered (Fig. 9-4). They lock in place with levers, latches, or buttons. Bed rails are half, three quarters, or the full length of the bed. When half-length rails are used, each side may have two rails. One is for the upper part of the bed, the other for the lower part.

The nurse and care plan tell you when to raise bed rails. They are needed by persons who are unconscious or sedated with drugs. Some confused or disoriented people need them. If a person needs bed rails, keep them up at all times except when giving bedside nursing care.

Bed rails present hazards. The person can fall when trying to climb over them or the person cannot get out of bed or use the bathroom. Entrapment is a risk. That is, the person can get caught, trapped, entangled, or strangled (Chapter 14).

Bed rails are considered to be restraints (Chapter 10) if:

- The person cannot get out of bed.
- The person cannot lower them without help.

Bed rails cannot be used unless needed to treat a person's medical symptoms. They must be in the person's best interests. Some people feel safer with bed rails up. Others use them to change positions in bed. The person or legal representative must give consent for raised bed rails. The need for bed rails is carefully noted in the person's medical record and the care plan.

The procedures in this book include using bed rails. This helps you learn to use them correctly. The nurse, the care plan, and your assignment sheet tell you which people use bed rails. If a person does not use them, omit the "raise bed rails" or "lower bed rails" steps.

If a person uses bed rails, check the person often. Report to the nurse that you checked the person. If you are allowed to chart, record when you check the person and your observations.

See *Promoting Safety and Comfort: Bed Rails.*

HAND RAILS AND GRAB BARS

Hand rails are in hallways and stairways (Fig. 9-5). They give support to persons who are weak or unsteady when walking.

Grab bars (safety bars) are in bathrooms and in shower/tub rooms (Fig. 9-6). They provide support for sitting down or getting up from a toilet. They also are used for getting in and out of the shower or tub.

WHEEL LOCKS

Bed legs have wheels. Each wheel has a lock to prevent the bed from moving (Fig. 9-7). Wheels are locked at all times except when moving the bed. Make sure bed wheels are locked:

- When giving bedside care
- When you transfer a person to and from the bed

Wheelchair and stretcher wheels also are locked during transfers (Chapter 13). You or the person can be injured if the bed, wheelchair, or stretcher moves.

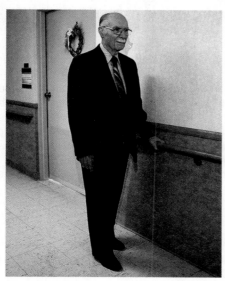

FIGURE 9-5 Hand rails provide support when walking.

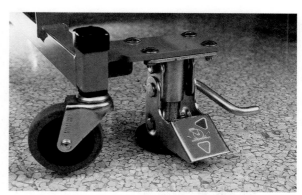

FIGURE 9-7 Lock on a bed wheel.

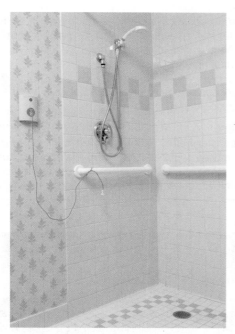

FIGURE 9-6 Grab bars in a shower.

❖ TRANSFER/GAIT BELTS

A **transfer belt (gait belt)** is a device used to support a person who is unsteady or disabled (Fig. 9-8, p. 126). It helps prevent falls and injuries. When used to transfer a person (Chapter 13), it is called a *transfer belt*. When used to help a person walk, it is called a *gait belt*. Many agencies require staff to use a belt when transferring or walking a person.

The belt goes around the person's waist. Grasp under the belt to support the person during the transfer or when assisting the person to walk.

See *Promoting Safety and Comfort: Transfer/Gait Belts*, p. 126.

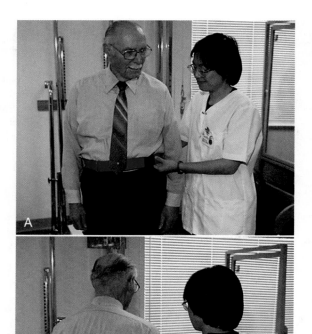

FIGURE 9-8 Transfer/gait belt. Note the different types of belts. **A,** The belt buckle is positioned off center. The nursing assistant grasps the belt from underneath. **B,** The belt buckle is not over the spine.

PROMOTING SAFETY AND COMFORT
Transfer/Gait Belts

Safety

Transfer/gait belts are routinely used in nursing centers. If the person needs help, a belt is required. To use one safely, always follow the manufacturer's instructions.

Some transfer/gait belts have a quick-release buckle. Position the quick-release buckle at the person's back where he or she cannot reach it. This prevents the person from releasing the buckle during the procedure. Injury could result if the buckle is released.

Do not leave excess strap dangling. Tuck the excess strap under the belt.

Remove the belt after the procedure. Do not leave the person alone while he or she is wearing a transfer/gait belt.

Using a transfer/gait belt is unsafe for some persons. The belt could cause pressure or rub against care equipment. Check with the nurse and the care plan before using a transfer/gait belt if the person has:

- An ostomy—colostomy, ileostomy, gastrostomy (Chapters 17 and 18)
- A gastric tube (Chapter 19)
- Chronic obstructive pulmonary disease (Chapter 26)
- An abdominal wound, incision, or drainage tube
- A chest wound, incision, or drainage tube
- Monitoring equipment
- A hernia
- Other conditions or care equipment involving the chest or abdomen

Comfort

A transfer belt is always applied over clothing. It is never applied over bare skin. Also, it is applied under the breasts. Breasts must not be caught under the belt. The belt buckle is never positioned over the person's spine.

APPLYING A TRANSFER/GAIT BELT

QUALITY OF LIFE

Remember to:
- Knock before entering the person's room.
- Address the person by name.
- Introduce yourself by name and title.

- Explain the procedure to the person before beginning and during the procedure.
- Protect the person's rights during the procedure.
- Handle the person gently during the procedure.

PROCEDURE

1. See *Promoting Safety and Comfort: Transfer/Gait Belts.*
2. Practice hand hygiene.
3. Identify the person. Check the identification bracelet against the assignment sheet. Also call the person by name.
4. Provide for privacy.
5. Assist the person to a sitting position.
6. Apply the belt around the person's waist over clothing. Do not apply it over bare skin.
7. Secure the buckle. The buckle is in front.
8. Tighten the belt so it is snug. It should not cause discomfort or impair breathing. You should be able to slide your open, flat hand under the belt.
9. Make sure that a woman's breasts are not caught under the belt.
10. Turn the belt so the quick-release buckle is at the person's back. The buckle is not over the spine.
11. Tuck any excess strap under the belt.

THE FALLING PERSON

A person may start to fall when standing or walking. See p. 121 for the risk factors for falls.

Do not try to prevent the fall. You could injure yourself and the person while twisting and straining to prevent the fall. Head, wrist, arm, hip, and knee injuries could occur.

If a person starts to fall, ease him or her to the floor. This lets you control the direction of the fall. You can also protect the person's head. Do not let the person move or get up before the nurse checks for injuries.

If you find a person on the floor, do not move the person. Stay with the person, and call for the nurse.

See *Persons with Dementia: The Falling Person.*

PERSONS WITH DEMENTIA
The Falling Person

Some older persons are confused. A confused person may not understand why you do not want him or her to move or get up after a fall. Forcing a person not to move may injure the person and you. You may need to let the person move for his or her safety and your own. Never use force to hold a person down. Stay calm, and protect the person from injury. Talk to the person in a quiet, soothing voice. Call for help.

HELPING THE FALLING PERSON

PROCEDURE

1 Stand behind the person with your feet apart. Keep your back straight.
2 Bring the person close to your body as fast as possible. Use the transfer/gait belt (Fig. 9-9, *A*, p. 128). Or wrap your arms around the person's waist. If necessary (but not preferred), you can also hold the person under the arms.
3 Move your leg so the person's buttocks rest on it (Fig. 9-9, *B*, p. 128). Move the leg near the person.

4 Lower the person to the floor. The person slides down your leg to the floor (Fig. 9-9, *C*, p. 128). Bend at your hips and knees as you lower the person.
5 Call a nurse to check the person. Stay with the person.
6 Help the nurse return the person to bed. Ask other staff to help if needed.

POST-PROCEDURE

7 Provide for comfort. (See the inside of the front book cover.)
8 Place the signal light within reach.
9 Raise or lower bed rails. Follow the care plan.
10 Complete a safety check of the room. (See the inside of the front book cover.)

11 Report and record the following:
 • How the fall occurred
 • How far the person walked
 • How activity was tolerated before the fall
 • Complaints before the fall
 • How much help the person needed while walking
12 Complete an incident report.

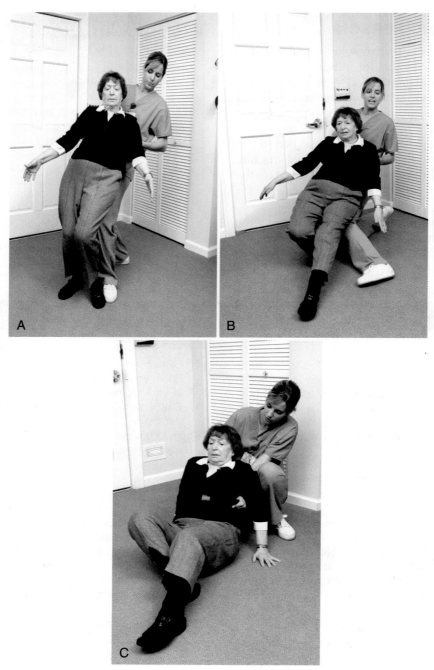

FIGURE 9-9 The falling person. **A,** The falling person is supported. **B,** The person's buttocks rest on the nursing assistant's leg. **C,** The person is eased to the floor on the nursing assistant's leg.

Focus on P R I D E
The Person, Family, and Yourself

Personal and Professional Responsibility—
Sometimes providing safety measures is time consuming. Perhaps you cannot find a transfer belt. Or you need to get a walker. Or you must put on the person's shoes. Resist the urge to take short cuts. Take the time to:

- Find and use assistive devices.
- Put proper footwear on the person.
- Raise or lower the bed and side rails as appropriate.
- Lock wheels on beds, stretchers, and wheelchairs.
- Ask others to help if needed.

You are responsible for providing safe care. This includes taking measures to prevent falls. See Box 9-2. Hurrying is never an excuse for causing harm. Take time for safety. Take pride in doing the right thing by providing safe care.

Rights and Respect—Patients and residents have the right to feel safe. Safety and security are not only rights but basic needs (Chapter 5). Fear of falling does not make a person feel safe. Before moving a person, explain what you are going to do and what he or she needs to do. Also give step-by-step instructions as you progress. Do not move the person without telling him or her first. These measures help increase the person's comfort. See Chapter 13 for safely handling, moving, and transferring the person. Good communication promotes comfort. It supports the person's right to safety and security.

Independence and Social Interaction—Some persons may feel restricted by the use of safety devices. They may feel it limits their independence. For example, Ms. Mills does not like having her bed rails up. She says: "I feel trapped. Do those have to be up?" Ms. Mills has fallen out of bed at night. The care plan includes having bed rails up while she is in bed.

Listen to the person's concerns. Kindly explain the reason for the safety device. If the person still refuses, tell the nurse. Do not let the person talk you out of performing a safety measure or using a safety device. Safety is always a priority.

Delegation and Teamwork—Helping co-workers with their patients or residents is an important part of teamwork. However, you may not be familiar with the person and his or her care plan. You must promote safety. Communication is essential. When assisting with the transfer of a co-worker's patient or resident, you must have information about the person. Ask the nurse or co-worker:

- Is the person at risk for falls?
- Is the person weak? Can he or she bear weight?
- Are there any activity limits?
- How many persons are needed for the transfer?
- Are any assistive devices needed? A cane, transfer belt, wheelchair, and walker are examples.
- Is any other equipment needed? Oxygen and braces are examples.

Ethics and Laws—The Joint Commission (TJC) certifies and accredits health care programs and organizations nationally. Its mission is to improve safety and quality of care. To earn The Joint Commission's approval, ethical and safety standards must be met. On-site surveys are done to evaluate compliance with the standards.

Every year The Joint Commission develops National Patient Safety Goals. Goals are made for hospitals, long-term care centers, and other agencies. The goals focus on ways to solve health care safety problems. Preventing falls is an example. Agencies must determine a person's fall risk. Some agencies use a form or screening tool to assess fall risk. Agencies must take action to prevent falls and reduce the risk of harm resulting from falls. Know your agency's policies and procedures for preventing harm from falls.

REVIEW QUESTIONS

Circle the BEST answer.

1 Most falls occur in
  a Patient and resident rooms and bathrooms
  b Dining rooms
  c Lounges
  d Hallways

2 Most falls occur
  a In the morning
  b At lunch time
  c In the afternoon
  d During the evening

3 A person's care plan includes fall prevention measures. Which should you question?
  a Assist with elimination needs.
  b Keep phone, lamp, and TV controls within reach.
  c Check the person every 2 hours.
  d Complete a safety check of the room after visitors leave.

4 You observe the following in the person's room. Which is *not* safe?
  a The lamp cord is by the chair.
  b The chair has armrests.
  c The night-light works.
  d The bed is in the lowest horizontal position.

5 You note the following after a person got dressed. Which is safe?
  a The person is wearing non-skid shoes.
  b Pant cuffs are dragging on the floor.
  c The belt is not fastened.
  d The shirt is too big.

6 A co-worker is helping Mr. Polk today. His chair alarm goes off. What should you do?
  a Find your co-worker.
  b Tell the nurse.
  c Assist Mr. Polk.
  d Wait for someone to respond to the alarm.

7 To help prevent falls, you need to report
  a Equipment and supplies being on one side of the hallway
  b A mattress on the floor beside the bed
  c A co-worker pulling a wheelchair through a doorway
  d Clutter on stairways

8 Bed rails are used
  a When you think they are needed
  b When the bed is raised
  c According to the care plan
  d To support persons who are weak or unsteady

9 You are going to transfer a person from the bed to a chair. Bed wheels must be locked.
  a True
  b False

10 A transfer/gait belt is applied
  a To the skin
  b Over clothing
  c Over the breasts
  d Under the robe

11 To safely use a transfer/gait belt, you must
  a Follow the manufacturer's instructions
  b Raise the bed rails
  c Lock the bed wheels
  d Set the bed alarm

12 You apply a transfer/gait belt. What should you do with the excess strap?
  a Cut it off.
  b Wrap it around the person's waist.
  c Tuck it under the belt.
  d Let it dangle.

13 A person starts to fall. Your first action is to
  a Try to prevent the fall
  b Call for help
  c Bring the person close to your body as fast as possible
  d Lower the person to the floor

14 You found a person lying on the floor. What should you do?
  a Call for the nurse.
  b Help the person back to bed.
  c Apply a transfer belt.
  d Lock the bed wheels.

Answers to these questions are on p. 527.

10

RESTRAINT ALTERNATIVES AND SAFE RESTRAINT USE

PROCEDURE

- Applying Restraints

OBJECTIVES

- Define the key terms and key abbreviations listed in this chapter.
- Describe the purpose and complications of restraints.
- Identify restraint alternatives.
- Explain how to use restraints safely.
- Explain how to promote PRIDE in the person, the family, and yourself.
- Perform the procedure described in this chapter.

KEY TERMS

chemical restraint Any drug that is used for discipline or convenience and not required to treat medical symptoms

freedom of movement Any change in place or position of the body or any part of the body that the person is physically able to control

medical symptom An indication or characteristic of a physical or psychological condition

physical restraint Any manual method or physical or mechanical device, material, or equipment attached to or near the person's body that he or she cannot remove easily and which restricts freedom of movement or normal access to one's body

remove easily The manual method device, material, or equipment used to restrain the person that can be removed intentionally by the person in the same manner it was applied by the staff

KEY ABBREVIATIONS

CMS Centers for Medicare & Medicaid Services

FDA Food and Drug Administration

TJC The Joint Commission

OBRA Omnibus Budget Reconciliation Act of 1987

Chapters 8 and 9 have many safety measures. However, some persons need extra protection. They may present dangers to themselves or others (including staff). Some need restraints.

The Centers for Medicare & Medicaid Services (CMS) have rules for using restraints. Like the Omnibus Budget Reconciliation Act of 1987 (OBRA), CMS rules protect the person's rights and safety. This includes the right to be free from restraint or seclusion. Restraints may only be used to treat a medical symptom (p. 134) or for the immediate physical safety of the person or others. Restraints may only be used when less restrictive measures fail to protect the person or others. They must be discontinued at the earliest possible time.

The CMS uses these terms in its rules for long-term care agencies:

- **Physical restraint**—is any manual method or physical or mechanical device, material, or equipment attached to or near the person's body that he or she cannot remove easily and which restricts freedom of movement or normal access to one's body.

- **Chemical restraint**—any drug that is used for discipline or convenience and not required to treat medical symptoms. The drug or dosage is not a standard treatment for the person's condition.
- **Freedom of movement**—is any change in place or position of the body or any part of the body that the person is physically able to control.
- **Remove easily**—means that the manual method device, material, or equipment used to restrain the person that can be removed intentionally by the person in the same manner it was applied by the staff. For example, the person can put bed rails down, untie a knot, unclasp a buckle.

HISTORY OF RESTRAINT USE

Restraints were once thought to *prevent* falls. Research shows that restraints *cause* falls. Falls occur when persons try to get free of the restraints. Injuries are more serious from falls in restrained persons than in those not restrained.

Restraints also were used to prevent wandering or interfering with treatment. They were often used for persons who showed confusion, poor judgment, or behavior problems. Older persons were restrained more often than were younger persons. Restraints were viewed as necessary devices to protect a person. However, they can cause serious harm (Box 10-1). They can even cause death.

Besides the CMS, the Food and Drug Administration (FDA), state agencies, and The Joint Commission (TJC—an accrediting agency) have guidelines for the use of restraints. They do not forbid the use of restraints. However, *they require considering or trying all other appropriate alternatives first.*

BOX 10-1 Risks of Restraint Use

- Agitation
- Anger
- Constipation
- Cuts and bruises
- Dehydration
- Depression
- Embarrassment and humiliation
- Fractures
- Incontinence (Chapters 17 and 18)
- Infections: pneumonia and urinary tract
- Mistrust
- Nerve injuries
- Pressure ulcers (Chapter 23)
- Strangulation

Every agency has policies and procedures about restraints. They include identifying persons at risk for harm, harmful behaviors, restraint alternatives, and proper restraint use. Staff training is required.

RESTRAINT ALTERNATIVES

Often there are causes and reasons for harmful behaviors. Knowing and treating the cause can prevent restraint use. The nurse tries to find out what the behavior means.

- Is the person in pain, ill, or injured?
- Is the person short of breath? Are cells getting enough oxygen? (See Chapter 24.)
- Is the person afraid in a new setting?
- Does the person need to use the bathroom?
- Is clothing or a dressing (Chapter 23) tight or causing other discomfort?
- Is the person's position uncomfortable?
- Are body fluids, secretions, or excretions causing skin irritation?
- Is the person too hot or too cold? Hungry or thirsty?
- What are the person's life-long habits at this time of day?
- Does the person have problems communicating?
- Is the person seeing, hearing, or feeling things that are not real (Chapter 27)?
- Is the person confused or disoriented (Chapter 28)?
- Are drugs causing the behaviors?

Restraint alternatives for the person are identified (Box 10-2). They become part of the care plan. Care plan changes are made as needed. Restraint alternatives may not protect the person. The doctor may need to order restraints.

SAFE RESTRAINT USE

Restraints can cause serious injury and even death. CMS, OBRA, FDA, and TJC guidelines are followed. So are state laws. They are part of your agency's policies and procedures for restraint use.

BOX 10-2   Alternatives to Restraint Use

- Diversion is provided—TV, videos, music, games, relaxation tapes, and so on.
- Life-long habits and routines are in the care plan. For example, showers before breakfast; reads in the bathroom; walks outside before lunch; watches TV after lunch; and so on.
- Family and friends make videos of themselves for the person to watch.
- Videos are made of visits with family and friends for the person to watch.
- Time is spent in supervised areas (dining room, lounge, near the nurses' station).
- Pillows, wedge cushions, and posture and positioning aids are used.
- The signal light is within reach.
- Signal lights are answered promptly.
- Food, fluid, hygiene, and elimination needs are met.
- The bedpan, urinal, or commode is within the person's reach.
- Back massages are given.
- Family, friends, and volunteers visit.
- The person has companions or sitters.
- Time is spent with the person.
- Extra time is spent with a person who is restless.
- Reminiscing is done with the person.
- A calm, quiet setting is provided.
- The person wanders in safe areas.
- The entire staff is aware of persons who tend to wander. This includes staff in housekeeping, maintenance, the business office, dietary, and so on.
- Exercise programs are provided.
- Outdoor time is planned during nice weather.
- The person does jobs or tasks he or she consents to.
- Warning devices are used on beds, chairs, and doors.
- Knob guards are used on doors.
- Padded hip protectors are worn under clothing (Fig. 10-1, p. 134).
- Floor cushions are placed next to beds (Chapter 9).
- Roll guards are attached to the bed frame (Fig. 10-2, p. 134).
- Falls are prevented (Chapter 9).
- The person's furniture meets his or her needs (lower bed, reclining chair, rocking chair).
- Walls and furniture corners are padded.
- Observations and visits are made at least every 15 minutes. Or as often as noted in the care plan.
- The person is moved to a room close to the nurses' station.
- Procedures and care measures are explained.
- Frequent explanations are given about equipment or devices.
- Confused persons are oriented to person, time, and place. Calendars and clocks are provided.
- Light is adjusted to meet the person's basic needs and preferences.
- Staff assignments are consistent.
- Sleep is not interrupted.
- Noise levels are reduced.

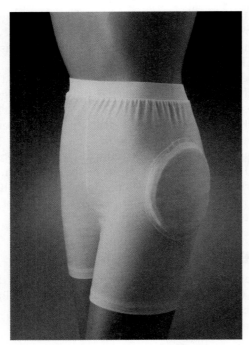

FIGURE 10-1 Hip protector. (*Image courtesy J. T. Posey Co., Arcadia, Calif.*)

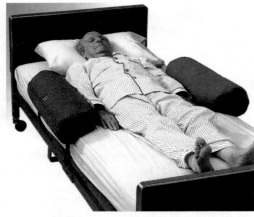

FIGURE 10-2 Roll guard. (*Image courtesy J. T. Posey Co., Arcadia, Calif.*)

Restraints are not used to discipline a person. They are not used for staff convenience. *Discipline* is any action that punishes or penalizes a person. *Convenience* is any action that:

- Controls or manages the person's behavior
- Requires less effort by the agency
- Is not in the person's best interests

Restraints are used only when necessary to treat a person's medical symptoms. The CMS defines a **medical symptom** as an indication or characteristic of a physical or psychological condition. Symptoms may relate to physical, emotional, or behavioral problems. Sometimes restraints are needed to protect the person or others. That is, a person may have violent or aggressive behaviors that are harmful to self or others.

Imagine being restrained:

- Your nose itches. But your wrists are restrained. You cannot scratch your nose.
- You need to use the bathroom. Your wrists are restrained. You cannot get up. You cannot reach your signal light. You soil yourself with urine and a bowel movement.
- Your phone is ringing. You cannot answer it because your wrists are restrained.
- You are not wearing your eyeglasses. You cannot identify people coming into and going out of your room. And you cannot speak because of a stroke. You have a vest restraint. You cannot move or turn in bed.
- You are thirsty. The water cup is within your reach but your wrists are restrained.
- You hear the fire alarm. You have on a restraint. You cannot get up to move to a safe place. You must wait to be rescued.

What would you try to do? Would you calmly lie or sit there? Would you try to get free from the restraint? Would you cry out for help? What would the nursing staff think? Would they think that you are uncomfortable? Or would they think that you are agitated and uncooperative? Would they think your behavior is improving or getting worse? Would you feel angry, embarrassed, or humiliated?

Try to put yourself in the person's situation. That will help you understand how the person feels. Treat the person like you would want to be treated—with kindness, caring, respect, and dignity.

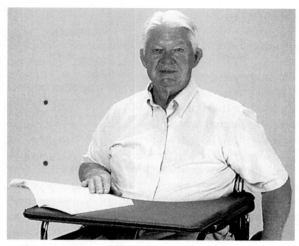

FIGURE 10-3 This lap-top tray is a restraint alternative. It is a restraint when used to prevent freedom of movement. *(Image courtesy J. T. Posey Co., Arcadia, Calif.)*

Physical and Chemical Restraints

According to the CMS, *physical restraints* include these points:
- May be any manual method, physical or mechanical device, material, or equipment
- Is attached to or next to the person's body
- Cannot be easily removed by the person
- Restricts freedom of movement or normal access to one's body

Physical restraints are applied to the chest, waist, elbows, wrists, hands, or ankles. They confine the person to a bed or chair. Or they prevent movement of a body part. Some furniture or barriers also prevent freedom of movement:
- A device used with a chair that the person cannot remove easily. The device prevents the person from rising. Trays, tables, bars, and belts are examples (Fig. 10-3).
- Any chair that prevents the person from rising.
- Any bed or chair placed so close to the wall that the person cannot get out of the bed or chair.
- Bed rails (Chapter 9) that prevent the person from getting out of bed. For example, four half-length bed rails are raised. They are restraints if the person cannot lower them.
- Tucking in or using Velcro to hold a sheet, fabric, or clothing so tightly that freedom of movement is restricted.
- Wheelchair locks if the person cannot release them.

Drugs or drug dosages are *chemical restraints* if they:
- Control behavior or restrict movement
- Are not standard treatment for the person's condition

Drugs cannot be used if they affect physical or mental function. Sometimes drugs can help persons who are confused or disoriented. They may be anxious, agitated, or aggressive. The doctor may order drugs to control these behaviors. The drugs should not make the person sleepy and unable to function at his or her highest level.

Complications of Restraint Use

Box 10-1 lists the many complications from restraints. Injuries occur as the person tries to get free of the restraint. Injuries also occur from using the wrong restraint, applying it wrong, or keeping it on too long. Cuts, bruises, and fractures are common. *The most serious risk is death from strangulation.*

There are also mental effects. Restraints affect dignity and self-esteem. See Box 10-1.

Restraints are medical devices. The Safe Medical Device Act applies if a restraint causes illness, injury, or death. Also, CMS requires the reporting of any death that occurs:
- While a person is in a restraint.
- Within 24 hours after a restraint was removed.
- Within 1 week after a restraint was removed. This is done if the restraint may have contributed directly or indirectly to the person's death.

Legal Aspects

Laws applying to restraint use must be followed. Remember the following:

- *Restraints must protect the person.* A restraint is used only when it is the best safety measure for the person. Restraining someone is not easier than properly supervising and observing the person. A restrained person requires more staff time for care, supervision, and observation.
- *A doctor's order is required.* The doctor gives the medical symptom for the restraint, what body part to restrain, what to use, and how long to use it. This information is on the care plan and your assignment sheet.
- *The least restrictive method is used.* It allows the greatest amount of movement or body access possible. Some restraints attach to the person's body and to a fixed (non-movable) object. They restrict freedom of movement or body access. Vest, jacket, ankle, wrist, hand, and some belt restraints are examples. Other restraints are near but not directly attached to the person's body (bed rails or wedge cushions). They do not totally restrict freedom of movement and are less restrictive.
- *Restraints are used only if other measures fail to protect the person* (see Box 10-2). Some people can harm themselves or others. The care plan must include measures to protect the person and prevent harm to others. Many fall prevention measures are restraint alternatives (Chapter 9).
- *Unnecessary restraint is false imprisonment* (Chapter 2). You must clearly understand the reason for the restraint and its risk. If not, politely ask about its use. If you apply an unneeded restraint, you could face false imprisonment charges. See *Focus on Communication: Legal Aspects.*
- *Consent is required.* The person must understand the reason for the restraint. The person is told how the restraint will help the planned medical treatment. The person is told about the risks of restraint use. If the person cannot give consent, his or her legal representative is given the information. Either the person or legal representative must give consent before a restraint can be used. The doctor or nurse provides the necessary information and obtains the consent. However, using restraints cannot be refused if used as a last resort because the person's behavior causes an immediate threat to self or others.

FOCUS ON COMMUNICATION
Legal Aspects

You may not know the reason for a restraint. If so, politely ask the nurse why it is needed. For example:
- "Why does Mr. Reed need a restraint?"
- "I don't understand. Why did the doctor order the restraint?"

Safety Guidelines

The restrained person must be kept safe. Follow the safety measures in Box 10-3. Also remember these key points:

- *Observe for increased confusion and agitation.* Restraints can increase confusion and agitation. Whether confused or alert, people are aware of restricted movements. They may try to get out of the restraint or struggle or pull at it. Some restrained persons beg others to free or to help release them. These behaviors often are viewed as signs of confusion. Some people become more confused because they do not understand what is happening to them. Restrained persons need repeated explanations and reassurance. Spending time with them has a calming effect. See *Focus on Communication: Safety Guidelines.*
- *Protect the person's quality of life.* Restraints are used for as short a time as possible. The care plan must show how to reduce restraint use. The person's needs are met with as little restraint as possible. You must meet the person's physical, emotional, and social needs. Visit with the person and explain the reason for the restraints.
- *Follow the manufacturer's instructions.* They explain how to apply and secure the restraint for the person's safety. The restraint must be snug and firm, but not tight. Tight restraints affect circulation and breathing. The person must be comfortable and able to move the restrained part to a limited and safe extent. You could be negligent if you do not apply or secure a restraint properly.

- *Apply restraints with enough help to protect the person and staff from injury.* Persons in immediate danger of harming themselves or others are restrained quickly. Combative and agitated people can hurt themselves and the staff when restraints are applied. Enough staff members are needed to complete the task safely and quickly.
- *Observe the person at least every 15 minutes or as often as noted in the care plan.* Restraints are dangerous. Injuries and deaths can result from improper restraint use and poor observation. Prevent complications. Interferences with breathing and circulation are examples.
- *Remove or release the restraint, reposition the person, and meet basic needs at least every 2 hours or as often as noted in the care plan.* The restraint is removed or released for at least 10 minutes. Provide for food, fluid, comfort, safety, hygiene, and elimination needs and give skin care. Perform range-of-motion exercises or help the person walk (Chapter 22). Follow the care plan.

Text continued on p. 141

FOCUS ON COMMUNICATION
Safety Guidelines

Restraints can increase confusion. Remind the person why the restraint is necessary and to call for help when it is needed. Repeat the following as often as needed:

- "Dr. Monroe ordered this restraint so you don't hurt yourself. If you need to get up, please call for help. I'll check on you every 15 minutes. Other staff will check on you too."
- "Please put your signal light on. I want to make sure that you can reach and use it with the restraint on."
- "Please call for help right away if the restraint is too tight."
- "Please call for help right away if you feel pain in your fingers or hands. Also call for me if you feel numbness or tingling."
- "Please call for help right away if you are having problems breathing."

BOX 10-3   Safety Measures for Using Restraints

Before Applying Restraints

- Do not use sheets, towels, tape, rope, straps, bandages, Velcro, or other items to restrain a person.
- Apply a restraint only after being instructed about its proper use.
- Demonstrate proper application of the restraint before applying it.
- Use the restraint noted in the care plan. Use the correct size. Small restraints are tight. They cause discomfort and agitation. They also restrict breathing and circulation. Strangulation is a risk from big or loose restraints.
- Use only restraints that have manufacturer instructions and warning labels.
- Read the manufacturer's warning labels. Note the front and back of the restraint.
- Follow the manufacturer's instructions. Some restraints are safe for bed, chair, and wheelchair use. Others are used only with certain equipment.
- Use intact restraints. Look for tears, cuts, or frayed fabric or straps. Look for missing or loose hooks, loops, or straps or other damage.
- Do not use a restraint near a fire, a flame, or smoking materials.

Applying Restraints

- Do not use restraints to position a person on a toilet.
- Do not use restraints to position a person on furniture that does not allow for correct application. Follow the manufacturer's instructions.
- Follow agency policies and procedures.
- Position the person in good alignment before applying the restraint (Chapter 12).
- Pad bony areas and the skin as instructed by the nurse. This prevents pressure and injury from the restraint.
- Secure the restraint. It should be snug but allow some movement of the restrained part. Follow the manufacturer's instructions to check for snugness. For example:
  - If applied to the chest or waist—Make sure that the person can breathe easily. A flat hand should slide between the restraint and the person's body (Fig. 10-4, p. 139). Check with the nurse if you have very small or very large hands. Small or large hands could cause the restraint to be too tight or too loose.
  - For wrist and mitt restraints—You should be able to slide 1 finger under the restraint. Check with the nurse if you have very small or very large fingers. Small or large fingers could cause the restraint to be too tight or too loose.

Continued

BOX 10-3 Safety Measures for Using Restraints—cont'd

Applying Restraints—cont'd

- Criss-cross vest or jacket restraints in front (Fig. 10-5). Do not criss-cross restraints in the back unless part of the manufacturer's instructions (Fig. 10-6). Criss-crossing vests or jackets in the back can cause death from strangulation.
- Buckle or tie restraints according to agency policy. The policy should follow the manufacturer's instructions and allow for quick release in an emergency. Quick-release buckles or airline type buckles are used (Fig. 10-7). So are quick-release ties (Fig. 10-8).
- Secure straps out of the person's reach.
- Leave 1 to 2 inches of slack in the straps (if directed to do so by the nurse). This allows some movement of the part.
- Secure the restraint to the movable part of the bed frame at waist level (see Fig. 10-8). The restraint will not tighten or loosen when the head or foot of the bed is raised or lowered. For chairs, secure straps under the seat of the wheelchair or chair (Fig. 10-9, p. 140).
- Make sure that straps will not slide in any direction. If straps slide, they change the restraint's position. The person can get suspended off the mattress or chair (Figs. 10-10 and 10-11, p. 140). Strangulation can result.
- Never secure restraints to the bed rails. The person can reach bed rails to release knots or buckles. Also, injury to the person is likely when raising or lowering bed rails.
- Use bed rail covers or gap protectors according to the nurse's instructions (Fig. 10-12, p. 141). They prevent entrapment between the rails or the bed rail bars (see Fig. 10-10). Entrapment can occur between:
  - The bars of a bed rail
  - The space between half-length (split) bed rails
  - The bed rail and mattress
  - The headboard or footboard and mattress
- Position the person in semi-Fowler's position (Chapter 12) when using a vest, jacket, or belt restraint.
- Position the person in a chair so the hips are well to the back of the chair.
- Apply a belt restraint at a 45-degree angle over the thighs (Fig. 10-13, p. 141).

After Applying Restraints

- Keep full bed rails up when using a vest, jacket, or belt restraint. Also use bed rail covers or gap protectors. Otherwise the person could fall off the bed and strangle on the restraint. If half-length bed rails are used, the person can get caught between them.
- Do not use back cushions when a person is restrained in a chair. If the cushion moves out of place, slack occurs in the straps. Strangulation could result if the person slides forward or down from the extra slack (see Fig. 10-11).
- Do not cover the person with a sheet, blanket, bedspread, or other covering. The restraint must be within plain view at all times.
- Check the person at least every 15 minutes for safety, comfort, and signs of injury.

After Applying Restraints—cont'd

- Check the person's circulation at least every 15 minutes if mitt, wrist, or ankle restraints are applied. You should feel a pulse at a pulse site below the restraint. Fingers or toes should be warm and pink. Tell the nurse at once if:
  - You cannot feel a pulse.
  - Fingers or toes are cold, pale, or blue in color.
  - The person complains of pain, numbness, or tingling in the restrained part.
  - The skin is red or damaged.
- Check the person at least every 15 minutes if a belt, jacket, or vest restraint is used. The person should be able to breathe easily. Also check the position of the restraint, especially in the front and back.
- Monitor persons in the supine position constantly. They are at great risk for aspiration if vomiting occurs (Chapter 19). Call for the nurse at once.
- Keep scissors in your pocket. In an emergency, cutting the tie may be faster than untying a knot. Never leave scissors at the bedside where the person can reach them. Make sure the person cannot reach the scissors in your pocket.
- Remove or release the restraint and reposition the person every 2 hours or as often as noted in the care plan. The restraint is removed or released for at least 10 minutes. Meet the person's basic needs. You need to:
  - Measure vital signs.
  - Meet elimination needs.
  - Offer food and fluids.
  - Meet hygiene needs.
  - Give skin care.
  - Perform range-of-motion exercises or help the person walk. Follow the care plan.
  - Provide for physical and emotional comfort. (See the inside of the front book cover.)
- Keep the signal light within the person's reach. Chart that this was done.
- Complete a safety check before leaving the room. (See the inside of the front book cover.)
- Report to the nurse every time you checked the person and removed or released the restraint. Report your observations and the care given. Follow agency policy for recording.

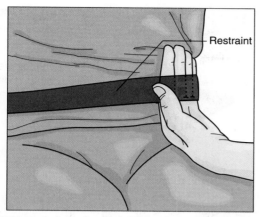

FIGURE 10-4 A flat hand slides between the restraint and the person.

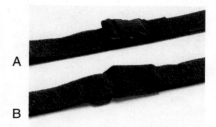

FIGURE 10-7 A, Quick-release buckle. **B,** Airline-type buckle. (*Images courtesy J. T. Posey Co., Arcadia, Calif.*)

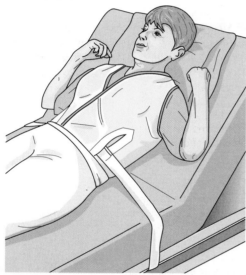

FIGURE 10-5 Vest restraint criss-crosses in front. (Note: The bed rails are raised after the restraint is applied.)

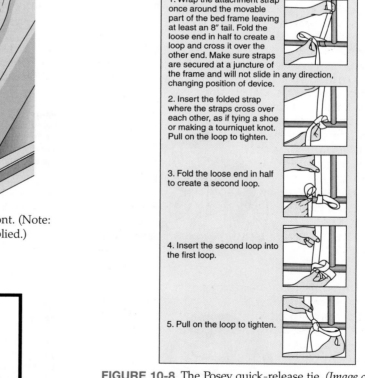

How to Tie the Posey Quick-Release Tie

1. Wrap the attachment strap once around the movable part of the bed frame leaving at least an 8" tail. Fold the loose end in half to create a loop and cross it over the other end. Make sure straps are secured at a juncture of the frame and will not slide in any direction, changing position of device.

2. Insert the folded strap where the straps cross over each other, as if tying a shoe or making a tourniquet knot. Pull on the loop to tighten.

3. Fold the loose end in half to create a second loop.

4. Insert the second loop into the first loop.

5. Pull on the loop to tighten.

FIGURE 10-8 The Posey quick-release tie. (*Image courtesy J. T. Posey Co., Arcadia, Calif.*)

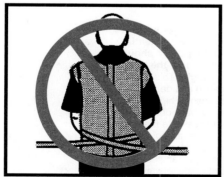

FIGURE 10-6 Never criss-cross vest or jacket straps in back. (*Image courtesy J. T. Posey Co., Arcadia, Calif.*)

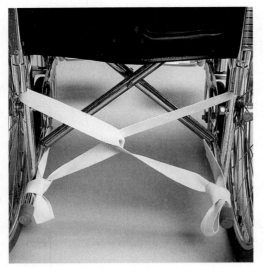

FIGURE 10-9 The restraint straps are secured to the wheelchair frame with quick-release ties. (*Image courtesy J. T. Posey Co., Arcadia, Calif.*)

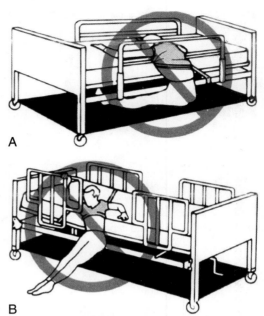

A

B

FIGURE 10-10 A, A person can get suspended and caught between bed rail bars. **B,** The person can get suspended and caught between half-length bed rails. (*Images courtesy J. T. Posey Co., Arcadia, Calif.*)

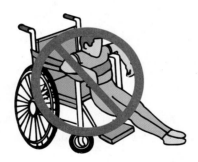

Straps to prevent sliding should always be over the thighs—NOT around the waist or chest. Straps should be at a 45° angle and secured to the chair under the seat, not behind the back. They should be snug but comfortable and not restrict breathing. If a belt or vest is too loose or applied around the waist, the person may slide partially off the seat—resulting in possible suffocation and death.

Tray tables (with or without a belt or vest) pose potential danger if the person should slide partly under the table and become caught. This could result in suffocation and death. Make sure the person's hips are positioned at the back of the chair—this may necessitate the use of an anti-slide material (Posey Grip), a pommel cushion, or a restrictive device if the person shows any tendency to slide forward.

FIGURE 10-11 Strangulation could result if the person slides forward or down because of extra slack in the restraint. (*Images courtesy J. T. Posey Co., Arcadia, Calif.*)

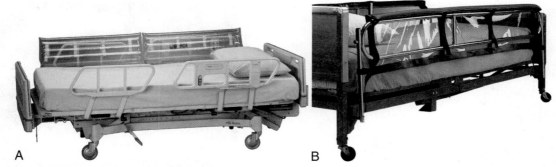

FIGURE 10-12 A, Bed rail protector. **B,** Guard rail pads. *(Images courtesy J. T. Posey Co., Arcadia, Calif.)*

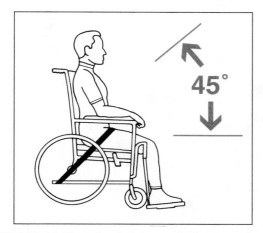

FIGURE 10-13 The safety belt is at a 45-degree angle over the thighs. *(Image courtesy J. T. Posey Co., Arcadia, Calif.)*

Reporting and Recording

Information about restraints is recorded in the person's medical record. You might apply restraints or care for a restrained person. Report and record the following:
- The type of restraint applied
- The body part or parts restrained
- The reason for the application
- Safety measures taken (for example, bed rails padded and up, signal light within reach)
- The time you applied the restraint
- The time you removed or released the restraint and for how long
- The person's vital signs
- The care given when the restraint was removed or released
- Skin color and condition
- Condition of the limbs
- The pulse felt in the restrained part

- Changes in the person's behavior
- Complaints of discomfort; a tight restraint; difficulty breathing; or pain, numbness, or tingling in the restrained part (Report these complaints to the nurse at once.)

Applying Restraints

Restraints are made of cloth or leather. Cloth restraints (soft restraints) are mitts, belts, straps, jackets, and vests. They are applied to the wrists, ankles, hands, waist, and chest. Leather restraints are applied to the wrists and ankles. Leather restraints are used for extreme agitation and combativeness.

Wrist Restraints Wrist restraints (limb holders) limit arm movement (Fig. 10-14, p. 142). They may be used when a person continually tries to pull out tubes used for life-saving treatment (intravenous [IV] infusion, feeding tube). Or the person scratches at, pulls at, or peels the skin, a wound, or a dressing. This can damage the skin or the wound.

Mitt Restraints Hands are placed in mitt restraints. They prevent finger use. They allow hand, wrist, and arm movements. They are used for the same reasons as wrist restraints. Most mitts are padded (Fig. 10-15, p. 142).

Belt Restraints The belt restraint (Fig. 10-16, p. 142) is used when injuries from falls are risks or for positioning during a medical treatment. The person cannot get out of bed. However, a roll belt allows the person to turn from side to side or sit up in bed.

The belt is applied around the waist and secured to the bed or chair (lap belt). It is applied over a garment. The person can release the quick-release type. It is less restrictive than those that only staff members can release.

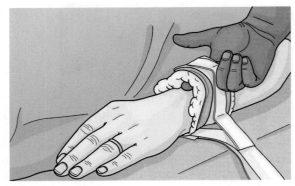

FIGURE 10-14 Wrist restraint. The soft part is toward the skin. Note that 1 finger fits between the restraint and the wrist.

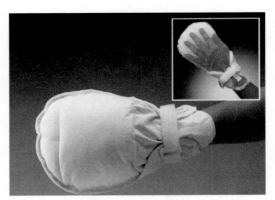

FIGURE 10-15 Mitt restraint. (*Images courtesy J. T. Posey Co., Arcadia, Calif.*)

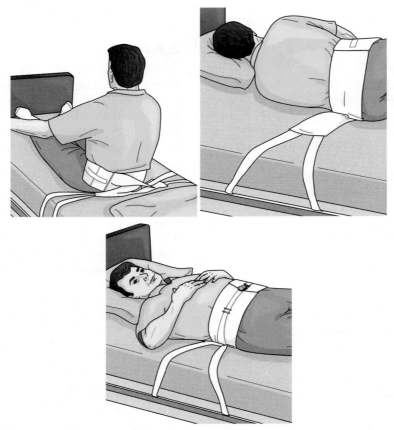

FIGURE 10-16 Belt restraint. (Note: The bed rails are raised after the restraint is applied.)

Vest Restraints and Jacket Restraints Vest and jacket restraints are applied to the chest. They may be used to prevent injuries from falls. And they may be used for persons who need positioning for a medical treatment. The person cannot turn in bed or get out of a chair.

A jacket restraint is applied with the opening in the back (Fig. 10-17). For a vest restraint, the vest crosses in front (see Fig. 10-5). *The straps of vest and jacket restraints always cross in the front.* They must *never* cross in the back. Vest and jacket restraints are never worn backward. Strangulation or other injury

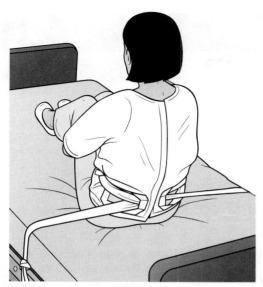

FIGURE 10-17 Jacket restraint. (Note: The bed rails are raised after the restraint is applied.)

could occur if the person slides down in the bed or chair. The restraint is always applied over a garment. *(Note: A vest or jacket restraint may have a positioning slot in the back. Criss-cross the straps following the manufacturer's instructions.)*

Vest and jacket restraints have life-threatening risks. Death can occur from strangulation. If the person gets caught in the restraint, it can become so tight that the person's chest cannot expand to inhale air. The person quickly suffocates and dies. Correctly applying vest and jacket restraints is critical. You are advised to only assist the nurse in applying them. The nurse should assume full responsibility for applying a vest or jacket restraint.

See *Persons With Dementia: Applying Restraints.*
See *Focus on Communication: Applying Restraints.*
See *Delegation Guidelines: Applying Restraints.*
See *Promoting Safety and Comfort: Applying Restraints*, p. 144.

PERSONS WITH DEMENTIA
Applying Restraints

Restraints may increase confusion and agitation in persons with dementia. They do not understand what you are doing. They may resist your efforts to apply a restraint. They may actively try to get free from the restraint. Serious injury and death are risks.

Never use force to apply a restraint. If a person is confused or agitated, ask a co-worker to help apply the restraint. Report problems to the nurse at once.

FOCUS ON COMMUNICATION
Applying Restraints

The nurse may ask you to apply a restraint you have not used before. If you do not know how to apply a certain restraint, do not do so. Tell the nurse. Ask him or her to show you the correct application. You can say: "I've never applied a restraint like this before. Would you please show me how and then watch me apply it?" Then thank the nurse for helping you.

When applying a restraint, explain to the person what you are going to do. Then tell the person what you are doing step-by-step. Always check for safety and comfort. You can ask: "How does the restraint feel? Is it too tight? Is it too loose?"

Make sure the person can communicate with you after you leave the room. Place the signal light in reach. Make sure the person can use it with the restraint on. Remind the person to call if he or she becomes uncomfortable or if anything is needed.

DELEGATION GUIDELINES
Applying Restraints

Before applying a restraint, you need this information from the nurse and the care plan:
- Why the doctor ordered the restraint
- What type and size to use
- Where to apply the restraint
- How to safely apply the restraint (Have the nurse show you how to apply it. Then show correct application back to the nurse.)
- How to correctly position the person
- What bony areas to pad and how to pad them
- If bed rail covers or gap protectors are needed
- If bed rails are up or down
- What special equipment is needed
- If the person needs to be checked more often than every 15 minutes
- When to apply and release the restraint
- What observations to report and record (p. 141)
- When to report observations
- What specific patient and resident concerns to report at once

PROMOTING SAFETY AND COMFORT
Applying Restraints

Safety

Restraints can cause serious harm, even death. Always follow the manufacturer's instructions. Manufacturers have many types of restraints. The instructions for one type may not apply to another. Also, the manufacturer may have instructions for applying restraints on persons who are agitated.

Never use force to apply a restraint. Ask a co-worker to help apply a restraint on a person who is confused and agitated. Report problems to the nurse at once.

Check the person at least every 15 minutes or more often as instructed by the nurse and the care plan. Make sure the signal light is within reach. Ask the person to use the signal light at the first sign of problems or discomfort.

Never use a restraint as a seat belt in a car or other vehicle.

Comfort

The person's comfort is always important. It is more so when restraints are used. Remember, restraints limit movement. This affects position changes and reaching needed items. Position the person in good alignment before applying a restraint (Chapter 12). Also make sure the person can reach needed items—signal light, water, tissues, phone, bed controls, and so on.

APPLYING RESTRAINTS

QUALITY OF LIFE

Remember to:
- Knock before entering the person's room.
- Address the person by name.
- Introduce yourself by name and title.

- Explain the procedure to the person before beginning and during the procedure.
- Protect the person's rights during the procedure.
- Handle the person gently during the procedure.

PRE-PROCEDURE

1   Follow *Delegation Guidelines: Applying Restraints,* p. 143. See *Promoting Safety and Comfort: Applying Restraints.*
2   Collect the following as instructed by the nurse:
   - Correct type and size of restraints
   - Padding for skin and bony areas
   - Bed rail pads or gap protectors (if needed)

3   Practice hand hygiene.
4   Identify the person. Check the ID (identification) bracelet against the assignment sheet. Also call the person by name.
5   Provide for privacy.

PROCEDURE

6   Make sure the person is comfortable and in good alignment.
7   Put the bed rail pads or gap protectors (if needed) on the bed if the person is in bed. Follow the manufacturer's instructions.
8   Pad bony areas. Follow the nurse's instructions and the care plan.
9   Read the manufacturer's instructions. Note the front and back of the restraint.

10   *For wrist restraints:*
   a   Apply the restraint following the manufacturer's instructions. Place the soft or foam part toward the skin.
   b   Secure the restraint so it is snug but not tight. Make sure you can slide 1 finger under the restraint (see Fig. 10-14). Follow the manufacturer's instructions. Adjust the straps if the restraint is too loose or too tight. Check for snugness again.
   c   Buckle or tie the straps to the movable part of the bed frame out of the person's reach. Use an agency-approved tie.
   d   Repeat steps 10 a, b, and c for the other wrist.

11 *For mitt restraints:*

  a Make sure the person's hands are clean and dry.

  b Apply the mitt restraint. Follow the manufacturer's instructions.

  c Secure the restraint to the bed if directed to do so by the nurse. Buckle or tie the straps to the movable part of the bed frame. Use an agency-approved tie.

  d Make sure the restraint is snug. Slide 1 finger between the restraint and the wrist. Follow the manufacturer's instructions. Adjust the straps if the restraint is too loose or too tight. Check for snugness again.

  e Repeat steps 11 b, c (if directed to do so), and d for the other hand.

12 *For a belt restraint:*

  a Assist the person to a sitting position.

  b Apply the restraint with your free hand. Follow the manufacturer's instructions.

  c Remove wrinkles or creases from the front and back of the restraint.

  d Bring the ties through the slots in the belt.

  e Help the person lie down if he or she is in bed.

  f Make sure the person is comfortable and in good alignment.

  g Buckle or tie the straps to the movable part of the bed frame out of the person's reach or to the chair or wheelchair. Use an agency-approved tie.

  h Make sure the belt is snug. Slide an open hand between the restraint and the person. Adjust the restraint if it is too loose or too tight. Check for snugness again.

13 *For a vest restraint:*

  a Assist the person to a sitting position.

  b Apply the restraint with your free hand. Follow the manufacturer's instructions. The "V" part of the vest crosses in front.

  c Bring the straps through the slots.

  d Make sure the vest is free of wrinkles in the front and back.

  e Help the person lie down if he or she is in bed.

  f Make sure the person is comfortable and in good alignment.

  g Buckle or tie the straps underneath the chair seat or to the movable part of the bed frame. Use an agency-approved tie. If secured to the bed frame, the straps are secured at waist level out of the person's reach.

  h Make sure the vest is snug. Slide an open hand between the restraint and the person. Adjust the restraint if it is too loose or too tight. Check for snugness again.

14 *For a jacket restraint:*

  a Assist the person to a sitting position.

  b Apply the restraint with your free hand. Follow the manufacturer's instructions. The jacket opening goes in the back.

  c Close the back with the zipper, ties, or hook and loop closures.

  d Make sure the side seams are under the arms. Remove any wrinkles in the front and back.

  e Help the person lie down if he or she is in bed.

  f Make sure the person is comfortable and in good alignment.

  g Buckle or tie the straps underneath the chair seat or to the movable part of the bed frame. Use an agency-approved knot. If secured to the bed frame, the straps are secured at waist level out of the person's reach.

  h Make sure the jacket is snug. Slide an open hand between the restraint and the person. Adjust the restraint if it is too loose or too tight. Check for snugness again.

POST-PROCEDURE

15 Position the person as the nurse directs.

16 Provide for comfort. (See the inside of the front book cover.)

17 Place the signal light within the person's reach.

18 Raise or lower bed rails. Follow the care plan and the manufacturer's instructions for the restraint.

19 Unscreen the person.

20 Complete a safety check of the room. (See the inside of the front book cover.)

21 Decontaminate your hands.

22 Check the person and the restraint at least every 15 minutes. Report and record your observations:

  a For wrist or mitt restraints: check the pulse, color, and temperature of the restrained parts.

  b For a vest, jacket, or belt restraint: check the person's breathing. *Call for the nurse at once if the person is not breathing or is having problems breathing.* Make sure the restraint is properly positioned in the front and back.

23 Do the following at least every 2 hours for at least 10 minutes:

  a Remove or release the restraint.

  b Measure vital signs.

  c Reposition the person.

  d Meet food, fluid, hygiene, and elimination needs.

  e Give skin care.

  f Perform range-of-motion exercises or help the person walk. Follow the care plan.

  g Provide for physical and emotional comfort. (See the inside of the front book cover.)

  h Re-apply the restraints.

24 Complete a safety check of the room. (See the inside of the front book cover.)

25 Report and record your observations and the care given.

Focus on P R I D E
The Person, Family, and Yourself

Personal and Professional Responsibility—Restraint use has many risks. See Box 10-1. Therefore, restraint use brings many responsibilities for you. They include:

- Monitoring for the person's safety
- Ensuring proper application
- Promoting the person's comfort
- Increasing supervision of the person
- Meeting the person's basic needs
- Reporting any concerns to the nurse

If you do not know how to apply a restraint, do not do so. Ask the nurse to show you. Always monitor restrained persons closely. To use restraints safely and responsibly, follow the guidelines in Box 10-3.

Rights and Respect—Every person has the right to freedom from restraint. Restraints are used only as a last resort to protect a person or others from harm. Other methods must be tried before restraints are used. You may be asked to assist with an alternative method (see Box 10-2). Make a genuine effort. Be honest. Do not tell the nurse you tried if you really did not. Do your best to allow the person the right to freedom from restraint.

Independence and Social Interaction—All restraint forms limit movement. Independence is restricted. You can promote independence even when restraints are used. To do so:

- Make sure the signal light is in reach at all times. Make sure the person is able to use it. Tell the person to press it if anything is needed. Answer the signal light and meet the person's needs promptly.
- Make sure needed items are within reach. This is especially important with restraints that allow hand and arm use. Belt, vest, and jacket restraints are examples.
- Check on the person at least every 15 minutes.
- Remove or release the restraint at least every 2 hours.
- Meet food, fluid, hygiene, and elimination needs.
- Assist the person with walks or range-of-motion exercises.
- Allow choice. For example, let the person choose where to walk or what to eat and drink.
- Let the person do as much for himself or herself as safely as possible.

Personal choice and freedom of movement promote independence, dignity, and self-esteem. Provide care that gives restrained persons the independence they deserve.

Delegation and Teamwork—You may not be assigned to a restrained person. However, you still must keep the person safe. Make sure you know who is restrained on your unit. Every time you walk past the person or the person's room, check to see if the person is safe and comfortable. Act right away if the person is at risk for harm. Take pride in promoting teamwork by assisting others with restrained persons.

Ethics and Laws—The CMS issues standards and rules for safe restraint use. They focus on maintaining the person's rights, promoting safety, and avoiding unnecessary restraint use. Surveys are conducted to monitor compliance. The following are included in the CMS standards:

- Restraints are only used to protect the safety of the person or others.
- Restraints are never to be used as a form of punishment or for staff's convenience.
- The restraint ordered must be the least restrictive method possible.
- The restraint must be removed as soon as is safely possible.

REVIEW QUESTIONS

Circle T if the statement is *true.* Circle F if the statement is *false.*

1 T (F) Restraint alternatives fail to protect a person. You can apply a restraint.
2 (T) F A restraint restricts a person's freedom of movement.
3 (T) F Some drugs are restraints.
4 T (F) Restraints can be used for staff convenience.
5 T (F) A device is a restraint only if it is attached to the person's body.
6 (T) F Bed rails are restraints if the person cannot lower them.
7 (T) F Restraints are used only for a person's specific medical symptom.
8 (T) F Unnecessary restraint is false imprisonment.
9 T (F) You can apply restraints when you think they are needed.
10 T (F) Restraints are secured within the person's reach.
11 T (F) You can use a vest restraint to position a person on the toilet.
12 (T) F Restraints are removed or released at least every 2 hours to reposition the person and give skin care.
13 T (F) Restraints are tied to bed rails.
14 (T) F A vest restraint crosses in front.
15 T (F) Bed rails are left down when vest restraints are used.

Circle the BEST answer.

16 Which is *not* a restraint alternative?
   (a) Positioning the person's chair close to the wall
   b Answering signal lights promptly
   c Taking the person outside in nice weather
   d Padding walls and corners of furniture
17 Physical restraints
   a Control mental function
   (b) Control a behavior
   c Confine a person to a bed or chair
   d Decrease care needs

18 The following can occur because of restraints. Which is the *most* serious?
   a Fractures
   (b) Strangulation
   c Pressure ulcers
   d Urinary tract infections
19 A belt restraint is applied to a person in bed. Where should you secure the straps?
   a To the bed rails
   b To the headboard
   (c) To the movable part of the bed frame
   d To the footboard
20 A person has a restraint. You should check the person and the position of the restraint at least every
   (a) 15 minutes
   b 30 minutes
   c Hour
   d 2 hours
21 A person has mitt restraints. Which of these is especially important to report to the nurse?
   a The heart rate
   b The respiratory rate
   c Why the restraints were applied
   (d) If you felt a pulse in the restrained extremities
22 The doctor ordered mitt restraints for a person. You need the following information from the nurse *except*
   a What size to use
   b What other equipment is needed
   (c) What drugs the person is taking
   d When to apply and release the restraints
23 A person has a vest restraint. It is not too tight or too loose if you can slide
   a A fist between the vest and the person
   b One finger between the vest and the person
   (c) An open hand between the vest and the person
   d Two fingers between the vest and the person
24 The correct way to apply any restraint is to follow the
   a Nurse's directions
   b Doctor's orders
   c Care plan
   (d) Manufacturer's instructions

Answers to these questions are on p. 527.

11

PREVENTING INFECTION

PROCEDURES

 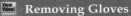 Hand Washing
Removing Gloves
Donning and Removing a Gown
Donning and Removing a Mask

OBJECTIVES

- Define the key terms and key abbreviations listed in this chapter.
- Identify what microbes need to live and grow.
- List the signs and symptoms of infection.
- Explain the chain of infection.
- Describe health care–associated infections and the persons at risk.
- Describe the practices of medical asepsis.
- Describe disinfection and sterilization methods.
- Explain how to care for equipment and supplies.
- Describe Standard Precautions and Transmission-Based Precautions.
- Explain the Bloodborne Pathogen Standard.
- Explain how to promote PRIDE in the person, the family, and yourself.
- Perform the procedures described in this chapter.

KEY TERMS

asepsis Being free of disease-producing microbes

biohazardous waste Items contaminated with blood, body fluids, secretions, or excretions; *bio* means life, and *hazardous* means dangerous or harmful

carrier A human or animal that is a reservoir for microbes but does not have the signs and symptoms of infection

clean technique See "medical asepsis"

communicable disease A disease caused by pathogens that spread easily; a contagious disease

contagious disease See "communicable disease"

contamination The process of becoming unclean

disinfection The process of destroying pathogens

healthcare-associated infection (HAI) An infection that develops in a person cared for in any setting where health care is given; the infection is related to receiving health care

infection A disease state resulting from the invasion and growth of microbes in the body

medical asepsis Practices used to remove or destroy pathogens and to prevent their spread from one person or place to another person or place; clean technique

microbe See "microorganism"

microorganism A small *(micro)* living plant or animal *(organism)* seen only with a microscope; a microbe

non-pathogen A microbe that does not usually cause an infection

pathogen A microbe that is harmful and can cause an infection

sterile The absence of *all* microbes

sterilization The process of destroying *all* microbes

KEY ABBREVIATIONS

AIIR Airborne infection isolation room

CDC Centers for Disease Control and Prevention

HAI Healthcare-associated infection

HBV Hepatitis B virus

HIV Human immunodeficiency virus

MDRO Multidrug-resistant organism

MRSA Methicillin-resistant *Staphylococcus aureus*

OPIM Other potentially infectious materials

OSHA Occupational Safety and Health Administration

PPE Personal protective equipment

TB Tuberculosis

VRE Vancomycin-resistant *Enterococcus*

Infection is a major safety and health hazard. Minor infections cause short illnesses. Some infections are serious and can cause death. Older and disabled persons are at risk. The health team follows certain practices and procedures to protect patients, residents, visitors, and staff from infection.

MICROORGANISMS

A **microorganism (microbe)** is a small *(micro)* living plant or animal *(organism)*. It is seen only with a microscope. Microbes are everywhere—in the mouth, nose, respiratory tract, stomach, and intestines. They are on the skin and in the air, soil, water, and food. They are on animals, clothing, and furniture.

Some microbes are harmful and can cause infections. They are called **pathogens. Non-pathogens** are microbes that do not usually cause an infection.

Microbes need a *reservoir (host)* to live and grow. The reservoir is the environment where the microbe lives and grows. People, plants, animals, the soil, food, and water are common reservoirs. Microbes need *water* and *nourishment* from the reservoir. Most need *oxygen* to live. A *warm* and *dark* environment is needed. Most grow best at body temperature. They are destroyed by heat and light.

Multidrug-Resistant Organisms

Multidrug-resistant organisms (MDROs) can resist the effects of antibiotics. *Antibiotics* are drugs that kill microbes that cause infections. Some microbes can change their structures. This makes them harder to kill. They can survive in the presence of antibiotics. Therefore the infections they cause are hard to treat.

MDROs are caused by doctors prescribing antibiotics when they are not needed (over-prescribing). Not taking antibiotics for the prescribed length of time is a cause.

Two common MDROs are:
* *Methicillin-resistant Staphylococcus aureus (MRSA)*—is commonly called "staph." MRSA is normally found in the nose and on the skin. It can cause serious wound and bloodstream infections and pneumonia.
* *Vancomycin-resistant Enterococcus (VRE)*—is normally found in the intestines and is present in feces. VRE can be transmitted to others by contaminated hands, toilet seats, care equipment, and other items that the hands touch. When not in its natural site (the intestines), VRE can cause an infection. It can cause urinary tract, wound, pelvic, and other infections.

INFECTION

An **infection** is a disease state resulting from the invasion and growth of microbes in the body. A *local infection* is in a body part. A *systemic infection* involves the whole body. (Systemic means entire.) The person has some or all of the signs and symptoms listed in Box 11-1.

The chain of infection is a process (Fig. 11-1). It begins with a *source*—a pathogen. It must have a *reservoir* where it can grow and multiply. Humans and animals are reservoirs. If they do not have signs and symptoms of infection, they are **carriers.** Carriers can pass the pathogen to others. To leave the reservoir, the pathogen needs a *portal of exit*. Exits are the respiratory, gastro-intestinal, urinary, and reproductive tracts; breaks in the skin; and the blood.

After leaving the reservoir, the pathogen must be *transmitted* to another host (Fig. 11-2). The pathogen enters the body through a *portal of entry*. Portals of entry and exit are the same. A *susceptible host* is needed for the microbe to grow and multiply. Susceptible hosts are persons at risk for infection.

The human body can protect itself from infection. The ability to resist infection relates to age, nutrition, stress, fatigue, and health. Drugs, disease, and injury also are factors.

BOX 11-1	Signs and Symptoms of Infection

- Fever (elevated body temperature)
- Chills
- Pulse and respiratory rates: increased
- Pain or tenderness
- Fatigue and loss of energy
- Appetite: loss of (*anorexia*)
- Nausea
- Vomiting
- Diarrhea
- Rash
- Sores on mucous membranes
- Redness and swelling of a body part
- Discharge or drainage from the infected area
- Heat or warmth in a body part
- Limited use of a body part
- Headache
- Muscle aches
- Joint pain
- Confusion

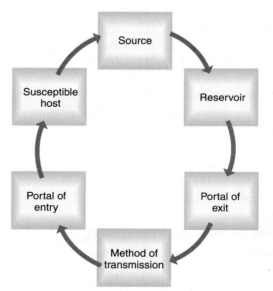

FIGURE 11-1 The chain of infection. (*Redrawn from Potter PA, Perry AG:* Fundamentals of nursing: concepts, process, and practice, *ed 7, St Louis, 2009, Mosby.*)

Healthcare-Associated Infection

A **healthcare-associated infection (HAI)** is an infection that develops in a person cared for in any setting where health care is given. The infection is related to receiving health care. HAIs were once called *nosocomial infections.* (*Nosocomial* comes from the Greek word for hospital.) HAIs are caused by microbes

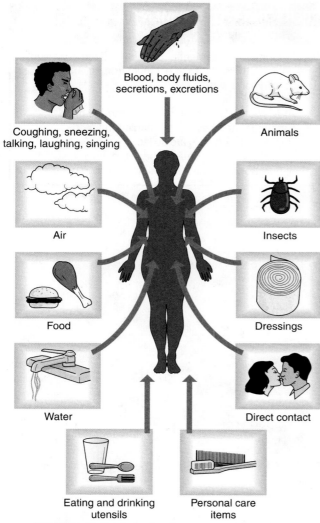

Blood, body fluids, secretions, excretions

Coughing, sneezing, talking, laughing, singing

Animals

Air

Insects

Food

Dressings

Water

Direct contact

Eating and drinking utensils

Personal care items

FIGURE 11-2 Methods of transmitting microbes.

normally found in the body. Or they are caused by microbes transmitted to the person from other sources.

For example, *Escherichia coli* is normally in the colon. Feces (bowel movements) contain *E. coli*. Poor wiping after bowel movements can cause *E. coli* to enter the urinary system. The hands can transmit *E. coli* to other body areas. If hand washing is poor, *E. coli* spreads to any body part or anything the hands touch. It also can be transmitted to other people.

Microbes can enter the body through equipment and supplies. Such items must be free of microbes. Staff can transfer microbes from one person to another and from themselves to others. The urinary and respiratory systems, wounds, and bloodstream are common sites for HAIs.

HAIs are prevented by:
- Medical asepsis. This includes hand hygiene.
- Standard Precautions and Transmission-Based Precautions (p. 157).
- The Bloodborne Pathogen Standard (p. 168).

Infection in Older Persons

The immune system protects the body from disease and infection (Chapter 6). Changes occur in the immune system with aging. Older persons may not show the signs and symptoms (see Box 11-1). The person may have only a slight fever or no fever at all. Redness and swelling may be very slight. The person may not complain of pain. Confusion and delirium may occur (Chapter 28).

An infection can become life-threatening before the older person has obvious signs and symptoms. Stay alert to the most minor changes in the person's behavior or condition. Report any concerns to the nurse at once.

MEDICAL ASEPSIS

Asepsis is being free of disease-producing microbes. Microbes are everywhere. Measures are needed to achieve asepsis. **Medical asepsis (clean technique)** is the practices used to:
- Remove or destroy pathogens. The number of pathogens is reduced.
- Prevent pathogens from spreading from one person or place to another person or place.

Contamination is the process of becoming unclean. In medical asepsis, an item or area is *clean* when it is free of pathogens. The item or area is contaminated if pathogens are present. A sterile item or area is contaminated when pathogens or non-pathogens are present. **Sterile** means the absence of *all* microbes—pathogens and non-pathogens.

Common Aseptic Practices

Aseptic practices break the chain of infection. To prevent the spread of microbes, wash your hands:
- After urinating or having a bowel movement.
- After changing tampons or sanitary pads.
- After contact with your own or another person's blood, body fluids, secretions, or excretions. This includes saliva, vomitus, urine, feces, vaginal discharge, mucus, semen, wound drainage, pus, and respiratory secretions.
- After coughing, sneezing, or blowing your nose.
- Before and after handling, preparing, or eating food.
- After smoking a cigarette, cigar, or pipe.

Also do the following:

- Provide all persons with their own linens and personal care items.
- Cover your nose and mouth when coughing, sneezing, or blowing your nose.
- Bathe, wash hair, and brush your teeth regularly.
- Wash fruits and raw vegetables before eating or serving them.
- Wash cooking and eating utensils with soap and water after use.

See *Persons With Dementia: Common Aseptic Practices.*

PERSONS WITH DEMENTIA

Common Aseptic Practices

Persons with dementia do not understand aseptic practices. Others must protect them from infection. Assist them with hand washing:

- After elimination
- After coughing, sneezing, or blowing the nose
- Before or after they eat or handle food
- Any time their hands are soiled

Check and clean their hands and fingernails often. They may not or cannot tell you when soiling occurs.

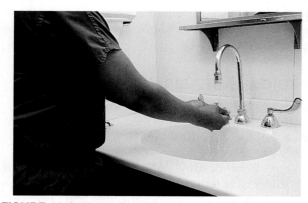

FIGURE 11-3 The uniform does not touch the sink. Soap and water are within reach. Hands are lower than the elbows. Hands do not touch the inside of the sink.

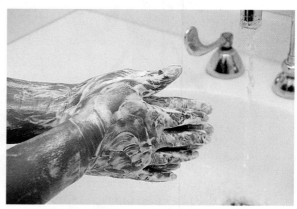

FIGURE 11-4 The palms are rubbed together to work up a good lather.

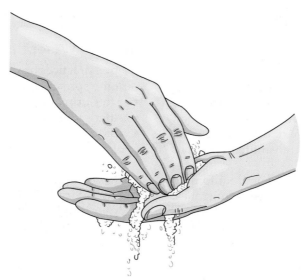

FIGURE 11-5 The fingertips are rubbed against the palms to clean under the fingernails.

Hand Hygiene

Hand hygiene is the easiest and most important way to prevent the spread of infection. You use your hands for almost everything. They are easily contaminated. They can spread microbes to other persons or items. *Practice hand hygiene before and after giving care.* See Box 11-2 for the rules of hand hygiene.

See *Promoting Safety and Comfort: Hand Hygiene.*

PROMOTING SAFETY AND COMFORT
Hand Hygiene

Safety

You use your hands in almost every task. They can pick up microbes from one person, place, or thing. Your hands transfer microbes to other people, places, and things. That is why hand hygiene is so very important. You must practice hand hygiene before and after giving care.

Comfort

You will practice hand hygiene very often during your shift. Hand lotions and hand creams help prevent chapping and dry skin. Apply hand lotion or cream as often as needed. Use an agency-approved lotion or cream.

BOX 11-2   Rules of Hand Hygiene

- Wash your hands (with soap and water) when they are visibly dirty or soiled with blood, body fluids, secretions, or excretions.
- Wash your hands (with soap and water) before eating and after using a restroom.
- Wash your hands (with soap and water) if exposure to the anthrax spore is suspected or proven.
- Use an alcohol-based hand rub to decontaminate your hands if they are not visibly soiled. (If an alcohol-based hand rub is not available, wash your hands with soap and water.) Follow this rule in the following clinical situations:
  - Before having direct contact with a person.
  - After contact with the person's intact skin. For example, after taking a pulse or blood pressure or after moving a person.
  - After contact with body fluids or excretions, mucous membranes, non-intact skin, and wound dressings if hands are not visibly soiled.
  - When moving from a contaminated body site to a clean body site during care activities.
  - After contact with objects (including equipment) in the person's care setting.
  - After removing gloves.
- Follow these rules for washing your hands with soap and water. See procedure: *Hand Washing* (p. 154).
  - Wash your hands under warm running water. Do not use hot water.
  - Stand away from the sink. Do not let your hands, body, or uniform touch the sink. The sink is contaminated (Fig. 11-3).
  - Do not touch the inside of the sink at any time.
  - Keep your hands and forearms lower than your elbows. Your hands are dirtier than your elbows and forearms. If you hold your hands and forearms up, dirty water runs from your hands to your elbows. Those areas become contaminated.
  - Rub your palms together to work up a good lather (Fig. 11-4). The rubbing action helps remove microbes and dirt.
  - Pay attention to areas often missed during hand washing—thumbs, knuckles, sides of the hands, little fingers, and under the nails.
  - Clean fingernails by rubbing the fingertips against your palms (Fig. 11-5).
  - Use a nail file or orange stick to clean under fingernails (Fig. 11-6, p. 154). Microbes easily grow under the fingernails.
  - Wash your hands for at least 15 to 20 seconds. Wash your hands longer if they are dirty or soiled with blood, body fluids, secretions, or excretions. Use your judgment, and follow agency policy.
  - Use a clean, dry paper towel to dry your hands.
  - Dry your hands starting at the fingertips. Work up to your forearms. You will dry the cleanest area first.
  - Use a clean, dry paper towel for each faucet to turn the water off (Fig. 11-7, p. 154). Faucets are contaminated. The paper towels prevent clean hands from becoming contaminated again.
- Follow these rules when decontaminating your hands with an alcohol-based hand rub:
  - Apply the product to the palm of one hand. Follow the manufacturer's instructions for the amount to use.
  - Rub your hands together.
  - Make sure you cover all surfaces of your hands and fingers.
  - Continue rubbing your hands together until your hands are dry.
- Apply hand lotion or cream after hand hygiene. This prevents the skin from chapping and drying. Skin breaks can occur in chapped and dry skin. Skin breaks are portals of entry for microbes.

Modified from Centers for Disease Control and Prevention: Guideline for hand hygiene in health-care settings, *Morbidity and Mortality Report,* 51(RR-16), October 25, 2002.

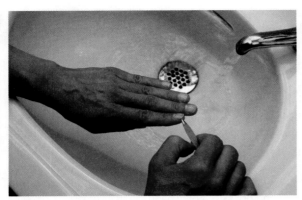

FIGURE 11-6 A nail file is used to clean under the fingernails.

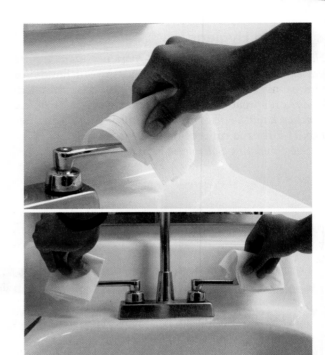

FIGURE 11-7 A paper towel is used to turn off each faucet.

HAND WASHING

PROCEDURE

1. See *Promoting Safety and Comfort: Hand Hygiene,* p. 153.
2. Make sure you have soap, paper towels, an orange stick or nail file, and a wastebasket. Collect missing items.
3. Push your watch up your arm 4 to 5 inches. If your uniform sleeves are long, push them up too.
4. Stand away from the sink so your clothes do not touch the sink. Stand so the soap and faucet are easy to reach (see Fig. 11-3). Do not touch the inside of the sink at any time.
5. Turn on and adjust the water until it feels warm.
6. Wet your wrists and hands. Keep your hands lower than your elbows. Be sure to wet the area 3 to 4 inches above your wrists.
7. Apply about 1 teaspoon of soap to your hands.
8. Rub your palms together and interlace your fingers to work up a good lather (see Fig. 11-4). This step should last at least 15 to 20 seconds. (NOTE: Some state competency tests require that you wash your hands for 20 or 30 seconds. Others require that you wash your hands for 1 to 2 minutes.)
9. Wash each hand and wrist thoroughly. Clean well between the fingers.
10. Clean under the fingernails. Rub your fingertips against your palms (see Fig. 11-5).
11. Clean under the fingernails with a nail file or orange stick (see Fig. 11-6). This step is done for the first hand washing of the day and when your hands are highly soiled.
12. Rinse your wrists and hands well. Water flows from the arms to the hands.
13. Repeat steps 7 through 12, if needed.
14. Dry your wrists and hands with a clean, dry paper towel. Pat dry starting at your fingertips.
15. Discard the paper towels into the wastebasket.
16. Turn off faucets with clean, dry paper towels. This prevents you from contaminating your hands (see Fig. 11-7). Use a clean paper towel for each faucet.
17. Discard the paper towels into the wastebasket.

Supplies and Equipment

Most health care equipment is disposable. Single-use items are discarded after use. A person uses multi-use items many times. They include bedpans, urinals, wash basins, and water pitchers and drinking cups and glasses. Label such items with the person's name and room and bed number. Do not "borrow" them for another person.

Non-disposable items are cleaned and then disinfected. Then they are sterilized.

Cleaning Cleaning reduces the number of microbes present. It also removes organic matter such as blood, body fluids, secretions, and excretions. When cleaning equipment:

- Wear personal protective equipment (PPE)—gloves, mask, gown, and goggles or a face shield—when cleaning items contaminated with blood, body fluids, secretions, or excretions.
- Rinse the item in cold water first. Rinsing removes organic matter. Heat causes organic matter to become thick, sticky, and hard to remove.
- Wash the item with soap and hot water.
- Scrub thoroughly. Use a brush if necessary.
- Rinse the item in warm water. Then dry the item.
- Disinfect or sterilize the item.
- Disinfect equipment and the sink used in the cleaning procedure.
- Discard PPE.
- Practice hand hygiene.

Disinfection **Disinfection** is the process of destroying pathogens. *Germicides* are disinfectants applied to skin, tissues, and non-living objects. Alcohol is a common germicide.

Chemical disinfectants are used to clean surfaces. Counters, tubs, and showers are examples. They also are used to clean re-usable items. Such items include:

- Blood pressure cuffs
- Commodes and metal bedpans
- Wheelchairs and stretchers
- Furniture
  See *Promoting Safety and Comfort: Disinfection.*

PROMOTING SAFETY AND COMFORT
Disinfection

Safety

Chemical disinfectants can burn and irritate the skin. Wear utility gloves or rubber household gloves to prevent skin irritation. These gloves are *waterproof*. Do not wear disposable gloves.

Some chemical disinfectants have special measures for use and storage. Check the material safety data sheet (MSDS) before handling a disinfectant. See Chapter 8.

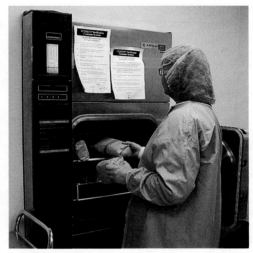

FIGURE 11-8 An autoclave.

Sterilization **Sterilization** is the process of destroying *all* microbes (non-pathogens and pathogens). Very high temperatures are used. Microbes are destroyed by heat.

Boiling water, radiation, liquid or gas chemicals, dry heat, and *steam under pressure* are sterilization methods. An *autoclave* (Fig. 11-8) is a pressure steam sterilizer. It is used for glass, surgical items, and metal objects. High temperatures destroy plastic and rubber items. They are not autoclaved.

Other Aseptic Measures

Hand hygiene, cleaning, disinfection, and sterilization are important aseptic measures. So are the measures listed in Box 11-3, p. 156.

BOX 11-3 | Aseptic Measures

Controlling Reservoirs (Hosts—You or the Person)

- Provide for the person's hygiene needs (Chapter 15).
- Wash contaminated areas with soap and water. Feces, urine, and blood can contain microbes. So can body fluids, secretions, and excretions.
- Use leak-proof plastic bags for soiled tissues, linens, and other materials.
- Keep tables, counters, wheelchair trays, and other surfaces clean and dry.
- Label bottles with the person's name and the date the bottle was opened.
- Keep bottles and fluid containers tightly capped or covered.
- Keep drainage containers below the drainage site.
- Empty drainage containers and dispose of drainage following agency policy. Usually drainage containers are emptied every shift. Follow the nurse's directions.

Controlling Portals of Exit

- Cover your nose and mouth when coughing or sneezing.
- Provide the person with tissues to use when coughing or sneezing.
- Wear PPE as needed (p. 159).

Controlling Transmission

- Make sure all persons have their own personal care equipment. This includes wash basins, bedpans, urinals, commodes, and eating and drinking utensils.
- Do not take equipment from one person's room to use for another person. Even if the item is unused, do not take it from one room to another.
- Hold equipment and linens away from your uniform (Fig. 11-9).
- Practice hand hygiene. See Box 11-2.
- Assist the person with hand washing:
  - Before and after eating
  - After elimination
  - After changing tampons, sanitary napkins, or other personal hygiene products
  - After contact with blood, body fluids, secretions, or excretions
- Prevent dust movement. Do not shake linens or equipment. Use a damp cloth for dusting.
- Clean from the cleanest area to the dirtiest. This prevents soiling a clean area.

Controlling Transmission—cont'd

- Clean away from your body. Do not dust, brush, or wipe toward yourself. Otherwise you transmit microbes to your skin, hair, and clothing.
- Flush urine and feces down the toilet. Avoid splatters and splashes.
- Pour contaminated liquids directly into sinks or toilets. Avoid splashing onto other areas.
- Do not sit on the person's bed. You will pick up microbes. You will transfer them to the next surface that you sit on.
- Do not use items that are on the floor. The floor is contaminated.
- Clean tubs, showers, and shower chairs after each use. Follow the agency's disinfection procedures.
- Clean bedpans, urinals, and commodes after each use. Follow the agency's disinfection procedures.
- Report pests—ants, spiders, mice, and so on.

Controlling Portals of Entry

- Provide for good skin care (Chapter 15). This promotes intact skin.
- Provide for good oral hygiene (Chapter 15). This promotes intact mucous membranes.
- Do not let the person lie on tubes or other items. This protects the skin from injury.
- Make sure linens are dry and wrinkle-free (Chapter 14). This protects the skin from injury.
- Turn and reposition the person as directed by the nurse and care plan (Chapters 12 and 13). This protects the skin from injury.
- Assist with or clean the genital area after elimination (Chapter 15). Wipe and clean from the urethra (the cleanest area) to the rectum (the dirtiest area). This helps prevent urinary tract infections.
- Make sure drainage tubes are properly connected. This prevents microbes from entering the drainage system.

Protecting the Susceptible Host

- Follow the care plan to meet hygiene needs. This protects the skin and mucous membranes.
- Follow the care plan to meet nutrition and fluid needs (Chapter 19). This helps prevent infection.
- Assist with deep-breathing and coughing exercises as directed (Chapter 24). This helps prevent respiratory infections.

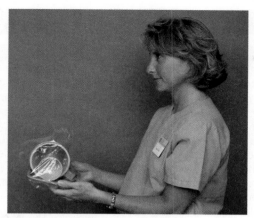

FIGURE 11-9 Hold equipment away from your uniform.

ISOLATION PRECAUTIONS

Blood, body fluids, secretions, and excretions can transmit pathogens. Sometimes barriers are needed to prevent their escape. The pathogens are kept within a certain area, usually the person's room. This requires isolation procedures.

The *Guideline for Isolation Precautions: Preventing Transmission of Infectious Agents in Healthcare Settings 2007* is followed. The guideline was issued by the Centers for Disease Control and Prevention (CDC). Isolation precautions prevent the spread of **communicable diseases (contagious diseases).** They are diseases caused by pathogens that spread easily.

Isolation precautions are based on *clean* and *dirty.* *Clean* areas or objects are free of pathogens. They are not contaminated. *Dirty* areas or objects are contaminated with pathogens. If a *clean* area or object has contact with something *dirty,* the clean area is now dirty. *Clean* and *dirty* also depend on how the pathogen is spread.

The CDC's isolation precautions guideline has two tiers of precautions:
* Standard Precautions
* Transmission-Based Precautions
  See *Focus on Communication: Isolation Precautions.*
  See *Delegation Guidelines: Isolation Precautions.*
  See *Promoting Safety and Comfort: Isolation Precautions.*

Standard Precautions

Standard Precautions are part of the CDC's isolation precautions (Box 11-4, p. 158). They reduce the risk of spreading pathogens. They also reduce the risk of

FOCUS ON COMMUNICATION
Isolation Precautions

Some agencies require visitors to wear PPE when visiting a person needing isolation precautions. Visitors may question the need for PPE. They do not wear PPE around the person in his or her home or outside the agency. They do not understand why it is needed. Some visitors ignore signs or requests to wear PPE. It is important to communicate with the person and visitors about PPE. You can politely say:
* "Your visitors will need to wear a gown and gloves while in your room."
* "Please wear this mask. It is our policy to protect you, your family member, and others."

Tell the nurse if the person or visitors have more questions. Also tell the nurse if someone refuses to follow isolation precautions.

DELEGATION GUIDELINES
Isolation Precautions

If a person requires isolation precautions, review the type used with the nurse. Also check with the nurse and the care plan about:
* What PPE to use
* What special safety measures are needed

PROMOTING SAFETY AND COMFORT
Isolation Precautions

Safety
Preventing the spread of infection is important. Isolation precautions protect everyone—patients, residents, visitors, staff, and you. If you are careless, everyone's safety is at risk.

spreading known and unknown infections. *Standard Precautions are used for all persons whenever care is given.* They prevent the spread of infection from:
* Blood.
* All body fluids, secretions, and excretions (except sweat) even if blood is not visible. Sweat is not known to spread infection.
* Non-intact skin (skin with open breaks).
* Mucous membranes.

BOX 11-4 Standard Precautions

Hand Hygiene

- Follow the rules for hand hygiene. See Box 11-2.
- Avoid unnecessary touching of surfaces close to the person. This prevents contamination of clean hands from environmental surfaces. It also prevents the transmission of pathogens from contaminated hands to other surfaces.
- Do not wear fake nails or nail extenders if you will have contact with persons at risk for infection or other adverse outcomes.

Personal Protective Equipment (PPE)

- Wear PPE when contact with blood or body fluids is likely.
- Do not contaminate your clothing or skin when removing PPE.
- Remove and discard PPE before leaving the person's room or care setting.

Gloves

- Wear gloves when contact with the following is likely:
  - Blood
  - Potentially infectious materials (body fluids, secretions, and excretions are examples)
  - Mucous membranes
  - Non-intact skin
  - Skin that may be contaminated (for example, a person is incontinent of stool or urine)
- Wear gloves that fit and are appropriate for the task:
  - Wear disposable gloves to provide direct care to the person.
  - Wear disposable gloves or utility gloves for cleaning equipment or care settings.
- Remove gloves after contact with the person or the person's care setting. The care setting includes equipment used in the person's care.
- Remove gloves after contact with care equipment.
- Do not wear the same pair of gloves to care for more than one person. Remove gloves after contact with a person and before going to another person.
- Do not wash gloves for re-use with different persons.
- Change gloves during care if your hands will move from a contaminated body site to a clean body site.

Gowns

- Wear a gown that is appropriate to the task.
- Wear a gown to protect your skin and clothing when contact with blood, body fluids, secretions, or excretions is likely.
- Wear a gown for direct contact with a person if he or she has uncontained secretions or excretions.
- Remove the gown and perform hand hygiene before leaving the person's room or care setting.
- Do not re-use gowns, even for repeat contacts with the same person.

Mouth, Nose, and Eye Protection

- Wear PPE—masks, goggles, face shields—for procedures and tasks that are likely to cause splashes and sprays of blood, body fluids, secretions, or excretions.
- Wear PPE—mask, goggles, face shield—appropriate for the procedure or task.
- Wear gloves, a gown, and one of the following for procedures that are likely to cause sprays of respiratory secretions:
  - A face shield that fully covers the front and sides of the face
  - A mask with attached shield
  - A mask and goggles

Respiratory Hygiene/Cough Etiquette

- Instruct persons with respiratory symptoms to:
  - Cover the nose and mouth when coughing or sneezing.
  - Use tissues to contain respiratory secretions.
  - Dispose of tissues in the nearest waste container after use.
  - Perform hand hygiene after contact with respiratory secretions.
- Provide visitors with masks according to agency policy.

Care Equipment

- Wear appropriate PPE when handling care equipment that is visibly soiled with blood, body fluids, secretions, or excretions.
- Wear appropriate PPE when handling care equipment that may have been in contact with blood, body fluids, secretions, or excretions.
- Remove organic material before disinfection and sterilization procedures. Use cleaning agents according to agency policy.

BOX 11-4 Standard Precautions—cont'd

Care of the Environment

- Follow agency policies and procedures for cleaning and maintaining surfaces. Environmental surfaces and care equipment are examples. Surfaces near the person may need more frequent cleaning and maintenance—door knobs, bed rails, overbed tables, toilet surfaces and areas, and so on.
- Clean and disinfect multi-use electronic equipment according to agency policy. This includes:
  - Items used by patients and residents
  - Items used to give care
  - Mobile devices that are moved in and out of patient or resident rooms
- Follow these rules for toys used by children or child play toys in waiting areas:
  - Select play toys that can be easily cleaned and disinfected.
  - Do not allow the use of stuffed or furry toys if they will be shared.
  - Clean and disinfect large stationary toys (for example, climbing equipment) at least weekly and whenever visibly soiled.
  - Rinse toys with water after disinfection if they are likely to be mouthed by children. Or wash them in a dishwasher.
  - Clean and disinfect a toy immediately when it requires cleaning. Or store the toy in a labeled container away from toys that are clean and ready for use.

Textiles and Laundry

- Handle used textiles and fabrics (linens) with minimum agitation. This is done to avoid contamination of air, surfaces, and other persons.

Worker Safety

- Protect yourself and others from exposure to bloodborne pathogens. This includes how to handle needles and other sharps. Follow federal and state standards and guidelines. See the Bloodborne Pathogen Standard (p. 168).
- Use a mouthpiece, resuscitation bag, or other ventilation device during resuscitation to prevent contact with the person's mouth and oral secretions. See Chapter 29.

Patient or Resident Placement

- A private room is preferred if the person is at risk for transmitting the infection to others.
- Follow the nurse's instructions if a private room is not available.

Modified from Siegel JD, Rhinehart E, Jackson M, Chiarello L, and the Healthcare Infection Control Practices Advisory Committee: *Guideline for isolation precautions: preventing transmission of infectious agents in healthcare settings 2007,* Centers for Disease Control and Prevention, June 2007.

Transmission-Based Precautions

Some infections require Transmission-Based Precautions (Box 11-5, p. 160). You must understand how certain infections are spread (see Fig. 11-2). This helps you understand the 3 types of Transmission-Based Precautions.

Agency policies may differ from those in this text. The rules in Box 11-6, p. 161 are a guide for giving safe care when using isolation precautions.

Protective Measures

Isolation precautions involve wearing PPE—gloves, a gown, a mask, and goggles or a face shield. Removing linens, trash, and equipment from the room may require double-bagging. Follow agency procedures when collecting specimens and transporting persons.

See *Promoting Safety and Comfort: Protective Measures,* p. 161.

Text continued on p. 163

BOX 11-5   Transmission-Based Precautions

Contact Precautions

- Used for persons with known or suspected infections or conditions that increase the risk of contact transmission.
- Patient or resident placement:
  - A single room is preferred.
  - Do the following if a room is shared with another person who is not infected with the same agent:
    - Keep the privacy curtain between the beds closed.
    - Change PPE and perform hand hygiene between contact with persons in the same room. Do so regardless of whether one or both persons are on Contact Precautions.
- Gloves:
  - Don gloves upon entering the person's room or care setting.
  - Wear gloves whenever touching the person's intact skin.
  - Wear gloves whenever touching surfaces or items near the person.
- Gowns:
  - Wear a gown whenever clothing may have direct contact with the person.
  - Wear a gown whenever contact is likely with surfaces or equipment near the person.
  - Don the gown upon entering the person's room or care setting.
  - Remove the gown and perform hand hygiene before leaving the person's room or care setting.
  - After removing the gown, make sure your clothing and skin do not touch potentially contaminated surfaces.
- Patient or resident transport:
  - Limit transport and movement of the person outside of the room to medically-necessary purposes.
  - Cover the area of the person's body that is infected.
  - Remove and discard contaminated PPE and perform hand hygiene before transporting the person.
  - Don clean PPE to handle the person at the transport destination.
- Care equipment:
  - Follow Standard Precautions.
  - Use disposable equipment when possible. If possible, leave non-disposable equipment in the person's room.
  - Clean and disinfect non-disposable and multiple-use equipment before use on another person.
  - For home care settings:
    - Limit the amount of non-disposable care items brought into the home. Leave them in the home as long as they are needed.
    - Clean and disinfect items that cannot be left in the home. Stethoscopes and blood pressure cuffs are examples. Clean and disinfect care items before taking them from the home. Or place them in a plastic bag for transport for later cleaning and disinfection.

Droplet Precautions

- Used for persons known or suspected to be infected with pathogens transmitted by respiratory droplets. Such droplets are generated by a person who is coughing, sneezing, or talking.
- Patient or resident placement:
  - A single room is preferred.
  - Do the following if a room is shared with another person who is not infected with the same agent:
    - Keep the privacy curtain between the beds closed.
    - Change PPE and perform hand hygiene between contact with persons in the same room. Do so regardless of whether one or both persons are on Droplet Precautions.
- Personal protective equipment:
  - Don a mask upon entering the person's room or care setting.
- Patient or resident transport:
  - Limit transport and movement of the person outside of the room to medically-necessary purposes.
  - Have the person wear a mask.
  - Instruct the person to follow Respiratory Hygiene/Cough Etiquette (see Box 11-4).
  - No mask is required for health team members transporting the person.

Airborne Precautions

- Used for persons known or suspected to be infected with pathogens transmitted person-to-person by the airborne route. Tuberculosis (TB), measles, chickenpox, smallpox, and severe acute respiratory syndrome (SARS) are examples.
- The patient or resident is placed in an airborne infection isolation room (AIIR). If one is not available, the person is transferred to an agency with an AIIR.
- Health team members susceptible to the infection are restricted from entering the room. This is if immune staff members are available.
- Personal protective equipment:
  - An approved respirator is worn on entering the room or home of a person with TB.
  - Respiratory protection is recommended for all health team members when caring for persons with smallpox.
- Patient or resident transport:
  - Limit transport and movement of the person outside of the room to medically-necessary purposes.
  - Have the person wear a surgical mask.
  - Instruct the person to follow Respiratory Hygiene/Cough Etiquette (see Box 11-4).
  - Cover skin lesions infected with the microbe.
  - No mask or respirator is required for health team members transporting the person.

Modified from Siegel JD, Rhinehart E, Jackson M, Chiarello L, and the Healthcare Infection Control Practices Advisory Committee: *Guideline for isolation precautions: preventing transmission of infectious agents in healthcare settings 2007,* Centers for Disease Control and Prevention, June 2007.

BOX 11-6 Rules for Isolation Precautions

- Collect all needed items before entering the room.
- Prevent contamination of equipment and supplies. Floors are contaminated. So is any object on the floor or that falls to the floor.
- Use mops wetted with a disinfectant solution to clean floors. Floor dust is contaminated.
- Prevent drafts. Some microbes are carried in the air by drafts.
- Use paper towels to handle contaminated items.
- Remove items from the room in leak-proof plastic bags.
- Double-bag items if the outer part of the bag is or can be contaminated (p. 167).
- Follow agency policy for removing and transporting disposable and re-usable items.
- Return re-usable dishes, drinking vessels, eating utensils, and trays to the food service (dietary) department. Discard disposable dishes, drinking vessels, eating utensils, and trays in the waste container in the person's room.
- Do not touch your hair, nose, mouth, eyes, or other body parts.
- Do not touch any clean area or object if your hands are contaminated.
- Wash your hands if they are visibly dirty or contaminated with blood, body fluids, secretions, or excretions.
- Place clean items on paper towels.
- Do not shake linens.
- Use paper towels to turn faucets on and off.
- Use a paper towel to open the door to the person's room. Discard it as you leave.
- Tell the nurse if you have any cuts, open skin areas, a sore throat, vomiting, or diarrhea.

PROMOTING SAFETY AND COMFORT
Protective Measures

Safety

The PPE needed for Standard Precautions depends on what tasks, procedures, and care measures you will do while in the room. The PPE needed also depends on the type of Transmission-Based Precautions ordered for the person. Sometimes only gloves are needed. The nurse tells you when other PPE are needed.

Gloves are always worn when gowns are worn. Sometimes other PPE are needed when gowns are worn. The CDC's isolation guideline shows PPE donned and removed in the following order:

- Donning PPE (Fig. 11-10, *A*, p. 162)
  - Gown
  - Mask or respirator
  - Eyewear (goggles or face shield)
  - Gloves
- Removing PPE (removed at the doorway before leaving the person's room) (Fig. 11-10, *B*, p. 162)
  - Gloves
  - Goggles or face shield
  - Gown
  - Mask or respirator

SEQUENCE FOR DONNING PERSONAL PROTECTIVE EQUIPMENT (PPE)

The type of PPE used will vary based on the level of precautions required; e.g., Standard and Contact, Droplet or Airborne Infection Isolation.

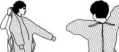

1. GOWN
- Fully cover torso from neck to knees, arms to end of wrists, and wrap around the back
- Fasten in back of neck and waist

2. MASK OR RESPIRATOR
- Secure ties or elastic bands at middle of head and neck
- Fit flexible band to nose bridge
- Fit snug to face and below chin
- Fit-check respirator

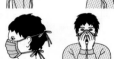

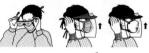

3. GOGGLES OR FACE SHIELD
- Place over face and eyes and adjust to fit

4. GLOVES
- Extend to cover wrist of isolation gown

USE SAFE WORK PRACTICES TO PROTECT YOURSELF AND LIMIT THE SPREAD OF CONTAMINATION

- Keep hands away from face
- Limit surfaces touched
- Change gloves when torn or heavily contaminated
- Perform hand hygiene

SECUENCIA PARA PONERSE EL EQUIPO DE PROTECCIÓN PERSONAL (PPE)

El tipo de PPE que se debe utilizar depende del nivel de precaución que sea necesario; por ejemplo, equipo Estándar y de Contacto o de Aislamiento de infecciones transportadas por gotas o por aire.

1. BATA
- Cubra con la bata todo el torso desde el cuello hasta las rodillas, los brazos hasta la muñeca y dóblela alrededor de la espalda
- Átesela por detrás a la altura del cuello y la cintura

2. MÁSCARA O RESPIRADOR
- Asegúrese los cordones o la banda elástica en la mitad de la cabeza y en el cuello
- Ajústese la banda flexible en el puente de la nariz
- Acomódesela en la cara y por debajo del mentón
- Verifique el ajuste del respirador

3. GAFAS PROTECTORAS O CARETAS
- Colóquesela sobre la cara y los ojos y ajústela

4. GUANTES
- Extienda los guantes para que cubran la parte del puño en la bata de aislamiento

UTILICE PRÁCTICAS DE TRABAJO SEGURAS PARA PROTEGERSE USTED MISMO Y LIMITAR LA PROPAGACIÓN DE LA CONTAMINACIÓN

- Mantenga las manos alejadas de la cara
- Limite el contacto con superficies
- Cambie los guantes si se rompen o están demasiado contaminados
- Realice la higiene de las manos

A

SEQUENCE FOR REMOVING PERSONAL PROTECTIVE EQUIPMENT (PPE)

Except for respirator, remove PPE at doorway or in anteroom. Remove respirator after leaving patient room and closing door.

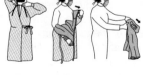

1. GLOVES
- Outside of gloves is contaminated!
- Grasp outside of glove with opposite gloved hand; peel off
- Hold removed glove in gloved hand
- Slide fingers of ungloved hand under remaining glove at wrist
- Peel glove off over first glove
- Discard gloves in waste container

2. GOGGLES OR FACE SHIELD
- Outside of goggles or face shield is contaminated!
- To remove, handle by head band or ear pieces
- Place in designated receptacle for reprocessing or in waste container

3. GOWN
- Gown front and sleeves are contaminated!
- Unfasten ties
- Pull away from neck and shoulders, touching inside of gown only
- Turn gown inside out
- Fold or roll into a bundle and discard

4. MASK OR RESPIRATOR
- Front of mask/respirator is contaminated — DO NOT TOUCH!
- Grasp bottom, then top ties or elastics and remove
- Discard in waste container

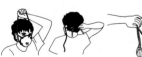

PERFORM HAND HYGIENE IMMEDIATELY AFTER REMOVING ALL PPE

SECUENCIA PARA QUITARSE EL EQUIPO DE PROTECCIÓN PERSONAL (PPE)

Con la excepción del respirador, quítese el PPE en la entrada de la puerta o en la antesala. Quítese el respirador después de salir de la habitación del paciente y de cerrar la puerta.

1. GUANTES
- ¡El exterior de los guantes está contaminado!
- Agarre la parte exterior del guante con la mano opuesta en la que todavía tiene puesto el guante y quíteselo
- Sostenga el guante que se quitó con la mano enguantada
- Deslice los dedos de la mano sin guante por debajo del otro guante que no se ha quitado todavía a la altura de la muñeca
- Quítese el guante de manera que acabe cubriendo el primer guante
- Arroje los guantes en el recipiente de deshechos

2. GAFAS PROTECTORAS O CARETA
- ¡El exterior de las gafas protectoras o de la careta está contaminado!
- Para quitárselas, tómelas por la parte de la banda de la cabeza o de las piezas de las orejas
- Colóquelas en el recipiente designado para reprocesar materiales o de materiales de deshecho

3. BATA
- ¡La parte delantera de la bata y las mangas están contaminadas!
- Desate los cordones
- Tocando solamente el interior de la bata, pásela por encima del cuello y de los hombros
- Voltee la bata al revés
- Dóblela o enróllela y deséchela

4. MÁSCARA O RESPIRADOR
- La parte delantera de la máscara o respirador está contaminada — ¡NO LA TOQUE!
- Primero agarre la parte de abajo, luego los cordones o banda elástica de arriba y por último quítese la máscara o respirador
- Arrójela en el recipiente de deshechos

EFECTÚE LA HIGIENE DE LAS MANOS INMEDIATAMENTE DESPUÉS DE QUITARSE CUALQUIER EQUIPO DE PROTECCIÓN PERSONAL

B

FIGURE 11-10 A, Donning personal protective equipment. **B,** Removing personal protective equipment. *(From Centers for Disease Control and Prevention—Division of Healthcare Quality Promotion (DHQP):* Personal protective equipment (PPE) in healthcare settings: sequence for donning and removing personal protective equipment (PPE), *Atlanta, GA, October 2004.)*

◆ Gloves Small skin breaks on the hands and fingers are common. Disposable gloves act as a barrier. They protect you from pathogens in the person's blood, body fluids, secretions, and excretions. They also protect the person from microbes on your hands.

Wear gloves whenever contact with blood, body fluids, secretions, excretions, mucous membranes, and non-intact skin is likely. Contact may be direct. Or contact may be with items or surfaces contaminated with blood, body fluids, secretions, or excretions.

Wearing gloves is the most common protective measure used with Standard Precautions and Transmission-Based Precautions. Remember the following when using gloves:

* The outside of gloves is contaminated.
* Gloves are easier to put on when your hands are dry.
* Do not tear gloves when putting them on. Carelessness, long fingernails, and rings can tear gloves. Blood, body fluids, secretions, and excretions can enter the glove through the tear. This contaminates your hand.
* You need a new pair for every person.
* Remove and discard torn, cut, or punctured gloves at once. Practice hand hygiene. Then put on a new pair.
* Wear gloves once. Discard them after use.
* Put on clean gloves just before touching mucous membranes or non-intact skin.
* Put on new gloves whenever gloves become contaminated with blood, body fluids, secretions, or excretions. A task may require more than one pair of gloves.
* Change gloves whenever moving from a contaminated body site to a clean body site.
* Change gloves if interacting with the person involves touching portable computer keyboards or other mobile equipment that is transported from room to room.
* Put on gloves last when they are worn with other PPE.
* Make sure gloves cover your wrists. If you wear a gown, gloves cover the cuffs (Fig. 11-11).
* Remove gloves so the inside part is on the outside. The inside is *clean.*
* Decontaminate your hands after removing gloves.

See *Promoting Safety and Comfort: Gloves.*

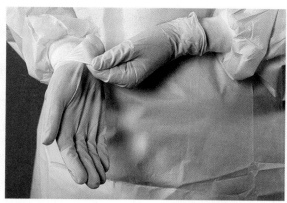

FIGURE 11-11 The gloves cover the cuffs of the gown.

PROMOTING SAFETY AND COMFORT
Gloves

Safety

No special method is needed to put on non-sterile gloves. To remove gloves, see procedure: *Removing Gloves,* p. 164.

Some gloves are made of latex (a rubber product). Latex allergies are common. They can cause skin rashes. Asthma and shock are more serious problems. Report skin rashes and breathing problems to the nurse at once.

You may have a latex allergy. Some patients and residents are allergic to latex. This information is on the care plan and your assignment sheet. Latex-free gloves are worn for latex allergies.

Comfort

You do not need to wear gloves for every patient or resident contact. Gloves are needed whenever contact with blood, body fluids, secretions, excretions, mucous membranes, and non-intact skin is likely. You do not need to wear gloves when such contact is not likely. Back massages and brushing and combing hair are examples. Wearing gloves only when needed helps reduce exposure to latex.

REMOVING GLOVES

NNAAP™

PROCEDURE

1 See *Promoting Safety and Comfort: Gloves*, p. 163.
2 Make sure that glove touches only glove.
3 Grasp a glove just below the cuff (Fig. 11-12, *A*). Grasp it on the outside.
4 Pull the glove down over your hand so it is inside out (Fig. 11-12, *B*).
5 Hold the removed gloved with your other gloved hand.

6 Reach inside the other glove. Use the first two fingers of the ungloved hand (Fig. 11-12, *C*).
7 Pull the glove down (inside out) over your hand and the other glove (Fig. 11-12, *D*).
8 Discard the gloves into the wastebasket.
9 Decontaminate your hands.

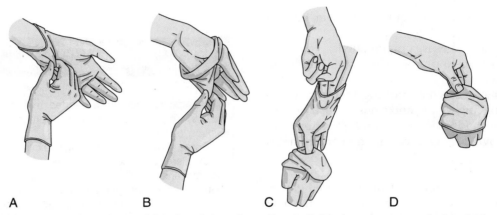

A   B   C   D

FIGURE 11-12 Removing gloves. **A,** Grasp the glove below the cuff. **B,** Pull the glove down over the hand. The glove is inside out. **C,** Insert the fingers of the ungloved hand inside the other glove. **D,** Pull the glove down and over the other hand and glove. The glove is inside out.

Gowns Gowns prevent the spread of microbes. They protect your clothes and body from contact with blood, body fluids, secretions, and excretions. They also protect against splashes and sprays.

Gowns must completely cover you from your neck to your knees. The long sleeves have tight cuffs. The gown opens at the back. It is tied at the neck and waist. The front of the gown and sleeves are considered to be *contaminated*.

Gowns are used once. They are discarded after use. A wet gown is contaminated. It is removed and a dry one put on.

View Video!

DONNING AND REMOVING A GOWN

NNAAP™

PROCEDURE

1 Remove your watch and all jewelry.
2 Roll up uniform sleeves.
3 Practice hand hygiene.
4 Hold a clean gown out in front of you. Let it unfold. Do not shake the gown.
5 Put your hands and arms through the sleeves (see Fig. 11-10, *A*).
6 Make sure the gown covers you from your neck to your knees. It must cover your arms to the end of your wrists.
7 Tie the strings at the back of the neck (see Fig. 11-10, *A*).
8 Overlap the back of the gown. Make sure it covers your uniform. The gown should be snug, not loose.
9 Tie the waist strings. Tie them at the back or the side. Do not tie them in front.
10 Put on other PPE.
    a Mask or respirator (if needed).
    b Goggles or face shield (if needed).
    c Gloves. Make sure the gloves cover the gown cuffs.

11 Provide care.
12 Remove and discard the gloves.
13 Remove and discard the goggles or face shield if worn.
14 Remove the gown. Do not touch the outside of the gown.
    a Untie the neck and waist strings (see Fig. 11-10, *B*).
    b Pull the gown down from each shoulder toward the same hand (see Fig. 11-10, *B*).
    c Turn the gown inside out as it is removed. Hold it at the inside shoulder seams, and bring your hands together (Fig. 11-13).
15 Hold and roll up the gown away from you (see Fig. 11-10, *B*). Keep it inside out.
16 Discard the gown.
17 Remove and discard the mask if worn.
18 Decontaminate your hands.

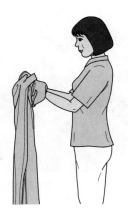

FIGURE 11-13 The gown is turned inside out as it is removed.

Masks and Respiratory Protection Masks prevent contact with infectious materials from the patient or resident. Respiratory secretions and sprays of blood or body fluids are examples.

Masks are disposable. A wet or moist mask is contaminated. Breathing can cause masks to become wet or moist. Apply a new mask when contamination occurs.

A mask fits snugly over your nose and mouth. Practice hand hygiene before putting on a mask. When removing a mask, touch only the ties or the elastic bands. The front of the mask is contaminated.

DONNING AND REMOVING A MASK

PROCEDURE

1 Practice hand hygiene.
2 Put on a gown if required.
3 Pick up a mask by its upper ties. Do not touch the part that will cover your face.
4 Place the mask over your nose and mouth (Fig. 11-14, *A*).
5 Place the upper strings above your ears. Tie them at the back in the middle of your head (Fig. 11-14, *B*).
6 Tie the lower strings at the back of your neck (Fig. 11-14, *C*). The lower part of the mask is under your chin.
7 Pinch the metal band around your nose. The top of the mask must be snug over your nose. If you wear eyeglasses, the mask must be snug under the bottom of the eyeglasses.
8 Make sure the mask is snug over your face and under your chin.

9 Put on goggles or a face shield if needed and if not part of the mask.
10 Put on gloves.
11 Provide care. Avoid coughing, sneezing, and unnecessary talking.
12 Change the mask if it becomes wet or contaminated.
13 Remove the mask (see Fig. 11-10, *B*).
  a Remove the gloves.
  b Remove the goggles or face shield and gown if worn.
  c Untie the lower strings of the mask.
  d Untie the top strings.
  e Hold the top strings. Remove the mask.
14 Discard the mask.
15 Decontaminate your hands.

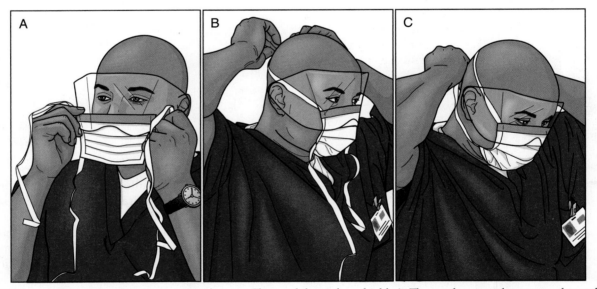

FIGURE 11-14 Donning and removing a mask. NOTE: The mask has a face shield. **A,** The mask covers the nose and mouth. **B,** Upper strings are tied at the back of the head. **C,** Lower strings are tied at the back of the neck.

Goggles and Face Shields Goggles and face shields protect your eyes, mouth, and nose from splashing or spraying of blood, body fluids, secretions, and excretions (see Fig. 11-14). Splashes and sprays can occur when giving care, cleaning items, or disposing of fluids.

The outside of goggles or a face shield is contaminated. The ties, ear pieces, or headband used to secure the device are considered "clean." Use them to remove the device. They are safe to touch with bare hands.

Discard disposable goggles or face shields after use. Re-usable eyewear is cleaned with soap and water before re-use. Then a disinfectant is used.

See *Promoting Safety and Comfort: Goggles and Face Shields.*

Bagging Items Contaminated items are bagged to remove them from the person's room. Leak-proof plastic bags are used. They have the BIOHAZARD symbol (Fig. 11-15). **Biohazardous waste** is items contaminated with blood, body fluids, secretions, or excretions. (*Bio* means life. *Hazardous* means dangerous or harmful.)

Bag and transport linens following agency policy. Laundry bags with contaminated linen need a BIOHAZARD symbol. Melt-away bags are common. They dissolve in hot water. Once soiled linen is bagged, no one needs to handle it. Do not overfill the bag. Tie the bag securely. Then place it in a laundry hamper lined with a biohazard plastic bag.

Trash is placed in a container labeled with the BIOHAZARD symbol. Follow agency policy for bagging and transporting trash, equipment, and supplies.

Usually one bag is needed. Double-bagging involves two bags. Double-bagging is not needed unless the outside of the bag is soiled. Two staff members are needed. One is inside the room. The other is at the doorway outside the room. The person in the room places contaminated items into a bag. Then the bag is sealed. The person outside the room holds open another bag. This bag is clean. A wide cuff is made on the clean bag to protect the hands from contamination (Fig. 11-16). The contaminated bag is placed into the clean bag at the doorway.

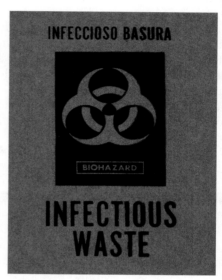

FIGURE 11-15 BIOHAZARD symbol.

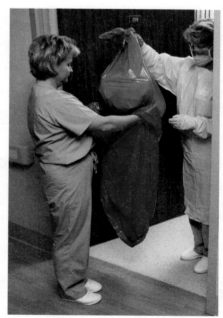

FIGURE 11-16 Double-bagging. One nursing assistant is in the room by the doorway. The other is outside the doorway. The "dirty" bag is placed inside the "clean" bag.

PROMOTING SAFETY AND COMFORT
Goggles and Face Shields

Safety

Eyeglasses and contact lenses do not provide adequate eye protection. If you wear eyeglasses, use a face shield that fits over your glasses with minimal gaps.

Goggles do not provide splash or spray protection to other parts of your face.

Meeting Basic Needs

The person has love, belonging, and self-esteem needs. Often they are unmet when Transmission-Based Precautions are used. Visitors and staff often avoid the person. Putting on PPE takes extra effort before entering the room. Some are not sure what they can touch. They may fear getting the disease.

The person may feel lonely, unwanted, and rejected. The person knows the disease can be spread to others. He or she may feel dirty and undesirable. Without intending to, visitors and staff can make the person feel ashamed and guilty for having a contagious disease. Remember, the *pathogen* is undesirable, not the *person.*

You can help meet love, belonging, and self-esteem needs. See *Focus on PRIDE: The Person, Family, and Yourself* (p. 170).

See *Persons With Dementia: Meeting Basic Needs.*

PERSONS WITH DEMENTIA
Meeting Basic Needs

Persons with dementia do not understand the need for isolation precautions. Masks, gowns, goggles, and face shields may increase confusion and cause fear and agitation. These measures can help:

- Let the person see your face before putting on PPE.
- Tell the person who you are and what you are going to do.
- Use a calm, soothing voice.
- Do not hurry the person.
- Use touch to reassure the person.
- Follow the care plan and the nurse's instructions for other measures to help the person.
- Report signs of increased confusion or behavior changes.

BLOODBORNE PATHOGEN STANDARD

The Bloodborne Pathogen Standard protects against the human immunodeficiency virus (HIV) and the hepatitis B virus (HBV). It is a regulation of the Occupational Safety and Health Administration (OSHA).

HIV and HBV are found in the blood. They are bloodborne pathogens. They exit the body through blood. They are spread to others by blood and other potentially infectious materials (OPIM). OPIM are contaminated with blood or with a body fluid that may contain blood. This includes semen, vaginal secretions, and saliva. OPIM also includes needles, suction equipment, soiled linens, dressings, and other care items.

Staff at risk for exposure to blood or OPIM receive free training. Training occurs upon employment and yearly. Training is also required for new or changed tasks involving exposure to bloodborne pathogens.

Hepatitis B Vaccination

Hepatitis B is a liver disease. It is caused by HBV. HBV is spread by blood and sexual contact.

The hepatitis B vaccine produces immunity against hepatitis B. *Immunity* means that a person has protection against a certain disease. He or she will not get the disease.

A *vaccination* involves giving a vaccine to produce immunity against an infectious disease. A vaccine contains dead or weakened microbes. You can receive the hepatitis B vaccination within 10 working days of being hired. The agency pays for it. You can refuse the vaccination. If so, you must sign a statement refusing the vaccine. You can have the vaccination at a later date.

Engineering and Work Practice Controls

Engineering controls reduce employee exposure in the workplace. Special containers for contaminated sharps (needles, broken glass) and specimens remove and isolate the hazard from staff. Containers are closeable puncture-resistant, leak-proof, and color-coded in red. They have the BIOHAZARD symbol.

Work practice controls also reduce exposure risks. All tasks involving blood or OPIM are done in ways to limit splatters, splashes, and sprays. Producing droplets also is avoided. OSHA requires these work practice controls:

- Do not eat, drink, smoke, apply cosmetics or lip balm, or handle contact lenses in areas of occupational exposure.
- Do not store food or drinks where blood or OPIM are kept.
- Practice hand hygiene after removing gloves.
- Wash hands as soon as possible after skin contact with blood or OPIM.
- Never recap, bend, or remove needles by hand. When recapping, bending, or removing contaminated needles is required, use mechanical means (forceps) or a one-handed method.
- Never shear or break contaminated needles.
- Discard contaminated needles and sharp instruments (such as razors) in containers that are closable, puncture-resistant, and leak-proof. Containers are color-coded in red and have the BIOHAZARD symbol. Containers must be upright and not allowed to overfill.

Personal Protective Equipment (PPE)

This includes gloves, goggles, face shields, masks, laboratory coats, gowns, shoe covers, and surgical caps. Blood or OPIM must not pass through them. They protect your clothes, undergarments, skin, eyes, mouth, and hair.

PPE is free to employees. OSHA requires these measures for the safe handling and use of PPE:

- Remove PPE before leaving the work area.
- Remove PPE when a garment becomes contaminated.
- Place used PPE in marked areas or containers when being stored, washed, decontaminated, or discarded.
- Wear gloves when you expect contact with blood or OPIM.
- Wear gloves when handling or touching contaminated items or surfaces.
- Replace worn, punctured, or contaminated gloves.
- Never wash or decontaminate disposable gloves for re-use.
- Discard utility gloves that show signs of cracking, peeling, tearing, or puncturing. Utility gloves are decontaminated for re-use if the process will not ruin them.

Equipment

Contaminated equipment is cleaned and decontaminated. Decontaminate work surfaces with a proper disinfectant:

- Upon completing tasks
- At once when there is obvious contamination
- After any spill of blood or OPIM
- At the end of the work shift when surfaces became contaminated since the last cleaning

Use a brush and dustpan or tongs to clean up broken glass. Never pick up broken glass with your hands, not even with gloves. Discard broken glass into a puncture-resistant container.

Laundry

OSHA requires these measures for contaminated laundry:

- Handle it as little as possible.
- Wear gloves or other needed PPE.
- Bag contaminated laundry where it is used.
- Mark laundry bags or containers with the BIOHAZARD symbol for laundry sent off-site.
- Place wet, contaminated laundry in leak-proof containers before transport. The containers are color-coded in red or have the BIOHAZARD symbol.

Exposure Incidents

An *exposure incident* is any eye, mouth, other mucous membrane, non-intact skin, or parenteral contact with blood or OPIM. *Parenteral* means piercing the mucous membranes or the skin barrier. Piercing occurs through needle sticks, human bites, cuts, and abrasions.

Report exposure incidents at once. Medical evaluation and follow-up are free. Your blood is tested for HIV and HBV. If you refuse testing, the blood sample is kept for at least 90 days. Testing is done later if you change your mind.

You are told of any medical conditions that may need treatment. You receive a written opinion of the medical evaluation within 15 days after its completion.

The *source individual* is the person whose blood or body fluids are the source of an exposure incident. His or her blood is tested for HIV or HBV. State laws vary about releasing the results. The agency informs you about laws affecting the source's identity and test results.

Focus on P R I D E
The Person, Family, and Yourself

Personal and Professional Responsibility—You have an important role in preventing the spread of infection. Your actions increase or decrease a person's risk for an infection. You are responsible for following the guidelines in this chapter. Practice good hand hygiene. Wash your hands before and after giving care. Follow Standard and Transmission-Based Precautions.

When assisting with or performing a procedure, remove items that become contaminated. If necessary, stop and get new supplies. Do not use a contaminated item. You may be alone. Be honest with yourself. Be responsible. Do the right thing, even if other staff are not present. Take pride in providing care that reduces the risk of spreading infection.

Rights and Respect—Without intending to, people can make a person feel ashamed and guilty for having a contagious disease. Avoid statements or actions that make the person feel embarrassed or guilty. For example, do not say:

- "How did you get that?"
- "What were you doing?"
- "I'm afraid to touch you."
- "Don't breathe on me."

Do not judge a person for having a disease. Treat all persons with respect, kindness, and dignity.

Independence and Social Interaction—Persons requiring isolation precautions usually must stay in their rooms. They cannot go into the hallway or go to the nurses' station, dining room, or lounge. The person may feel lonely, especially if visitors are few. To help the person, you can:

- Remember that the pathogen is undesirable, not the person.
- Treat the person with respect, kindness, and dignity.
- Provide newspapers, magazines, books, and other reading matter. (Items brought into the person's room become contaminated. Disinfect or discard the items according to agency policy.)
- Provide hobby materials if possible.
- Place a clock in the room.
- Urge the person to call family and friends.
- Provide a current TV guide.
- Organize your work so you can stay to visit with the person.
- Say "hello" from the doorway often.

Delegation and Teamwork—Caring for a person needing isolation precautions requires teamwork. Once in the room, the nursing team member cannot easily leave the room to answer signal lights or obtain needed care items. When a person requires isolation, offer to help your co-worker. Do so willingly and pleasantly. Bring items to the room as needed. Also, answer signal lights for your co-worker. Be sure to report what you did for the person and what you observed. Likewise, ask a co-worker to help you if you are going to be with a person needing isolation precautions. Ask politely and thank your co-worker for helping you.

Ethics and Laws—The Centers for Disease Control and Prevention (CDC) is a federal agency. It serves to protect the health and safety of people in the United States. The CDC develops guidelines and standards to improve health. The CDC's *Hand Hygiene Guideline* and *Guideline for Isolation Precautions: Preventing Transmission of Infectious Agents in Healthcare Settings 2007* are examples. Survey teams check to make sure that the agency complies with CDC guidelines and standards. They also observe how care is given.

REVIEW QUESTIONS

Circle T if the statement is *true.* Circle F if the statement is *false.*

1 **T** F A pathogen can cause an infection.
2 T **F** An item is sterile if non-pathogens are present.
3 T **F** You hold your hands and forearms up during hand washing.
4 T **F** Unused items in the person's room are used for another person.
5 T **F** A person received the hepatitis B vaccine. The person will develop the disease.
6 **T** F Hand hygiene helps prevent healthcare-associated infections.

Circle the BEST answer.

7 Most pathogens need the following to grow *except*
   a Water
   b Light
   c Oxygen
   d Nourishment
8 Signs and symptoms of infection include the following *except*
   a Fever, nausea, vomiting, rash, and/or sores
   b Pain or tenderness, redness, and/or swelling
   c Fatigue, loss of appetite, and/or a discharge
   d A wound and/or bleeding
9 Which is *not* a portal of exit?
   a Respiratory tract
   b Blood
   c Reproductive system
   d Intact skin
10 Your hands are soiled with blood. What should you do?
   a Wash your hands.
   b Decontaminate your hands.
   c Rinse your hands.
   d Tell the nurse.
11 You move from a contaminated body site to a clean body site. What should you do?
   a Wash your hands.
   b Sterilize your hands.
   c Rinse your hands.
   d Use an alcohol-based hand rub.

12 You are going to use an alcohol-based hand rub. Which action is *not* correct?
   a Wash your hands before applying the hand rub.
   b Rub your hands together.
   c Cover all surfaces of your hands and fingers.
   d Rub your hands together until your hands are dry.
13 When cleaning equipment, do the following *except*
   a Rinse the item in cold water before cleaning
   b Wash the item with soap and hot water
   c Use a brush if necessary
   d Work from dirty to clean areas
14 Standard Precautions
   a Are used for all persons
   b Prevent the spread of pathogens through the air
   c Require gowns, masks, gloves, and goggles
   d Require a doctor's order
15 A mask
   a Can be re-used
   b Is clean on the front
   c Is contaminated when moist
   d Should fit loosely for breathing
16 These statements are about personal protective equipment (PPE). Which is *false?*
   a Wash disposable gloves for re-use.
   b Remove PPE before leaving the work area.
   c Discard cracked or torn utility gloves.
   d Wear gloves when touching contaminated items or surfaces.
17 Contaminated surfaces are cleaned at the following times *except*
   a After completing a task
   b When there is obvious contamination
   c After blood is spilled
   d After removing gloves
18 The Bloodborne Pathogen Standard involves the following *except*
   a Wearing gloves
   b Discarding sharp items into a biohazard container
   c Storing food and blood in different places
   d Eating and drinking in care settings

Answers to these questions are on p. 527.

12

BODY MECHANICS

OBJECTIVES

- Define the key terms and key abbreviations listed in this chapter.
- Explain the purpose and rules of body mechanics.
- Explain how ergonomics can prevent work-related injuries.
- Identify the causes, signs, and symptoms of back injuries.
- Position persons in the basic bed positions and in a chair.
- Explain how to promote PRIDE in the person, the family, and yourself.

KEY TERMS

base of support The area on which an object rests

body alignment The way the head, trunk, arms, and legs are aligned with one another; posture

body mechanics Using the body in an efficient and careful way

dorsal recumbent position See "supine position"

ergonomics The science of designing a job to fit the worker

Fowler's position A semi-sitting position; the head of the bed is raised between 45 and 60 degrees

lateral position The person lies on one side or the other; side-lying position

posture See "body alignment"

prone position Lying on the abdomen with the head turned to one side

semi-prone side position See "Sims' position"

side-lying position See "lateral position"

Sims' position A left side-lying position in which the upper leg is sharply flexed so it is not on the lower leg and the lower arm is behind the person; semi-prone side position

supine position The back-lying position; dorsal recumbent position

KEY ABBREVIATIONS

MSD Musculoskeletal disorder

OSHA Occupational Safety and Health Administration

Body mechanics means using the body in an efficient and careful way. It involves good posture, balance, and using your strongest and largest muscles for work. Fatigue, muscle strain, and injury can result from improper use and positioning of the body during activity or rest.

PRINCIPLES OF BODY MECHANICS

Body alignment (posture) is the way the head, trunk, arms, and legs are aligned with one another. Good alignment lets the body move and function with strength and efficiency. Standing, sitting, and lying down require good alignment.

Base of support is the area on which an object rests. A good base of support is needed for balance (Fig. 12-1, p. 174). When standing, your feet are your base of support. Stand with your feet apart for a wider base of support and more balance.

Our strongest and largest muscles are in the shoulders, upper arms, hips, and thighs. Use these muscles to handle and move persons and heavy objects. Otherwise, you strain and exert smaller and weaker muscles. This causes fatigue and injury. *Back injuries are a major risk.* For good body mechanics:

- Bend your knees and squat to lift a heavy object (Fig. 12-2, p. 174). Do not bend from your waist. That places strain on small back muscles.
- Hold items close to your body and base of support (see Fig. 12-2). This involves upper arm and shoulder muscles. Holding objects away from your body places strain on small muscles in your lower arms.

All activities require good body mechanics. Follow the rules in Box 12-1, p. 175.

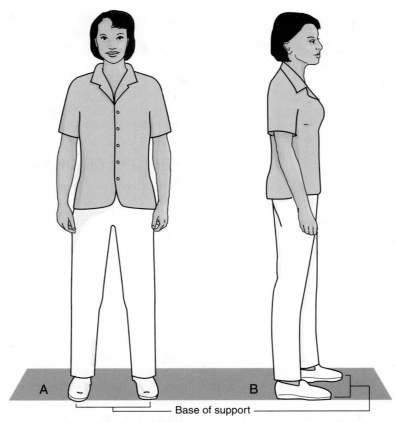

FIGURE 12-1 **A,** Anterior (front) view of an adult in good body alignment. The feet are apart for a wide base of support. **B,** Lateral (side) view of an adult with good posture and alignment.

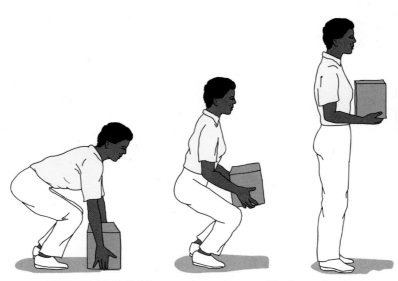

FIGURE 12-2 Picking up a box using good body mechanics.

BOX 12-1	Rules for Body Mechanics

- Keep your body in good alignment with a wide base of support.
- Use an upright working posture. Bend your legs. Do not bend your back.
- Use the stronger and larger muscles in your shoulders, upper arms, thighs, and hips.
- Keep objects close to your body when you lift, move, or carry them (see Fig. 12-2).
- Avoid unnecessary bending and reaching. Raise the bed so it is close to your waist. Adjust the overbed table so it is at your waist level.
- Face your work area. This prevents unnecessary twisting.
- Push, slide, or pull heavy objects whenever you can rather than lifting them. Pushing is easier than pulling.
- Widen your base of support when pushing or pulling. Move your front leg forward when pushing. Move your rear leg back when pulling (Fig. 12-3).

- Use both hands and arms to lift, move, or carry objects.
- Turn your whole body when changing the direction of your movement. Move and turn your feet in the direction of the turn instead of twisting your body.
- Work with smooth and even movements. Avoid sudden or jerky motions.
- Do not lean over a person to give care.
- *Get help from a co-worker to move heavy objects. Do not lift or move them by yourself.*
- Bend your hips and knees to lift heavy objects from the floor (see Fig. 12-2). Straighten your back as the object reaches thigh level. Your leg and thigh muscles work to raise the item off the floor and to waist level.
- Do not lift objects higher than chest level. Do not lift above your shoulders. Use a step stool or ladder to reach an object higher than chest level.

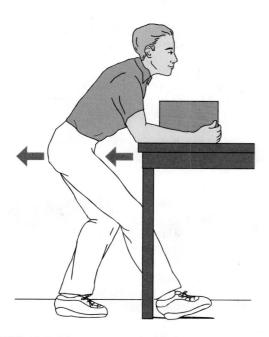

FIGURE 12-3 Move your rear leg back when pulling an item.

ERGONOMICS

Ergonomics is the science of designing a job to fit the worker. (*Ergo* means work. *Nomos* means law.) The task, work station, equipment, and tools are changed to help reduce stress on the worker's body. The goal is to prevent a serious and disabling work-related musculoskeletal disorder (MSD).

MSDs are injuries and disorders of the muscles, tendons, ligaments, joints, and cartilage. They also can involve the nervous system. The arms and back are often affected. So are the hands, fingers, neck, wrists, legs, and shoulders. MSDs are painful and disabling. They can develop slowly over weeks, months, and years. Or they can occur from one event. Pain, numbness, tingling, stiff joints, difficulty moving, and muscle loss can occur. So can paralysis.

Early signs and symptoms of MSDs include pain, limited joint movement, or soft tissue swelling. Always report a work-related injury as soon as possible. Early attention can help prevent the problem from becoming worse. In later stages, the problem can become more serious and harder and more costly to treat.

The Occupational Safety and Health Administration (OSHA) has identified risk factors for MSDs in nursing team members. The risk of an MSD increases if risk factors are combined. For example, a task involves both force and repeating actions.

- *Force*—the amount of effort needed to perform a task. Lifting or transferring heavy persons, preventing falls, and unexpected or sudden motions are examples.
- *Repeating action*—performing the same motion or series of motions continually or frequently. Repositioning patients and residents and transfers to and from beds, chairs, and commodes without adequate rest breaks are examples.
- *Awkward postures*—assuming positions that place stress on the body. Examples include reaching above shoulder height, kneeling, squatting, leaning over a bed, bending, or twisting the torso while lifting.
- *Heavy lifting*—manually lifting persons who cannot move themselves.

See *Promoting Safety and Comfort: Ergonomics.*

POSITIONING THE PERSON

The person must be properly positioned at all times. Regular position changes and good alignment promote comfort and well-being. Breathing is easier. Circulation is promoted. Contractures (Chapter 22) and pressure ulcers (Chapter 23) are prevented.

Whether in bed or in a chair, the person is repositioned at least every 2 hours. Some people are repositioned more often. You must follow the nurse's instructions and the care plan.

Follow these guidelines to safely position a person:

- Use good body mechanics.
- Ask a co-worker to help you if needed.
- Explain the procedure to the person.
- Be gentle when moving the person.
- Provide for privacy.
- Use pillows as directed by the nurse for support and alignment.
- Provide for comfort after positioning. (See the inside of the front book cover.)
- Place the signal light within reach after positioning.
- Complete a safety check before leaving the room. (See the inside of the front book cover.)

See *Focus on Communication: Positioning the Person.*
See *Delegation Guidelines: Positioning the Person.*
See *Promoting Safety and Comfort: Positioning the Person.*

PROMOTING SAFETY AND COMFORT
Ergonomics

Safety

Back injuries can occur from repeated activities or from one event. Use good body mechanics to protect yourself from injury. Do not work alone. Avoid lifting whenever possible. Have a co-worker help you handle, move, or transfer a person. Follow the rules in Box 12-1. Signs and symptoms of a back injury include:

- Pain when trying to assume a normal posture
- Decreased mobility
- Pain when standing or rising from a seated position

FOCUS ON COMMUNICATION
Positioning the Person

Moving is painful for many persons. Some older persons have painful joints. Most persons have pain after surgery or an injury. You must make sure that you are not causing pain when positioning the person. Tell the person what you are going to do before and during the procedure. Move the person slowly and gently. Allow the person time to tell you if a movement is painful. Make sure the person is comfortable. You can say:

- "Am I hurting you?"
- "Please tell me if I'm moving you too fast."
- "Please tell me if you feel pain or discomfort."
- "Do you need a pillow adjusted?"
- "Are you comfortable?"
- "How can I help make you more comfortable?"

DELEGATION GUIDELINES
Positioning the Person

You are often delegated tasks that involve positioning and repositioning. You need this information from the nurse and the care plan:

- Position or positioning limits ordered by the doctor
- How often to turn and reposition the person
- How many staff members need to help you
- What assist devices to use (Chapter 13)
- What skin care measures to perform (Chapter 15)
- What range-of-motion exercises to perform (Chapter 22)
- Where to place pillows
- What positioning devices are needed and how to use them (Chapter 22)
- What observations to report and record
- When to report observations
- What specific patient or resident concerns to report at once

PROMOTING SAFETY AND COMFORT
Positioning the Person

Safety

Pressure ulcers (Chapter 23) are serious threats from lying or sitting too long in one place. Wet, soiled, and wrinkled linens are other causes. Whenever you reposition a person, make sure linens are clean, dry, and wrinkle-free. Change or straighten linens as needed.

Contractures can develop from staying in one position too long (Chapter 22). A *contracture* is the lack of joint mobility caused by abnormal shortening of a muscle. Repositioning, exercise, and activity help prevent contractures.

Comfort

Pillows and positioning devices are used to position the person. They support body parts and keep the person in good alignment. This promotes comfort. Place pillows and positioning devices as directed by the nurse and the care plan.

Fowler's Position

Fowler's position is a semi-sitting position. The head of the bed is raised between 45 and 60 degrees (Fig. 12-4). The knees may be slightly elevated. For good alignment:

- The spine is straight.
- The head is supported with a small pillow.
- The arms are supported with pillows.

Supine Position

The **supine position (dorsal recumbent position)** is the back-lying position (Fig. 12-5).

For good alignment:
- The bed is flat.
- The head and shoulders are supported on a pillow.
- Arms and hands are at the sides. You can support the arms with regular pillows. Or you can support the hands on small pillows with the palms down.

Prone Position

A person in the **prone position** lies on the abdomen with the head turned to one side. For good alignment (Fig. 12-6, p. 178):
- The bed is flat.
- Small pillows are placed under the head, abdomen, and lower legs.
- Arms are flexed at the elbows with the hands near the head.

You also can position a person with the feet hanging over the end of the mattress (Fig. 12-7, p. 178). A pillow is not needed under the feet.

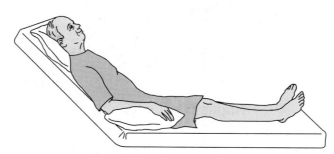

Figure 12-4 Fowler's position.

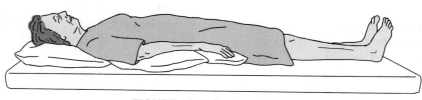

FIGURE 12-5 Supine position.

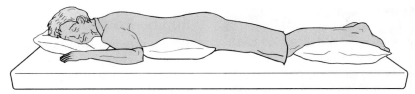

FIGURE 12-6 Prone position.

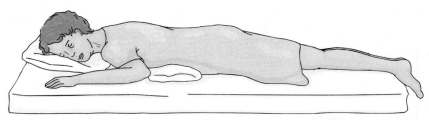

FIGURE 12-7 Prone position with the feet hanging over the edge of the mattress.

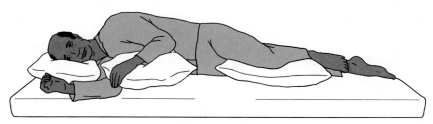

FIGURE 12-8 Lateral position.

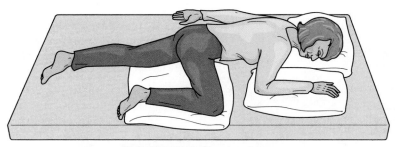

FIGURE 12-9 Sims' position.

Lateral Position

A person in the **lateral position (side-lying position)** lies on one side or the other (Fig. 12-8):

- The bed is flat.
- A pillow is under the head and neck.
- The upper leg is in front of the lower leg. (The nurse may ask you to position the upper leg behind the lower leg, not on top of it.)
- The ankle, upper leg, and thigh are supported with pillows.
- A small pillow is positioned against the person's back.
- A small pillow is under the upper hand and arm.

Sims' Position

The **Sims' position (semi-prone side position)** is a left side-lying position. The upper leg is sharply flexed so it is not on the lower leg. The lower arm is behind the person (Fig. 12-9). For good alignment:

- The bed is flat.
- A pillow is under the person's head and shoulder.
- The upper leg is supported with a pillow.
- A pillow is under the upper arm and hand.

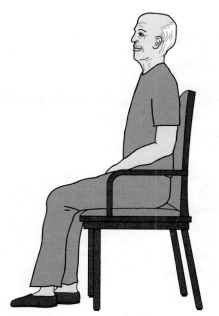

FIGURE 12-10 The person is positioned in a chair. The person's feet are flat on the floor; the calves do not touch the chair. The back is straight and against the back of the chair.

Chair Position

Persons who sit in chairs must hold their upper bodies and heads erect. If not, poor alignment results. For good alignment (Fig. 12-10):

- The person's back and buttocks are against the back of the chair.
- Feet are flat on the floor or wheelchair footplates. Never leave feet unsupported.
- Backs of the knees and calves are slightly away from the edge of the seat.

The nurse may ask you to put a small pillow between the person's lower back and the chair. This supports the lower back. *Remember, a pillow is not used behind the back if restraints are used* (Chapter 10).

Paralyzed arms are supported on pillows. Some persons have positioners (Fig. 12-11). Ask the nurse about their proper use. Wrists are positioned at a slight upward angle.

Some people require postural supports if they cannot keep their upper bodies erect (Fig. 12-12). They help maintain good alignment.

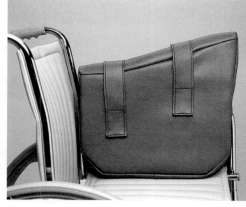
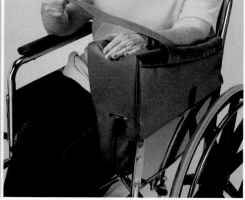

FIGURE 12-11 Elevated armrest. *(Images courtesy J. T. Posey Co., Arcadia, Calif.)*

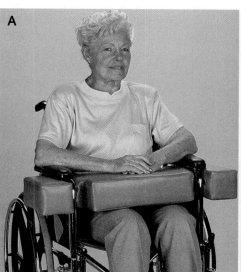
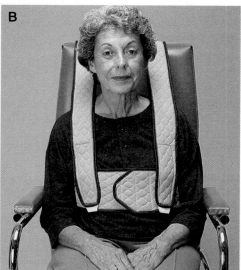

FIGURE 12-12 Postural supports. **A,** Pelvic holder. **B,** Torso support. *(Images courtesy J. T. Posey Co., Arcadia, Calif.)*

Focus on P R I D E
The Person, Family, and Yourself

Personal and Professional Responsibility—Moving persons causes strain on your body. Injuries can occur. Some factors increase your risk for injury. For example:

- Poor physical condition—not having the strength or endurance to perform tasks
- Fatigue
- Poor posture when sitting or standing
- Poor body mechanics when lifting, pushing, pulling, or carrying objects
- Repeated lifting of awkward items, equipment, or persons
- Twisting or bending while lifting or maintaining a bent posture
- Reaching over raised bed rails
- Trying to lift or move an object or person alone

You must protect yourself from injury. Avoid the factors listed above. Also, follow the rules for body mechanics in Box 12-1. Use good judgment when moving, repositioning, and transferring patients and residents. Ask for help when needed. Take responsibility for protecting yourself from harm.

Rights and Respect—OSHA requires that employers provide employees with a safe work setting. You have the right to ask potential or current employers about safety plans to reduce your risk of injury. Ask about training or orientation programs related to body mechanics, safe handling of persons, and workplace hazards. Know and follow agency procedures for reporting potential problems.

Independence and Social Interaction—Remaining independent to the extent possible promotes dignity, self-esteem, and pride. Let the person help as much as safely possible. Let the person choose such things as bed positioning or where the wheelchair or chair is placed. Talk with the person while moving him or her. Ask about his or her preferences. Doing so promotes comfort, independence, and social interaction.

Delegation and Teamwork—Transferring and positioning a person are always safer when done by two or more workers. Willingly help others when asked. If you cannot stop what you are doing, tell your co-worker when you will be available. Then help the person when you said that you would. Work as a team to protect yourself and others from injury.

Ethics and Laws—OSHA requires employers to provide a workplace that is free from recognized hazards that may cause serious harm or death. Employers must make reasonable attempts to prevent or reduce hazards. OSHA inspection teams enforce this law.

OSHA identifies handling, transferring, and repositioning persons as a potential hazard. OSHA provides guidelines and recommendations to prevent or reduce work-related injuries from moving persons. Recommendations include:

- Minimizing manual lifting of person in all cases
- Avoiding manual lifting if possible

REVIEW QUESTIONS

Circle the BEST answer.

1 Good body mechanics involves the following *except*
   a Good posture
   b Balance
   c Using the strongest and largest muscles
   d Having the job fit the worker

2 Good alignment means
   a The area on which an object rests
   b Having the head, trunk, arms, and legs aligned with one another
   c Using muscles, tendons, ligaments, and joints correctly
   d The back-lying or supine position

3 These actions are about body mechanics. Which action is *not* correct?
   a Hold objects away from your body when lifting, moving, or carrying them.
   b Face the direction you are working to prevent twisting.
   c Push, pull, or slide heavy objects.
   d Use both hands and arms to lift, move, or carry heavy objects.

4 The purpose of ergonomics is to
   a Reduce stress on the worker's body
   b Safely position a person
   c Promote quality of life
   d Use good body mechanics

5 Risk factors for work-related musculoskeletal disorders include the following *except*
   a Repeating actions
   b Awkward postures
   c Bending your hips and knees
   d Force

6 Patients and residents are repositioned at least every
   a 30 minutes
   b 1 hour
   c 2 hours
   d 3 hours

7 The back-lying position is called
   a Fowler's position
   b The supine position
   c The prone position
   d Sims' position

8 For Fowler's position
   a The bed is flat
   b The head of the bed is raised between 45 and 60 degrees
   c The person's head is turned toward one side
   d The person's feet hang over the edge of the mattress

9 A pillow is placed against the person's back in
   a Fowler's position
   b The prone position
   c The lateral position
   d Sims' position

10 A person is positioned in a chair. The feet
   a Must be flat on the floor
   b Are positioned on footplates
   c Dangle
   d Are positioned on pillows

Answers to these questions are on p. 527.

13

SAFELY HANDLING, MOVING, AND TRANSFERRING THE PERSON

PROCEDURES

- Moving the Person Up in Bed
- Moving the Person Up in Bed With an Assist Device
- Moving the Person to the Side of the Bed
- Turning and Repositioning the Person
- Logrolling the Person
- Sitting on the Side of the Bed (Dangling)
- Transferring the Person to a Chair or Wheelchair
- Transferring the Person From a Chair or Wheelchair to a Bed
- Transferring the Person Using a Mechanical Lift
- Transferring the Person to and From the Toilet

OBJECTIVES

- Define the key terms and key abbreviations listed in this chapter.
- Identify comfort and safety measures for handling, moving, and transferring the person.
- Explain how to prevent work-related injuries when handling, moving, and transferring persons.
- Describe four levels of dependence.
- Identify the information needed from the nurse and care plan before handling, moving, and transferring persons.
- Explain how to promote PRIDE in the person, the family, and yourself.
- Perform the procedures described in this chapter.

KEY TERMS

friction The rubbing of one surface against another

logrolling Turning the person as a unit, in alignment, with one motion

shearing When skin sticks to a surface while muscles slide in the direction the body is moving

transfer Moving the person from one place to another

KEY ABBREVIATIONS

ID Identification

OSHA Occupational Safety and Health Administration

You will turn and reposition persons often. You move them in bed. You transfer them to and from beds, chairs, wheelchairs, stretchers, and toilets. To **transfer** a person means moving the person from one place to another. Use your body correctly to protect you and the person from injury.

See *Focus on Communication: Safely Handling, Moving, and Transferring the Person.*

See *Promoting Safety and Comfort: Safely Handling, Moving, and Transferring the Person.*

FOCUS ON COMMUNICATION
Safely Handling, Moving, and Transferring the Person

Some persons may be afraid of moving and transferring. Fear of pain and falling is common. Always explain what you are going to do before starting the procedure. Then explain what you are doing step-by-step. This promotes comfort. When giving step-by-step directions:
- Speak slowly and clearly.
- Talk loudly enough for the person to hear you.
- Give directions calmly and kindly. Do not yell at or insult the person.
- Face the person and use eye contact when possible.
- Give one direction at a time.

PROMOTING SAFETY AND COMFORT
Safely Handling, Moving, and Transferring the Person

Safety

Many older persons have fragile bones and joints. To prevent injuries:
- Follow the rules of body mechanics (Chapter 12).
- Always have help when moving a person.
- Be aware of equipment and tubings involved in the person's care. Urinary catheters and oxygen, intravenous, drainage, and naso-gastric tubes are examples.
- Move the person carefully to prevent injury or pain.
- Keep the person in good alignment during the procedure.
- Position the person in good alignment after the procedure.
- Make sure his or her face, nose, and mouth are not obstructed by a pillow or other device.

Comfort

To promote mental comfort when handling, moving, or transferring the person:
- Always explain what you are going to do and how the person can help.
- Always screen and cover the person to protect the right to privacy.
To promote physical comfort:
- Keep the person in good alignment.
- Make sure the person's head does not hit the headboard when he or she is moved up in bed. If the person can be without a pillow, place it upright against the headboard.
- Use pillows to position the person as directed by the nurse and the care plan. If a pillow is allowed under the person's head, make sure it is under the head and shoulders.
- Use other positioning devices as directed by the nurse and the care plan.

PREVENTING WORK-RELATED INJURIES

You must prevent work-related injuries when handling, moving, and transferring patients and residents. *For all of the procedures, practice good body mechanics (Chapter 12) and follow the rules in Box 13-1.* The Occupational Safety and Health Administration (OSHA) recommends that:

- Manual lifting be minimized in all cases.
- Manual lifting be eliminated when possible.

To safely handle, move, and transfer the person, the nurse and health team determine:

- The person's dependence level. See Box 13-2.
- The amount of assistance and how many staff members are needed.
- What procedure to use.
- The equipment needed.

See *Persons With Dementia: Preventing Work-Related Injuries,* p. 187.

See *Delegation Guidelines: Preventing Work-Related Injuries,* p. 187.

See *Promoting Safety and Comfort: Preventing Work-Related Injuries,* p. 187.

Text continued on p. 187

BOX 13-1 Preventing Work-Related Injuries

General Guidelines

- Wear shoes that provide good traction. Avoid shoes with worn-down soles.
- Use assist equipment and devices (p. 186) whenever possible. Follow the person's care plan.
- Get help from other staff. The nurse and care plan tell you how many staff members are needed to complete the task.
- Plan and prepare for the task. For example, know what equipment is needed, where to place chairs or wheelchairs, and what side of the bed to work on.
- Schedule harder tasks early in your shift.
- Balance lighter and harder tasks. Plan your work to complete a lighter task after a harder one.
- Lock bed wheels and wheelchair or stretcher wheels.
- Tell the person what he or she can do to help. Give clear, simple instructions. Give the person time to respond.
- Do not hold or grab the person under the underarms.
- Do not let the person hold or grasp you around your neck.

Manual Lifting

- Use good body mechanics.
  - Stand with good posture. Keep your back straight.
  - Bend your legs, not your back.
  - Use your legs to do the work.
  - Face the person.
  - Do not twist or turn. Pick up your feet, and pivot your whole body in the direction of the move.
- Keep what you are moving close to you—the person, equipment, or supplies.
- Move the person toward you, not away from you.
- Use slides and lateral transfers instead of manual lifting.
- Use a wide, balanced base of support. Stand with one foot slightly ahead of the other.
- Lower the person slowly by bending your legs. Do not bend your back. Return to an erect position as soon as possible.
- Use smooth, even movements. Avoid jerking movements.
- Lift on the "count of 3" when lifting with others. Everyone should lift at the same time.

Lateral Transfers

- Position surfaces as close as possible to each other (bed and chair; bed and stretcher).
- Adjust surfaces to about waist height. The receiving surface should be slightly lower to take advantage of gravity. For example, for a bed to a chair transfer, the chair surface is lower than the bed.
- Lower bed rails and stretcher side rails.
- Use drawsheets (Chapter 14), turning pads (p. 190), large incontinence pads (Chapter 17), or other friction-reducing devices. Such devices include slide boards, slide sheets, and low-friction mattress covers.
- Get a good hand-hold. Roll up drawsheets, turning pads, and incontinence pads. Or use assist devices with handles.
- Kneel on the bed or stretcher. This helps prevent extended reaches and bending the back.
- Have staff on both sides of the bed or other surface. Move the person on the "count of 3." Use a smooth, push-pull motion. Do not reach across the person.

Gait/Transfer Belts

- Keep the person as close to you as possible.
- Avoid bending, reaching, or twisting when:
  - Attaching or removing a belt
  - Lowering the person to a chair, the bed, toilet, or the floor
  - Assisting the person with walking
- Use a gentle rocking motion to assist the person to stand. The rocking motion gives strength and force as you pull the person to standing position.
- See Chapter 9.

BOX 13-1   Preventing Work-Related Injuries—cont'd

Stand-Pivot Transfers

- Use assist devices as directed. Follow the care plan.
- Use a gait/transfer belt with handles.
- Keep your feet at least shoulder width apart.
- Lower the bed so the person can place his or her feet on the floor.
- Plan the transfer so that the person moves his or her strong side first.
- Get the person close to the edge of the bed or the chair. Ask the person to lean forward as he or she stands.
- Block the person's weak leg with your legs or knees. If the position is awkward, do the following:
  - Use a transfer belt with handles.
  - Straddle your legs around the person's weak leg.
- Bend your legs. Do not bend your back.
- Pivot with your feet to turn.
- Use a gentle rocking motion to assist the person to stand. The rocking motion gives strength and force as you pull the person to a standing position.

Lifting or Moving the Person in Bed

- Adjust the height of the bed, stretcher, or other surface to waist level.
- Lower the bed rail or the stretcher side rail.
- Work on the side where the person will be closest to you.
- Place equipment or other items close to you and at waist level.
- Use drawsheets, turning pads, large incontinence pads, or slide sheets.

Transporting Patients, Residents, and Equipment

- Push, do not pull.
- Keep the load close to your body.
- Use an up-right posture.
- Push with your whole body, not just your arms.
- Move down the center of the hallway. This helps avoid collisions.
- Watch out for door handles and high thresholds on floors. These can cause abrupt stops.

Transferring the Person From the Floor

- Use a mechanical lift if possible (p. 205). If not, place a sling, blanket, drawsheet, cot, or other assist device under the person as directed by the nurse.
- Position at least two staff members on each side of the person. More staff is needed if the person is large.
- Bend at your knees, not your back. Do not twist.
- Roll the person onto his or her side to position the assist device. Do not reach across the person.
- Lower the hoist (if using a mechanical lift) to attach the sling. The hoist should be low enough to easily attach the sling.
- Do the following for a manual lift:
  - Kneel on one knee.
  - Grasp the blanket, drawsheet, cot, or other device.
  - Lift smoothly with your legs as you stand on the "count of 3." Do not bend your back.

Modified from *A back injury prevention guide for health care providers,* Cal/OSHA, revised November 1997, Sacramento, Calif, as referenced in *Ergonomics: guidelines for nursing homes,* Occupational Safety and Health Administration, revised March, 2009.

BOX 13-2   Levels of Dependence

Code 4: Total Dependence. The person cannot help with the transfer. The task or procedure is done by the staff. The person should be lifted and transferred using a full-sling mechanical lift (Fig. 13-1, p. 186).

Code 3: Extensive Assistance. The person can bear some weight, can sit up with help, and may be able to pivot to transfer. The person should be lifted and transferred using a full-sling mechanical lift or stand-assist lift (Fig. 13-2, p. 186).

Code 2: Limited Assistance. The person is highly involved in the moving or transfer procedure. He or she needs some help moving the legs. The person can stand (bear weight). The person has upper body strength and can sit up. He or she is able to pivot transfer.

- Stand-assist devices may be needed. These can be attached to the bed or chair (Fig. 13-3, p. 186). Others include walkers (Chapter 22) and gait/transfer belts with handles (Chapter 9).
- Sliding boards are useful for transfers to and from beds and chairs (Fig. 13-4, p. 186).

Code 1: Supervision. The staff needs to look after, encourage, or remind the person what to do. The devices for Code 2 may be needed.

Code 0: Independent. The person can walk without help. Sometimes the person may need limited assistance. Mechanical assistance is not normally required for transferring, lifting, or repositioning.

Modified from Nelson AL: *Patient care ergonomics resource guide: safe patient handling and movement,* Patient Safety Center of Inquiry, Tampa, Fla, Veterans Health Administration and Department of Defense, April 2005.

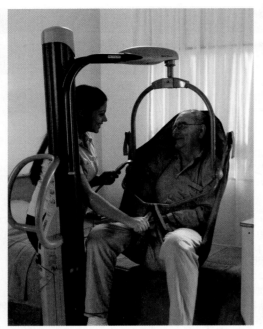

FIGURE 13-1 Full-sling mechanical lift. (*Courtesy ARJO, Inc., Roselle, Ill. [800]323-1245.*)

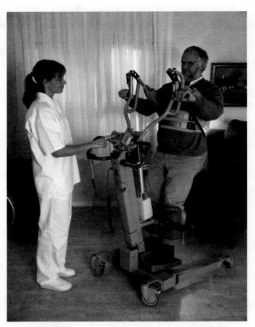

FIGURE 13-2 Stand-assist lift. (*Courtesy ARJO, Inc., Roselle, Ill. [800]323-1245.*)

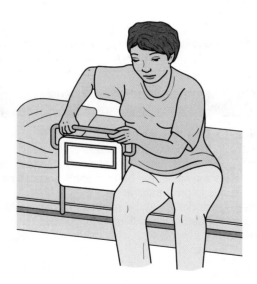

FIGURE 13-3 Stand-assist bed attachment.

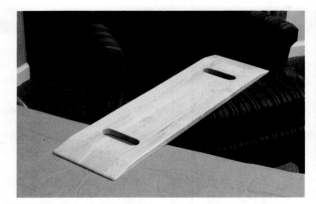

FIGURE 13-4 Slide board for transferring to and from surfaces.

PERSONS WITH DEMENTIA
Preventing Work-Related Injuries

Some older persons have dementia. They may not understand what you are doing. They may resist your handling, moving, and transfer efforts. The person may shout at you, grab you, or try to hit you. Always get a co-worker to help you. Do not force the person. The person's care plan also has measures for providing safe care. For example:
- Proceed slowly.
- Use a calm, pleasant voice.
- Divert the person's attention.

Tell the nurse at once if you have problems handling, moving, or transferring the person.

DELEGATION GUIDELINES
Preventing Work-Related Injuries

Many delegated tasks involve handling, moving, and transferring persons. Before doing so, you need this information from the nurse and the care plan:
- The person's height and weight.
- The person's dependence level (see Box 13-2).
- The person's physical abilities. For example, can the person sit up, stand up, or walk without help? Does the person have strength in his or her arms?
- If the person has a weak side. If yes, what side?
- If the person has a medical condition that increases the risk of injury. Dizziness, confusion, hearing or vision problems, recent surgery, and fragile skin are examples.
- Any doctor's orders for handling, moving, or transferring the person.
- The person's ability to follow directions.
- If behavior problems are likely. Combative, agitated, uncooperative, and unpredictable behaviors are examples.
- The amount of assistance needed.
- How many staff members are needed to complete the task safely.
- What procedure to use.
- What equipment to use.

PROMOTING SAFETY AND COMFORT
Preventing Work-Related Injuries

Safety

Decide how to move the person before starting the procedure. If you need help from other staff members, ask them to help before you begin. Also plan how to protect drainage tubes or containers connected to the person.

Beds are raised to move persons in bed (Chapter 14). This reduces bending and reaching. You must:
- Use the bed correctly.
- Protect the person from falling when the bed is raised.
- Follow the rules of body mechanics (Chapter 12).

PROTECTING THE SKIN

Protect the person's skin during handling, moving, and transfer procedures. Friction and shearing injure the skin. Both cause infection and pressure ulcers (Chapter 23).
- **Friction** is the rubbing of one surface against another. When moved in bed, the person's skin rubs against the sheet.
- **Shearing** is when the skin sticks to a surface while muscles slide in the direction the body is moving (Fig. 13-5). It occurs when the person slides down in bed or is moved in bed.

To reduce friction and shearing:
- Roll the person.
- Use friction-reducing devices. Such devices include a lift sheet (turning sheet). A cotton draw-sheet (Chapter 14) serves as a lift sheet (turning sheet). Turning pads, large incontinence products (Chapter 17), slide boards, and slide sheets are other friction-reducing devices.

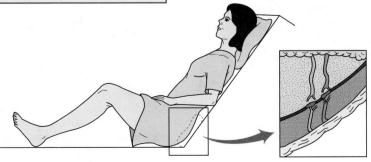

FIGURE 13-5 Shearing. When the head of the bed is raised to a sitting position, skin on the buttocks stays in place. However, internal structures move forward as the person slides down in bed. This causes the skin to be pinched between the mattress and the hip bones.

MOVING PERSONS IN BED

Some persons need help moving and turning in bed. Those who are weak, unconscious, paralyzed, or in casts need help. Sometimes 2 or 3 people or a mechanical lift is needed. OSHA recommends the following:

- Dependence level of *Code 4: Total Dependence*—a mechanical lift or friction-reducing device and at least 2 staff members
- Dependence level of *Code 3: Extensive Assistance*—a mechanical lift or friction-reducing device and at least 2 staff members
- The person weighs less than 200 pounds—2 to 3 staff members and a friction-reducing device
- The person weighs more than 200 pounds—at least 3 staff members and a friction-reducing device

See *Delegation Guidelines: Moving Persons in Bed.*

DELEGATION GUIDELINES
Moving Persons in Bed

Before moving a person in bed, you need this information from the nurse and the care plan:
- What procedure to use
- How many workers are needed to safely move the person
- Position limits and restrictions
- How far you can lower the head of the bed
- Any limits in the person's ability to move or be repositioned
- What pillows can be removed before moving the person
- What equipment is needed—trapeze, lift sheet, slide sheet, mechanical lift
- How to position the person
- If the person uses bed rails
- What observations to report and record:
  - Who helped you with the procedure
  - How much help the person needed
  - How the person tolerated the procedure
  - How you positioned the person
  - Complaints of pain or discomfort
- When to report observations
- What specific patient or resident concerns to report at once

---

 ## Moving the Person Up in Bed

When the head of the bed is raised, it is easy to slide down toward the middle and foot of the bed (Fig. 13-6). The person is moved up in bed for good alignment and comfort.

You can sometimes move lightweight adults up in bed alone if they assist and use a trapeze. However, it is best to have help and to use an assist device (p. 190). Two or more staff members are needed to move heavy, weak, and very old persons up in bed. Always protect the person and yourself from injury.

See *Promoting Safety and Comfort: Moving the Person Up in Bed.*

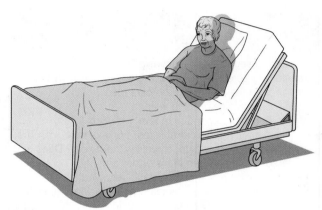

FIGURE 13-6 A person in poor alignment after sliding down in bed.

PROMOTING SAFETY AND COMFORT
Moving the Person Up in Bed

Safety

This procedure is best done with at least two staff members. Assist devices are used as directed by the nurse and the care plan.

Perform this procedure alone *only if:*
- The person is small in size.
- The person can follow directions.
- The person can assist with much of the moving.
- The person uses a trapeze.
- The person can push against the mattress with his or her feet.
- The nurse says it is safe to do so.
- You are comfortable doing so.

Follow the nurse's directions and the care plan. Ask any questions before you begin the procedure.

MOVING THE PERSON UP IN BED

QUALITY OF LIFE

Remember to:
- Knock before entering the person's room.
- Address the person by name.
- Introduce yourself by name and title.

- Explain the procedure to the person before beginning and during the procedure.
- Protect the person's rights during the procedure.
- Handle the person gently during the procedure.

PRE-PROCEDURE

1 Follow *Delegation Guidelines:*
  a *Preventing Work-Related Injuries,* p. 187
  b *Moving Persons in Bed.*
  See *Promoting Safety and Comfort:*
  a *Safely Handling, Moving, and Transferring the Person,* p. 183
  b *Preventing Work-Related Injuries,* p. 187
  c *Moving the Person Up in Bed*
2 Ask a co-worker to help you.

3 Practice hand hygiene.
4 Identify the person. Check the ID (identification) bracelet against the assignment sheet. Also call the person by name.
5 Provide for privacy.
6 Lock the bed wheels.
7 Raise the bed for body mechanics. Bed rails are up if used.

PROCEDURE

8 Lower the head of the bed to a level appropriate for the person. It is as flat as possible.
9 Stand on one side of the bed. Your co-worker stands on the other side.
10 Lower the bed rails if up.
11 Remove pillows as directed by the nurse. Place a pillow upright against the headboard if the person can be without it.
12 Stand with a wide base of support. Point the foot near the head of the bed toward the head of the bed. Face the head of the bed.
13 Bend your hips and knees. Keep your back straight.

14 Place one arm under the person's shoulder and one arm under the thighs. Your co-worker does the same. Grasp each other's forearms (Fig. 13-7).
15 Ask the person to grasp the trapeze.
16 Have the person flex both knees.
17 Explain the following:
  a You will count "1, 2, 3."
  b The move will be on "3."
  c On "3," the person pushes against the bed with the feet if able and pulls up with the trapeze.
18 Move the person to the head of the bed on the count of "3." Shift your weight from your rear leg to your front leg. Your co-worker does the same.
19 Repeat steps 12 through 18 if necessary.

POST-PROCEDURE

20 Put the pillow under the person's head and shoulders. Straighten linens.
21 Position the person in good alignment.
22 Provide for comfort. (See the inside of the front book cover.)
23 Place the signal light within reach.
24 Raise the head of the bed to a level appropriate for the person.

25 Lower the bed to its lowest position.
26 Raise or lower bed rails. Follow the care plan.
27 Unscreen the person.
28 Complete a safety check of the room. (See the inside of the front book cover.)
29 Decontaminate your hands.
30 Report and record your observations.

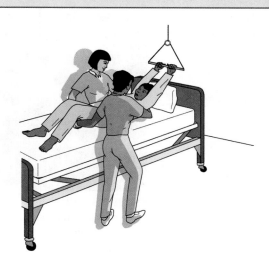

FIGURE 13-7 A person is moved up in bed by two nursing assistants. Each has one arm under the person's shoulders and the other under the thighs. They have locked arms under the person. The person grasps the trapeze and flexes the knees. The nursing assistants shift their weight from the rear leg to the front leg as the person is moved up in bed.

❖ Moving the Person Up in Bed With an Assist Device

Assist devices are used to move some persons up in bed. Such assist devices include a drawsheet (lift sheet), flat sheet folded in half, turning pad (Fig. 13-8), slide sheet (Fig. 13-9), and large incontinence product. With these devices, the person is moved more evenly. And shearing and friction are reduced.

The device is placed under the person from the head to above the knees or lower. At least two staff members are needed. This procedure is used for most patients and residents. It is used:

- Following OSHA recommendations (p. 188)
- For persons recovering from spinal cord surgery or spinal cord injuries
- For older persons

See *Promoting Safety and Comfort: Moving the Person Up in Bed With an Assist Device.*

PROMOTING SAFETY AND COMFORT
Moving the Person Up in Bed With an Assist Device

Safety

For use as an assist device, incontinence products must:

- Be strong enough to support the person's weight. Disposable, single use underpads are not strong enough.
- Extend from under the person's head to above the knees or lower.
- Be wide enough for you and other staff to get a firm grip for the move.

Ask the nurse if the person's underpad is safe to use as an assist device.

To use a slide sheet, you need to place it under the person. See procedure: *Making an Occupied Bed* in Chapter 14 for this step. After the procedure, remove the slide sheet. Otherwise the person is in danger of sliding down in bed or off the bed.

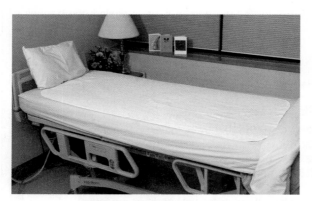

FIGURE 13-8 Turning pad.

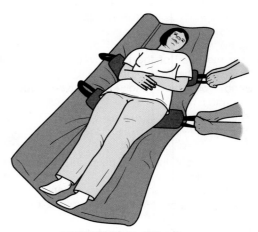

FIGURE 13-9 Slide sheet.

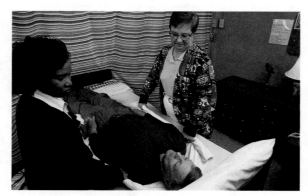

FIGURE 13-10 A drawsheet is used to move the person up in bed. It extends from the person's head to above the knees. Rolled close to the person, the drawsheet is held near the shoulders and hips.

MOVING THE PERSON UP IN BED WITH AN ASSIST DEVICE

QUALITY OF LIFE

Remember to:
- Knock before entering the person's room.
- Address the person by name.
- Introduce yourself by name and title.

- Explain the procedure to the person before beginning and during the procedure.
- Protect the person's rights during the procedure.
- Handle the person gently during the procedure.

PRE-PROCEDURE

1 Follow *Delegation Guidelines:*
   a *Preventing Work-Related Injuries,* p. 187
   b *Moving Persons in Bed,* p. 188
   See *Promoting Safety and Comfort:*
   a *Safely Handling, Moving, and Transferring the Person,* p. 183
   b *Preventing Work-Related Injuries,* p. 187
   c *Moving the Person Up in Bed,* p. 188
   d *Moving the Person Up in Bed With an Assist Device*

2 Ask a co-worker to help you.
3 Practice hand hygiene.
4 Identify the person. Check the ID bracelet against the assignment sheet. Also call the person by name.
5 Provide for privacy.
6 Lock the bed wheels.
7 Raise the bed for body mechanics. Bed rails are up if used.

PROCEDURE

8 Lower the head of the bed to a level appropriate for the person. It is as flat as possible.
9 Stand on one side of the bed. Your co-worker stands on the other side.
10 Lower the bed rails if up.
11 Remove pillows as directed by the nurse. Place a pillow upright against the headboard if the person can be without it.
12 Stand with a broad base of support. Point the foot near the head of the bed toward the head of the bed. Face that direction.

13 Roll the sides of the assist device up close to the person. (NOTE: Omit this step if the device has handles.)
14 Grasp the rolled-up assist device firmly near the person's shoulders and hips (Fig. 13-10). Or grasp it by the handles. Support the head.
15 Bend your hips and knees.
16 Move the person up in bed on the count of "3." Shift your weight from your rear leg to your front leg.
17 Repeat steps 12 through 16 if necessary.
18 Unroll the assist device. (NOTE: Omit this step if the device has handles.)

POST-PROCEDURE

19 Put the pillow under the person's head and shoulders.
20 Position the person in good alignment.
21 Provide for comfort. (See the inside of the front book cover.)
22 Place the signal light within reach.
23 Raise the head of the bed to a level appropriate for the person.

24 Lower the bed to its lowest position.
25 Raise or lower bed rails. Follow the care plan.
26 Unscreen the person.
27 Complete a safety check of the room. (See the inside of the front book cover.)
28 Decontaminate your hands.
29 Report and record your observations.

Moving the Person to the Side of the Bed

Repositioning and care procedures require moving the person to the side of the bed. The person is moved to the side of the bed before turning. Otherwise, after turning, the person lies on the side of the bed—not in the middle.

Sometimes you have to reach over the person. You reach less if the person is close to you.

One method involves moving the person in segments (Fig. 13-11). Sometimes one person can do this. Use a mechanical lift (p. 205) or the assist device method:

- Following OSHA recommendations (p. 188)
- For older persons
- For persons with arthritis
- For persons recovering from spinal cord injuries or spinal cord surgery

Use an assist device as directed by the nurse and care plan (see *Delegation Guidelines: Moving Persons in Bed*, p. 188). An assist device helps prevent pain and skin damage, and injury to the bones, joints, and spinal cord.

See *Promoting Safety and Comfort: Moving the Person to the Side of the Bed.*

PROMOTING SAFETY AND COMFORT
Moving the Person to the Side of the Bed

Safety

The nurse and care plan tell you how to move the person to the side of the bed (see *Delegation Guidelines: Moving Persons in Bed*, p. 188). Many tasks involve moving the person to the side of the bed. They include repositioning, bedmaking, bathing, and range-of-motion exercises.

The wrong method could seriously injure a person. This is very important for persons who are very old, have arthritis, or have spinal cord involvement.

To use an assist device, you need at least 1 co-worker to help you. Depending on the person's size, 3 staff members may be needed.

A slide board or slide sheet is placed under the person. After moving the person up in bed, remove the device.

To move the person in segments, move the person toward you, not away from you. This helps protect you from injury.

Comfort

After moving the person to the side of the bed, move the pillow too (if the person uses one). Position the pillow correctly. It should be under the person's head and shoulders.

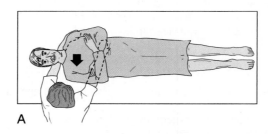

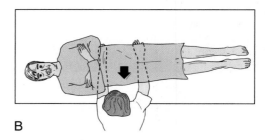

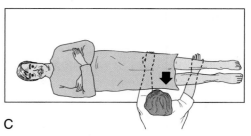

FIGURE 13-11 Moving the person to the side of the bed in segments. **A,** The upper part of the body is moved. **B,** The lower part of the body is moved. **C,** The legs and feet are moved.

MOVING THE PERSON TO THE SIDE OF THE BED

QUALITY OF LIFE

Remember to:
- Knock before entering the person's room.
- Address the person by name.
- Introduce yourself by name and title.

- Explain the procedure to the person before beginning and during the procedure.
- Protect the person's rights during the procedure.
- Handle the person gently during the procedure.

PRE-PROCEDURE

1 Follow *Delegation Guidelines:*
   a *Preventing Work-Related Injuries,* p. 187
   b *Moving Persons in Bed,* p. 188
   See *Promoting Safety and Comfort:*
   a *Safely Handling, Moving, and Transferring the Person,* p. 183
   b *Preventing Work-Related Injuries,* p. 187
   c *Moving the Person to the Side of the Bed,* p. 188

2 Ask a co-worker to help you if using an assist device.
3 Practice hand hygiene.
4 Identify the person. Check the ID bracelet against the assignment sheet. Also call the person by name.
5 Provide for privacy.
6 Lock the bed wheels.
7 Raise the bed for body mechanics. Bed rails are up if used.

PROCEDURE

8 Lower the head of the bed to a level appropriate for the person. It is as flat as possible.
9 Stand on the side of the bed to which you will move the person.
10 Lower the bed rail near you if bed rails are used. (Both bed rails are lowered for step 15.)
11 Remove pillows as directed by the nurse.
12 Stand with your feet about 12 inches apart. One foot is in front of the other. Flex your knees.
13 Cross the person's arms over the person's chest.
14 *Method 1—Moving the person in segments:*
   a Place your arm under the person's neck and shoulders. Grasp the far shoulder.
   b Place your other arm under the mid-back.
   c Move the upper part of the person's body toward you. Rock backward and shift your weight to your rear leg (see Fig. 13-11, *A*).
   d Place one arm under the person's waist and one under the thighs.

   e Rock backward to move the lower part of the person toward you (see Fig. 13-11, *B*).
   f Repeat the procedure for the legs and feet (see Fig. 13-11, *C*). Your arms should be under the person's thighs and calves.
15 *Method 2—Moving the person with a drawsheet:*
   a Roll up the drawsheet close to the person (see Fig. 13-10).
   b Grasp the rolled-up drawsheet near the person's shoulder's and hips. Your co-worker does the same. Support the person's head.
   c Rock backward on the count of "3" moving the person toward you. Your co-worker rocks backward slightly and then forward toward you while keeping the arms straight.
   d Unroll the drawsheet. Remove any wrinkles.

POST-PROCEDURE

16 Position the person in good alignment.
17 Provide for comfort. (See the inside of the front book cover.)
18 Place the signal light within reach.
19 Lower the bed to its lowest position.
20 Raise or lower bed rails. Follow the care plan.

21 Unscreen the person.
22 Complete a safety check of the room. (See the inside of the front book cover.)
23 Decontaminate your hands.
24 Report and record your observations.

❖ TURNING PERSONS

Turning persons onto their sides helps prevent complications from bedrest (Chapter 22). Certain procedures and care measures also require the side-lying position.

Many older persons suffer from arthritis in their spines, hips, and knees. To turn these persons, logrolling is preferred (p. 196). Logrolling may be less painful for these persons.

See *Delegation Guidelines: Turning Persons.*
See *Promoting Safety and Comfort: Turning Persons.*

DELEGATION GUIDELINES
Turning Persons

Before turning and repositioning a person, you need this information from the nurse and the care plan:
- The person's dependency level (see Box 13-2)
- How much help the person needs
- How many staff members are needed to safely complete the procedure
- The person's comfort level and what body parts are painful
- Which procedure to use
- What assist devices to use
- What supportive devices are needed for positioning (Chapter 22)
- Where to place pillows
- What observations to report and record:
  - Who helped you with the procedure
  - How much help the person needed
  - How the person tolerated the procedure
  - How you positioned the person
  - Complaints of pain or discomfort
- When to report observations
- What specific patient or resident concerns to report at once

---

PROMOTING SAFETY AND COMFORT
Turning Persons

Safety

To safely turn a person:
- Keep the person in good alignment.
- Ask a co-worker to help you.
- Make sure the person's face, nose, and mouth are not obstructed by a pillow or other device.

Comfort

After turning, position the person in good alignment. Use pillows as directed to support the person in the side-lying position (Chapter 12).

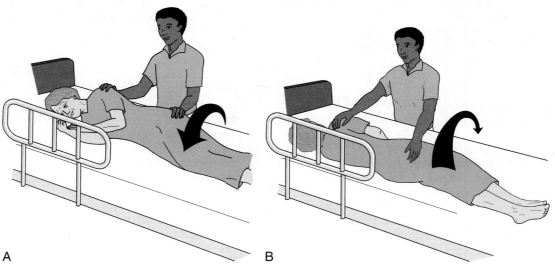

A   B

FIGURE 13-12 Turning the person. **A,** Turning the person away from you. **B,** Turning the person toward you. Note: Non-standard bed rails are used to show positioning and hand placement.

TURNING AND REPOSITIONING THE PERSON

QUALITY OF LIFE

Remember to:
- Knock before entering the person's room.
- Address the person by name.
- Introduce yourself by name and title.

- Explain the procedure to the person before beginning and during the procedure.
- Protect the person's rights during the procedure.
- Handle the person gently during the procedure.

PRE-PROCEDURE

1 Follow *Delegation Guidelines:*
   a *Preventing Work-Related Injuries,* p. 187
   b *Moving Persons in Bed,* p. 188
   c *Turning Persons.*
   See *Promoting Safety and Comfort:*
   a *Safely Handling, Moving, and Transferring the Person,* p. 183
   b *Preventing Work-Related Injuries,* p. 187
   c *Moving the Person to the Side of the Bed,* p. 192
   d *Turning Persons*

2 Practice hand hygiene.
3 Identify the person. Check the ID bracelet against the assignment sheet. Also call the person by name.
4 Provide for privacy.
5 Lock the bed wheels.
6 Raise the bed for body mechanics. Bed rails are up.

PROCEDURE

7 Lower the head of the bed to a level appropriate for the person. It is as flat as possible.
8 Stand on the side of the bed opposite to where you will turn the person.
9 Lower the bed rail near you.
10 Move the person to the side near you. (See procedure: *Moving the Person to the Side of the Bed,* p. 193.)
11 Cross the person's arms over the person's chest. Cross the leg near you over the far leg.
12 *Turning the person away from you:*
   a Stand with a wide base of support. Flex the knees.
   b Place one hand on the person's shoulder. Place the other on the hip near you.
   c Roll the person gently away from you toward the raised bed rail (Fig. 13-12, *A*). Shift your weight from your rear leg to your front leg.
13 *Turning the person toward you:*
   a Raise the bed rail.
   b Go to the other side of the bed. Lower the bed rail.

   c Stand with a wide base of support. Flex your knees.
   d Place one hand on the person's far shoulder. Place the other on the far hip.
   e Roll the person toward you gently (Fig. 13-12, *B*).
14 Position the person. Follow the nurse's directions and the care plan. The following is common:
   a Place a pillow under the head and neck.
   b Adjust the shoulder. The person should not lie on an arm.
   c Place a small pillow under the upper hand and arm.
   d Position a pillow against the back.
   e Flex the upper knee. Position the upper leg in front of the lower leg.
   f Support the upper leg and thigh on pillows. Make sure the ankle is supported.

POST-PROCEDURE

15 Provide for comfort. (See the inside of the front book cover.)
16 Place the signal light within reach.
17 Lower the bed to its lowest position.
18 Raise or lower bed rails. Follow the care plan.

19 Unscreen the person.
20 Complete a safety check of the room. (See the inside of the front book cover.)
21 Decontaminate your hands.
22 Report and record your observations.

Logrolling

Logrolling is turning the person as a unit, in alignment, with one motion. The spine is kept straight. The procedure is used to turn:

- Older persons with arthritic spines or knees
- Persons recovering from hip fractures
- Persons with spinal cord injuries (the spine is kept straight at all times after spinal cord injury)
- Persons recovering from spinal surgery (the spine is kept straight at all times after spinal surgery)
  See *Promoting Safety and Comfort: Logrolling.*

PROMOTING SAFETY AND COMFORT
Logrolling

Safety

Two or three staff members are needed to logroll a person. Three are needed if the person is tall or heavy. Sometimes an assist device is needed (see *Delegation Guidelines: Moving Persons in Bed*, p. 188).

If the person has a spinal cord injury, assist the nurse as directed. The nurse holds the neck during moving or repositioning. This is known as *cervical spine immobilization*. It prevents further injury to the neck. The nurse tells you what to do step-by-step.

Comfort

After spinal cord injury or surgery, the spine must be kept straight. This includes the person's neck. Therefore, *usually a pillow is not allowed under the head and neck.* Follow the nurse's directions and the care plan for positioning the person and using pillows.

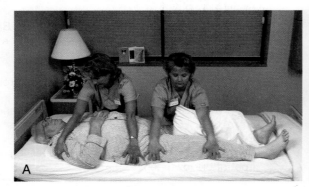
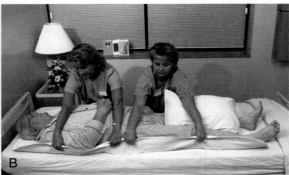

FIGURE 13-13 Logrolling. **A,** A pillow is between the person's legs. The arms are crossed on the chest. The person is on the far side of the bed. **B,** The assist device is used to logroll the person.

LOGROLLING THE PERSON

QUALITY OF LIFE

Remember to:
- Knock before entering the person's room.
- Address the person by name.
- Introduce yourself by name and title.

- Explain the procedure to the person before beginning and during the procedure.
- Protect the person's rights during the procedure.
- Handle the person gently during the procedure.

PRE-PROCEDURE

1 Follow *Delegation Guidelines:*
   a *Preventing Work-Related Injuries*, p. 187
   b *Moving Persons in Bed*, p. 188
   c *Turning Persons*, p. 194
   See *Promoting Safety and Comfort:*
   a *Safely Handling, Moving, and Transferring the Person*, p. 183
   b *Preventing Work-Related Injuries*, p. 187
   c *Turning Persons*, p. 194
   d *Logrolling*

2 Ask a co-worker to help you.
3 Practice hand hygiene.
4 Identify the person. Check the ID bracelet against the assignment sheet. Also call the person by name.
5 Provide for privacy.
6 Lock the bed wheels.
7 Raise the bed for body mechanics. Bed rails are up if used.

PROCEDURE

8 Make sure the bed is flat.
9 Stand on the side opposite to which you will turn the person. Your co-worker stands on the other side.
10 Lower the bed rails if used.
11 Move the person as a unit to the side of the bed near you. Use the assist device. (If the person has a spinal cord injury, assist the nurse as directed.)
12 Place the person's arms across the chest. Place a pillow between the knees.
13 Raise the bed rail if used.
14 Go to the other side.
15 Stand near the shoulders and chest. Your co-worker stands near the hips and thighs.
16 Stand with a broad base of support. One foot is in front of the other.

17 Ask the person to hold his or her body rigid.
18 Roll the person toward you (Fig. 13-13, *A*). Or use the assist device (Fig. 13-13, *B*). Turn the person as a unit.
19 Position the person in good alignment. Use pillows as directed by the nurse and the care plan. The following is common (unless the spinal cord is involved):
   a One pillow against the back for support
   b One pillow under the head and neck if allowed
   c One pillow or a folded bath blanket between the legs
   d A small pillow under the upper arm and hand

POST-PROCEDURE

20 Provide for comfort. (See the inside of the front book cover.)
21 Place the signal light within reach.
22 Lower the bed to its lowest position.
23 Raise or lower bed rails. Follow the care plan.

24 Unscreen the person.
25 Complete a safety check of the room. (See the inside of the front book cover.)
26 Decontaminate your hands.
27 Report and record your observations.

SITTING ON THE SIDE OF THE BED (DANGLING)

Patients and residents may become dizzy or faint when getting out of bed too fast. They may need to sit on the side of the bed for 1 to 5 minutes before walking or transferring. Some persons increase activity in stages—bedrest, to sitting on the side of the bed, and then to sitting in a chair. Walking is the next step. Surgical patients sit on the side of the bed some time after surgery.

While dangling the legs, the person coughs and deep breathes. He or she moves the legs back and forth in circles. This stimulates circulation.

Two staff members may be needed. Persons with balance and coordination problems need support. If dizziness or fainting occurs, lay the person down.

See *Delegation Guidelines: Dangling*, p. 198.
See *Promoting Safety and Comfort: Dangling*, p. 198.

Text continued on p. 200

DELEGATION GUIDELINES
Dangling

The nurse may ask you to help a person sit on the side of the bed. The procedure is part of other tasks—assisting the person to stand, transferring from bed to chair, partial bath, and others. When delegated the dangling procedure or tasks that involve dangling, you need this information from the nurse and the care plan:

- Areas of weakness. For example, if the person's arms are weak, he or she cannot hold onto the side of the mattress for support. If the left side is weak, turn the person onto the stronger right side. The person can use the right arm to help move from the lying to sitting position.
- The person's dependence level (see Box 13-2).
- The amount of help the person needs.
- If you need a co-worker to help you.
- If the bed is raised or in its lowest position.
- How long the person needs to sit on the side of the bed.
- What exercises the person needs to perform while dangling:
  - Range-of-motion exercises (Chapter 22)
  - Deep breathing and coughing exercises (Chapter 24)
- If the person will walk or transfer to a chair after dangling. If yes, the bed is in its lowest position.
- What observations to report and record:
  - Pulse and respiratory rates (Chapter 20)
  - Pale or bluish skin color (cyanosis)
  - Complaints of dizziness, light-headedness, or difficulty breathing
  - Who helped you with the procedure
  - How well the activity was tolerated
  - The length of time the person dangled
  - The amount of help needed
  - Other observations and complaints
- When to report observations.
- What specific patient or resident concerns to report at once.

PROMOTING SAFETY AND COMFORT
Dangling

Safety

This procedure is not used for persons with these dependence levels:
- Code 4: Total Dependence
- Code 3: Extensive Assistance

Problems with sitting and balance often occur after illness, injury, surgery, and bedrest. Some persons who are disabled also have problems sitting and with balance. Provide support when the person is sitting on the side of the bed. It is best to have a co-worker help you. This protects the person from falling and other injuries.

Comfort

Provide for the person's warmth during the dangling procedure. Help the person put on a robe. Or cover the person's shoulders and back with a bath blanket.

The person may want to perform simple hygiene measures while sitting on the side of the bed. Oral hygiene and washing the face and hands are examples (Chapter 15). These measures refresh the person and stimulate circulation. Follow the nurse's directions and the care plan.

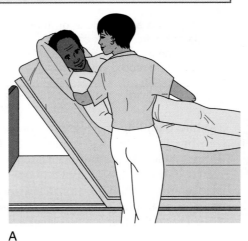
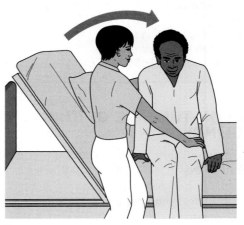

A   B

FIGURE 13-14 Helping the person sit on the side of the bed. **A,** The person's shoulders and thighs are supported. **B,** The person sits upright as the legs and feet are pulled over the edge of the bed.

SITTING ON THE SIDE OF THE BED (DANGLING)

QUALITY OF LIFE

Remember to:
- Knock before entering the person's room.
- Address the person by name.
- Introduce yourself by name and title.

- Explain the procedure to the person before beginning and during the procedure.
- Protect the person's rights during the procedure.
- Handle the person gently during the procedure.

PRE-PROCEDURE

1 Follow *Delegation Guidelines:*
   a *Preventing Work-Related Injuries,* p. 187
   b *Dangling*
   See *Promoting Safety and Comfort:*
   a *Safely Handling, Moving, and Transferring the Person,* p. 183
   b *Preventing Work-Related Injuries,* p. 187
   c *Dangling*
2 Ask a co-worker to help you if the person will dangle.

3 Practice hand hygiene.
4 Identify the person. Check the ID bracelet against the assignment sheet. Also call the person by name.
5 Provide for privacy.
6 Decide what side of the bed to use.
7 Move furniture to provide moving space.
8 Lock the bed wheels.
9 Raise the bed for body mechanics. Bed rails are up if used.

PROCEDURE

10 Lower the bed rail if up.
11 Position the person in a side-lying position facing you. The person lies on the strong side.
12 Raise the head of the bed to a sitting position.
13 Stand by the person's hips. Face the foot of the bed.
14 Stand with your feet apart. The foot near the head of the bed is in front of the other foot.
15 Slide one arm under the person's neck and shoulders. Grasp the far shoulder. Place your other hand over the thighs near the knees (Fig. 13-14, *A*).
16 Pivot toward the foot of the bed while moving the person's legs and feet over the side of the bed. As the legs go over the edge of the mattress, the trunk is upright (Fig. 13-14, *B*).
17 Ask the person to hold onto the edge of the mattress. This supports the person in the sitting position. If possible, raise a half-length bed rail for the person to grasp. Raise the bed rail on the person's strong side. Have your co-worker support the person at all times.

18 Do not leave the person alone. Provide support at all times.
19 Check the person's condition:
   a Ask how the person feels. Ask if the person feels dizzy or light-headed.
   b Check the pulse and respirations.
   c Check for difficulty breathing.
   d Note if the skin is pale or bluish in color *(cyanosis).*
20 Reverse the procedure to return the person to bed. (Or prepare to transfer the person to a chair or wheelchair. Lower the bed to its lowest position so the person's feet are flat on the floor. Support the person at all times.)
21 Lower the head of the bed after the person returns to bed. Help him or her move to the center of the bed.
22 Position the person in good alignment.

POST-PROCEDURE

23 Provide for comfort. (See the inside of the front book cover.)
24 Place the signal light within reach.
25 Lower the bed to its lowest position.
26 Raise or lower bed rails. Follow the care plan.
27 Return furniture to its proper place.

28 Unscreen the person.
29 Complete a safety check of the room. (See the inside of the front book cover.)
30 Decontaminate your hands.
31 Report and record your observations.

TRANSFERRING PERSONS

Patients and residents are moved to and from beds, chairs, wheelchairs, shower chairs, commodes, and toilets. The amount of help needed and the method used vary with the person's dependency level (see Box 13-2).

Arrange the room so there is enough space for a safe transfer. Correct placement of the chair, wheelchair, or other device also is needed for a safe transfer.

See *Delegation Guidelines: Transferring Persons.*
See *Promoting Safety and Comfort: Transferring Persons.*

Transfer Belts

Transfer belts (gait belts) are discussed in Chapter 9. They are used to:
- Support patients and residents during transfers
- Reposition persons in chairs and wheelchairs (p. 209)

Wider belts have padded handles. They are easier to grip and allow better control should the person fall.

DELEGATION GUIDELINES
Transferring Persons

When delegated transferring procedures, you need this information from the nurse and the care plan:
- What procedure to use.
- The person's dependency level (see Box 13-2).
- The amount of help the person needs.
- What equipment to use—transfer belt, wheelchair, mechanical assist device, positioning devices, wheelchair cushion, and so on.
- The person's height and weight.
- How many staff members are needed to complete the task safely.
- Areas of weakness. For example, if the person's arms are weak, the person cannot hold onto the mattress for support. If the person has a weak left side, he or she gets out of bed on the stronger right side. The person uses the right arm to help move from the lying to sitting position.
- What observations to report and record:
  - Pulse rate before and after the transfer (Chapter 20)
  - Complaints of light-headedness, pain, discomfort, difficulty breathing, weakness, or fatigue
  - The amount of help needed to transfer the person
  - Who helped you with the procedure
  - How the person helped with the transfer
  - How you positioned the person
- When to report observations.
- What specific patient or resident concerns to report at once.

PROMOTING SAFETY AND COMFORT
Transferring Persons

Safety

The person wears non-skid footwear for transfers. Such footwear protects the person from falls. Slipping and sliding are prevented. Tie shoelaces securely. Otherwise the person can trip and fall.

Check the length of the person's gown or robe if necessary. Long gowns and robes can cause falls. Also, avoid robes with long ties. The person can trip and fall.

Lock bed, wheelchair, and wheels on other devices. This prevents the bed and the device from moving during the transfer. Otherwise, the person can fall. You also are at risk for injury.

Comfort

After the transfer, position the person in good alignment. Make sure needed items are within reach.

Bed to Chair or Wheelchair Transfers

Safety is important for chair, wheelchair, commode, and shower chair transfers. Help the person out of bed on his or her strong side. If the left side is weak and the right side strong, get the person out of bed on the right side. In transferring, the strong side moves first. It pulls the weaker side along. Transfers from the weak side are awkward and unsafe.

The following stand and pivot transfers are used if:
- The person's legs are strong enough to bear some or all of his or her weight.
- The person is cooperative and can follow directions.
- The person can assist with the transfer.

See *Promoting Safety and Comfort: Bed to Chair or Wheelchair Transfers.*

Text continued on p. 204

PROMOTING SAFETY AND COMFORT
Bed to Chair or Wheelchair Transfers

Safety

The chair, wheelchair, or other device must support the person's weight. The number of staff members needed for a transfer depends on the person's abilities, condition, and size. For some persons, you will use mechanical assist devices (p. 205).

The person must not put his or her arms around your neck. Otherwise the person can pull you forward or cause you to lose your balance. Neck, back, and other injuries from falls are possible.

If not using a mechanical assist device, using a gait/ transfer belt is the preferred method for chair or wheelchair transfers. It is safer for the person and you. Putting your arms around the person and grasping the shoulder blades is the other method. It can cause the person discomfort. And it can be stressful for you. Use this method *only* if instructed to do so by the nurse and the care plan.

Wheelchair wheels are locked for a safe transfer. After the transfer, unlock the wheels to position the wheelchair as the person prefers. After positioning the chair, lock the wheels or keep them unlocked according to the care plan. Locked wheels may be viewed as restraints if the person cannot unlock them to move the wheelchair (Chapter 10). However, falls and other injuries are risks if the person tries to stand when the wheelchair wheels are unlocked.

Comfort

Most wheelchairs and bedside chairs have vinyl seats and backs. Vinyl holds body heat. The person becomes warm and perspires more. You can cover the back and seat with a folded bath blanket. This increases the person's comfort in the chair. Some people have wheelchair cushions or positioning devices. Ask the nurse how to use and place the devices. Also follow the manufacturer's instructions.

TRANSFERRING THE PERSON TO A CHAIR OR WHEELCHAIR

QUALITY OF LIFE

Remember to:
- Knock before entering the person's room.
- Address the person by name.
- Introduce yourself by name and title.

- Explain the procedure to the person before beginning and during the procedure.
- Protect the person's rights during the procedure.
- Handle the person gently during the procedure.

PRE-PROCEDURE

1 Follow *Delegation Guidelines:*
  a *Preventing Work-Related Injuries,* p. 187
  b *Transferring Persons*
  See *Promoting Safety and Comfort:*
  a *Transfer/Gait Belts* (Chapter 11)
  b *Safely Handling, Moving, and Transferring the Person,* p. 183
  c *Preventing Work-Related Injuries,* p. 187
  d *Transferring Persons*
  e *Bed to Chair or Wheelchair Transfers*
2 Collect:
  - Wheelchair or arm chair
  - Bath blanket

  - Lap blanket
  - Robe and non-skid footwear
  - Paper or sheet
  - Transfer belt (if needed)
  - Seat cushion (if needed)
3 Practice hand hygiene.
4 Identify the person. Check the ID bracelet against the assignment sheet. Also call the person by name.
5 Provide for privacy.
6 Decide which side of the bed to use. Move furniture for a safe transfer.

Continued

PROCEDURE

7 Position the chair:
  a The chair is near the head of the bed on the person's strong side.
  b The chair faces the foot of the bed.
  c The arm of the chair almost touches the bed.
8 Place a folded bath blanket or cushion on the seat (if needed).
9 Lock the wheelchair wheels. Raise the footplates. Remove or swing the front rigging out of the way.
10 Lower the bed to its lowest position. Lock the bed wheels.
11 Fan-fold top linens to the foot of the bed.
12 Place the paper or sheet under the person's feet. (This protects the person's linens from the footwear.) Put footwear on the person.
13 Help the person sit on the side of the bed (p. 197). His or her feet touch the floor.
14 Help the person put on a robe.
15 Apply the transfer belt if needed (Chapter 9).
16 *Method 1: Using a transfer belt:*
  a Stand in front of the person.
  b Have the person hold onto the mattress.
  c Make sure the person's feet are flat on the floor.
  d Have the person lean forward.
  e Grasp the transfer belt at each side. Grasp the handles or grasp the belt from underneath. See Chapter 9.
  f Prevent the person from sliding or falling by doing one of the following:
    (1) Brace your knees against the person's knees. Block his or her feet with your feet (Fig. 13-15).
    (2) Use the knee and foot of one leg to block the person's weak leg or foot. Place your other foot slightly behind you for balance.
    (3) Straddle your legs around the person's weak leg.
  g Explain the following:
    (1) You will count "1, 2, 3."
    (2) The move will be on "3."
    (3) On "3," the person pushes down on the mattress and stands.
  h Ask the person to push down on the mattress and to stand on the count of "3." Pull the person to a standing position as you straighten your knees (Fig. 13-16).

17 *Method 2: No transfer belt:* (NOTE: Use this method only if directed by the nurse and the care plan.)
  a Follow steps 16, a–c.
  b Place your hands under the person's arms. Your hands are around the person's shoulder blades (Fig. 13-17).
  c Have the person lean forward.
  d Prevent the person from sliding or falling by doing one of the following:
    (1) Brace your knees against the person's knees. Block his or her feet with your feet.
    (2) Use the knee and foot of one leg to block the person's weak leg or foot. Place your other foot slightly behind you for balance.
    (3) Straddle your legs around the person's weak leg.
  e Explain the "count of 3." See step 16-g.
  f Ask the person to push down on the mattress and to stand on the count of "3." Pull the person up into a standing position as you straighten your knees.
18 Support the person in the standing position. Hold the transfer belt, or keep your hands around the person's shoulder blades. Continue to prevent the person from sliding or falling.
19 Turn the person so he or she can grasp the far arm of the chair. The legs will touch the edge of the chair (Fig. 13-18).
20 Continue to turn the person until the other armrest is grasped.
21 Lower him or her into the chair as you bend your hips and knees. The person assists by leaning forward and bending the elbows and knees (Fig. 13-19).
22 Make sure the hips are to the back of the seat. Position the person in good alignment.
23 Attach the wheelchair front rigging. Position the person's feet on the wheelchair footplates.
24 Cover the person's lap and legs with a lap blanket. Keep the blanket off the floor and the wheels.
25 Remove the transfer belt if used.
26 Position the chair as the person prefers. Lock the wheelchair wheels according to the care plan.

POST-PROCEDURE

27 Provide for comfort. (See the inside of the front book cover.)
28 Place the signal light and other needed items within reach.
29 Unscreen the person.
30 Complete a safety check of the room. (See the inside of the front book cover.)
31 Decontaminate your hands.
32 Report and record your observations.
33 See procedure: *Transferring the Person From a Chair or Wheelchair to a Bed,* p. 204 to return the person to bed.

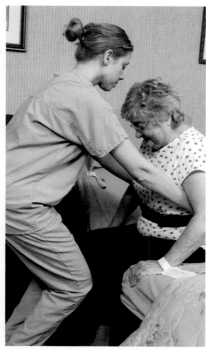

FIGURE 13-15 Transferring the person to a chair using a transfer belt. The person's feet and knees are blocked by the nursing assistant's feet and knees. This prevents the person from sliding or falling.

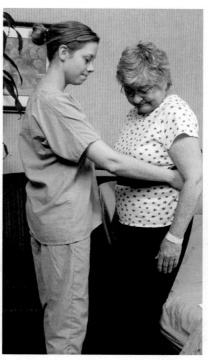

FIGURE 13-16 The person is pulled up to a standing position and supported by holding the transfer belt and blocking the person's knees and feet.

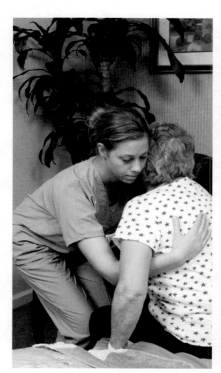

FIGURE 13-17 The person is being prepared to stand. The hands are placed under the person's arms and around the shoulder blades.

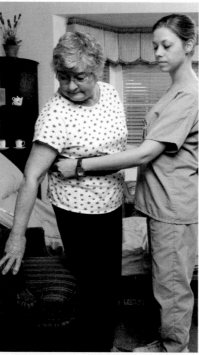

FIGURE 13-18 The person is supported as he or she grasps the far arm of the chair. The legs are against the chair.

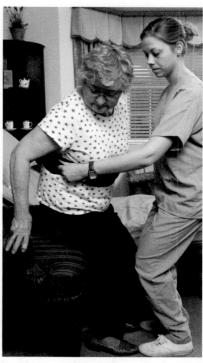

FIGURE 13-19 The person holds the armrests, leans forward, and bends the elbows and knees while being lowered into the chair.

Chair or Wheelchair to Bed Transfers

Chair or wheelchair to bed transfers have the same rules as bed to chair transfers. If the person is weak on one side, transfer the person so the strong side moves first. The chair or wheelchair is positioned so the person's strong side is near the bed.

For example, Mrs. Lee's right side is weak. Her left side is strong. To transfer her from bed to chair, the chair was on the left side of the bed. This allowed her left side (strong side) to move first. Now you will transfer Mrs. Lee back to bed. If the chair is on the left side of the bed, her right side—the weak side—is near the bed. It is unsafe to move the weak side first. You need to move the chair to the other side of the bed or turn the chair around. Mrs. Lee's stronger left side will be near the bed. The stronger side moves first for a safe transfer.

TRANSFERRING THE PERSON FROM A CHAIR OR WHEELCHAIR TO A BED

QUALITY OF LIFE

Remember to:
- Knock before entering the person's room.
- Address the person by name.
- Introduce yourself by name and title.

- Explain the procedure to the person before beginning and during the procedure.
- Protect the person's rights during the procedure.
- Handle the person gently during the procedure.

PRE-PROCEDURE

1 Follow *Delegation Guidelines:*
  a *Preventing Work-Related Injuries*, p. 187
  b *Transferring Persons*, p. 200
  See *Promoting Safety and Comfort:*
  a *Transfer/Gait Belts* (Chapter 9)
  b *Safely Handling, Moving, and Transferring the Person*, p. 183
  c *Preventing Work-Related Injuries*, p. 187

  d *Transferring Persons*, p. 200
  e *Bed to Chair or Wheelchair Transfers*, p. 201
2 Collect a transfer belt if needed.
3 Practice hand hygiene.
4 Identify the person. Check the ID bracelet against the assignment sheet. Also call the person by name.
5 Provide for privacy.

PROCEDURE

6 Move furniture for moving space.
7 Raise the head of the bed to a sitting position. The bed is in the lowest position.
8 Move the signal light so it is on the strong side when the person is in bed.
9 Position the chair or wheelchair so the person's strong side is next to the bed (Fig. 13-20). Have a co-worker help you if necessary.
10 Lock the wheelchair and bed wheels.
11 Remove and fold the lap blanket.
12 Remove the person's feet from the footplates. Raise the footplates. Remove or swing the front rigging out of the way. (The person has on non-skid footwear.)
13 Apply the transfer belt (if needed).
14 Make sure the person's feet are flat on the floor.
15 Stand in front of the person.
16 Ask the person to hold onto the armrests. (If the nurse directs you to do so, place your arms under the person's arms. Your hands are around the shoulder blades.)
17 Have the person lean forward.
18 Grasp the transfer belt on each side if using it. Grasp underneath the belt.

19 Prevent the person from sliding or falling by doing one of the following:
  a Brace your knees against the person's knees. Block his or her feet with your feet.
  b Use the knee and foot of one leg to block the person's weak leg or foot. Place your other foot slightly behind you for balance.
  c Straddle your legs around the person's weak leg.
20 Explain the "count of 3." (See procedure: *Transferring the Person to a Chair or Wheelchair*, p. 201.)
21 Ask the person to push down on the armrests on the count of "3." Pull the person into a standing position as you straighten your knees.
22 Support the person in the standing position. Hold the transfer belt, or keep your hands around the person's shoulder blades. Continue to prevent the person from sliding or falling.
23 Turn the person so he or she can reach the edge of the mattress. The legs will touch the mattress.
24 Continue to turn the person until he or she can reach the mattress with both hands.

25 Lower him or her onto the bed as you bend your hips and knees. The person assists by leaning forward and bending the elbows and knees.
26 Remove the transfer belt.

27 Remove the robe and footwear.
28 Help the person lie down.

POST-PROCEDURE

29 Provide for comfort. (See the inside of the front book cover.)
30 Place the signal light and other needed items within reach.
31 Raise or lower bed rails. Follow the care plan.
32 Arrange furniture to meet the person's needs.

33 Unscreen the person.
34 Complete a safety check of the room. (See the inside of the front book cover.)
35 Decontaminate your hands.
36 Report and record your observations.

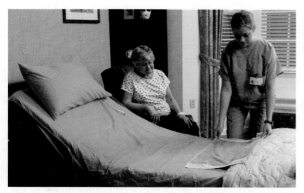

FIGURE 13-20 To transfer the person from chair to bed, the chair is positioned so the person's strong side is near the bed.

Mechanical Lifts

Persons who cannot help themselves are transferred with mechanical lifts. So are persons too heavy for the staff to transfer. The devices are used for transfers to and from beds, chairs, stretchers, tubs, shower chairs, toilets, commodes, whirlpools, or vehicles.

There are manual, battery-operated, and electric lifts. Some lifts are mounted on the ceiling. Before using a lift:

- You must be trained in its use.
- It must work.
- The sling, straps, hooks, and chains must be in good repair. The type of sling used depends on the person's size, condition, and other needs. Slings are padded, unpadded, or made of mesh.
- The person's weight must not exceed the lift's capacity.
- At least two staff members are needed.

There are different types of mechanical lifts. Always follow the manufacturer's instructions. The following procedure is used as a guide.

See *Delegation Guidelines: Using Mechanical Lifts.*

See *Promoting Safety and Comfort: Using Mechanical Lifts.*

DELEGATION GUIDELINES
Using Mechanical Lifts

When delegated tasks that involve using a mechanical lift, you need this information from the nurse and the care plan:

- The person's dependency level (see Box 13-2)
- What lift to use
- What sling to use—full, extended length, bathing, toileting, amputee
- If you should use a padded, unpadded, or mesh sling
- How many staff members are needed to perform the task safely

---

PROMOTING SAFETY AND COMFORT
Using Mechanical Lifts

Safety

Always follow the manufacturer's instructions. Knowing how to use one lift does not mean that you know how to use others.

If you have questions, ask the nurse. If you have not used a certain lift before, ask for needed training. Ask the nurse to help you until you are comfortable using the lift.

Mechanical lifts must be in good working order. Tell the nurse when a lift needs repair or is not working properly.

Some mechanical lifts are powered by batteries. The batteries must be well-charged. Follow the manufacturer's instructions.

Comfort

The person will be lifted up and off the bed or chair. Falling from the lift is a common fear. To promote the person's mental comfort, always explain the procedure before you begin. Also show the person how the lift works.

View Video!

TRANSFERRING THE PERSON USING A MECHANICAL LIFT

QUALITY OF LIFE

Remember to:
- Knock before entering the person's room.
- Address the person by name.
- Introduce yourself by name and title.

- Explain the procedure to the person before beginning and during the procedure.
- Protect the person's rights during the procedure.
- Handle the person gently during the procedure.

PRE-PROCEDURE

1 Follow *Delegation Guidelines:*
   a *Preventing Work-Related Injuries,* p. 187
   b *Transferring Persons,* p. 200
   c *Using Mechanical Lifts,* p. 205
   See *Promoting Safety and Comfort:*
   a *Safely Handling, Moving, and Transferring the Person,* p. 183
   b *Preventing Work-Related Injuries,* p. 187
   c *Transferring Persons,* p. 200
   d *Using Mechanical Lifts,* p. 205
2 Ask a co-worker to help you.

3 Collect:
   - Mechanical lift
   - Arm chair or wheelchair
   - Footwear
   - Bath blanket or cushion
   - Lap blanket
4 Practice hand hygiene.
5 Identify the person. Check the ID bracelet against the assignment sheet. Also call the person by name.
6 Provide for privacy.

PROCEDURE

7 Raise the bed for body mechanics. Bed rails are up if used.
8 Lower the head of the bed to a level appropriate for the person. It is as flat as possible.
9 Stand on one side of the bed. Your co-worker stands on the other side.
10 Lower the bed rails if up.
11 Center the sling under the person (Fig. 13-21, *A*). To position the sling, turn the person from side to side as if making an occupied bed (Chapter 14). Position the sling according to the manufacturer's instructions.
12 Position the person in semi-Fowler's position.
13 Place the chair at the head of the bed. It is even with the headboard and about 1 foot away from the bed. Place a folded bath blanket or cushion in the chair.
14 Lock the bed wheels. Lower the bed to its lowest position.
15 Raise the lift so you can position it over the person.
16 Position the lift over the person (Fig. 13-21, *B*).
17 Lock the lift wheels in position.
18 Attach the sling to the swivel bar (Fig. 13-21, *C*).
19 Raise the head of the bed to a sitting position.

20 Cross the person's arms over the chest. He or she can hold onto the straps or chains but not the swivel bar.
21 Raise the lift high enough until the person and sling are free of the bed (Fig. 13-21, *D*).
22 Have your co-worker support the person's legs as you move the lift and the person away from the bed (Fig. 13-21, *E*).
23 Position the lift so the person's back is toward the chair.
24 Position the chair so you can lower the person into it.
25 Lower the person into the chair. Guide the person into the chair (Fig. 13-21, *F*).
26 Lower the swivel bar to unhook the sling. Remove the sling from under the person unless otherwise indicated.
27 Put footwear on the person. Position the person's feet on the wheelchair footplates.
28 Cover the person's lap and legs with a lap blanket. Keep it off the floor and wheels.
29 Position the chair as the person prefers. Lock the wheelchair wheels according to the care plan.

POST-PROCEDURE

30 Provide for comfort. (See the inside of the front book cover.)
31 Place the signal light and other needed items within the person's reach.
32 Unscreen the person.

33 Complete a safety check of the room. (See the inside of the front book cover.)
34 Decontaminate your hands.
35 Report and record your observations.
36 Reverse the procedure to return the person to bed.

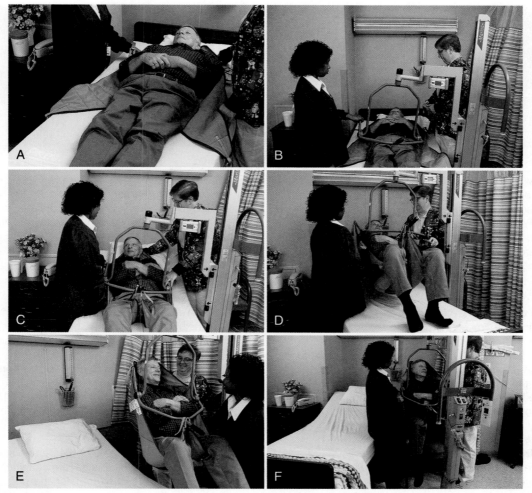

FIGURE 13-21 Using a mechanical lift. **A,** The sling is positioned under the person. **B,** The lift is over the person. **C,** The sling is attached to a swivel bar. **D,** The lift is raised until the sling and person are off of the bed. **E,** The person's legs are supported as the person and lift are moved away from the bed. **F,** The person is guided into a chair.

Transferring the Person to and From the Toilet

Using the bathroom for elimination promotes dignity, self-esteem, and independence. It also is more private than using a bedpan, urinal, or bedside commode. However, getting to the toilet is hard for persons who use wheelchairs. Bathrooms are often small. There is little room for you or a wheelchair. Therefore transfers involving wheelchairs and toilets are often hard. Falls and work-related injuries are risks.

Sometimes mechanical lifts are used for a transfer to and from a toilet. The following procedure can be used if the person can stand and pivot from the wheelchair to the toilet.

See *Promoting Safety and Comfort: Transferring the Person to and From the Toilet.*

TRANSFERRING THE PERSON TO AND FROM THE TOILET

QUALITY OF LIFE

Remember to:
- Knock before entering the person's room.
- Address the person by name.
- Introduce yourself by name and title.
- Explain the procedure to the person before beginning and during the procedure.
- Protect the person's rights during the procedure.
- Handle the person gently during the procedure.

PRE-PROCEDURE

1 Follow *Delegation Guidelines:*
  a *Preventing Work-Related Injuries,* p. 187
  b *Transferring Persons,* p. 200
  See *Promoting Safety and Comfort:*
  a *Transfer/Gait Belts* (Chapter 9)
  b *Safely Handling, Moving, and Transferring the Person,* p. 183

  c *Preventing Work-Related Injuries,* p. 187
  d *Transferring Persons,* p. 200
  e *Bed to Chair or Wheelchair Transfers,* p. 201
  f *Transferring the Person to and From the Toilet,* p. 207
2 Practice hand hygiene.

PROCEDURE

3 Have the person wear non-skid footwear.
4 Position the wheelchair next to the toilet if there is enough room. If not, position the chair at a right angle (90-degree angle) to the toilet (Fig. 13-22). It is best if the person's strong side is near the toilet.
5 Lock the wheelchair wheels.
6 Raise the footplates. Remove or swing the front rigging out of the way.
7 Apply the transfer belt.
8 Help the person unfasten clothing.
9 Use the transfer belt to help the person stand and to turn to the toilet. (See procedure: *Transferring the Person to a Chair or Wheelchair,* p. 201.) The person uses the grab bars to turn to the toilet.
10 Support the person with the transfer belt while he or she lowers clothing. Or have the person hold onto the grab bars for support. Lower the person's pants and undergarments.
11 Use the transfer belt to lower the person onto the toilet seat. Make sure he or she is properly positioned on the toilet.
12 Remove the transfer belt.
13 Tell the person you will stay nearby. Remind the person to use the signal light or call for you when help is needed. Stay with the person if required by the care plan.

14 Close the bathroom door to provide for privacy.
15 Stay near the bathroom. Complete other tasks in the person's room. Check on the person every 5 minutes.
16 Knock on the bathroom door when the person calls for you.
17 Help with wiping, perineal care (Chapter 15), flushing, and hand washing as needed. Wear gloves, and practice hand hygiene after removing the gloves.
18 Apply the transfer belt.
19 Use the transfer belt to help the person stand.
20 Help the person raise and secure clothing.
21 Use the transfer belt to transfer the person to the wheelchair. (See procedure: *Transferring the Person to a Chair or Wheelchair,* p. 201).
22 Make sure the person's buttocks are to the back of the seat. Position the person in good alignment.
23 Position the person's feet on the footplates.
24 Cover the person's lap and legs with a lap blanket. Keep the blanket off the floor and wheels.
25 Position the chair as the person prefers. Lock the wheelchair wheels according to the care plan.

POST-PROCEDURE

26 Provide for comfort. (See the inside of the front book cover.)
27 Place the signal light and other needed items within the person's reach.
28 Unscreen the person.

29 Complete a safety check of the room. (See the inside of the front book cover.)
30 Practice hand hygiene.
31 Report and record your observations.

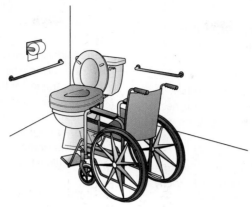

FIGURE 13-22 The wheelchair is placed at a right angle (90-degree angle) to the toilet.

REPOSITIONING IN A CHAIR OR WHEELCHAIR

The person can slide down into the chair. For good alignment and safety, the person's back and buttocks must be against the back of the chair.

Some persons can help with repositioning. If the person cannot help, a mechanical lift is used. Follow the nurse's directions and the care plan for the best way to reposition a person in a chair or wheelchair. *Do not pull the person from behind the chair or wheelchair.*

If the person's chair reclines, do the following:
• Ask a co-worker to help you.
• Lock the wheels.
• Recline the chair.
• Position a friction-reducing device (drawsheet or slide sheet) under the person.
• Use the device to move the person up. See procedure: *Moving the Person Up in Bed With an Assist Device*, p. 191.

The following method can be used if the person is alert and cooperative. The person must be able to follow directions. And the person must have the strength to help.
• Lock the wheelchair wheels.
• Remove or swing the front rigging out of the way.
• Position the person's feet flat on the floor.
• Apply a transfer belt.
• Position the person's arms on the armrests.

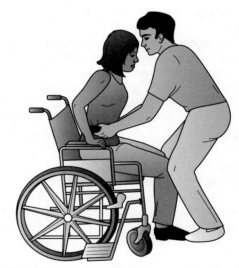

FIGURE 13-23 Repositioning the person in a wheelchair. A transfer belt is used to move the person to the back of the chair.

• Stand in front of the person. Block his or her knees and feet with your knees and feet.
• Grasp the transfer belt on each side while the person leans forward.
• Ask the person to push with his or her feet and arms on the count of "3."
• Move the person back into the chair on the count of "3" as the person pushes with his or her feet and arms (Fig. 13-23).

Focus on P R I D E
The Person, Family, and Yourself

Personal and Professional Responsibility—You are responsible for handling, moving, and transferring persons safely. This includes the person's safety and your own. Follow the rules of body mechanics in Chapter 12 to protect yourself. Ask the nurse if you are unsure how to safely transfer a person. Never be afraid to ask for help. Take pride in safely assisting patients and residents with their mobility.

Rights and Respect—When moving or transferring a person, remember to respect his or her privacy. Properly cover the person. For example, a person is wearing a gown that is open in the back. The person's back is exposed. You can apply a robe or another gown to cover the person's backside. Use a covering that is safe during the transfer. Avoid long robes or robes with long ties. These could get caught or cause the person to fall.

Independence and Social Interaction—Persons who need help moving and transferring have limited independence. They cannot turn or move in bed alone, sit up in a chair alone, or go to the bathroom alone. This can cause feelings of embarrassment and helplessness.

To promote pride and independence while handling, moving, and transferring the person:
- Focus on the person's abilities.
- Encourage the person.
- Let him or her help as much as safely possible.
- Tell the person when you notice even small improvements. Such motivation can improve self-esteem and aid in healing.

Delegation and Teamwork—Patients and residents need to be moved, turned, transferred, and repositioned. These tasks and procedures are best done by at least 2 staff members.

Friendships are common among co-workers. And some working relationships are better than others. Do not just ask your friends or those with whom you work well to help you. Include all co-workers. In return, do not just help your friends or those with whom you work well. Assist anyone who asks for your help. This includes new staff members and those from other units. Take pride in forming positive work relationships with all team members.

Ethics and Laws—Ethics involves right and wrong conduct. The following are examples of wrong ways to handle, move, or transfer a person. *Do not:*
- Pull on a person's arm, underarm, or other body part
- Move the person alone when help is needed
- Position the chair or wheelchair farther away from the bed than necessary
- Move a person without the proper equipment such as a transfer belt or mechanical lift
- Use broken or damaged equipment

REVIEW QUESTIONS

Circle the BEST answer.

1 A person's skin rubs against the sheet. This is called
   a Shearing
   b Friction
   c Ergonomics
   d Posture

2 Which occurs when a person slides down in bed?
   a Shearing
   b Friction
   c Ergonomics
   d Posture

3 Which protects the skin when moving the person in bed?
   a Rolling the person
   b Sliding the person up in bed
   c Moving the mattress
   d Using ergonomics

4 Whenever you handle, move, or transfer a person, you must
   a Allow personal choice
   b Protect the person's privacy
   c Use pillows for support
   d Get help from a co-worker

5 You are delegated tasks that involve moving persons in bed. Which is *true?*
   a The nurse tells you how to position the person.
   b You decide which procedure to use.
   c Bed rails are used at all times.
   d Three workers are needed to complete the task safely.

6 You are using a drawsheet as an assist device. It is placed so that it
   a Covers the person's body
   b Is under the person from the head to above the knees
   c Extends from the mid-back to mid-thigh level
   d Covers the entire mattress

7 Before turning a person onto his or her side, you
   a Move the person to the side of the bed
   b Move the person to the middle of the bed
   c Raise the head of the bed
   d Position pillows for comfort

8 The logrolling procedure
   a Is used after spinal cord injuries or surgeries
   b Requires a transfer belt
   c Requires a mechanical lift
   d Involves a wheelchair and a drawsheet

9 When getting ready to dangle a person, you need to know
   a Which side is stronger
   b If bed rails are used
   c If a mechanical lift is needed
   d If a transfer belt is needed

10 For chair and wheelchair transfers, the person must
    a Wear non-skid footwear
    b Have the bed rails up
    c Use a mechanical lift
    d Have a drawsheet or other assist device

11 Before transferring a person to or from a bed, you must
    a Raise the bed rails
    b Lock the bed wheels
    c Apply a transfer belt
    d Position pillows for support

12 When transferring the person to bed, a chair, or the toilet
    a The person's strong side moves first
    b The weak side moves first
    c Pillows are used for support
    d The transfer belt is removed

13 You are going to use a mechanical lift. You must do the following *except*
    a Follow the manufacturer's instructions
    b Make sure the lift works
    c Compare the person's weight to the lift's weight limit
    d Use a transfer belt

14 To safely transfer a person with a mechanical lift, at least
    a 1 worker is needed
    b 2 workers are needed
    c 3 workers are needed
    d 4 workers are needed

15 These statements are about transfers to and from a toilet. Which is *false?*
    a The person wears non-skid footwear.
    b Wheelchair wheels must be locked.
    c The person uses the towel bars for support.
    d A transfer belt is used.

Answers to these questions are on p. 527.

14

ASSISTING WITH COMFORT

PROCEDURES

 Making a Closed Bed

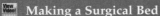 Making an Occupied Bed

Making a Surgical Bed

OBJECTIVES

- Define the key terms and key abbreviations listed in this chapter.
- Describe how to control temperature, odors, noise, and lighting for the person's comfort.
- Describe the basic bed positions.
- Identify the persons at risk for entrapment in the hospital bed system.
- Identify hospital bed system entrapment zones.
- Explain how to use the furniture and equipment in the person's unit.
- Describe four ways to make beds.
- Handle linens following the rules of medical asepsis.
- Explain how to assist the nurse with relieving pain.
- Explain how to assist the nurse with promoting sleep.
- Explain how to promote PRIDE in the person, the family, and yourself.
- Perform the procedures described in this chapter.

KEY TERMS

Fowler's position A semi-sitting position; the head of the bed is raised between 45 and 60 degrees

full visual privacy Having the means to be completely free from public view while in bed

high-Fowler's position A semi-sitting position; the head of the bed is raised 60 to 90 degrees

insomnia A chronic condition in which the person cannot sleep or stay asleep all night

pain To ache, hurt, or be sore

reverse Trendelenburg's position The head of the bed is raised and the foot of the bed is lowered

semi-Fowler's position The head of the bed is raised 30 degrees; or the head of the bed is raised 30 degrees and the knee portion is raised 15 degrees

sleep deprivation The amount and quality of sleep are decreased

sleep-walking The sleeping person leaves the bed and walks about

Trendelenburg's position The head of the bed is lowered and the foot of the bed is raised

KEY ABBREVIATIONS

F Fahrenheit

OBRA Omnibus Budget Reconciliation Act of 1987

Comfort is a state of well-being. Many factors affect comfort. Sleep is promoted when the person is comfortable and pain free.

THE PERSON'S UNIT

Patient and resident rooms are designed to provide comfort, safety, and privacy. In nursing centers, resident rooms are as personal and home-like as possible.

The *person's unit* is the personal space, furniture, and equipment provided for the person by the agency (Fig. 14-1). This area is a private area. Like a person's home, it is treated with respect.

You need to help keep the person's unit clean, neat, safe, and comfortable. Follow the rules in Box 14-1.

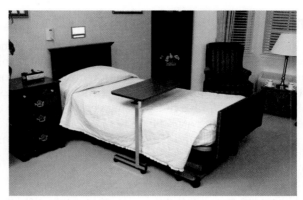

FIGURE 14-1 Furniture and equipment in a resident's unit.

BOX 14-1   Maintaining the Person's Unit

- Keep the signal light within the person's reach at all times.
- Meet the needs of persons who cannot use the call system.
- Place the overbed table and the bedside stand within the person's reach.
- Arrange personal items as the person prefers. They are within easy reach.
- Place the phone and TV, bed, and light controls within the person's reach.
- Provide the person with enough tissues and toilet paper.
- Adjust lighting, temperature, and ventilation for the person's comfort.
- Handle equipment carefully to prevent noise.
- Explain the causes of strange noises.
- Use room deodorizers according to agency policy.
- Empty the person's wastebaskets at least once a day. In some agencies they are emptied every shift.
- Respect the person's belongings. An item may not have importance or value to you. Yet it has great meaning for the person. Even a scrap of paper can have great meaning to the person.
- Do not throw away any items belonging to the person.
- Do not move furniture or the person's belongings. Persons with poor vision rely on memory or feel to find items.
- Straighten bed linens and towels as often as needed.
- Complete a safety check before leaving the room. (See the inside of the front book cover.)

Temperature and Ventilation

Most healthy people are comfortable when the temperature is 68° F (Fahrenheit) to 74° F. Older persons and ill persons may need higher temperatures for comfort. The Omnibus Budget Reconciliation Act of 1987 (OBRA) requires that nursing centers maintain a temperature range of 71° F to 81° F.

To protect older and ill persons from cool areas and drafts:
* Keep room temperatures warm.
* Make sure they wear the correct clothing.
* Offer lap robes to those in chairs and wheelchairs. Lap robes cover the legs.
* Provide enough blankets for warmth.
* Cover them with bath blankets when giving care.
* Move them from drafty areas.

Odors

Many odors occur in health care agencies. Bowel movements and urine have embarrassing odors. So do draining wounds and vomitus. Body, breath, and smoking odors may offend others. To reduce odors:
* Empty, clean, and disinfect bedpans, urinals, commodes, and kidney basins promptly.
* Make sure toilets are flushed.
* Check incontinent persons often (Chapters 17 and 18).
* Clean persons who are wet or soiled from urine, feces, vomitus, or wound drainage.
* Change wet or soiled linens and clothing promptly.
* Keep laundry containers closed.
* Follow agency policy for wet or soiled linens and clothing.
* Dispose of incontinence and ostomy products promptly (Chapters 17 and 18).
* Provide good hygiene to prevent body and breath odors (Chapter 15).
* Use room deodorizers as needed and allowed by agency policy. Sometimes odors remain after removing the cause. Do not use sprays around persons with breathing problems. Ask the nurse if you are unsure.

If you smoke, follow the agency's policy. Practice hand washing after handling smoking materials and before giving care. Give careful attention to your uniforms, hair, and breath because of smoke odors.

PERSONS WITH DEMENTIA
Noise

Persons with dementia do not understand what is happening around them. They do not react to common, every day sounds as other people do. For example, a ringing phone may frighten a person with dementia. The person may not know or understand the sound. He or she may have an extreme reaction to the sound (Chapter 28). The reaction may be more severe at night. This is likely when the sound awakens the person suddenly. A dark, strange room can make the problem worse.

PERSONS WITH DEMENTIA
Lighting

In dementia care units, lighting is adjusted to help control agitated and aggressive behaviors. Soft, non-glare lights are relaxing. They can decrease agitation. Brighter lighting may improve orientation. The person can see surroundings more clearly.

Noise

Common health care sounds may disturb patients and residents. The clatter and clanging of equipment, dishes, and meal trays are examples. So are loud voices, TVs, music, and phones. Intercom systems and signal lights are annoying. So is noise from equipment needing repair and wheels needing oil.

To decrease noise:
* Control your voice.
* Handle equipment carefully.
* Keep equipment in good working order.
* Answer phones, signal lights, and intercoms promptly.

See *Persons With Dementia: Noise.*

Lighting

Good lighting is needed for safety and comfort. Glares, shadows, and dull lighting can cause falls, headaches, and eyestrain. A bright room is cheerful. Dim light is better for relaxing and rest.

Adjust lighting and window coverings to meet the person's changing needs. The overbed light can provide soft, medium, or bright lighting. Keep light controls within the person's reach. This protects the right to personal choice.

See *Persons With Dementia: Lighting.*

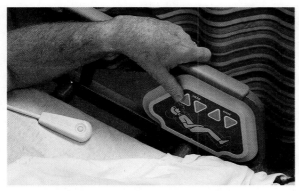

FIGURE 14-2 Bed controls in the bed rail.

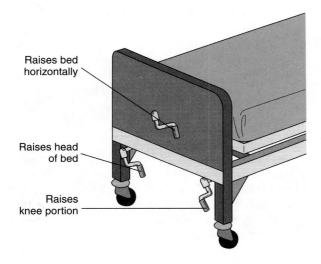

Raises bed
horizontally

Raises head
of bed

Raises
knee portion

FIGURE 14-3 Manually operated hospital bed.

Room Furniture and Equipment

Rooms are furnished and equipped to meet basic needs. The right to privacy is considered.

The Bed Beds have electrical or manual controls. Beds are raised horizontally to reduce bending and reaching when giving care. The lowest horizontal position lets the person get out of bed with ease. The head of the bed is flat or raised varying degrees.

Electric beds have controls that are on a side panel, bed rail, or the footboard (Fig. 14-2). Or they have hand-held devices. Patients and residents are taught to use the controls safely. They are warned not to raise the bed to the high position or to adjust the bed to harmful positions. They are told of any position limits or restrictions.

Manual beds have cranks at the foot of the bed (Fig. 14-3). The cranks are pulled up for use. They are kept down at all other times. Cranks in the "up" position are safety hazards. Anyone walking past may bump into them.

See *Promoting Safety and Comfort: The Bed.*

Bed Positions The six basic bed positions are:
* *Flat*—This is the usual sleeping position.
* *Fowler's position*—**Fowler's position** is a semi-sitting position. The head of the bed is raised between 45 and 60 degrees (Fig. 14-4, p. 216).
* High-Fowler's position—**High-Fowler's position** is a semi-sitting position. The head of the bed is raised 60 to 90 degrees (Fig. 14-5, p. 216).
* *Semi-Fowler's position*—In **semi-Fowler's position,** the head of the bed is raised 30 degrees (Fig. 14-6, p. 216). Some agencies define semi-Fowler's position as when the head of the bed is raised 30 degrees and the knee portion is raised 15 degrees. Know the definition used by your agency.
* *Trendelenburg's position*—In **Trendelenburg's position,** the head of the bed is lowered and the foot of the bed is raised (Fig. 14-7, p. 216). A doctor orders the position. Blocks are placed under the legs at the foot of the bed. Or the bed frame is tilted.
* *Reverse Trendelenburg's position*—In **reverse Trendelenburg's position,** the head of the bed is raised and the foot of the bed is lowered (Fig. 14-8, p. 216). Blocks are placed under the legs at the head of the bed. Or the bed frame is tilted. This position requires a doctor's order.

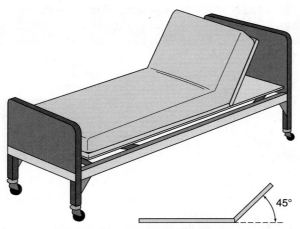

FIGURE 14-4 Fowler's position.

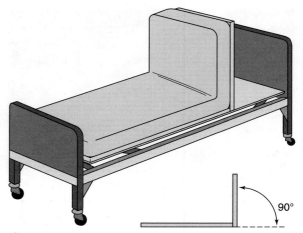

FIGURE 14-5 High-Fowler's position.

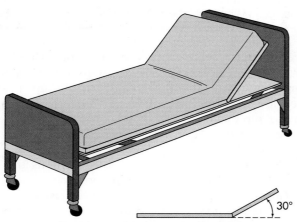

FIGURE 14-6 Semi-Fowler's position.

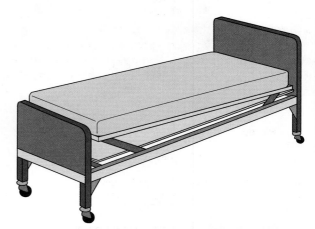

FIGURE 14-7 Trendelenburg's position.

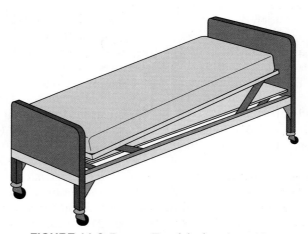

FIGURE 14-8 Reverse Trendelenburg's position.

Bed Safety Bed safety involves the *hospital bed system*—the bed frame and its parts. The parts include the mattress, bed rails, headboards and footboards, and bed attachments.

Hospital bed systems have seven entrapment zones (Figs. 14-9 below and 14-10, p. 218). *Entrapment* means that the person can get caught, trapped, or entangled in spaces created by bed rails, the mattress, the bed frame, the headboard, or the footboard. Serious injuries and deaths have occurred from head, neck, and chest entrapment. Arm and leg entrapment also can occur. Persons at greatest risk include persons who:

• Are older
• Are frail
• Are confused or disoriented
• Are restless
• Have uncontrolled body movements
• Have poor muscle control
• Are small in size
• Are restrained (Chapter 10)

Always check the person for entrapment. If a person is caught, trapped, or entangled in the bed or any of its parts, try to release the person. Also call for the nurse at once.

The Overbed Table   The overbed table (see Fig. 14-1) is placed over the bed by sliding the base under the bed. It is raised or lowered for the person in bed or in a chair. The table is used for meals, writing, reading, and other activities.

The nursing team uses the overbed table as a work area. Only clean and sterile items are placed on the table. Never place bedpans, urinals, or soiled linen on the overbed table. Clean the table after using it for a work surface.

The Bedside Stand   The bedside stand has a top drawer and a lower cabinet with shelves or drawers (Fig. 14-11, p. 219). The top drawer is used for money, eyeglasses, books, and other items.

The top shelf or middle drawer is used for the wash basin. The wash basin can hold personal items—soap and soap dish, powder, lotion, deodorant, towels, washcloth, bath blanket, and a clean gown or pajamas. An emesis basin or kidney basin (shaped like a kidney) can hold oral hygiene items. The kidney basin is stored in the top drawer, middle drawer, or on the top shelf. The bedpan and its cover, the urinal, and toilet paper are stored on the lower shelf or in the bottom drawer.

Zone 1: Within the rail

Zone 2: Between the top of the compressed mattress and the bottom of the rail, between the supports

Zone 3: Between the rail and the mattress

Zone 4: Between the top of the compressed mattress and the bottom of the rail, at the end of the rail

Zone 5: Between the split bed rails

Zone 6: Between the end of the rail and the side edge of the headboard or footboard

Zone 7: Between the head or footboard and the mattress end

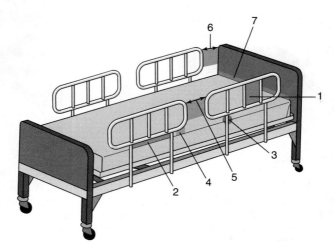

FIGURE 14-9 Hospital bed system entrapment zones. (*Redrawn from* Guidance for industry and FDA staff: hospital bed system dimensional and assessment guidance to reduce entrapment, *updated August 19, 2009, Food and Drug Administration.*)

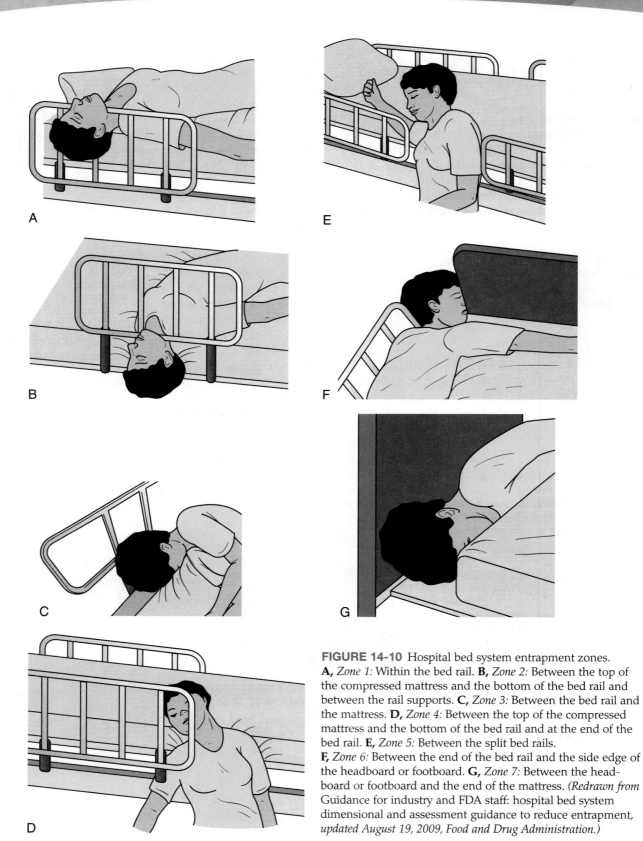

FIGURE 14-10 Hospital bed system entrapment zones.
A, *Zone 1:* Within the bed rail. **B,** *Zone 2:* Between the top of
the compressed mattress and the bottom of the bed rail and
between the rail supports. **C,** *Zone 3:* Between the bed rail and
the mattress. **D,** *Zone 4:* Between the top of the compressed
mattress and the bottom of the bed rail and at the end of the
bed rail. **E,** *Zone 5:* Between the split bed rails.
F, *Zone 6:* Between the end of the bed rail and the side edge of
the headboard or footboard. **G,** *Zone 7:* Between the headboard or footboard and the end of the mattress. *(Redrawn from*
Guidance for industry and FDA staff: hospital bed system
dimensional and assessment guidance to reduce entrapment,
updated August 19, 2009, Food and Drug Administration.)

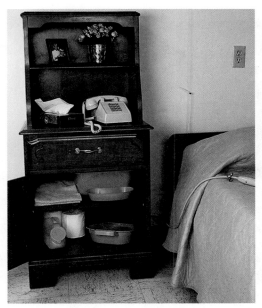

FIGURE 14-11 The bedside stand.

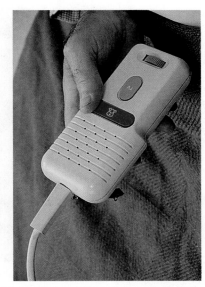

FIGURE 14-12 A signal light. The signal light button is pressed when help is needed.

The top of the stand is often used for tissues, the phone, and personal items. The person may put a radio, clock, photos, phone, flowers, cards, gifts, or other things there.

Place only clean and sterile items on top of the bedside stand. Never place bedpans, urinals, or soiled linen on the top of the stand. If you use the bedside stand for a work surface, clean it when you are done.

Chairs The person's unit always has at least one chair. It must be comfortable, sturdy, and not move or tip during transfers. The person should be able to get in and out of the chair with ease.

Privacy Curtains Each person has the right to **full visual privacy**—the means to be completely free from public view while in bed. The privacy curtain is pulled around the bed to provide privacy. *Always* pull it completely around the bed before giving care.

Privacy curtains do not block sounds or conversations. Others in the room can hear sounds or talking behind the curtain.

The Call System The call system lets the person signal for help. The signal light is at the end of a long cord (Fig. 14-12). It attaches to the bed or chair. *Always keep the signal light within the person's reach—in the room, bathroom, and shower or tub room.*

To get help, the person presses a button at the end of the signal light. The signal light connects to a light above the room door. The signal light also connects to a light panel or intercom system at the nurses' station (Fig. 14-13, p. 220). These tell the nursing team that the person needs help.

An intercom system lets a nursing team member talk with the person from the nurses' station. The person tells what is needed. Hard-of-hearing persons may have problems using an intercom. Be careful when using an intercom. Remember confidentiality. Persons nearby can hear what you and the person say.

Some persons have limited hand mobility. They may need a signal light that is turned on by tapping it with a hand or fist (Fig. 14-14, p. 220).

Some people cannot use signal lights. Examples are persons who are confused or in a coma. Check the care plan for special communication measures. Check these persons often. Make sure their needs are met. You must:

• Keep the signal light within the person's reach. Even if the person cannot use the signal light, keep it within reach for use by visitors and staff. They may need to signal for help.
• Place the signal light on the person's strong side.
• Remind the person to signal when help is needed.
• Answer signal lights promptly. Remember, the person signals when help is needed.
• Answer bathroom and shower or tub room signal lights at once.

See *Focus on Communication: The Call System,* p. 220.

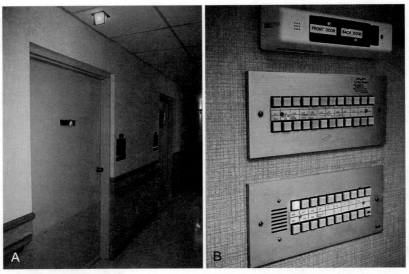

FIGURE 14-13 A, Light above the room door. **B,** Light panel and intercom at the nurses' station.

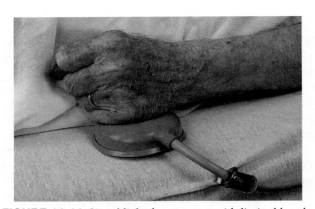

FIGURE 14-14 Signal light for a person with limited hand mobility.

The Bathroom A toilet, sink, call system, and mirror are standard equipment in bathrooms. Some bathrooms have showers.

For safety, grab bars are by the toilet. The person uses them for support when lowering to or raising from the toilet. Some bathrooms have raised toilet seats. They make wheelchair transfers easier and are helpful for persons with joint problems.

Towel racks, toilet paper, soap, paper towel dispenser, and a wastebasket are in the bathroom. They are placed within easy reach of the person.

Usually the signal light is by the toilet. The bathroom signal light flashes above the room door and at the nurses' station. The sound at the nurses' station is different from signal lights in rooms. Someone must respond at once when a person needs help in a bathroom.

Closet and Drawer Space Closet and drawer space are provided. OBRA requires closet space for each nursing center resident. Such closet space must have shelves and a clothes rack. The person must have free access to the closet and its contents. Items in closets and drawers are the person's private property.

Some people hoard items—drugs, napkins, straws, food, sugar, salt, pepper, and so on. Hoarding can cause safety or health risks. The nurse may ask you to inspect a person's closet, drawers, or personal items. If so, the person must be present. Also have a co-worker with you. Your co-worker is a witness to what you are doing. This protects you if the person claims that something was stolen or damaged.

Other Equipment

Many agencies furnish rooms with other equipment. A TV, radio, and clock provide comfort and relaxation. Many rooms have phones, a computer, and Internet access. Residents may bring some furniture and other items from home.

See *Promoting Safety and Comfort: Other Equipment.*

BEDMAKING

Beds are made every day. Clean, dry, and wrinkle-free linens promote comfort. They also prevent skin breakdown and pressure ulcers (Chapter 23).

To keep beds neat and clean:
- Straighten linens whenever loose or wrinkled and at bedtime.
- Check for and remove food and crumbs after meals.
- Check linens for dentures, eyeglasses, hearing aids, sharp objects, and other items.
- Change linens whenever they become wet, soiled, or damp.
- Follow Standard Precautions and the Bloodborne Pathogen Standard. Contact with blood, body fluids, secretions, or excretions is likely.

Types of Beds

Beds are made in these ways:
- A *closed bed* is not in use. Top linens are not folded back (Fig. 14-15). The bed is ready for a new patient or resident. In nursing centers, closed beds are made for residents who are up during the day.
- An *open bed* is in use. Top linens are fan-folded back so the person can get into bed. A closed bed becomes an open bed by fan-folding back the top linens (Fig. 14-16).
- An *occupied bed* is made with the person in it (Fig. 14-17, p. 222).
- A *surgical bed* is made to transfer a person from a stretcher (Fig. 14-18, p. 222). This bed also is made for persons who arrive by ambulance.

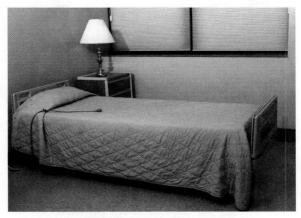

FIGURE 14-15 Closed bed.

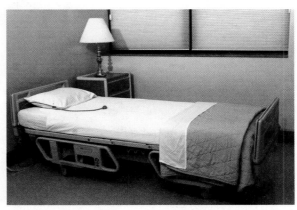

FIGURE 14-16 Open bed. Top linens are fan-folded to the foot of the bed.

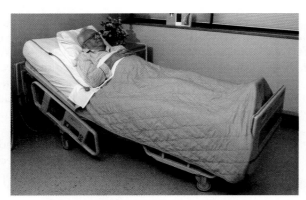

FIGURE 14-17 Occupied bed.

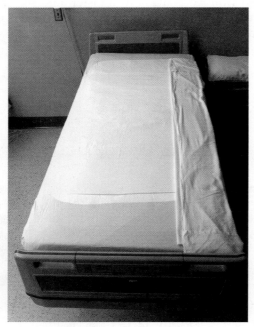

FIGURE 14-18 Surgical bed.

Linens

Collect linens in the order you will use them:
- Mattress pad (if needed)
- Bottom sheet (flat or fitted)
- Plastic (waterproof) drawsheet or waterproof pad (if needed)
- Cotton drawsheet (if needed)
- Top sheet
- Blanket
- Bedspread
- Pillowcase(s)
- Bath towel(s)
- Hand towel
- Washcloth
- Gown or pajamas
- Bath blanket

Use one arm to hold the linens. Use your other hand to pick them up. The item you will use first is at the bottom of your stack. (You picked up the mattress pad first. It is at the bottom. The bath blanket is on top.) You need the mattress pad first. To get it on top, place your arm over the bath blanket. Then turn the stack over onto the arm on the bath blanket (Fig. 14-19). The arm that held the linens is now free. Place the clean linen on a clean surface.

Remove dirty linen one piece at a time. Roll each piece away from you. The side that touched the person is inside the roll and away from you (Fig. 14-20). Discard each piece into the laundry bag.

In hospitals, top and bottom sheets, the cotton drawsheet, and pillowcases are changed daily. The mattress pad, plastic drawsheet, blanket, and bedspread are re-used for the same person.

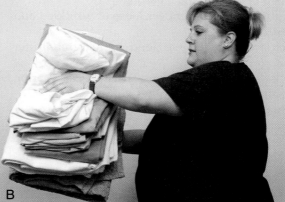
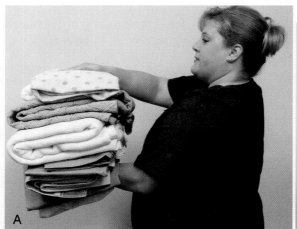

FIGURE 14-19 Collecting linens. **A,** The arm is placed over the top of the stack of linens. **B,** The stack of linens is turned onto the arm. Note that the linens are held away from the body.

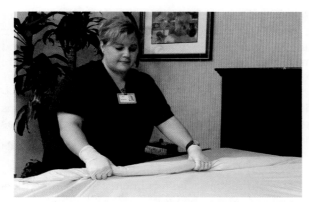

FIGURE 14-20 Roll dirty linen away from you.

In nursing centers, linens are not changed every day. A complete linen change is done on the person's bath day. Pillowcases, top and bottom sheets, and drawsheets (if used) may be changed twice a week.

Linens are not re-used if soiled, wet, or wrinkled. Wet, damp, or soiled linens are changed right away. Wear gloves and follow Standard Precautions and the Bloodborne Pathogen Standard.

Drawsheets A *drawsheet* is a small sheet placed over the middle of the bottom sheet.
- A *cotton drawsheet* is made of cotton. It helps keep the mattress and bottom linens clean.
- A *waterproof drawsheet* is made of plastic or rubber. It is placed between the bottom sheet and cotton drawsheet. It protects the mattress and bottom linens from dampness and soiling.

The cotton drawsheet protects the person from contact with plastic and absorbs moisture. However, discomfort and skin breakdown may occur. Plastic retains heat. Waterproof drawsheets are hard to keep tight and wrinkle-free. Many agencies use incontinence products (Chapter 17) to keep the person and linens dry. Others use waterproof pads or disposable bed protectors.

Cotton drawsheets are often used without waterproof drawsheets. Plastic-covered mattresses cause some persons to perspire heavily. This increases discomfort. A cotton drawsheet reduces heat retention and absorbs moisture. Cotton drawsheets are often used as assist devices to move and transfer persons in bed (Chapter 13). When used for this purpose, do not tuck them in at the sides.

The bedmaking procedures that follow include waterproof and cotton drawsheets. This is so you learn how to use them. Ask the nurse about their use in your agency.

Making Beds

When making beds, follow the rules in Box 14-2.
See *Delegation Guidelines: Making Beds,* p. 224
See *Promoting Safety and Comfort: Making Beds,* p. 224.

BOX 14-2   Rules for Bedmaking

- Use good body mechanics at all times (Chapter 12).
- Follow the rules in Chapter 13 to safely handle, move, and transfer the person.
- Follow the rules of medical asepsis.
- Follow Standard Precautions and the Bloodborne Pathogen Standard.
- Practice hand hygiene before handling clean linen.
- Wear gloves to remove used linen from a bed.
- Practice hand hygiene after handling dirty linen.
- Bring enough linen to the person's room. Bring only the linens that you will need. Extra linens cannot be used for another person.
- Place clean linen on a clean surface. You can use the bedside chair, overbed table, or bedside stand. Place a barrier (towel, paper towels) between the clean surface and the linens if required by agency policy.
- Do not use extra linen in the person's room for another patient or resident. Extra linen is considered contaminated. Put it with the dirty laundry.
- Do not use torn or frayed linen.
- Never shake linens. Shaking linens spreads microbes.
- Hold linens away from your body and uniform. Dirty and clean linen must not touch your uniform.
- Never put dirty linens on the floor or on clean linens. Follow agency policy for dirty linen.
- Keep bottom linens tucked in and wrinkle-free.
- Cover a waterproof drawsheet with a cotton drawsheet. A waterproof drawsheet must not touch the person's body.
- Straighten and tighten loose sheets, blankets, and bedspreads as needed.
- Make as much of one side of the bed as possible before going to the other side. This saves time and energy.
- Change wet, damp, and soiled linens right away.

The Closed Bed The closed bed is made after a person is discharged. It is made for a new patient or resident. The bed is made after the bed frame and mattress are cleaned and disinfected. Clean linens are needed for the entire bed.

In nursing centers, closed beds are made for residents who are up for most or all of the day. Top linens are folded back at bedtime. Clean linens are used as needed.

The Open Bed A closed bed becomes an open bed by fan-folding back the top linen. The open bed lets the person get into bed with ease. Make this bed for:
- Newly admitted persons arriving by wheelchair
- Persons who are getting ready for bed
- Persons who are out of bed for a short time

Text continued on p. 228

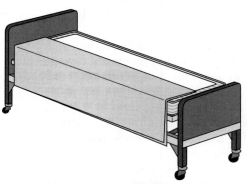

FIGURE 14-21 The bottom sheet is on the bed with the center crease in the middle. The lower edge of the sheet is even with the bottom of the mattress.

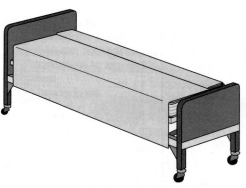

FIGURE 14-22 The bottom sheet is fan-folded to the other side of the bed.

MAKING A CLOSED BED

QUALITY OF LIFE

Remember to:
- Knock before entering the person's room.
- Address the person by name.
- Introduce yourself by name and title.

- Explain the procedure to the person before beginning and during the procedure.
- Protect the person's rights during the procedure.
- Handle the person gently during the procedure.

PRE-PROCEDURE

1 Follow *Delegation Guidelines: Making Beds.*
  See *Promoting Safety and Comfort: Making Beds.*
2 Practice hand hygiene.
3 Collect clean linen:
  - Mattress pad (if needed)
  - Bottom sheet (flat sheet or fitted sheet)
  - Waterproof drawsheet or waterproof pad (if needed)
  - Cotton drawsheet (if needed)
  - Top sheet
  - Blanket
  - Bedspread
  - A pillowcase for each pillow
  - Bath towel(s)

  - Hand towel
  - Washcloth
  - Gown or pajamas
  - Bath blanket
  - Gloves
  - Laundry bag
  - Paper towels (if a barrier is needed for clean linens)
4 Place linen on a clean surface. Use the paper towels as a barrier between the clean surface and clean linen if required by agency policy.
5 Raise the bed for body mechanics. Bed rails are down.

PROCEDURE

6 Put on the gloves.
7 Remove linen. Roll each piece away from you. Place each piece in a laundry bag. (NOTE: Discard incontinence products or disposable bed protectors in the trash. Do not put them in the laundry bag.)
8 Clean the bed frame and mattress (if this is your job).
9 Remove and discard gloves. Decontaminate your hands.
10 Move the mattress to the head of the bed.
11 Put the mattress pad on the mattress. It is even with the top of the mattress.
12 Place the bottom sheet on the mattress pad (Fig. 14-21):
  a Unfold it length-wise.
  b Place the center crease in the middle of the bed.
  c Position the lower edge even with the bottom of the mattress.
  d Place the large hem at the top and the small hem at the bottom.
  e Face hem-stitching downward, away from the person.
13 Open the sheet. Fan-fold it to the other side of the bed (Fig. 14-22).
14 Tuck the top of the sheet under the mattress. The sheet is tight and smooth.
15 Make a mitered corner if using a flat sheet (Fig. 14-23, p. 226).

16 Place the waterproof drawsheet on the bed. It is in the middle of the mattress. Or put the waterproof pad on the bed.
17 Open the waterproof drawsheet. Fan-fold it to the other side of the bed.
18 Place a cotton drawsheet over the waterproof drawsheet. It covers the entire waterproof drawsheet (Fig. 14-24, p. 227).
19 Open the cotton drawsheet. Fan-fold it to the other side of the bed.
20 Tuck both drawsheets under the mattress. Or tuck each in separately.
21 Go to the other side of the bed.
22 Miter the top corner of the flat bottom sheet.
23 Pull the bottom sheet tight so there are no wrinkles. Tuck in the sheet.
24 Pull the drawsheets tight so there are no wrinkles. Tuck both in together or separately (Fig. 14-25, p. 227).
25 Go to the other side of the bed.
26 Put the top sheet on the bed:
  a Unfold it length-wise.
  b Place the center crease in the middle.
  c Place the large hem even with the top of the mattress.
  d Open the sheet. Fan-fold it to the other side.
  e Face hem-stitching outward, away from the person.
  f Do not tuck the bottom in yet.
  g Never tuck top linens in on the sides.

Continued

MAKING A CLOSED BED—cont'd

PROCEDURE—cont'd

27 Place the blanket on the bed:
   a Unfold it so the center crease is in the middle.
   b Put the upper hem about 6 to 8 inches from the top of the mattress.
   c Open the blanket. Fan-fold it to the other side.
   d If steps 33 and 34 are not done, turn the top sheet down over the blanket. Hem-stitching is down, away from the person.

28 Place the bedspread on the bed:
   a Unfold it so the center crease is in the middle.
   b Place the upper hem even with the top of the mattress.
   c Open and fan-fold the bedspread to the other side.
   d Make sure the bedspread facing the door is even. It covers all top linens.

29 Tuck in top linens together at the foot of the bed. They should be smooth and tight. Make a mitered corner.

30 Go to the other side.

31 Straighten all top linen. Work from the head of the bed to the foot.

32 Tuck in top linens together at the foot of the bed. Make a mitered corner.

33 Turn the top hem of the bedspread under the blanket to make a cuff (Fig. 14-26).

34 Turn the top sheet down over the bedspread. Hem-stitching is down. (Steps 33 and 34 are not done in some agencies. The bedspread covers the pillow. If so, tuck the bedspread under the pillow.)

35 Put the pillowcase on the pillow as in Figure 14-27 or Figure 14-28, p. 228. Fold extra material under the pillow at the seam end of the pillowcase.

36 Place the pillow on the bed. The open end of the pillowcase is away from the door. The seam is toward the head of the bed.

POST-PROCEDURE

37 Provide for comfort. (See the inside of the front book cover.) NOTE: Omit this step if the bed is prepared for a new patient or resident.

38 Attach the signal light to the bed. Or place it within the person's reach.

39 Lower the bed to its lowest position. Lock the bed wheels.

40 Put the towels, washcloth, gown or pajamas, and bath blanket in the bedside stand.

41 Complete a safety check of the room. (See the inside of the front book cover.)

42 Follow agency policy for dirty linen.

43 Decontaminate your hands.

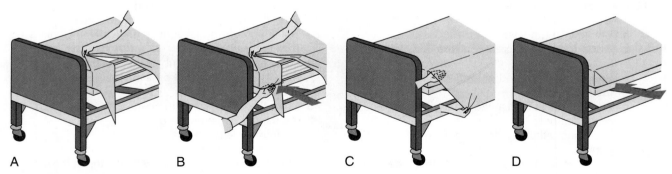

A   B   C   D

FIGURE 14-23 Making a mitered corner. **A,** The bottom sheet is tucked under the mattress at the head of the bed. The side of the sheet is raised onto the mattress. **B,** The remaining portion of the sheet is tucked under the mattress. **C,** The raised portion of the sheet is brought off the mattress. **D,** The entire side of the sheet is tucked under the mattress.

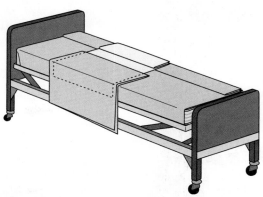

FIGURE 14-24 A cotton drawsheet is over the waterproof drawsheet. The cotton drawsheet completely covers the waterproof drawsheet.

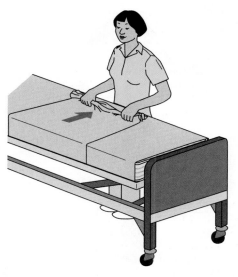

FIGURE 14-25 The drawsheet is pulled tight to remove wrinkles.

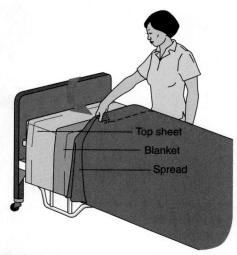

FIGURE 14-26 The top hem of the bedspread is turned under the top hem of the blanket to make a cuff.

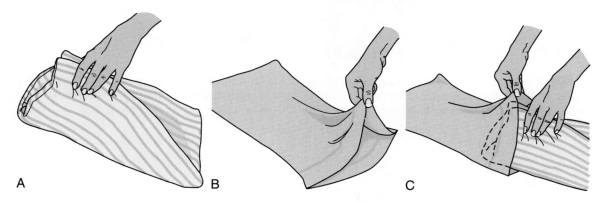

A   B   C

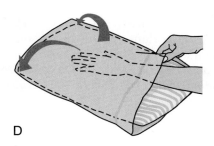

D

FIGURE 14-27 Putting a pillowcase on a pillow. **A,** Grasp the corners of the pillow at the seam end and form a "V" with the pillow. **B,** Open the pillowcase with your free hand. **C,** Guide the "V" end of the pillow into the pillowcase. **D,** Let the "V" end of the pillow fall into the corners of the pillowcase.

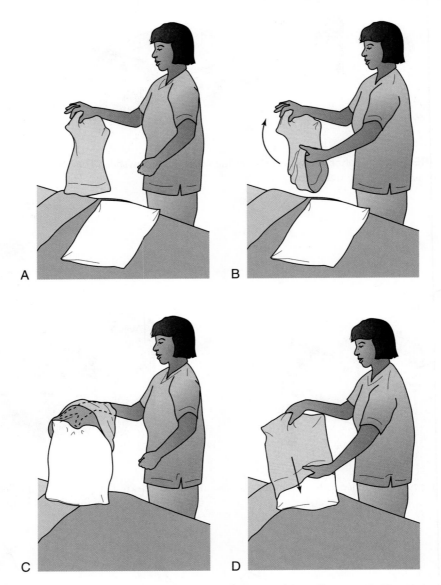

FIGURE 14-28 Putting a pillowcase on a pillow. **A,** Grasp the closed end of the pillowcase. **B,** Using your other hand, gather up the pillowcase. The pillowcase should cover your hand holding the closed end. **C,** Grasp the pillow with the hand covered by the pillowcase. **D,** Pull the pillowcase down over the pillow with your other hand.

The Occupied Bed You make an occupied bed when the person stays in bed. Keep the person in good alignment. Follow restrictions or limits in the person's movement or position.

Explain each procedure step to the person before it is done. This is important even if the person cannot respond to you or is in a coma.

See *Focus on Communication: The Occupied Bed.*

See *Promoting Safety and Comfort: The Occupied Bed.*

FOCUS ON COMMUNICATION
The Occupied Bed

After making an occupied bed, make sure the person is comfortable. You can ask:
- "Are you comfortable?"
- "What can I do to make you more comfortable?"
- "Are you warm enough?"
- "Can I adjust your pillow?"

After making the bed, thank the person for cooperating.

PROMOTING SAFETY AND COMFORT
The Occupied Bed

Safety

The person lies on one side of the bed and then the other. Protect the person from falling out of bed. If the person uses bed rails, the far bed rail is up. If the person does not use bed rails, have a co-worker help you. You work on one side of the bed. Your co-worker works on the other.

Comfort

To make an occupied bed, the person lies on his or her side. You tuck dirty bottom linens under the person. Then you put clean linens on the bed. These, too, are tucked under the person. The tucked linens create a "bump" in the middle of the bed. To make the other side, the person rolls over the "bump" to the other side of the bed. For the person's comfort, try to make the "bump" as low as possible. Do this by fan-folding dirty and clean bottom linens neatly and flatly.

MAKING AN OCCUPIED BED

QUALITY OF LIFE

Remember to:
- Knock before entering the person's room.
- Address the person by name.
- Introduce yourself by name and title.

- Explain the procedure to the person before beginning and during the procedure.
- Protect the person's rights during the procedure.
- Handle the person gently during the procedure.

PRE-PROCEDURE

1 Follow *Delegation Guidelines: Making Beds,* p. 224. See *Promoting Safety and Comfort:*
   a *Making Beds,* p. 224
   b *The Occupied Bed*
2 Practice hand hygiene.
3 Collect the following:
   - Gloves
   - Laundry bag
   - Clean linen (see procedure: *Making a Closed Bed,* p. 225)
   - Paper towels (if a barrier is needed for clean linens)

4 Place linen on a clean surface. Use the paper towels as a barrier between the clean surface and clean linen if required by agency policy.
5 Identify the person. Check the ID (identification) bracelet against the assignment sheet. Also call the person by name.
6 Provide for privacy.
7 Remove the signal light.
8 Raise the bed for body mechanics. Bed rails are up if used.
9 Lower the head of the bed. It is as flat as possible.

PROCEDURE

10 Decontaminate your hands. Put on gloves.
11 Loosen top linens at the foot of the bed.
12 Lower the bed rail near you if up.
13 Remove the bedspread (Fig. 14-29, p. 231). Then remove the blanket. Place each over the chair.
14 Cover the person with a bath blanket. Use the blanket in the bedside stand.
   a Unfold a bath blanket over the top sheet.

   b Ask the person to hold onto the bath blanket. If he or she cannot, tuck the top part under the person's shoulders.
   c Grasp the top sheet under the bath blanket at the shoulders. Bring the sheet down to the foot of the bed. Remove the sheet from under the blanket (Fig. 14-30, p. 231).

Continued

MAKING AN OCCUPIED BED—cont'd

PROCEDURE—cont'd

15 Position the person on the side of the bed away from you. Adjust the pillow for comfort.

16 Loosen bottom linens from the head to the foot of the bed.

17 Fan-fold bottom linens one at a time toward the person. Start with the cotton drawsheet (Fig. 14-31, p. 231). If re-using the mattress pad, do not fan-fold it.

18 Place a clean mattress pad on the bed. Unfold it length-wise. The center crease is in the middle. Fan-fold the top part toward the person. If re-using the mattress pad, straighten and smooth any wrinkles.

19 Place the bottom sheet on the mattress pad. Hem-stitching is away from the person. Unfold the sheet so the crease is in the middle. The small hem is even with the bottom of the mattress. Fan-fold the top part toward the person.

20 Make a mitered corner at the head of the bed. Tuck the sheet under the mattress from the head to the foot.

21 Pull the waterproof drawsheet toward you over the bottom sheet. Tuck excess material under the mattress. Do the following for a clean plastic drawsheet (Fig. 14-32, p. 232).
   a Place the waterproof drawsheet on the bed. It is in the middle of the mattress.
   b Fan-fold the top part toward the person.
   c Tuck in excess fabric.

22 Place the cotton drawsheet over the waterproof drawsheet. It covers the entire waterproof drawsheet. Fan-fold the top part toward the person. Tuck in excess fabric.

23 Explain to the person that he or she will roll over a "bump." Assure the person that he or she will not fall.

24 Help the person turn to the other side. Adjust the pillow for comfort.

25 Raise the bed rail. Go to the other side, and lower the bed rail.

26 Loosen bottom linens. Remove one piece at a time. Place each piece in the laundry bag. (NOTE: Discard disposable bed protectors and incontinence prod-ucts in the trash. Do not put them in the laundry bag.)

27 Remove and discard the gloves. Decontaminate your hands.

28 Straighten and smooth the mattress pad.

29 Pull the clean bottom sheet toward you. Make a mitered corner at the top. Tuck the sheet under the mattress from the head to the foot of the bed.

30 Pull the drawsheets tightly toward you. Tuck both under together or separately.

31 Position the person supine in the center of the bed. Adjust the pillow for comfort.

32 Put the top sheet on the bed. Unfold it length-wise. The crease is in the middle. The large hem is even with the top of the mattress. Hem-stitching is on the outside.

33 Ask the person to hold onto the top sheet so you can remove the bath blanket. Or tuck the top sheet under the person's shoulders. Remove the bath blanket.

34 Place the blanket on the bed. Unfold it so the crease is in the middle and it covers the person. The upper hem is 6 to 8 inches from the top of the mattress.

35 Place the bedspread on the bed. Unfold it so the center crease is in the middle and it covers the person. The top hem is even with the mattress top.

36 Turn the top hem of the bedspread under the blanket to make a cuff.

37 Bring the top sheet down over the bedspread to form a cuff.

38 Go to the foot of the bed.

39 Make a toe pleat. Make a 2-inch pleat across the foot of the bed. The pleat is about 6 to 8 inches from the foot of the bed.

40 Lift the mattress corner with one arm. Tuck all top linens under the mattress. Make a mitered corner.

41 Raise the bed rail. Go to the other side, and lower the bed rail.

42 Straighten and smooth top linens.

43 Tuck all top linens under the mattress. Make a mitered corner.

44 Change the pillowcase(s).

POST-PROCEDURE

45 Provide for comfort. (See the inside of the front book cover.)

46 Place the signal light within reach.

47 Lower the bed to its lowest position. Lock the bed wheels.

48 Raise or lower bed rails. Follow the care plan.

49 Put the towels, washcloth, gown or pajamas, and bath blanket in the bedside stand.

50 Unscreen the person.

51 Complete a safety check of the room. (See the inside of the front book cover.)

52 Follow agency policy for dirty linen.

53 Decontaminate your hands.

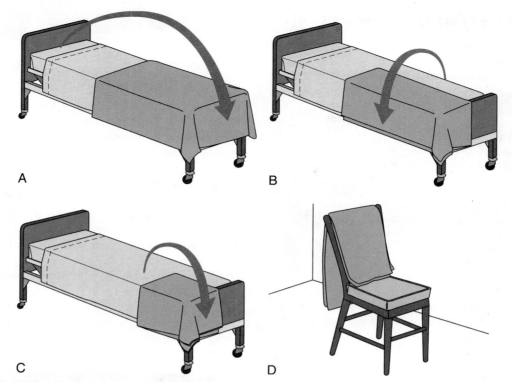

A

B

C

D

FIGURE 14-29 Folding linen for re-use. **A,** Fold the top edge of the bedspread down to the bottom edge. **B,** Fold the bedspread from the far side of the bed to the near side. **C,** Fold the top edge of the bedspread down to the bottom edge again. **D,** Place the folded bedspread over the back of the chair.

FIGURE 14-30 The person holds onto the bath blanket. The top sheet is removed from under the bath blanket.

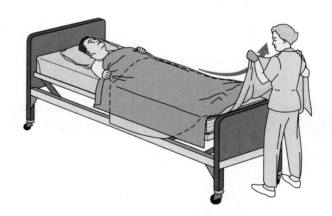

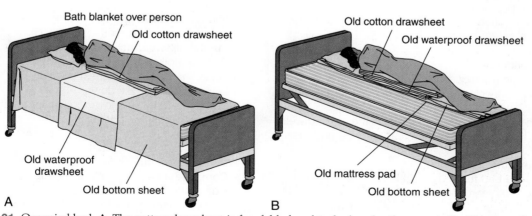

Bath blanket over person

Old cotton drawsheet

Old waterproof drawsheet

Old bottom sheet

A

Old cotton drawsheet

Old waterproof drawsheet

Old mattress pad

Old bottom sheet

B

FIGURE 14-31 Occupied bed. **A,** The cotton drawsheet is fan-folded and tucked under the person. **B,** All bottom linens are tucked under the person.

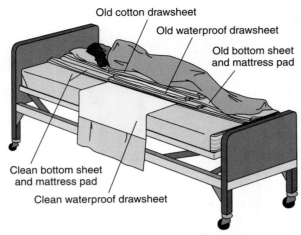

Old cotton drawsheet

Old waterproof drawsheet

Old bottom sheet and mattress pad

Clean bottom sheet and mattress pad

Clean waterproof drawsheet

FIGURE 14-32 A clean bottom sheet and waterproof drawsheet are on the bed with both fan-folded and tucked under the person.

 The Surgical Bed

The surgical bed also is called a *recovery bed* or *postoperative bed.* Top linens are folded to transfer the person from a stretcher to the bed. These beds are made for persons:

- Returning to their rooms from surgery. A complete linen change is needed.
- Who arrive at the agency by ambulance. A complete linen change is needed if the person is:
  - A new patient or resident
  - A resident returning to the nursing center from the hospital
- Who are taken by stretcher to treatment or therapy areas. A complete linen change is not needed.
- Using portable tubs. Because the person will have a bath, a complete linen change is needed.
  See *Promoting Safety and Comfort: The Surgical Bed.*

PROMOTING SAFETY AND COMFORT
The Surgical Bed

Safety
Follow the rules for stretcher safety (Chapter 8). After the transfer, lower the bed to its lowest position. Make sure the bed wheels are locked. Raise or lower bed rails according to the care plan.

View Video!

MAKING A SURGICAL BED

PROCEDURE

1 Follow *Delegation Guidelines: Making Beds, p. 224.* See *Promoting Safety and Comfort:*
  a *Making Beds,* p. 224
  b *The Surgical Bed*
2 Practice hand hygiene.
3 Collect the following:
- Clean linen (see procedure: *Making a Closed Bed,* p. 225)
- Gloves
- Laundry bag
- Equipment requested by the nurse
- Paper towels (if a barrier is needed for clean linens)
4 Place linen on a clean surface. Use the paper towels as a barrier between the clean surface and clean linen if required by agency policy.
5 Remove the signal light.
6 Raise the bed for body mechanics.
7 Remove all linen from the bed. Wear gloves. Decontaminate your hands after removing them.

8 Make a closed bed (see procedure: *Making a Closed Bed,* p. 225). Do not tuck top linens under the mattress.
9 Fold all top linens at the foot of the bed back onto the bed. The fold is even with the edge of the mattress (Fig. 14-33, *A*)
10 Fan-fold linen length-wise to the side of the bed farthest from the door (Fig. 14-33, *B*).
11 Put the pillowcase(s) on the pillow(s).
12 Place the pillow(s) on a clean surface.
13 Leave the bed in its highest position.
14 Leave both bed rails down.
15 Put the towels, washcloth, gown or pajamas, and bath blanket in the bedside stand.
16 Move furniture away from the bed. Allow room for the stretcher and the staff.
17 Do not attach the signal light to the bed.
18 Complete a safety check of the room. (See the inside of the front book cover.)
19 Follow agency policy for soiled linen.
20 Decontaminate your hands.

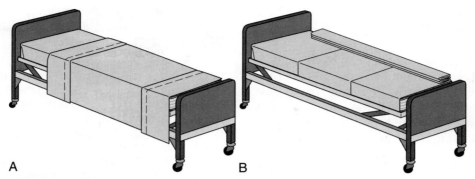

FIGURE 14-33 Surgical bed. **A,** The bottom of the top linens is folded back onto the bed. The fold is even with the bottom edge of the mattress. **B,** Top linens are fan-folded length-wise to the opposite side of the bed.

ASSISTING WITH PAIN RELIEF

Pain means to ache, hurt, or be sore. Pain is subjective (Chapter 4). That is, you cannot see, hear, touch, or smell pain or discomfort. You must rely on what the person says.

The nurse uses the nursing process to promote comfort and relieve pain. The types, signs, and symptoms of pain are described in Chapter 20. Report the person's complaints and your observations to the nurse. The person's care plan may include the measures in Box 14-3.

See *Focus on Communication: Assisting With Pain Relief.*

FOCUS ON COMMUNICATION
Assisting With Pain Relief

Communicating with persons about pain promotes comfort. You can say:
- "I want you to be comfortable. Please tell me if you are having any pain."
- "I will tell the nurse about your pain."

If a person complains of pain, the person has pain. You must rely on what the person tells you. Promptly report any complaints of pain to the nurse.

BOX 14-3   Nursing Measures to Promote Comfort and Relieve Pain

- Position the person in good alignment. Use pillows for support.
- Keep bed linens tight and wrinkle-free.
- Make sure the person is not lying on drainage tubes.
- Assist with elimination needs.
- Provide blankets for warmth and to prevent chilling.
- Use correct handling, moving, and turning procedures.
- Wait 30 minutes after pain-relief drugs are given before giving care or starting activities.
- Give a back massage.
- Provide soft music to distract the person.
- Talk softly and gently.
- Use touch to provide comfort.
- Allow family and friends at the bedside as requested by the person.
- Avoid sudden or jarring movements of the bed or chair.
- Handle the person gently.
- Practice safety measures if the person takes strong pain drugs or sedatives:
  - Keep the bed in the low position.
  - Raise bed rails as directed. Follow the care plan.
  - Check on the person every 10 to 15 minutes.
  - Provide help when the person needs to get up and when he or she is up and about.
- Apply warm or cold applications as directed by the nurse (Chapter 23).
- Provide a calm, quiet, darkened setting.

Factors Affecting Pain

Many factors affect pain.

- *Past experience.* The severity of pain, its cause, how long it lasted, and if relief occurred all affect the person's response to pain. Knowing what to expect can help or hinder how the person handles pain. Some people have not had pain. When it occurs, pain can cause fear and anxiety. They can make pain worse.
- *Anxiety.* Anxiety relates to feelings of fear, dread, worry, and concern. The person is uneasy and tense. Pain and anxiety are related. Pain can cause anxiety. Anxiety increases how much pain the person feels. Reducing anxiety helps lessen pain.
- *Rest and sleep.* Pain seems worse when tired or restless. Also, the person tends to focus on pain when tired and unable to rest or sleep.
- *Personal and family duties.* Often pain is ignored when there are children to care for. Some people go to work with pain. Others deny pain if a serious illness is feared. The illness can interfere with a job, going to school, or caring for children, a partner, or ill parents.
- *The value or meaning of pain.* To some people, pain is a sign of weakness. It may mean a serious illness and the need for painful tests and treatments. Sometimes pain gives pleasure. The pain of childbirth is one example. For some persons, pain is used to avoid certain people or things. Some people like doting and pampering by others. The person values and wants such attention.
- *Support from others.* Dealing with pain is often easier when family and friends offer comfort and support. The use of touch by a valued person is very comforting. Just being nearby also helps. Some people do not have caring family or friends. Dealing with pain alone can increase anxiety.
- *Culture.* Culture affects pain responses. Non-English speaking persons may have problems describing pain. The agency uses interpreters to communicate with the person. See *Caring About Culture: Pain Reactions.*
- *Illness.* Some diseases cause decreased pain sensations. Central nervous system disorders are examples. The person may not feel pain. Or it may not feel severe.
- *Age.* Older persons may have decreased pain sensations. They may not feel pain or it may not feel severe. See *Persons With Dementia: Factors Affecting Pain.*

CARING ABOUT CULTURE
Pain Reactions

People of *Mexico* and the *Philippines* may appear stoic in reaction to pain. To be stoic means to show no reaction to joy, sorrow, pleasure, or pain. In the *Philippines*, pain is viewed as the will of God. It is believed that God will give strength to bear the pain.

In *Vietnam*, pain may be severe before pain-relief measures are requested. The people of *India* accept pain quietly. They accept pain-relief measures.

In *China*, showing emotion is a weakness of character. Therefore pain is often suppressed.

From D'Avanzo CE, Geissler EM: *Pocket guide to cultural health assessment*, ed 4, St Louis, 2008, Mosby.

PERSONS WITH DEMENTIA
Factors Affecting Pain

Persons with dementia may not be able to complain of pain. Changes in usual behavior may signal pain. A person who moans and groans may become quiet and withdrawn. A person who is friendly and outgoing may become agitated and aggressive. One who is nonverbal and quiet may become restless and cry easily. Loss of appetite also signals pain.

Report any changes in a person's usual behavior to the nurse. All persons have the right to correct pain management. The nurse needs to do a pain assessment when the person's behavior changes.

PROMOTING SLEEP

Sleep is a basic need. The mind and body rest. The body saves energy. Body functions slow. Vital signs (temperature, pulse, respirations, and blood pressure) are lower than when awake. Tissue healing and repair occur. Sleep lowers stress, tension, and anxiety. It refreshes and renews the person. The person regains energy and mental alertness. The person thinks and functions better after sleep.

The nurse uses the nursing process to promote sleep. Report your observations about how the person slept. The person's care plan may include the measures in Box 14-4.

See *Persons With Dementia: Promoting Sleep.*

BOX 14-4   Nursing Measures to Promote Sleep

- Plan care for uninterrupted rest.
- Avoid physical activity before bedtime.
- Allow a flexible bedtime. Bedtime is when the person is tired, not a certain time.
- Provide a comfortable room temperature.
- Let the person take a warm bath or shower.
- Provide a bedtime snack.
- Avoid caffeine (coffee, tea, colas, chocolate) and alcoholic beverages.
- Have the person urinate before going to bed.
- Make sure incontinent persons are clean and dry.
- Follow bedtime routines. Hygiene, elimination, and prayer are examples.
- Have the person wear loose-fitting sleepwear.
- Provide for warmth (blankets, socks) for those who tend to be cold.
- Reduce noise.
- Darken the room—close window coverings and the privacy curtain. Shut off or dim lights.
- Make sure linens are clean, dry, and wrinkle-free.
- Position the person in good alignment and in a comfortable position.
- Support body parts as ordered.
- Give a back massage.
- Follow the care plan to relieve pain.
- Let the person read, listen to music, or watch TV.
- Assist with relaxation exercises as ordered.
- Sit and talk with the person.
- Dim lights in hallways and the nursing unit.

PERSONS WITH DEMENTIA
Promoting Sleep

Sleep problems are common in persons with Alzheimer's disease and other dementias. Night wandering is common. Restlessness and confusion often increase at night. This increases the risk of falls. It often helps to quietly and calmly direct the person to his or her room. Allowing night-time wandering in a safe and supervised setting is the best approach for some persons. The measures listed in Box 14-4 are tried. Follow the care plan.

Factors Affecting Sleep

Many factors affect the amount and quality of sleep.

- *Illness.* Illness increases the need for sleep. However, pain, nausea, vomiting, coughing, difficulty breathing, diarrhea, frequent voiding, and itching can interfere with sleep. So can treatments and therapies. Often the person is awakened for treatments or drugs. Care devices can cause uncomfortable positions. Fear, anxiety, and worry also affect sleep.
- *Nutrition.* Foods with caffeine (chocolate, coffee, tea, or colas) prevent sleep. Caffeine is a stimulant. The protein tryptophan tends to help sleep. It is found in milk, cheese, red meat, fish, poultry, and peanuts.
- *Exercise.* Exercise causes the release of substances into the bloodstream that stimulate the body. Exercise is avoided 2 hours before bedtime.
- *Environment.* People adjust to their usual sleep settings. They get used to the bed, pillows, noises, lighting, and a sleeping partner. Any change in the usual setting can affect sleep.
- *Drugs and other substances.* Sleeping pills promote sleep. Drugs for anxiety, depression, and pain may cause the person to sleep. Alcohol interferes with sleep. Some drugs contain caffeine. The side effects of some drugs cause frequent urination and nightmares.
- *Emotional problems.* Fear, worry, depression, and anxiety affect sleep. People may have problems falling asleep, or they awaken often. Some have problems getting back to sleep.

Sleep Disorders

Sleep disorders involve repeated sleep problems. The amount and quality of sleep are affected. Physical and behavioral problems may result.

- **Insomnia** is a chronic condition in which the person cannot sleep or stay asleep all night. The person:
  - Cannot fall asleep
  - Cannot stay asleep
  - Awakens early and cannot fall back asleep
- **Sleep deprivation** means that the amount and quality of sleep are decreased. Sleep is interrupted.
- **Sleep-walking** is when the person leaves the bed and walks about. The person is not aware of sleep-walking. He or she has no memory of the event on awakening. The event may last 3 to 4 minutes or longer. Protect the person from injury. Falling is a risk. Guide sleep-walkers back to bed. They startle easily. Awaken them gently.

Focus on P R I D E
The Person, Family, and Yourself

Personal and Professional Responsibility—Loud talking and laughter in hallways and at the nurses' station are common. Patients, residents, and visitors overhear this noise. They may think the staff is not working. Or they may think the staff is talking about or laughing at them. Some may find this irritating or upsetting. Some may become anxious, uncomfortable, or angry.

Reducing noise requires cooperation from all staff members. It is not your responsibility alone. But you can help. To do so:

- Avoid talking loudly in the hallways or nurses' station.
- If necessary, politely ask others to speak more softly.
- Avoid unnecessary conversation. Always be professional. Do not discuss inappropriate topics at work. Others overhear this and may become offended.

Do your part to reduce noise. Take pride in providing patients and residents with a quiet and comfortable setting.

Rights and Respect—Nursing center residents have the right to make their settings as home-like as possible. Some residents bring bedspreads, pillows, blankets, and quilts from home. Use them to make the bed. These items are the person's property. Handle them with care and respect. Label the items with the person's name. This prevents loss or confusion with another person's property.

Independence and Social Interaction—A person's comfort involves more than physical needs alone. Emotional, spiritual, and social needs must also be met. Time spent with friends and family provides comfort for patients and residents. For some, religious ceremonies or rituals promote peace and healing. Allow time and privacy for these needs.

Delegation and Teamwork—A person may use his or her signal light while you are with another person. The same may happen to other co-workers. If co-workers answer signal lights for each other, lights are answered promptly. Patients and residents receive quality care.

When answering signal lights for co-workers, you may not know the person. Also, the person may not know you. To promote safe and quality care, you can say:

- "My name is Kate. I'm a nursing assistant. How can I help you?"
- "Mrs. Miller, I'll need to check your care plan before I bring you more salt. I'll be right back."
- "Mrs. Palmer, do you use the bathroom or the bedpan?"
- "Mr. Duncan, I'll be happy to take your meal tray. I'll tell your nursing assistant what you ate. Is there anything else I can do before I leave?"

Ethics and Laws—OBRA has requirements for nursing center rooms. They include a clean, neat, and odor-free room. The noise level must be acceptable to the person. Temperature and lighting must be adequate and comfortable. Rooms must be free of hazards. Also, areas where residents walk or use wheelchairs must be free of clutter.

Remember these requirements when providing care. Show respect for the person's comfort and well-being. Take pride in promoting a safe and comfortable setting.

REVIEW QUESTIONS

Circle the BEST answer.

1 Which does *not* protect a person from drafts?
   a Wearing enough clothing
   b Being covered with enough blankets
   c Being moved from a drafty area
   d Sitting by a fan

2 To prevent odors, you need to do the following *except*
   a Check incontinent persons often
   b Dispose of ostomy products at the end of your shift
   c Keep laundry containers closed
   d Clean persons who are wet or soiled

3 Which does *not* control noise?
   a Using plastic items
   b Handling dishes with care
   c Speaking softly
   d Talking with others in the hallway

4 The head of the bed is raised 30 degrees. This is called
   a Fowler's position
   b Semi-Fowler's position
   c Trendelenburg's position
   d Reverse Trendelenburg's position

5 These statements are about hospital bed system entrapment. Which is *false*?
   a Serious injuries and death can occur.
   b Older, frail, and confused persons are at risk.
   c The head, neck, and chest are areas of entrapment.
   d Bed rails present the only risk for entrapment.

6 The overbed table is used for
   a A work surface   c The urinal
   b Soiled linen   d The telephone

7 The bedpan is stored in the
   a Closet   c Overbed table
   b Bedside stand   d Bathroom

8 Signal lights are answered
   a When you have time
   b At the end of your shift
   c Promptly
   d When you are near the person's room

9 Which requires a linen change?
   a The person will have visitors
   b Wet linen
   c Wrinkled linen
   d Loose linen

10 When handling linens
   a Put dirty linens on the floor
   b Hold linens away from your body and uniform
   c Shake linens to unfold them
   d Take extra linen to another person's room

11 A resident is out of the bed most of the day. Which bed should you make?
   a A closed bed   c An occupied bed
   b An open bed   d A surgical bed

12 You are using a waterproof drawsheet. Which is *true*?
   a A cotton drawsheet must completely cover the waterproof drawsheet.
   b Waterproof pads are needed.
   c The person's consent is needed.
   d The waterproof material is in contact with the person's skin.

13 When making an occupied bed, you do the following *except*
   a Cover the person with a bath blanket
   b Screen the person
   c Raise the far bed rail
   d Fan-fold top linens to the foot of the bed

14 A surgical bed is kept
   a In Fowler's position   **c In the highest position**
   b In the lowest position   d In the supine position

15 Measures to relieve pain are part of the person's care plan. Which should you question?
   a Give care before the nurse gives a drug for pain relief.
   b Provide blankets as needed.
   c Provide soft music.
   d Give a back massage.

16 Measures to promote sleep are part of person's care plan. Which should you question?
   a Let the person choose the bedtime.
   b Provide hot tea and a cheese sandwich at bedtime.
   c Position the person in good alignment.
   d Follow the person's bedtime rituals.

Circle T if the statement is *true*. Circle F if the statement is *false*.

17 **T** F   The person's unit is considered private.
18 **T** F   Persons with dementia may have extreme reactions to strange sounds.
19 T **F**   The privacy curtain prevents others from hearing conversations.
20 **T** F   Soft, dim lighting is relaxing.
21 **T** F   The signal light must always be within the person's reach.
22 **T** F   The overbed table and bedside stand should be within the person's reach.

Answers to these questions are on p. 527.

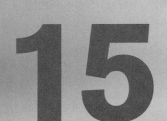

15

ASSISTING WITH HYGIENE

PROCEDURES

- Brushing and Flossing the Person's Teeth
- Providing Mouth Care for the Unconscious Person
- Providing Denture Care
- Giving a Complete Bed Bath
- Assisting With the Partial Bath
- Assisting With a Tub Bath or Shower
- Giving a Back Massage
- Giving Female Perineal Care
- Giving Male Perineal Care

OBJECTIVES

- Define the key terms and key abbreviations listed in this chapter.
- Describe the care given before and after breakfast, after lunch, and in the evening.
- Describe the rules for bathing.
- Identify safety measures for tub baths and showers.
- Explain the purposes of a back massage.
- Explain the purposes of perineal care.
- Identify the observations to report and record while assisting with hygiene.
- Explain how to promote PRIDE in the person, the family, and yourself.
- Perform the procedures described in this chapter.

KEY TERMS

aspiration Breathing fluid, food, vomitus, or an object into the lungs

denture An artificial tooth or a set of artificial teeth

oral hygiene Mouth care

perineal care Cleaning the genital and anal areas; peri-care

KEY ABBREVIATIONS

C Centigrade

F Fahrenheit

ID Identification

The skin is the body's first line of defense against disease. Intact skin prevents microbes from entering the body and causing an infection. Likewise, mucous membranes of the mouth, genital area, and anus must be clean and intact. Besides cleansing, good hygiene prevents body and breath odors. It is relaxing and increases circulation.

Culture and personal choice affect hygiene. (See *Caring About Culture: Personal Hygiene.*) The person's preferences are part of the care plan.

See *Persons With Dementia: Personal Hygiene.*

DAILY CARE

Most people have hygiene routines and habits. For example, teeth are brushed and face and hands washed after sleep. These and other hygiene measures are often done before and after meals and at bedtime.

Routine care is given during the day and evening. You assist with routine hygiene and whenever it is needed. Always protect the person's right to privacy and to personal choice.

⊘ CARING ABOUT CULTURE

Personal Hygiene

Personal hygiene is very important to *East Indian Hindus.* Their religion requires at least one bath a day. Some believe it is harmful to bathe after a meal. Another belief is that a cold bath prevents a blood disease. Some believe that eye injuries can occur if a bath is too hot. Hot water can be added to cold water. However, cold water is not added to hot water. After bathing, the body is carefully dried with a towel.

From Giger JN, Davidhizar RE: *Transcultural nursing: assessment and intervention*, ed 5, St Louis, 2008, Mosby.

PERSONS WITH DEMENTIA
Assisting With Hygiene

Persons with dementia may resist your efforts to assist with hygiene. Follow the care plan to meet the person's needs.

Before Breakfast

Routine care given before breakfast is called *early morning care* or *AM care.* The person gets ready for breakfast or morning tests. AM care includes:
- Assisting with elimination
- Cleaning incontinent persons
- Changing wet or soiled linens and garments
- Assisting with hygiene—face and hand washing and oral hygiene
- Assisting with dressing and hair care
- Positioning persons for breakfast—dining room, bedside chair, or in bed
- Making beds and straightening units

After Breakfast

Morning care is given after breakfast. Hygiene measures are thorough. They include:
- Assisting with elimination
- Cleaning incontinent persons
- Changing wet or soiled linens and garments
- Assisting with hygiene—face and hand washing, oral hygiene, bathing, back massage, and perineal care
- Assisting with grooming—hair care, shaving, dressing, and undressing
- Assisting with activity—range-of-motion exercises and ambulation
- Making beds and straightening units

Afternoon Care

Routine hygiene is done after lunch and before the evening meal. It is done before the person takes a nap, has visitors, or attends activity programs. Afternoon care involves:
- Assisting with elimination before and after naps
- Cleaning incontinent persons before and after naps
- Changing wet or soiled linen before and after naps
- Changing wet or soiled garments before and after naps
- Assisting with hygiene and grooming—face and hand washing, oral hygiene, and hair care
- Assisting with activity—range-of-motion exercises and ambulation
- Straightening beds and units

Evening Care

Care given in the evening at bedtime is called *evening care* or *PM care*. Evening care is relaxing and promotes comfort. Measures performed before sleep include:

- Assisting with elimination
- Cleaning incontinent persons
- Changing wet or soiled linens and garments
- Assisting with hygiene—face and hand washing, oral hygiene, and back massages
- Helping persons change into sleepwear
- Straightening beds and units

ORAL HYGIENE

Oral hygiene (mouth care) does the following:

- Keeps the mouth and teeth clean
- Prevents mouth odors and infections
- Increases comfort
- Makes food taste better
- Reduces the risk for *cavities (dental caries)* and *periodontal disease (gum disease, pyorrhea)*

Illness, disease, and some drugs often cause a bad taste in the mouth. They may cause a whitish coating in the mouth and on the tongue. Others cause redness and swelling in the mouth and on the tongue. Dry mouth also is common from oxygen, smoking, decreased fluid intake, anxiety, and some drugs.

See *Delegation Guidelines: Oral Hygiene.*
See *Promoting Safety and Comfort: Oral Hygiene.*

 Brushing and Flossing Teeth

Oral hygiene involves brushing and flossing teeth. Flossing removes food from between the teeth. It also removes *plaque* (a thin film that sticks to teeth) and *tartar* (hardened plaque). Plaque and tartar cause periodontal disease. Usually done after brushing, flossing can be done at other times. Some people floss after meals. If done once a day, bedtime is the best time to floss. You need to floss for persons who cannot do so themselves.

Some persons need help gathering and setting up equipment for oral hygiene. You may have to perform oral hygiene for persons who:

- Are very weak
- Cannot move or use their arms
- Are too confused to brush their teeth

DELEGATION GUIDELINES
Oral Hygiene

To assist with oral hygiene, you need this information from the nurse and the care plan:

- The type of oral hygiene to give:
  - See procedure: *Brushing and Flossing the Person's Teeth*
  - See procedure: *Providing Mouth Care for the Unconscious Person*, p. 244
  - See procedure: *Providing Denture Care*, p. 245
- If flossing is needed
- What cleaning agent and equipment to use
- If lubricant is applied to the lips; if so what lubricant to use
- How often to give oral hygiene
- How much help the person needs
- What observations to report and record:
  - Dry, cracked, swollen, or blistered lips
  - Mouth or breath odor
  - Redness, swelling, irritation, sores, or white patches in the mouth or on the tongue
  - Bleeding, swelling, or redness of the gums
  - Loose teeth
  - Rough, sharp, or chipped areas on dentures
- When to report observations
- What specific patient or resident concerns to report at once

PROMOTING SAFETY AND COMFORT
Oral Hygiene

Safety

Follow Standard Precautions and the Bloodborne Pathogen Standard when giving oral hygiene. You have contact with the person's mucous membranes. Gums may bleed during mouth care. Also, the mouth has many microbes. Pathogens spread through sexual contact may be in the mouths of some persons.

Comfort

Assist with oral hygiene after sleep, after meals, and at bedtime. Many people practice oral hygiene before meals. Some persons need mouth care every 2 hours or more often. Always follow the care plan.

BRUSHING AND FLOSSING THE PERSON'S TEETH

QUALITY OF LIFE

Remember to:
- Knock before entering the person's room.
- Address the person by name.
- Introduce yourself by name and title.

- Explain the procedure to the person before beginning and during the procedure.
- Protect the person's rights during the procedure.
- Handle the person gently during the procedure.

PRE-PROCEDURE

1 Follow *Delegation Guidelines: Oral Hygiene.*
   See *Promoting Safety and Comfort: Oral Hygiene.*
2 Practice hand hygiene.
3 Collect the following:
   - Toothbrush with soft bristles
   - Toothpaste
   - Mouthwash (or solution noted on the care plan)
   - Dental floss (if used)
   - Water glass with cool water
   - Straw
   - Kidney basin
   - Hand towel

   - Paper towels
   - Gloves
4 Place the paper towels on the overbed table. Arrange items on top of them.
5 Identify the person. Check the ID (identification) bracelet against the assignment sheet. Also call the person by name.
6 Provide for privacy.
7 Raise the bed for body mechanics. Bed rails are up if used.

PROCEDURE

8 Lower the bed rail near you if up.
9 Assist the person to a sitting position or to a side-lying position near you.
10 Place the towel across the person's chest.
11 Adjust the overbed table so you can reach it with ease.
12 Decontaminate your hands. Put on the gloves.
13 Hold the toothbrush over the kidney basin. Pour some water over the brush.
14 Apply toothpaste to the toothbrush.
15 Brush the teeth gently (Fig. 15-1, p. 242).
16 Brush the tongue gently.
17 Let the person rinse the mouth with water. Hold the kidney basin under the person's chin (Fig. 15-2, p. 242). Repeat this step as needed.
18 Floss the person's teeth (optional):
   a Break off an 18-inch piece of floss from the dispenser.

   b Hold the floss between the middle fingers of each hand (Fig. 15-3, *A*, p. 242).
   c Stretch the floss with your thumbs.
   d Start at the upper back tooth on the right side. Work around to the left side.
   e Move the floss gently up and down between the teeth (Fig. 15-3, *B*, p. 242). Move the floss up and down against the side of the tooth. Work from the top of the crown to the gum line.
   f Move to a new section of floss after every second tooth.
   g Floss the lower teeth. Use up and down motions as for the upper teeth. Start on the right side. Work around to the left side.
19 Let the person use mouthwash or other solution. Hold the kidney basin under the chin.
20 Wipe the person's mouth. Remove the towel.
21 Remove and discard the gloves. Decontaminate your hands.

POST-PROCEDURE

22 Provide for comfort. (See the inside of the front book cover.)
23 Place the signal light within reach.
24 Lower the bed to its lowest position.
25 Raise or lower bed rails. Follow the care plan.
26 Clean and return equipment to its proper place. Wear gloves.

27 Wipe off the overbed table with the paper towels. Discard the paper towels.
28 Unscreen the person.
29 Complete a safety check of the room. (See the inside of the front book cover.)
30 Follow agency policy for dirty linen.
31 Remove the gloves. Decontaminate your hands.
32 Report and record your observations.

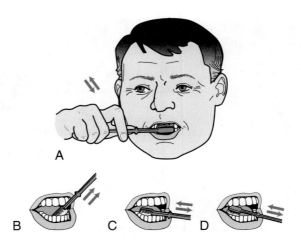

FIGURE 15-1 Brushing teeth. **A,** The brush is moved at a 45-degree angle to the gums. Teeth are brushed with short strokes. **B,** The brush is at a 45-degree angle against the inside of the front teeth. Teeth are brushed from the gum to the crown of the tooth with short strokes. **C,** The brush is held horizontally against the inner surfaces of the teeth. The teeth are brushed back and forth. **D,** The brush is positioned on the biting surfaces of the teeth. The teeth are brushed back and forth.

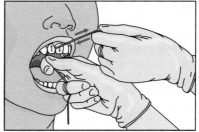

FIGURE 15-2 The kidney basin is held under the person's chin.

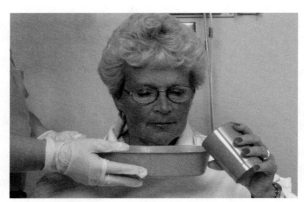

FIGURE 15-3 Flossing. **A,** Floss is wrapped around the middle fingers. **B,** Floss is moved in up-and-down motions between the teeth. Floss is moved up and down from the crown to the gum line.

Mouth Care for the Unconscious Person

Unconscious persons cannot eat or drink. They may breathe with their mouths open. Many receive oxygen. These factors cause mouth dryness. They also cause crusting on the tongue and mucous membranes. Oral hygiene keeps the mouth clean and moist. It also helps prevent infection.

The care plan tells you what cleaning agent to use. Use sponge swabs to apply the cleaning agent. Apply a lubricant (check the care plan) to the lips after cleaning. It prevents cracking of the lips.

Unconscious persons usually cannot swallow. Protect them from choking and aspiration. **Aspiration** is breathing fluid, food, vomitus, or an object into the lungs. It can cause pneumonia and death. To prevent aspiration:

- Position the person on one side with the head turned well to the side (Fig. 15-4). In this position, excess fluid runs out of the mouth.
- Use only a small amount of fluid to clean the mouth.
- Do not insert dentures. Dentures are not worn when the person is unconscious.

Keep the person's mouth open with a padded tongue blade (Fig. 15-5). Do not use your fingers. The person can bite down on them. The bite breaks the skin and creates a portal of entry for microbes. Infection is a risk.

Unconscious persons cannot speak or respond to you. However, some can hear. Always assume that unconscious persons can hear. Explain what you are doing step-by-step. Also tell the person when you are done, when you are leaving the room, and when you will return.

Mouth care is given at least every 2 hours. Follow the nurse's directions and the care plan.

See *Promoting Safety and Comfort: Mouth Care for the Unconscious Person.*

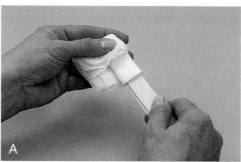

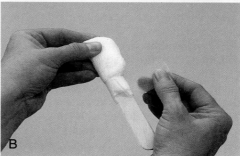

FIGURE 15-5 Making a padded tongue blade. **A,** Place two wooden tongue blades together. Wrap gauze around the top half. **B,** Tape the gauze in place.

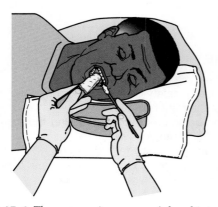

FIGURE 15-4 The unconscious person's head is turned well to the side to prevent aspiration. A padded tongue blade is used to keep the mouth open while cleaning the mouth with swabs.

PROMOTING SAFETY AND COMFORT
Mouth Care for the Unconscious Person

Safety

Use sponge swabs with care. Make sure the sponge pad is tight on the stick. The person could choke or aspirate on the sponge if it comes off the stick.

Comfort

Unconscious persons are repositioned at least every 2 hours. To promote comfort, combine mouth care with skin care, repositioning, and other comfort measures.

PROVIDING MOUTH CARE FOR THE UNCONSCIOUS PERSON

QUALITY OF LIFE

Remember to:
- Knock before entering the person's room.
- Address the person by name.
- Introduce yourself by name and title.

- Explain the procedure to the person before beginning and during the procedure.
- Protect the person's rights during the procedure.
- Handle the person gently during the procedure.

PRE-PROCEDURE

1 Follow *Delegation Guidelines: Oral Hygiene*, p. 240. See *Promoting Safety and Comfort:*
  a *Oral Hygiene*, p. 240
  b *Mouth Care for the Unconscious Person*, p. 243
2 Practice hand hygiene.
3 Collect the following:
- Cleaning agent (check the care plan)
- Sponge swabs
- Padded tongue blade
- Water glass or cup with cool water
- Hand towel
- Kidney basin

- Lip lubricant
- Paper towels
- Gloves
4 Place the towels on the overbed table. Arrange items on top of them.
5 Identify the person. Check the ID bracelet against the assignment sheet. Also call the person by name.
6 Provide for privacy.
7 Raise the bed for body mechanics. Bed rails are up if used.

PROCEDURE

8 Lower the bed rail near you if up.
9 Decontaminate your hands. Put on the gloves.
10 Position the person in a side-lying position near you. Turn his or her head well to the side.
11 Place the towel under the person's face.
12 Place the kidney basin under the chin.
13 Separate the upper and lower teeth. Use the padded tongue blade. Be gentle. Never use force. If you have problems, ask the nurse for help.
14 Clean the mouth using sponge swabs moistened with the cleaning agent (see Fig. 15-4).
  a Clean the chewing and inner surfaces of the teeth.

  b Clean the gums and outer surfaces of the teeth.
  c Swab the roof of the mouth, inside of the cheeks, and the lips.
  d Swab the tongue.
  e Moisten a clean swab with water. Swab the mouth to rinse.
  f Place used swabs in the kidney basin.
15 Remove the kidney basin and supplies.
16 Wipe the person's mouth. Remove the towel.
17 Apply lubricant to the lips.
18 Remove and discard the gloves. Decontaminate your hands.

POST-PROCEDURE

19 Provide for comfort. (See the inside of the front book cover.)
20 Place the signal light within reach.
21 Lower the bed to its lowest position.
22 Raise or lower bed rails. Follow the care plan.
23 Clean and return equipment to its proper place. Discard disposable items. (Wear gloves.)
24 Wipe off the overbed table with paper towels. Discard the paper towels.

25 Unscreen the person.
26 Complete a safety check of the room. (See the inside of the front book cover.)
27 Tell the person that you are leaving the room. Tell him or her when you will return.
28 Follow agency policy for dirty linen.
29 Remove the gloves. Decontaminate your hands.
30 Report and record your observations.

Denture Care

A **denture** is an artificial tooth or a set of artificial teeth (Fig. 15-6). Mouth care is given and dentures cleaned as often as natural teeth. Dentures are slippery when wet. They easily break or chip if dropped onto a hard surface (floors, sinks, counters). Hold them firmly. During cleaning, firmly hold them over a basin of water lined with a towel. This prevents them from falling onto a hard surface.

To use a cleaning agent, follow the manufacturer's instructions. They tell how to use the cleaning agent and what water temperature to use. Hot water causes

dentures to lose their shape (warp). If not worn after cleaning, store dentures in a container with cool water or a denture soaking solution. Otherwise they can dry out and warp.

Dentures are usually removed at bedtime. Some people do not wear their dentures. Others wear dentures for eating and remove them after meals. Remind them not to wrap dentures in tissues or napkins. Otherwise, they are easily discarded.

See *Promoting Safety and Comfort: Denture Care.*

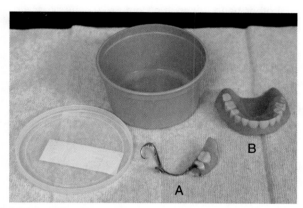

FIGURE 15-6 Dentures. **A,** Partial denture. **B,** Full denture.

PROMOTING SAFETY AND COMFORT
Denture Care

Safety

Dentures are the person's property. They are costly. Handle them very carefully. Label the denture cup with the person's name and room and bed number. Report lost or damaged dentures to the nurse at once. Losing or damaging dentures is negligent conduct.

Comfort

Many people do not like being seen without their dentures. Privacy is important. Allow privacy when the person cleans dentures. If you clean dentures, return them to the person as quickly as possible.

Persons with dentures may have some natural teeth. They need to brush and floss the natural teeth. See procedure: *Brushing and Flossing the Person's Teeth,* p. 241.

PROVIDING DENTURE CARE

QUALITY OF LIFE

Remember to:
- Knock before entering the person's room.
- Address the person by name.
- Introduce yourself by name and title.

- Explain the procedure to the person before beginning and during the procedure.
- Protect the person's rights during the procedure.
- Handle the person gently during the procedure.

PRE-PROCEDURE

1 Follow *Delegation Guidelines: Oral Hygiene,* p. 240. See *Promoting Safety and Comfort:*
   a *Oral Hygiene,* p. 240
   b *Denture Care*
2 Practice hand hygiene.
3 Collect the following:
   - Denture brush or toothbrush (for cleaning dentures)
   - Denture cup labeled with the person's name and room and bed number
   - Denture cleaning agent
   - Soft-bristled toothbrush or sponge swabs (for oral hygiene)
   - Toothpaste
   - Water glass with cool water

- Straw
- Mouthwash (or other noted solution)
- Kidney basin
- Two hand towels
- Gauze squares
- Paper towels
- Gloves

4 Place the paper towels on the overbed table. Arrange items on top of them.
5 Identify the person. Check the ID bracelet against the assignment sheet. Also call the person by name.
6 Provide for privacy.
7 Raise the bed for body mechanics.

Contin-

PROCEDURE—cont'd

8 Lower the bed rail near you if used.

9 Decontaminate your hands. Put on the gloves.

10 Place a towel over the person's chest.

11 Ask the person to remove the dentures. Carefully place them in the kidney basin.

12 Remove the dentures if the person cannot do so. Use gauze squares to get a good grip on the slippery dentures.

   a Grasp the denture with your thumb and index finger (Fig. 15-7). Move it up and down slightly to break the seal. Gently remove the denture. Place it in the kidney basin.

   b Grasp and remove the lower denture with your thumb and index finger. Turn it slightly, and lift it out of the person's mouth. Place it in the kidney basin.

13 Follow the care plan for raising bed rails.

14 Take the kidney basin, denture cup, denture brush, and denture cleaning agent to the sink.

15 Line the sink with a towel. Fill the sink half-way with water.

16 Rinse each denture under cool or warm running water. Follow agency policy for water temperature.

17 Return dentures to the kidney basin or denture cup.

18 Apply the denture cleaning agent to the brush.

19 Brush the dentures as in Figure 15-8.

20 Rinse the dentures under running water. Use warm or cool water as directed by the cleaning agent manufacturer. (Some state competency tests require cool water.)

21 Rinse the denture cup and lid. Place dentures in the denture cup. Cover the dentures with cool or warm water. Follow agency policy for water temperature.

22 Clean the kidney basin.

23 Take the denture cup and kidney basin to the overbed table.

24 Lower the bed rail if up.

25 Position the person for oral hygiene.

26 Clean the person's gums and tongue, using toothpaste and the toothbrush (or sponge swabs).

27 Have the person use mouthwash (or noted solution). Hold the kidney basin under the chin.

28 Ask the person to insert the dentures. Insert them if the person cannot.

   a Hold the upper denture firmly with your thumb and index finger. Raise the upper lip with the other hand. Insert the denture. Gently press on the denture with your index fingers to make sure it is in place.

   b Hold the lower denture with your thumb and index finger. Pull the lower lip down slightly. Insert the denture. Gently press down on it to make sure it is in place.

29 Place the denture cup in the top drawer of the bedside stand if the dentures are not worn. The dentures must be in water or in a denture soaking solution.

30 Wipe the person's mouth. Remove the towel.

31 Remove the gloves. Decontaminate your hands.

POST-PROCEDURE

32 Assist with hand washing.

33 Provide for comfort. (See the inside of the front book cover.)

34 Place the signal light within reach.

35 Lower the bed to its lowest position.

36 Raise or lower bed rails. Follow the care plan.

37 Remove the towel from the sink. Drain the sink.

38 Clean and return equipment to its proper place. Discard disposable items. Wear gloves for this step.

39 Wipe off the overbed table with the paper towels. Discard the paper towels.

40 Unscreen the person.

41 Complete a safety check of the room. (See the inside of the front book cover.)

42 Follow agency policy for dirty linen.

43 Remove the gloves. Decontaminate your hands.

44 Report and record your observations.

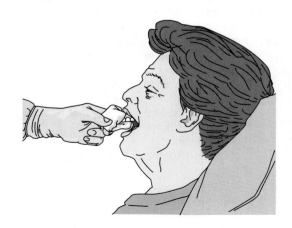

FIGURE 15-7 Remove the upper denture by grasping it with the thumb and index finger of one hand. Use a piece of gauze to grasp the slippery denture.

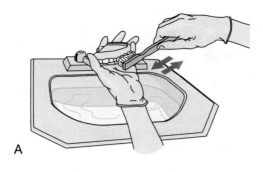

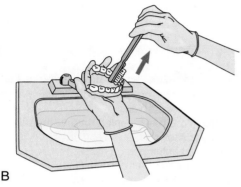

FIGURE 15-8 Cleaning dentures. **A,** Outer surfaces of the denture are brushed with back-and-forth motions. Note that the denture is held over the sink. The sink is filled half-way with water and is lined with a towel. **B,** Position the brush vertically to clean the inner surfaces of the denture. Use upward strokes.

BATHING

Bathing cleans the skin. It also cleans the mucous membranes of the genital and anal areas. Microbes, dead skin, perspiration, and excess oils are removed. A bath is refreshing and relaxing. Circulation is stimulated and body parts exercised. Observations are made, and you have time to talk to the person.

Complete or partial baths, tub baths, or showers are given. The method depends on the person's condition, self-care abilities, and personal choice. Bathing is common after breakfast. However, the person's choice of bath time is respected whenever possible.

Bathing frequency is a personal matter. Some people bathe daily. Others bathe once or twice a week. Personal choice, weather, activity, and illness affect bathing frequency. Ill persons may have fevers and perspire heavily. They need frequent bathing. Other illnesses and dry skin may limit bathing to every 2 or 3 days. The care plan tells you when to bathe the person.

The rules for bed baths, showers, and tub baths are listed in Box 15-1.

See *Persons With Dementia: Bathing,* p. 248.
See *Focus on Communication: Bathing,* p. 248.
See *Delegation Guidelines: Bathing,* p. 248.
See *Promoting Safety and Comfort: Bathing,* p. 249.

BOX 15-1   Rules for Bathing

- Follow the care plan for bathing method and skin care products.
- Allow personal choice whenever possible.
- Follow Standard Precautions and the Bloodborne Pathogen Standard.
- Collect needed items before starting the procedure.
- Provide for privacy. Screen the person. Close doors and window coverings—drapes, shades, blinds, shutters, and so on.
- Assist the person with elimination. Bathing stimulates the need to urinate. Comfort and relaxation increase if urination needs are met.
- Cover the person for warmth and privacy.
- Reduce drafts. Close doors and windows.
- Protect the person from falling.
- Use good body mechanics at all times.
- Follow the rules to safely handle, move, and transfer the person (Chapter 13).
- Know what water temperature to use. See *Delegation Guidelines: Bathing,* p. 248.
- Keep bar soap in the soap dish between latherings. This prevents soapy water. It also reduces the chances of slipping and falls in showers and tubs.
- Wash from the cleanest areas to the dirtiest areas.
- Encourage the person to help as much as is safely possible.
- Rinse the skin thoroughly. You must remove all soap.
- Pat the skin dry to avoid irritating or breaking the skin. Do not rub the skin.
- Dry under the breasts, between skin folds, in the perineal area, and between the toes.
- Bathe skin when urine or feces are present. This prevents skin breakdown and odors.

PERSONS WITH DEMENTIA
Bathing

Bathing procedures can threaten persons with dementia. They do not understand what is happening or why. And they may fear harm or danger. Confusion can increase. Therefore they may resist care and become agitated and combative. They may shout at you and cry out for help. You must be calm, patient, and soothing.

The nurse assesses the person's behaviors and routines. The person may be calmer and less confused or agitated during a certain time of the day. Bathing is scheduled for the person's calm times. The nurse decides the best bathing procedure for the person.

The rules in Box 15-1 apply when bathing these persons. The care plan also includes measures to help the person through the bath. Such measures may include:
- Use terms such as "cleaned up" or "washed" rather than "shower" or "bath."
- Complete pre-procedure activities. For example, ready supplies and linens. Make sure you have everything that you will need.
- Provide for warmth. Increase the room temperature before starting the bath or shower. Have extra towels and a robe nearby.
- Provide for safety. Use a hand-held shower nozzle. Have the person use a shower chair or shower bench. Do not leave the person alone in the tub or shower.
- Draw bath water ahead of time. Test the water temperature. Add more warm or cold water as necessary.
- Tell the person what you are doing step-by-step. Use clear, simple statements.
- Let the person help as much as possible. For example, give the person a washcloth. Ask him or her to wash the arms. If the person does not know what to do, still let the person hold the washcloth if it is safe to do so.
- Do not rush the person.
- Use a calm, pleasant voice.
- Divert the person's attention if necessary.
- Calm the person.
- Handle the person gently.
- Try giving a partial bath if a shower or tub bath agitates the person.
- Try the bath later if the person continues to resist care.

Persons with dementia often respond well to a *towel bath*. An over-sized towel is used. It covers the body from the neck to the feet. The towel is completely wet with a cleansing solution—water, cleaning agent, and skin-softening agent. It also has a drying agent so the person's body dries fast. The nurse and care plan tell you when to use a towel bath. To give a towel bath, follow agency policy.

FOCUS ON COMMUNICATION
Bathing

During bathing, you must make sure that the person is warm enough. You can ask:
- "Is the water warm enough?" "Is it too hot?" "Is it too cold?"
- "Are you warm enough?"
- "Do you need another bath blanket?"
- "Is the water starting to cool?"
- "Is the room warm enough?"

DELEGATION GUIDELINES
Bathing

To assist with bathing, you need this information from the nurse and the care plan:
- What bath to give—complete bed bath, partial bath, tub bath, or shower.
- How much help the person needs.
- The person's activity or position limits.
- What water temperature to use. Bath water cools rapidly. Heat is lost to the bath basin, overbed table, washcloth, and your hands. Therefore water temperature for complete bed baths and partial bed baths is usually between 110° and 115° F (Fahrenheit) (43.3° and 46.1° C [centigrade]) for adults. Infants and young children have fragile skin. So do older persons. They need lower water temperatures.
- What skin care products to use and what the person prefers.
- What observations to report and record:
  - The color of the skin, lips, nail beds, and sclera (whites of the eyes)
  - The location and description of rashes
  - Dry skin
  - Bruises or open skin areas
  - Pale or reddened areas, particularly over bony parts
  - Drainage or bleeding from wounds or body openings
  - Swelling of the feet and legs
  - Corns or calluses on the feet
  - Skin temperature
  - Complaints of pain or discomfort
- When to report observations.
- What specific patient or resident concerns to report at once.

PROMOTING SAFETY AND COMFORT
Bathing

Safety

Hot water can burn delicate and fragile skin. Measure water temperature according to agency policy. If unsure if the water is too hot, ask the nurse to check it.

Protect the person from falls and other injuries. Practice the safety measures presented in Chapters 8 and 9. Also protect the person from drafts.

Use caution when applying powder. Do not use powders near persons with respiratory disorders. Inhaling powder can irritate the airway and lungs. Before applying powder, check with the nurse and the care plan. Do not shake or sprinkle powder onto the person. To safely apply powder:

* Turn away from the person.
* Sprinkle a small amount of powder onto your hands or a cloth.
* Apply the powder in a thin layer.
* Make sure powder does not get on the floor. Powder is slippery and can cause falls.

Beds are made after baths. After making the bed, lower the bed to its lowest position. Then lock the bed wheels. For an occupied bed, raise or lower bed rails according to the care plan.

Protect the person and yourself from infection. When giving baths and making beds, contact with blood, body fluids, secretions, and excretions is likely. Follow Standard Precautions and the Bloodborne Pathogen Standard.

Comfort

Before bathing, allow the person to meet elimination needs (Chapters 17 and 18). Bathing stimulates the need to urinate. The person is more comfortable if his or her bladder is empty. Also, bathing is not interrupted.

Many people perform oral hygiene as part of their bathing routine. Some do so before the bathing procedure; others do so after. Allow personal choice and follow the person's care plan.

Provide for warmth. Cover the person with a bath blanket. Make sure the water is warm enough for the person. Cool water causes chilling.

Remove the person's gown or pajamas after washing the eyes, face, ears, and neck. Waiting to remove sleepwear at this time helps the person feel less exposed and more comfortable with the bath. If the person prefers, you can remove the sleepwear before washing the eyes, face, ears, and neck.

The Complete Bed Bath

The *complete bed bath* involves washing the person's entire body in bed. Bed baths are usually needed by persons who are:

* Unconscious
* Paralyzed
* In casts or traction
* Weak from illness or surgery

A bed bath is new to some people. Some are embarrassed to have others see their bodies. Some fear exposure. Explain how the bed bath is given. Also explain how you cover the body for privacy.

Text continued on

GIVING A COMPLETE BED BATH

QUALITY OF LIFE

Remember to:
- Knock before entering the person's room.
- Address the person by name.
- Introduce yourself by name and title.

- Explain the procedure to the person before beginning and during the procedure.
- Protect the person's rights during the procedure.
- Handle the person gently during the procedure.

PRE-PROCEDURE

1 Follow *Delegation Guidelines: Bathing,* p. 248. See *Promoting Safety and Comfort: Bathing,* p. 249.
2 Practice hand hygiene.
3 Identify the person. Check the ID bracelet against the assignment sheet. Also call the person by name.
4 Collect clean linen for a closed bed. See procedure: *Making a Closed Bed* in Chapter 14. Place linen on a clean surface.
5 Collect the following:
- Wash basin
- Soap
- Bath thermometer
- Orange stick or nail file
- Washcloth
- Two bath towels and two hand towels

- Bath blanket
- Clothing or sleepwear
- Lotion
- Powder
- Deodorant or antiperspirant
- Brush and comb
- Other grooming items as requested
- Paper towels
- Gloves

6 Cover the overbed table with paper towels. Arrange items on the overbed table. Adjust the height as needed.
7 Provide for privacy.
8 Raise the bed for body mechanics. Bed rails are up if used.

PROCEDURE

9 Remove the signal light.
10 Decontaminate your hands. Put on gloves.
11 Cover the person with a bath blanket. Remove top linens (see procedure: *Making an Occupied Bed* in Chapter 14).
12 Lower the head of the bed. It is as flat as possible. The person has at least one pillow.
13 Fill the wash basin two-thirds full with water. Water temperature is usually 110° to 115° F (43.3° to 46.1° C) for adults. Measure water temperature. Use the bath thermometer. Or test the water by dipping your elbow or inner wrist into the basin.
14 Lower the bed rail near you if up.
15 Ask the person to check the water temperature. Adjust the water temperature if it is too hot or too cold. Raise the bed rail before leaving the bedside. Lower it when you return.
16 Place the basin on the overbed table.
17 Remove the sleepwear. Do not expose the person.
18 Place a hand towel over the person's chest.
19 Make a mitt with the washcloth (Fig. 15-9). Use a mitt for the entire bath.
20 Wash around the person's eyes with water. Do not use soap.
   a Clean the far eye. Gently wipe from the inner to the outer aspect of the eye with a corner of the mitt (Fig. 15-10, p. 252).
   b Clean around the eye near you. Use a clean part of the washcloth for each stroke.
21 Ask the person if you should use soap to wash the face.
22 Wash the face, ears, and neck. Rinse and pat dry with the towel on the chest.

23 Help the person move to the side of the bed near you.
24 Expose the far arm. Place a bath towel length-wise under the arm. Apply soap to the washcloth.
25 Support the arm with your palm under the person's elbow. His or her forearm rests on your forearm.
26 Wash the arm, shoulder, and underarm. Use long, firm strokes (Fig. 15-11, p. 252). Rinse and pat dry.
27 Place the basin on the towel. Put the person's hand into the water (Fig. 15-12, p. 252). Wash it well. Clean under the fingernails with an orange stick or nail file.
28 Have the person exercise the hand and fingers.
29 Remove the basin. Dry the hand well. Cover the arm with the bath blanket.
30 Repeat steps 24 to 29 for the near arm.
31 Place a bath towel over the chest cross-wise. Hold the towel in place. Pull the bath blanket from under the towel to the waist. Apply soap to the washcloth.
32 Lift the towel slightly, and wash the chest (Fig. 15-13, p. 252). Do not expose the person. Rinse and pat dry, especially under the breasts.
33 Move the towel length-wise over the chest and abdomen. Do not expose the person. Pull the bath blanket down to the pubic area. Apply soap to the washcloth.
34 Lift the towel slightly, and wash the abdomen (Fig. 15-14, p. 252). Rinse and pat dry.
35 Pull the bath blanket up to the shoulders, covering both arms. Remove the towel.
36 Change soapy or cool water. Measure bath water temperature as in step 13. If bed rails are used, raise the bed rail near you before leaving the bedside. Lower it when you return.

PROCEDURE—cont'd

37 Uncover the far leg. Do not expose the genital area. Place a towel length-wise under the foot and leg. Apply soap to the washcloth.
38 Bend the knee, and support the leg with your arm. Wash it with long, firm strokes. Rinse and pat dry.
39 Place the basin on the towel near the foot.
40 Lift the leg slightly. Slide the basin under the foot.
41 Place the foot in the basin (Fig. 15-15, p. 253). Use an orange stick or nail file to clean under toenails if necessary. If the person cannot bend the knees:
   a Wash the foot. Carefully separate the toes. Rinse and pat dry.
   b Clean under the toenails with an orange stick or nail file if necessary.
42 Remove the basin. Dry the leg and foot. Apply lotion to the foot if directed by the nurse and care plan. Cover the leg with the bath blanket. Remove the towel.
43 Repeat steps 37 to 42 for the near leg.
44 Change the water. Measure water temperature as in step 13. If bed rails are used, raise the bed rail near you before leaving the bedside. Lower it when you return.
45 Turn the person onto the side away from you. The person is covered with the bath blanket.
46 Uncover the back and buttocks. Do not expose the person. Place a towel length-wise on the bed along the back. Apply soap to the washcloth.
47 Wash the back. Work from the back of the neck to the lower end of the buttocks. Use long, firm, continuous strokes (Fig. 15-16, p. 253). Rinse and dry well.

48 Give a back massage (p. 258). The person may want the back massage after the bath.
49 Turn the person onto his or her back.
50 Change the water for perineal care (p. 261). See step 13 for how to measure water temperature. (Some state competency tests also require changing gloves and hand hygiene at this time.) If bed rails are used, raise the bed rail near you before leaving the bedside. Lower it when you return.
51 Let the person wash the genital area. Adjust the overbed table so he or she can reach the wash basin, soap, and towels with ease. Place the signal light within reach. Ask the person to signal when finished. Make sure the person understands what to do.
52 Remove the gloves. Decontaminate your hands.
53 Answer the signal light promptly. Knock before entering the room. Provide perineal care if the person cannot do so (p. 261). (Decontaminate your hands and wear gloves for perineal care.)
54 Give a back massage if you have not already done so.
55 Apply deodorant or antiperspirant. Apply lotion and powder as requested. See *Promoting Safety and Comfort: Bathing.*
56 Put clean garments on the person.
57 Comb and brush the hair (Chapter 16).
58 Make the bed.

POST-PROCEDURE

59 Provide for comfort. (See the inside of the front book cover.)
60 Place the signal light within reach.
61 Lower the bed to its lowest position.
62 Raise or lower bed rails. Follow the care plan.
63 Put on clean gloves.
64 Empty, clean, and dry the wash basin. Return it and other supplies to their proper place.

65 Wipe off the overbed table with paper towels. Discard the paper towels.
66 Unscreen the person.
67 Complete a safety check of the room. (See the inside of the front book cover.)
68 Follow agency policy for dirty linen.
69 Remove the gloves. Decontaminate your hands.
70 Report and record your observations.

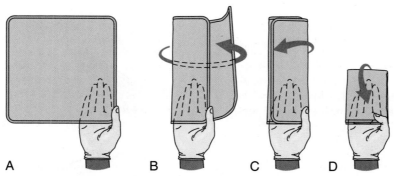

FIGURE 15-9 Making a mitted washcloth. **A,** Grasp the near side of the washcloth with your thumb. **B,** Bring the washcloth around and behind your hand. **C,** Fold the side of the washcloth over your palm as you grasp it with your thumb. **D,** Fold the top of the washcloth down and tuck it under next to your palm.

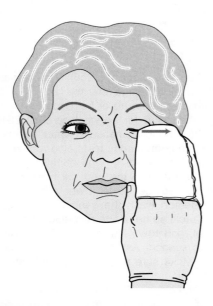

FIGURE 15-10 Wash the person's eyes with a mitted washcloth. Wipe from the inner to the outer aspect of the eye.

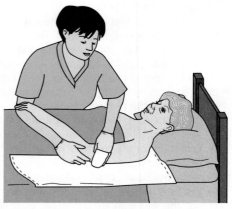

FIGURE 15-11 The person's arm is washed with firm, long strokes using a mitted washcloth.

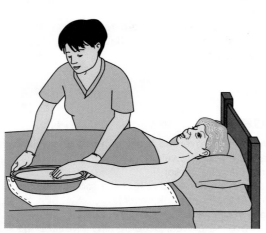

FIGURE 15-12 The person's hands are washed by placing the wash basin on the bed.

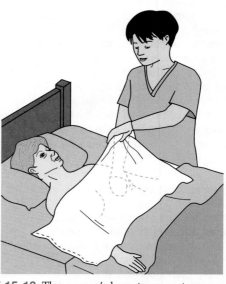

FIGURE 15-13 The person's breasts are not exposed during the bath. A bath towel is placed horizontally over the chest area. The towel is lifted slightly to reach under to wash the breasts and chest.

FIGURE 15-14 The bath towel is turned so that it is vertical to cover the breasts and abdomen. The towel is lifted slightly to bathe the abdomen. The bath blanket covers the pubic area.

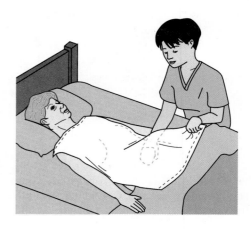

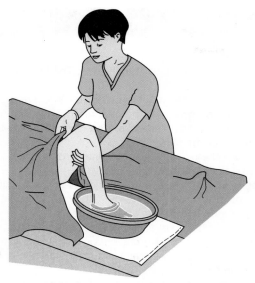

FIGURE 15-15 The foot is washed by placing it in the wash basin on the bed.

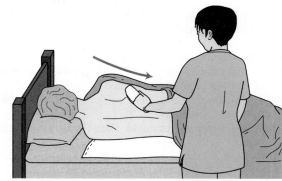

FIGURE 15-16 The back is washed with long, firm, continuous strokes. Note that the person is in a side-lying position. A towel is placed length-wise on the bed to protect the linens from water.

 ## The Partial Bath

The *partial bath* involves bathing the face, hands, axillae (underarms), back, buttocks, and perineal area. Odors or discomfort occurs if these areas are not clean. Some persons bathe themselves in bed or at the sink. You assist as needed. Most need help washing the back. You give partial baths to persons who cannot bathe themselves.

The rules for bathing apply (see Box 15-1). So do the complete bed bath considerations.

ASSISTING WITH THE PARTIAL BATH

QUALITY OF LIFE

Remember to:
- Knock before entering the person's room.
- Address the person by name.
- Introduce yourself by name and title.

- Explain the procedure to the person before beginning and during the procedure.
- Protect the person's rights during the procedure.
- Handle the person gently during the procedure.

PRE-PROCEDURE

1 Follow *Delegation Guidelines: Bathing*, p. 248. See *Promoting Safety and Comfort: Bathing*, p. 249.

2 Follow steps 2 through 7 in procedure: *Giving a Complete Bed Bath*, p. 250.

PROCEDURE

3 Make sure the bed is in the lowest position.
4 Decontaminate your hands. Put on gloves.
5 Cover the person with a bath blanket. Remove top linens.

6 Fill the wash basin two-thirds full with water. Water temperature is 110° to 115° F (43.3° to 46.1° C) or as directed by the nurse. Measure water temperature with the bath thermometer. Or test bath water by dipping your elbow or inner wrist into the basin.

Continued

ASSISTING WITH THE PARTIAL BATH—cont'd

PROCEDURE—cont'd

7   Ask the person to check the water temperature. Adjust the water temperature if it is too hot or too cold.
8   Place the basin on the overbed table.
9   Position the person in Fowler's position. Or assist him or her to sit at the bedside.
10 Adjust the overbed table so the person can reach the basin and supplies.
11 Help the person undress. Provide for privacy and warmth with the bath blanket.
12 Ask the person to wash easy to reach body parts (Fig. 15-17). Explain that you will wash the back and areas the person cannot reach.
13 Place the signal light within reach. Ask him or her to signal when help is needed or bathing is complete.
14 Leave the room after decontaminating your hands.
15 Return when the signal light is on. Knock before entering. Decontaminate your hands.
16 Change the bath water. Measure bath water temperature as in step 6.

17 Raise the bed for body mechanics. The far bed rail is up if used.
18 Ask what was washed. Put on gloves. Wash and dry areas the person could not reach. The face, hands, underarms, back, buttocks, and perineal area are washed for the partial bath.
19 Remove the gloves. Decontaminate your hands.
20 Give a back massage (p. 258).
21 Apply lotion, powder, and deodorant or antiperspirant as requested.
22 Help the person put on clean garments.
23 Assist with hair care and other grooming needs.
24 Assist the person to a chair. (Lower the bed if the person transfers to a chair.) Or turn the person onto the side away from you.
25 Make the bed. (Raise the bed for body mechanics.)

POST-PROCEDURE

26 Provide for comfort. (See the inside of the front book cover.)
27 Place the signal light within reach.
28 Lower the bed to its lowest position.
29 Raise or lower bed rails. Follow the care plan.
30 Put on clean gloves.
31 Empty, clean, and dry the bath basin. Return the basin and supplies to their proper place.

32 Wipe off the overbed table with the paper towels. Discard the paper towels.
33 Unscreen the person.
34 Complete a safety check of the room. (See the inside of the front book cover.)
35 Follow agency policy for dirty linen.
36 Remove the gloves. Decontaminate your hands.
37 Report and record your observations.

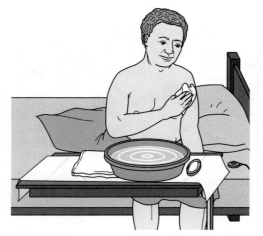

FIGURE 15-17 The person is bathing himself while sitting on the side of the bed. Necessary equipment is within his reach.

Tub Baths and Showers

Many people like tub baths or showers. Falls, burns, and chilling from water are risks. Safety is important (Box 15-2). The measures in Box 15-1 also apply. Follow the nurse's directions and the care plan.

Tub Baths Tub baths are relaxing. A tub bath can cause a person to feel faint, weak, or tired. These are greater risks for persons who were on bedrest. A tub bath lasts no longer than 20 minutes.

The agency may use these devices for tub baths:
• A tub with a side entry door (Fig. 15-18).
• Wheelchair or stretcher lift. The person is transferred to the tub room by wheelchair or stretcher. Then the device and person are lifted into the tub (Fig. 15-19).

Whirlpool tubs have a cleansing action. You wash the upper body. Carefully wash under the breasts and between skin folds. Also wash the perineal area. Pat dry the person with towels after the bath.

BOX 15-2   Safety Measures for Tub Baths and Showers

- Know what water temperature to use. See *Delegation Guidelines: Tub Baths and Showers,* p. 246.
- Clean and disinfect the tub or shower before and after use.
- Dry the tub or shower room floor.
- Check hand rails, grab bars, hydraulic lifts, and other safety aids. They must be in working order.
- Place a bath mat in the tub or on the shower floor. This is not needed if there are non-skid strips or a non-skid surface.
- Cover the person for warmth and privacy. This includes during transport to and from the shower or tub room.
- Place needed items within the person's reach.
- Show the person how to use the signal light in the shower or tub room. Place the signal light within the person's reach.
- Have the person use the grab bars when getting in and out of the tub. The person must not use towel bars for support.
- Turn cold water on first, then hot water. Turn hot water off first, then the cold water.
- Adjust water temperature and pressure to prevent chilling or burns. Do this before the person gets into the shower. If a shower chair is used, position it first.
- Direct water away from the person while adjusting water temperature and pressure.
- Fill the tub before the person gets into it.
- Measure the water temperature. For showers and tub baths, use the digital display. Or you can use a bath thermometer for a tub bath.
- Have the person check the water temperature. Adjust the temperature as needed.
- Keep the water spray directed toward the person during the shower. This helps keep him or her warm. (NOTE: Do not direct the water spray toward the person's face. This can frighten the person.)
- Avoid using bath oils. They make tub and shower surfaces slippery.
- Do not leave weak or unsteady persons unattended.
- Stay within hearing distance if the person can be left alone. Wait outside the shower curtain or door. You will be nearby if the person calls for you or has an accident.
- Drain the tub before the person gets out of the tub. Turn off the shower before the person gets out of the shower. Cover him or her to provide privacy and prevent chilling.

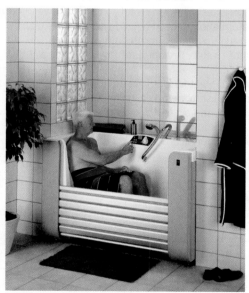

FIGURE 15-18 Tub with a side entry door. *(Courtesy ARJO, Inc., Roselle, Ill. [800]323-1245.)*

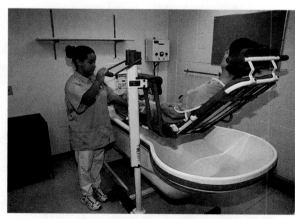

FIGURE 15-19 The stretcher and person are lowered into the tub.

Showers Some people can stand and use a regular shower. Have them use the grab bars for support during the shower. Like tubs, showers have non-skid surfaces. If not, provide a bath mat. Never let weak or unsteady persons stand in the shower. They may need one of the following:

- *Shower chair.* Water drains through an opening (Fig. 15-20). The chair is used to transport the person to and from the shower. The wheels are locked during the shower to prevent the chair from moving.
- *Shower trolley (portable tub).* This device allows the person to have a shower lying down (Fig. 15-21). The sides are lowered to transfer the person from the bed to the trolley. The sides are raised after the transfer. Then the person is transported to the tub or shower room. A hand-held nozzle is used to give the shower.

Some shower rooms have two or more stations. Protect the person's privacy. The person has the right not to have his or her body seen by others. Properly screen and cover the person. Also close doors and the shower curtain.

See *Delegation Guidelines: Tub Baths and Showers.*

See *Promoting Safety and Comfort: Tub Baths and Showers.*

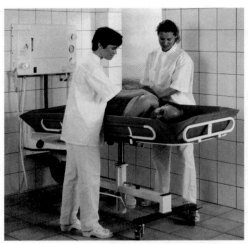

FIGURE 15-21 Shower trolley. The sides are lowered for transfers into and out of the trolley. *(Courtesy ARJO, Inc., Roselle, Ill. [800]323-1245.)*

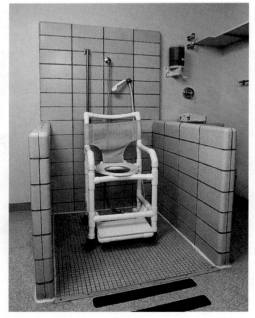

FIGURE 15-20 A shower chair in a shower stall.

DELEGATION GUIDELINES
Tub Baths and Showers

Before assisting with a tub bath or shower, you need this information from the nurse and the care plan:
- If the person takes a tub bath or shower
- What water temperature to use (usually 105° F; 40.5° C)
- What equipment is needed—shower chair, shower cabinet, shower trolley, and so on
- How much help the person needs
- If the person can bathe unattended
- What observations to report and record:
  - Dizziness
  - Light-headedness
  - See *Delegation Guidelines: Bathing*, p. 248
- When to report observations
- What specific patient or resident concerns to report at once

PROMOTING SAFETY AND COMFORT
Tub Baths and Showers

Safety

Some persons are very weak. At least two persons are needed to safely assist them with tub baths and showers. If the person is heavy, 3 staff members may be needed.

The person may use a tub with a side entry door, a shower chair, a shower trolley, or other device. Always follow the manufacturer's instructions.

Protect the person from falls, chilling, and burns. Follow the safety measures in Chapters 8 and 9. Remember to measure water temperature.

Clean and disinfect the tub or shower before and after use. This prevents the spread of microbes and infection.

Comfort

Warmth and privacy promote comfort during tub baths and showers. You need to:
- Make sure the tub or shower room is warm.
- Provide for privacy. Close the room door, screen the person, and close window coverings.
- Make sure water temperature is warm enough for the person.
- Have the person remove his or her clothing or robe and footwear just before getting into the tub or shower. Do not let the person remain exposed longer than necessary.
- Leave the room if the person can be alone.

ASSISTING WITH A TUB BATH OR SHOWER

QUALITY OF LIFE

Remember to:
- Knock before entering the person's room.
- Address the person by name.
- Introduce yourself by name and title.

- Explain the procedure to the person before beginning and during the procedure.
- Protect the person's rights during the procedure.
- Handle the person gently during the procedure.

PRE-PROCEDURE

1 Follow *Delegation Guidelines:*
  a *Bathing,* p. 248
  b *Tub Baths and Showers*
  See *Promoting Safety and Comfort:*
  a *Bathing,* p. 249
  b *Tub Baths and Showers*
2 Reserve the bathtub or shower.
3 Practice hand hygiene.
4 Identify the person. Check the ID bracelet against the assignment sheet. Also call the person by name.

5 Collect the following:
  - Washcloth and two bath towels
  - Soap
  - Bath thermometer (for a tub bath)
  - Clothing or sleepwear
  - Grooming items as requested
  - Robe and non-skid footwear
  - Rubber bath mat if needed
  - Disposable bath mat
  - Gloves
  - Wheelchair, shower chair, transfer bench, and so on as needed

PROCEDURE

6 Place items in the tub or shower room. Use the space provided or a chair.
7 Clean and disinfect the tub or shower.
8 Place a rubber bath mat in the tub or on the shower floor. Do not block the drain.
9 Place the disposable bath mat on the floor in the front of the tub or shower.
10 Put the OCCUPIED sign on the door.
11 Return to the person's room. Provide for privacy. Decontaminate your hands.
12 Help the person sit on the side of the bed.
13 Help the person put on a robe and non-skid footwear. Or the person can leave on clothing.

14 Assist or transport the person to the tub room or shower.
15 Have the person sit on a chair if he or she walked to the tub or shower room.
16 Provide for privacy.
17 *For a tub bath:*
  a Fill the tub half-way with warm water (usually 105° F; 40.5° C).
  b Measure water temperature with the bath thermometer. Or check the digital display.
  c Ask the person to check the water temperature. Adjust the water temperature if it is too hot or too cold.

Continued

ASSISTING WITH A TUB BATH OR SHOWER—cont'd

PROCEDURE—cont'd

18 *For a shower:*
   a Turn on the shower.
   b Adjust water temperature and pressure. Check the digital display.
   c Ask the person to check the water temperature. Adjust the water temperature if it is too hot or too cold.
19 Help the person undress and remove footwear.
20 Help the person into the tub or shower. Position the shower chair, and lock the wheels.
21 Assist with washing as necessary. Wear gloves.
22 Ask the person to use the signal light when done or when help is needed. Remind the person that a tub bath lasts no longer than 20 minutes.
23 Place a towel across the chair.
24 Leave the room if the person can bathe alone. If not, stay in the room or nearby. Remove the gloves and decontaminate your hands if you will leave the room.

25 Check the person at least every 5 minutes.
26 Return when he or she signals for you. Knock before entering. Decontaminate your hands.
27 Turn off the shower, or drain the tub. Cover the person while the tub drains.
28 Help the person out of the shower or tub and onto the chair.
29 Help the person dry off. Pat gently. Dry under the breasts, between skin folds, in the perineal area, and between the toes.
30 Assist with lotion and other grooming items as needed.
31 Help the person dress and put on footwear.
32 Help the person return to the room. Provide for privacy.
33 Assist the person to a chair or into bed.
34 Provide a back massage if the person returns to bed.
35 Assist with hair care and other grooming needs.

POST-PROCEDURE

36 Provide for comfort. (See the inside of the front book cover.)
37 Place the signal light within reach.
38 Raise or lower bed rails. Follow the care plan.
39 Unscreen the person.
40 Complete a safety check of the room. (See the inside of the front book cover.)

41 Clean and disinfect the tub or shower. Remove soiled linen. Wear gloves.
42 Discard disposable items. Put the UNOCCUPIED sign on the door. Return supplies to their proper place.
43 Follow agency policy for dirty linen.
44 Remove the gloves. Decontaminate your hands.
45 Report and record your observations.

❖ THE BACK MASSAGE

The back massage (back rub) relaxes muscles and stimulates circulation. Massages are given after the bath and with evening care. You also can give back massages at other times. Examples include after repositioning or helping the person to relax.

Back massages last 3 to 5 minutes. Observe the skin before the massage. Look for breaks in the skin, bruises, reddened areas, and other signs of skin breakdown.

Lotion reduces friction during the massage. It is warmed before being applied. To warm lotion, do one of the following:

• Rub some lotion between your hands.
• Place the bottle in the bath water.
• Hold the bottle under warm water.

Use firm strokes. Also keep your hands in contact with the person's skin. After the massage, apply some lotion to the elbows, knees, and heels. This keeps the skin soft. These bony areas are at risk for skin breakdown.

See *Delegation Guidelines: The Back Massage.*
See *Promoting Safety and Comfort: The Back Massage.*

DELEGATION GUIDELINES
The Back Massage

Before giving a back massage, you need this information from the nurse and the care plan:

- Can the person have a back massage (see *Promoting Safety and Comfort: The Back Massage*)
- How to position the person
- Does the person have position limits
- When should the person receive a back massage
- Does the person need frequent back massages for comfort and to relax
- What observations to report and record:
  - Breaks in the skin
  - Bruising
  - Reddened areas
  - Signs of skin breakdown
- When to report observations
- What specific patient or resident concerns to report at once

PROMOTING SAFETY AND COMFORT
The Back Massage

Safety

Back massages are dangerous for persons with certain heart and kidney diseases, back injuries, back and other surgeries, skin diseases, and lung disorders. Check with the nurse and the care plan before giving back massages to persons with these conditions.

Do not massage reddened bony areas. Reddened areas signal skin breakdown and pressure ulcers. Massage can lead to more tissue damage.

Wear gloves if the person's skin is not intact. Always follow Standard Precautions and the Bloodborne Pathogen Standard.

Comfort

The prone position is best for a massage. The side-lying position is often used. Older and disabled persons usually find the side-lying position more comfortable.

GIVING A BACK MASSAGE

QUALITY OF LIFE

Remember to:
- Knock before entering the person's room.
- Address the person by name.
- Introduce yourself by name and title.

- Explain the procedure to the person before beginning and during the procedure.
- Protect the person's rights during the procedure.
- Handle the person gently during the procedure.

PRE-PROCEDURE

1 Follow *Delegation Guidelines: The Back Massage.* See *Promoting Safety and Comfort: The Back Massage.*
2 Practice hand hygiene.
3 Identify the person. Check the ID bracelet against the assignment sheet. Also call the person by name.

4 Collect the following:
- Bath blanket
- Bath towel
- Lotion
5 Provide for privacy.
6 Raise the bed for body mechanics. Bed rails are up if used.

PROCEDURE

7 Lower the bed rail near you if up.
8 Position the person in the prone or side-lying position. The back is toward you.
9 Expose the back, shoulders, upper arms, and buttocks. Cover the rest of the body with the bath blanket.
10 Lay the towel on the bed along the back. (This step is done if the person is in a side-lying position.)
11 Warm the lotion.
12 Explain that the lotion may feel cool and wet.
13 Apply lotion to the lower back area.
14 Stroke up from the buttocks to the shoulders. Then stroke down over the upper arms. Stroke up the upper arms, across the shoulders, and down the back to the buttocks (Fig. 15-22, p. 260). Use firm strokes. Keep your hands in contact with the person's skin.
15 Repeat step 14 for at least 3 minutes.

16 Knead the back (Fig. 15-23, p. 260):
  a Grasp the skin between your thumb and fingers.
  b Knead half of the back. Start at the buttocks and move up to the shoulder. Then knead down from the shoulder to the buttocks.
  c Repeat on the other half of the back.
17 Apply lotion to bony areas. Use circular motions with the tips of your index and middle fingers. (Do not massage reddened bony areas.)
18 Use fast movements to stimulate. Use slow movements to relax the person.
19 Stroke with long, firm movements to end the massage. Tell the person you are finishing.
20 Straighten and secure clothing or sleepwear.
21 Cover the person. Remove the towel and bath blanket.

Continued

GIVING A BACK MASSAGE—cont'd

POST-PROCEDURE

22 Provide for comfort. (See the inside of the front book cover.)
23 Place the signal light within reach.
24 Lower the bed to its lowest position.
25 Raise or lower bed rails. Follow the care plan.
26 Return lotion to its proper place.

27 Unscreen the person.
28 Complete a safety check of the room. (See the inside of the front book cover.)
29 Follow agency policy for dirty linen.
30 Decontaminate your hands.
31 Report and record your observations.

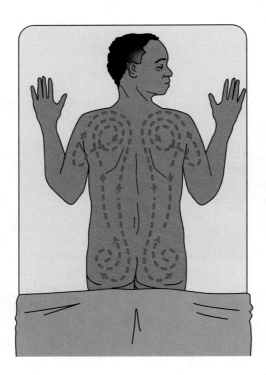

FIGURE 15-22 The person lies in the prone position for a back massage. Stroke upward from the buttocks to the shoulders, down over the upper arms, back up the upper arms, across the shoulders, and down the back to the buttocks.

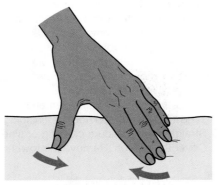
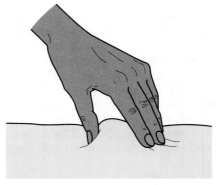

FIGURE 15-23 Kneading is done by picking up tissue between the thumb and fingers.

PERINEAL CARE

Perineal care (peri-care) involves cleaning the genital and anal areas. Cleaning prevents infection and odors, and it promotes comfort.

Perineal care is done daily during the bath. It also is done whenever the area is soiled with urine or feces. Perineal care is very important for persons who:
- Have urinary catheters (Chapter 17).
- Have had rectal or genital surgery.
- Have given birth.
- Are menstruating (Chapter 6).
- Are incontinent of urine or feces (Chapters 17 and 18).
- Are uncircumcised. Being *circumcised* means that the fold of skin (foreskin) covering the head of the penis was surgically removed. Being *uncircumcised* means that the person has foreskin covering the head of the penis.

The person does perineal care if able. Otherwise, it is given by the nursing staff. This procedure embarrasses many people and nursing staff.

Perineal and *perineum* are not common terms. Most people understand *privates, private parts, crotch, genitals,* or the *area between the legs.* Use terms the person understands. The term must be in good taste professionally.

Standard Precautions, medical asepsis, and the Bloodborne Pathogen Standard are followed. Work from the cleanest area to the dirtiest—commonly called from "front to back." The urethral area (the front) is the cleanest. The anal area (the back) is the dirtiest. Therefore clean from the urethra to the anal area.

The perineal area is delicate and easily injured. Use warm water, not hot. Use washcloths, towelettes, cotton balls, or swabs according to agency policy. Rinse thoroughly. Pat dry after rinsing. This reduces moisture and promotes comfort.

See *Focus on Communication: Perineal Care*
See *Delegation Guidelines: Perineal Care.*
See *Promoting Safety and Comfort: Perineal Care,* p. 262.

FOCUS ON COMMUNICATION
Perineal Care

Talking to the person about perineal care may be difficult. You may feel embarrassed. However, it is important to explain the procedure to the person.

When a person performs his or her own perineal care, you can say:
- "Mrs. Bell, I'll give you some privacy while you finish your bath. Can you reach everything you need? Please call me if you need help. Here is your signal light."
- "Mr. Monroe, I'll give you time to finish your bath. Please wash your genital and rectal areas. Signal for me when you're done or need help."

If you provide perineal care for the person, you can say:
- "Mrs. Allan, next I'll clean between your legs. I'll keep you covered with the bath blanket. I'll tell you before I touch you. Please tell me if you feel any pain or discomfort."
- "Mr. Scott, I'll clean your private parts now. Please let me know if you feel any pain or discomfort."

DELEGATION GUIDELINES
Perineal Care

Before giving perineal care, you need this information from the nurse and the care plan:
- When to give perineal care.
- What terms the person understands—perineum, privates, private parts, crotch, genitals, area between the legs, and so on.
- How much help the person needs.
- What water temperature to use—usually 105° to 109° F (40.5° to 42.7° C). Water in a basin cools rapidly.
- What cleaning agent to use.
- Any position restrictions or limits.
- What observations to report and record:
  - Odors
  - Redness, swelling, discharge, bleeding, or irritation
  - Complaints of pain, burning, or other discomfort
  - Signs of urinary or fecal incontinence
- When to report observations.
- What specific patient or resident concerns to report at once.

PROMOTING SAFETY AND COMFORT
Perineal Care

Safety

Hot water can burn delicate perineal tissues. To prevent burns, measure water temperature according to agency policy. If the water seems too hot, ask the nurse to check it.

Protect yourself and the person from infection. Contact with blood, body fluids, secretions, or excretions is likely during perineal care. Follow Standard Precautions and the Bloodborne Pathogen Standard.

Persons who are incontinent need perineal care. You must protect the person and dry garments and linens from the wet or soiled items. After cleaning and drying the perineal area, remove the wet or soiled incontinence products, garments, and linen. Then apply clean, dry ones.

Comfort

To avoid embarrassment, it is best if the person does perineal care. If you provide this care, explain how privacy is protected. Act in a professional manner at all times.

Perineal care involves touching the genital and anal areas. The person may prefer that someone of the same sex provide this care. Or the person may fear sexual assault. Always obtain the person's consent before providing perineal care. For mental comfort, the person may want a family member or another staff member present to witness the procedure. Ask if he or she wants someone present and that person's name.

GIVING FEMALE PERINEAL CARE

QUALITY OF LIFE

Remember to:
- Knock before entering the person's room.
- Address the person by name.
- Introduce yourself by name and title.

- Explain the procedure to the person before beginning and during the procedure.
- Protect the person's rights during the procedure.
- Handle the person gently during the procedure.

PRE-PROCEDURE

1. Follow *Delegation Guidelines: Perineal Care*, p. 261. See *Promoting Safety and Comfort: Perineal Care.*
2. Practice hand hygiene.
3. Collect the following:
   - Soap or other cleaning agent as directed
   - At least 4 washcloths
   - Bath towel
   - Bath blanket
   - Bath thermometer
   - Wash basin
   - Waterproof pad
   - Gloves
   - Paper towels
4. Cover the overbed table with paper towels. Arrange items on top of them.
5. Identify the person. Check the ID bracelet against the assignment sheet. Also call the person by name.
6. Provide for privacy.
7. Raise the bed for body mechanics. Bed rails are up if used.

PROCEDURE

8. Lower the bed rail near you if up.
9. Decontaminate your hands. Put on gloves.
10. Cover the person with a bath blanket. Move top linens to the foot of the bed.
11. Position the person on the back.
12. Drape the person as in Figure 15-24.
13. Raise the bed rail if used.
14. Fill the wash basin. Water temperature is usually 105° to 109° F (40.5° to 42.7° C). Measure water temperature according to agency policy.
15. Ask the person to check the water temperature. Adjust the water temperature if it is too hot or too cold. Raise the bed rail before leaving the bedside. Lower it when you return.
16. Place the basin on the overbed table.
17. Lower the bed rail if up.
18. Help the person flex her knees and spread her legs. Or help her spread her legs as much as possible with the knees straight.

PROCEDURE—cont'd

19 Place a waterproof pad under her buttocks. Protect the person and dry linen from the wet or soiled incontinence product.
20 Fold the corner of the bath blanket between her legs onto her abdomen.
21 Wet the washcloths.
22 Squeeze out excess water from a washcloth. Make a mitted washcloth. Apply soap.
23 Separate the labia. Clean downward from front to back with one stroke (Fig. 15-25, p. 264).
24 Repeat steps 22 and 23 until the area is clean. Use a clean part of the washcloth for each stroke. Use more than one washcloth if needed.
25 Rinse the perineum with a clean washcloth. Separate the labia. Stroke downward from front to back. Repeat as necessary. Use a clean part of the washcloth for each stroke. Use more than one washcloth if needed.
26 Pat the area dry with the towel. Dry from front to back.

27 Fold the blanket back between her legs.
28 Help the person lower her legs and turn onto her side away from you.
29 Apply soap to a mitted washcloth.
30 Clean the rectal area. Clean from the vagina to the anus with one stroke (Fig. 15-26, p. 264).
31 Repeat steps 29 and 30 until the area is clean. Use a clean part of the washcloth for each stroke. Use more than one washcloth if needed.
32 Rinse the rectal area with a washcloth. Stroke from the vagina to the anus. Repeat as necessary. Use a clean part of the washcloth for each stroke. Use more than one washcloth if needed.
33 Pat the area dry with the towel. Dry from front to back.
34 Remove any wet or soiled incontinence product. Remove the waterproof pad.
35 Remove and discard the gloves. Decontaminate your hands. Put on clean gloves.
36 Provide clean and dry linens and incontinence products as needed.

POST-PROCEDURE

37 Cover the person. Remove the bath blanket.
38 Provide for comfort. (See the inside of the front book cover.)
39 Place the signal light within reach.
40 Lower the bed to its lowest position.
41 Raise or lower bed rails. Follow the care plan.
42 Empty, clean, and dry the wash basin.
43 Return the basin and supplies to their proper place.

44 Wipe off the overbed table with the paper towels. Discard the paper towels.
45 Unscreen the person.
46 Complete a safety check of the room. (See the inside of the front book cover.)
47 Follow agency policy for dirty linen.
48 Remove the gloves. Decontaminate your hands.
49 Report and record your observations.

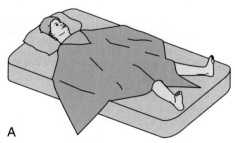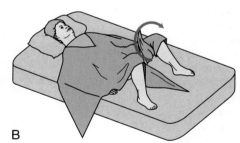

FIGURE 15-24 Draping for perineal care. **A,** Position the bath blanket like a diamond: one corner is at the neck, there is a corner at each side, and one corner is between the person's legs. **B,** Wrap the blanket around the leg by bringing the corner around under the leg and over the top. Tuck the corner under the hip.

FIGURE 15-25 Separate the labia with one hand. Use a mitted washcloth to cleanse between the labia with downward strokes.

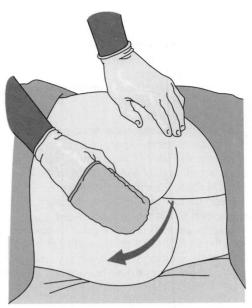

FIGURE 15-26 The rectal area is cleaned by wiping from the vagina to the anus. The side-lying position allows the anal area to be cleaned more thoroughly.

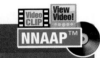

GIVING MALE PERINEAL CARE

QUALITY OF LIFE

Remember to:
- Knock before entering the person's room.
- Address the person by name.
- Introduce yourself by name and title.

- Explain the procedure to the person before beginning and during the procedure.
- Protect the person's rights during the procedure.
- Handle the person gently during the procedure.

PROCEDURE

1. Follow steps 1 through 17 in procedure: *Giving Female Perineal Care,* p. 262. Drape the person as in Figure 15-24.
2. Place a waterproof pad under his buttocks. Protect the person and dry linen from the wet or soiled incontinence product.
3. Retract the foreskin if the person is uncircumcised (Fig. 15-27).
4. Grasp the penis.
5. Clean the tip. Use a circular motion. Start at the meatus of the urethra, and work outward (Fig. 15-28). Repeat as needed. Use a clean part of the washcloth each time.
6. Rinse the area with another washcloth.
7. Return the foreskin to its natural position immediately after rinsing.
8. Clean the shaft of the penis. Use firm downward strokes. Rinse the area.
9. Help the person flex his knees and spread his legs. Or help him spread his legs as much as possible with his knees straight.
10. Clean the scrotum. Rinse well. Observe for redness and irritation of the skin folds.
11. Pat dry the penis and the scrotum. Use the towel.
12. Fold the bath blanket back between his legs.
13. Help him lower his legs and turn onto his side away from you.
14. Clean the rectal area. See procedure: *Giving Female Perineal Care,* p. 262). (Note: For males, clean from the scrotum to the anus.) Rinse and dry well.
15. Remove any wet or soiled incontinence product. Remove the waterproof pad.
16. Remove and discard the gloves. Decontaminate your hands. Put on clean gloves.
17. Provide clean and dry linens and incontinence products.

POST-PROCEDURE

18. Follow steps 37 through 49 in procedure: *Giving Female Perineal Care,* p. 262.

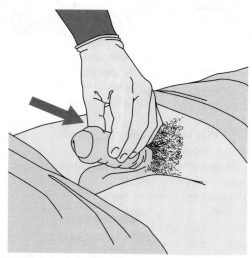

FIGURE 15-27 The foreskin of the uncircumcised male is pulled back for perineal care. It is returned to the normal position immediately after cleaning and rinsing.

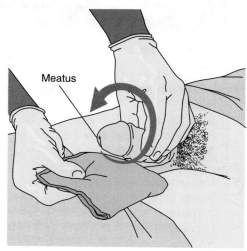

FIGURE 15-28 The penis is cleaned with circular motions starting at the meatus.

Focus on P R I D E
The Person, Family, and Yourself

Personal and Professional Responsibility—Persons depend on you to meet their hygiene needs. You are responsible for providing hygiene in a way that maintains or improves the person's quality of life, health, and safety. To do so, follow the guidelines and procedures presented in this chapter. Focus on the "Quality of Life" section at the beginning of each procedure. Take pride in providing care that benefits the person's overall well-being.

Rights and Respect—Privacy promotes dignity and respect. To protect the right to privacy:
- Do not expose the person.
- Ask visitors to leave the room before you give care.
- Close doors, privacy curtains, and window coverings before giving care.
- Cover the person when going to and from tubs or shower rooms.
- Expose only the body part involved in the procedure.

Independence and Social Interaction—Personal choice helps the person remain independent. Hygiene is a very personal matter. Allow choice in such matters as bath time, products used, and what to wear. Encourage the person to do as much self-care as safely possible. Doing so promotes independence and improves self-esteem.

Delegation and Teamwork—Many agencies do not have tubs, portable tubs, showers, and shower chairs for each person. You need to reserve the room and needed equipment for the person. Co-workers need to do the same for their patients or residents. Consider the needs of others. For example, you reserve the shower room from 0945 to 1030. Do your very best to follow the schedule. Also, make sure the shower room is clean and ready for the next person.

Ethics and Laws—Water gets soapy during a complete bed bath. It also cools. You must change the water when it is soapy or cool. It takes time to safely leave the bedside and change water. However, it is the right thing to do. Not changing the water is the wrong thing. Take pride in doing the right thing. Provide patients and residents with a warm, comforting bath.

REVIEW QUESTIONS

Circle T if the statement is *true*. Circle F if the statement is *false*.

1 **T** F Hygiene is needed for comfort, safety, and health.
2 **T** F After lunch Mrs. Bell asks for a back massage. You can give the back massage.
3 T F A toothbrush with hard bristles is used for oral hygiene.
4 **T** F Unconscious persons are supine for mouth care.
5 T **F** You use your fingers to keep an unconscious person's mouth open for oral hygiene.
6 T **F** A person has a lower denture. It is cleaned over a counter.
7 T **F** A tub bath lasts 30 minutes.
8 T **F** You can give permission for showers but not tub baths.
9 T **F** Weak persons are left alone in the shower if they are sitting.
10 **T** F A back massage relaxes muscles and stimulates circulation.
11 **T** F Perineal care helps prevent infection.
12 **T** F Foreskin is returned to its normal position immediately after cleaning.

Circle the BEST answer.

13 Oral hygiene does the following *except*
  a Prevent mouth odors
  b Prevent infection
  c Increase comfort
  d Coat and dry the mouth

14 You brush a person's teeth and note the following. Which is *not* reported to the nurse?
  a Bleeding, swelling, or redness of the gums
  b Irritations, sores, or white patches in the mouth or on the tongue
  c Lips that are dry, cracked, swollen, or blistered
  d Food between the teeth
15 Which is *not* a purpose of bathing?
  a Increasing circulation
  b Promoting drying of the skin
  c Exercising body parts
  d Refreshing and relaxing the person
16 Which action is *wrong* when bathing a person?
  a Covering the person for warmth and privacy
  b Rinsing the skin thoroughly to remove all soap
  c Washing from the dirtiest to the cleanest area
  d Patting the skin dry
17 Water for a complete bed bath is at least
  a 100° F
  b 105° F
  c 110° F
  d 120° F
18 You are going to give a back massage. Which is *false*?
  a It should last 3 to 5 minutes.
  b Lotion is warmed before being applied.
  c Your hands are always in contact with the skin.
  d The side-lying position is best.

Answers to these questions are on p. 527.

16

ASSISTING WITH GROOMING

PROCEDURES

- Brushing and Combing the Person's Hair
- Shampooing the Person's Hair
- Shaving the Person's Face With a Safety Razor
- Giving Nail and Foot Care
- Undressing the Person
- Dressing the Person
- Changing the Gown of the Person With an IV

OBJECTIVES

- Define the key terms and key abbreviations listed in this chapter.
- Explain why grooming is important.
- Describe how to provide grooming measures—hair care, shaving, nail and foot care.
- Describe the safety measures for shaving a person.
- Describe the rules for changing clothing and gowns.
- Explain how to promote PRIDE in the person, the family, and yourself.
- Perform the procedures described in this chapter.

KEY TERMS

alopecia Hair loss

dandruff Excessive amounts of dry, white flakes from the scalp

hirsutism Excessive body hair

lice See "pediculosis"

pediculosis Infestation with wingless insects; lice

scabies A skin disorder caused by a female mite—a very small spider-like organism

KEY ABBREVIATIONS

C Centigrade

F Fahrenheit

ID Identification

IV Intravenous

Hair care, shaving, nail and foot care, and fresh garments prevent infection and promote comfort. They also affect love, belonging, and self-esteem needs.

HAIR CARE

Many nursing centers have beauty and barber shops for residents. However, you assist patients and residents with brushing and combing hair and with shampooing according to the care plan. The nursing process reflects the person's culture, personal choice, skin and scalp condition, health history, and self-care ability.

Skin and Scalp Conditions

Skin and scalp conditions include:

- **Alopecia,** which means hair loss. Hair loss may be complete or partial. Male pattern baldness occurs with aging. It results from heredity. Hair also thins in some women with aging. Cancer treatments often cause alopecia in males and females.
- **Hirsutism,** which is excessive body hair. It can occur in women and children. It results from heredity and abnormal amounts of male hormones.
- **Dandruff,** which is the excessive amount of dry, white flakes from the scalp. Itching often occurs. Sometimes eyebrows and ear canals are involved.

- **Pediculosis (lice),** which is the infestation with wingless insects. *Infestation* means being in or on a host. Lice bites cause severe itching in the affected body area. Lice easily spread to others through clothing, head coverings, furniture, beds, towels, bed linen, and sexual contact. They also are spread by sharing combs and brushes. Medicated shampoos, lotions, and creams are used to treat lice. Thorough bathing is needed. So is washing clothing and linens in hot water.
  - *Pediculosis capitis* is the infestation of the scalp (*capitis*) with lice.
  - *Pediculosis pubis* is the infestation of the pubic (*pubis*) hair with lice.
  - *Pediculosis corporis* is the infestation of the body (*corporis*) with lice.
- **Scabies,** which is a skin disorder caused by a female mite. A *mite* is a very small spider-like organism. The female mite burrows into the skin and lays eggs. When the eggs hatch, the females produce more eggs. The person becomes infested with mites. The person has a rash and intense itching. Common sites are between the fingers, around the wrists, in the underarm area, on the thighs, and in the genital area. Other sites include the breasts, waist, and buttocks. Scabies is highly contagious. It is transmitted to others by close contact. Special creams are ordered to kill the mites. The person's room is cleaned. Clothing and linens are washed in hot water.

See *Focus on Communication: Skin and Scalp Conditions.*

FOCUS ON COMMUNICATION
Skin and Scalp Conditions

Some skin or scalp conditions may alarm you. Remain professional. Do not make statements that may embarrass the person.

Tell the nurse if you notice an abnormal skin or scalp condition. Describe what you saw as best as you can. For example:

- "I saw some small red spots on Mr. Martin's right underarm when I gave him his bath. Would you please take a look at them?"
- "I was getting ready to wash Ms. Miller's hair. I saw some small white specks. Would you please look at them before I wash her hair?"

Brushing and Combing Hair

Brushing and combing hair are part of early morning care, morning care, and afternoon care. They also are done whenever needed. Encourage patients and residents to do their own hair care. Assist as needed. The person chooses how to brush, comb, and style hair.

Long hair easily mats and tangles. Daily brushing and combing prevent the problem. So does braiding. Do not braid hair without the person's consent. *Never cut matted or tangled hair. Never cut hair for any reason.*

Special measures are needed for curly, coarse, and dry hair. The person may have certain hair care practices and hair care products. They are part of the care plan. Also, the person can guide you when giving hair care.

See *Caring About Culture: Brushing and Combing Hair.*

See *Delegation Guidelines: Brushing and Combing Hair.*

See *Promoting Safety and Comfort: Brushing and Combing Hair.*

 CARING ABOUT CULTURE

Brushing and Combing Hair

Styling hair in small braids is a common practice of some cultural groups. The braids are left intact for shampooing. To undo these braids, the nurse obtains the person's consent.

DELEGATION GUIDELINES
Brushing and Combing Hair

Before brushing and combing hair, you need this information from the nurse and the care plan:
- How much help the person needs
- What to do if hair is matted or tangled
- What measures are needed for curly, coarse, or dry hair
- What hair care products to use
- The person's preferences and routine hair care measures
- What observations to report and record:
  - Scalp sores
  - Flaking
  - Itching
  - The presence of nits or lice
    - Nits (lice eggs attached to hair shafts)—oval and yellow to white in color
    - Lice—about the size of a sesame seed and grayish-white in color
  - Patches of hair loss
  - Hair falling out in patches
  - Very dry or very oily hair
  - Matted or tangled hair
- When to report observations
- What specific patient or resident concerns to report at once

---

PROMOTING SAFETY AND COMFORT
Brushing and Combing Hair

Safety
Sharp bristles can injure the scalp. So can a comb with sharp or broken teeth. Tell the nurse if you have concerns about the person's brush or comb.

Comfort
When giving hair care, place a towel across the person's back and shoulders to protect garments from falling hair. If the person is in bed, give hair care before changing linens and the pillowcase. If done after a linen change, place a towel across the pillow to collect falling hair.

BRUSHING AND COMBING THE PERSON'S HAIR

QUALITY OF LIFE

Remember to:
- Knock before entering the person's room.
- Address the person by name.
- Introduce yourself by name and title.

- Explain the procedure to the person before beginning and during the procedure.
- Protect the person's rights during the procedure.
- Handle the person gently during the procedure.

PRE-PROCEDURE

1 Follow *Delegation Guidelines: Brushing and Combing Hair*, p. 269.
  See *Promoting Safety and Comfort: Brushing and Combing Hair*, p. 269.
2 Practice hand hygiene.
3 Identify the person. Check the ID (identification) bracelet against the assignment sheet. Also call the person by name.
4 Ask the person how to style hair.
5 Collect the following:
  - Comb and brush
  - Bath towel
  - Other hair care items as requested
6 Arrange items on the bedside stand.
7 Provide for privacy.

PROCEDURE

8 Lower the bed rail if up.
9 Help the person to the chair. The person puts on a robe and non-skid footwear when up. (If the person is in bed, raise the bed for body mechanics. Bed rails are up if used. Lower the bed rail near you. Assist the person to a semi-Fowler's position if allowed.)
10 Place a towel across the person's back and shoulders or across the pillow.
11 Ask the person to remove eyeglasses. Put them in the eyeglass case. Put the case inside the bedside stand.
12 *Brush and comb hair that is <u>not</u> matted or tangled:*
  a Use the comb to part the hair.
    (1) Part hair down the middle into 2 sides (Fig. 16-1, *A*).
    (2) Divide one side into 2 smaller sections (Fig. 16-1, *B*).

  b Brush one of the small sections of hair. Start at the scalp, and brush toward the hair ends (Fig. 16-2). Do the same for the other small section of hair.
  c Repeat steps 12 a(2) and b for the other side.
13 *Brush and comb matted and tangled hair:*
  a Take a small section of hair near the ends.
  b Comb or brush through to the hair ends.
  c Add small sections of hair as you work up to the scalp.
  d Comb or brush through each longer section to the hair ends.
  e Brush or comb from the scalp to the hair ends.
14 Style the hair as the person prefers.
15 Remove the towel.
16 Let the person put on the eyeglasses.

POST-PROCEDURE

17 Provide for comfort. (See the inside of the front book cover.)
18 Place the signal light within reach.
19 Lower the bed to its lowest position.
20 Raise or lower bed rails. Follow the care plan.
21 Clean and return hair care items to their proper place.
22 Unscreen the person.
23 Complete a safety check of the room. (See the inside of the front book cover.)
24 Follow agency policy for dirty linen.
25 Decontaminate your hands.

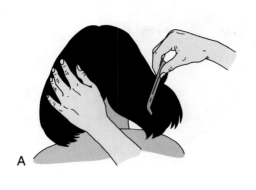

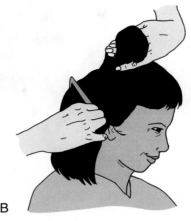

FIGURE 16-1 Part hair. **A,** Part hair down the middle. Divide it into two sides. **B,** Then part one side into two smaller sections.

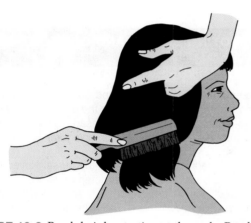

FIGURE 16-2 Brush hair by starting at the scalp. Brush down to the hair ends.

✤ SHAMPOOING

Most people shampoo 1, 2, or 3 times a week. Others shampoo every day. In nursing centers, shampooing usually is done on the person's bath or shower day. If a person's hair is done in the beauty shop, do not shampoo hair. Provide a shower cap for the bath or shower.

The shampoo method depends on the person's condition, safety factors, and personal choice. The nurse tells you what method to use.

* *Shampoo during the shower or tub bath.* The person shampoos in the shower. A hand-held nozzle is used for those using shower chairs or taking tub baths. A spray of water is directed to the hair.
* *Shampoo at the sink.* The person sits facing away from the sink. A folded towel is placed over the sink edge to protect the neck. The person's head is tilted back over the edge of the sink. A water pitcher or hand-held nozzle is used to wet and rinse the hair.
* *Shampoo on a stretcher.* The stretcher is in front of the sink. A towel is placed under the neck. The head is tilted over the edge of the sink (Fig. 16-3). A water pitcher or hand-held nozzle is used to wet and rinse the hair.
* *Shampoo in bed.* The person's head and shoulders are moved to the edge of the bed if possible. A shampoo tray placed under the head drains water into a basin placed on a chair by the bed (Fig. 16-4, p. 272). Use a water pitcher to wet and rinse the hair.

Hair is dried and styled as quickly as possible after the shampoo. Women may want hair curled or rolled up before drying. Check with the nurse before doing so.

See *Delegation Guidelines: Shampooing*, p. 272.

See *Promoting Safety and Comfort: Shampooing*, p. 272.

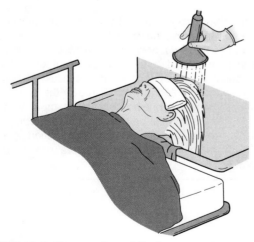

FIGURE 16-3 Shampooing while the person is on a stretcher. The stretcher is in front of the sink.

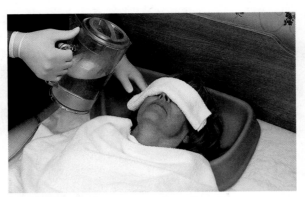

FIGURE 16-4 A shampoo tray is used to shampoo a person in bed. The tray is directed to the side of the bed so water drains into a collecting basin.

DELEGATION GUIDELINES
Shampooing

Before shampooing a person, you need this information from the nurse and the care plan:
- When to shampoo the person's hair
- What method to use
- What shampoo and conditioner to use
- The person's position restrictions or limits
- What water temperature to use—usually 105° F (Fahrenheit) (40.5° C [centigrade])
- If hair is curled or rolled up before drying
- What observations to report and record:
  - Scalp sores
  - Flaking
  - Itching
  - The presence of nits or lice
  - Patches of hair loss
  - Hair falling out in patches
  - Very dry or very oily hair
  - Matted or tangled hair
  - How the person tolerated the procedure
- When to report observations
- What specific patient or resident concerns to report at once

PROMOTING SAFETY AND COMFORT
Shampooing

Safety

Keep shampoo away from and out of the eyes. Have the person hold a washcloth over the eyes. When rinsing, cup your hand at the person's forehead. This keeps soapy water from running down the person's forehead and into the eyes.

Return medicated products to the nurse. Never leave them at the bedside unless instructed to do so.

Wear gloves if the person has scalp sores. Follow Standard Precautions and the Bloodborne Pathogen Standard.

For a shampoo on a stretcher, follow the rules for stretcher use (Chapter 8). Lock the stretcher wheels and use the safety straps and side rails. The far side rail is raised during the procedure.

Some people can shampoo themselves during a tub bath or shower. Place an extra towel, shampoo, and hair conditioner within the person's reach. Assist as needed.

Comfort

When shampooing during the tub bath or shower, the person tips his or her head back to keep shampoo and water out of the eyes. Support the back of the person's head with one hand. Shampoo with your other hand. Some persons cannot tip their heads back. They lean forward and hold a folded washcloth over the eyes. Support the forehead with one hand as you shampoo with the other. Make sure that the person can breathe easily.

Many people have limited range of motion in their necks. They are not shampooed at the sink or on a stretcher.

SHAMPOOING THE PERSON'S HAIR

QUALITY OF LIFE

Remember to:
- Knock before entering the person's room.
- Address the person by name.
- Introduce yourself by name and title.

- Explain the procedure to the person before beginning and during the procedure.
- Protect the person's rights during the procedure.
- Handle the person gently during the procedure.

PRE-PROCEDURE

1 Follow *Delegation Guidelines: Shampooing.*
See *Promoting Safety and Comfort: Shampooing.*
2 Practice hand hygiene.
3 Collect the following:
- Two bath towels
- Washcloth
- Shampoo
- Hair conditioner (if requested)
- Bath thermometer
- Pitcher or hand-held nozzle (if needed)
- Shampoo tray (if needed)
- Basin or pan (if needed)
- Waterproof pad (if needed)
- Gloves (if needed)
- Comb and brush
- Hair dryer
4 Arrange items nearby.
5 Identify the person. Check the ID bracelet against the assignment sheet. Also call the person by name.
6 Provide for privacy.
7 Raise the bed for body mechanics for a shampoo in bed. Bed rails are up if used.
8 Decontaminate your hands.

PROCEDURE

9 Lower the bed rail near you if up.
10 Cover the person's chest with a bath towel.
11 Brush and comb the hair to remove snarls and tangles.
12 Position the person for the method you will use. To shampoo the person in bed:
  a Lower the head of the bed and remove the pillow.
  b Place the waterproof pad and shampoo tray under the head and shoulders.
  c Support the head and neck with a folded towel if necessary.
13 Raise the bed rail if used.
14 Obtain water. Water temperature is usually 105° F (40.5° C). Test water temperature according to agency policy. Also ask the person to check the water. Adjust water temperature as needed. Raise the bed rail before leaving the bedside.
15 Lower the bed rail near you if up.
16 Put on gloves (if needed).
17 Ask the person to hold a washcloth over the eyes. It should not cover the nose and mouth. (NOTE: A damp washcloth is easier to hold. It will not slip. However, some state competency tests require a dry washcloth.)

18 Use the pitcher or nozzle to wet the hair.
19 Apply a small amount of shampoo.
20 Work up a lather with both hands. Start at the hairline. Work toward the back of the head.
21 Massage the scalp with your fingertips. Do not scratch the scalp.
22 Rinse the hair until the water runs clear.
23 Repeat steps 19 through 22.
24 Apply conditioner. Follow directions on the container.
25 Squeeze water from the person's hair.
26 Cover the hair with a bath towel.
27 Remove the shampoo tray, basin, and waterproof pad.
28 Dry the person's face with the towel. Use the towel on the person's chest.
29 Help the person raise the head if appropriate. For the person in bed, raise the head of the bed.
30 Rub the hair and scalp with the towel. Use the second towel if the first one is wet.
31 Comb the hair to remove snarls and tangles.
32 Dry and style hair as quickly as possible.
33 Remove and discard the gloves (if used). Decontaminate your hands.

POST-PROCEDURE

34 Provide for comfort. (See the inside of the front book cover.)
35 Place the signal light within reach.
36 Lower the bed to its lowest position.
37 Raise or lower bed rails. Follow the care plan.
38 Unscreen the person.
39 Complete a safety check of the room. (See the inside of the front book cover.)

40 Clean, dry, and return equipment to its proper place. Remember to clean the brush and comb. Discard disposable items.
41 Follow agency policy for dirty linen.
42 Decontaminate your hands.
43 Report and record your observations.

🔷 SHAVING

Many men shave for comfort and mental well-being. Many women shave their legs and underarms. Women with coarse facial hair may shave. Or they may use other hair removal methods. See Box 16-1 for shaving rules.

Safety razors or electric shavers are used. If the agency's shaver is used, clean it after every use. Follow the manufacturer's instructions and agency policy.

Safety razors (blade razors) involve razor blades. They can cause nicks and cuts. Do not use them on persons who have healing problems or for those who take anticoagulant drugs. An *anticoagulant* prevents or slows down *(anti)* blood clotting *(coagulate)*. Bleeding occurs easily and is hard to stop. A nick or cut can cause serious bleeding. Electric shavers are used.

Soften the beard before using an electric shaver or safety razor. Apply a moist, warm washcloth or towel for a few minutes. Then pat dry the face and apply talcum powder if using an electric shaver. If using a safety razor, lather the face with soap and water or shaving cream.

See *Persons With Dementia: Shaving.*
See *Delegation Guidelines: Shaving.*
See *Promoting Safety and Comfort: Shaving.*

Caring for Mustaches and Beards

Mustaches and beards need daily care. Food can collect in the whiskers. So can mouth and nose drainage. Daily washing and combing are needed. Ask the person how to groom his mustache or beard. *Never trim a mustache or beard without the person's consent.*

Shaving Legs and Underarms

Many women shave their legs and underarms. This practice varies among cultures.

Legs and underarms are shaved after bathing. The skin is soft at this time. Soap and water, shaving cream, or lotion is used for lather. Collect shaving items with bath items. Use the kidney basin to rinse the razor. Do not use the bath water. Follow the rules in Box 16-1.

PERSONS WITH DEMENTIA
Shaving

Safety razors are not used to shave persons with dementia. They may not understand what you are doing. They may resist care and move suddenly. Serious nicks and cuts can occur. Use electric shavers for these persons.

BOX 16-1 Rules for Shaving

- Use electric shavers for persons taking anticoagulant drugs. Never use safety razors.
- Protect bed linens. Place a towel under the part being shaved. Or place a towel across the person's chest and shoulders to protect clothing.
- Soften the skin before shaving. Apply a wet washcloth or towel to the face for a few minutes.
- Encourage the person to do as much as safely possible.
- Hold the skin taut as needed.
- Shave in the correct direction:
  - Shaving the face with a safety razor—shave in the direction of hair growth.
  - Shaving the underarms with a safety razor—shave in the direction of hair growth.
  - Shaving the legs with a safety razor—shave up from the ankles. This is against hair growth.
  - Using an electric shaver—shave against the direction of hair growth. If using a rotary-type shaver, move the shaver in small circles over the face.
- Do not cut, nick, or irritate the skin.
- Rinse the body part thoroughly.
- Apply direct pressure to nicks or cuts (Chapter 29).
- Report nicks, cuts, or irritation to the nurse at once.

DELEGATION GUIDELINES
Shaving

Before shaving a person, you need this information from the nurse and the care plan:
- What shaver to use—electric or safety
- If the person takes anticoagulant drugs
- When to shave the person
- What facial hair to shave
- The location of tender or sensitive areas on the person's face
- What observations to report and record:
  - Nicks (report at once)
  - Cuts (report at once)
  - Bleeding (report at once)
  - Irritation
- When to report observations
- What specific patient or resident concerns to report at once

PROMOTING SAFETY AND COMFORT
Shaving

Safety

Safety razors are very sharp. Protect the person and yourself from nicks or cuts. Prevent contact with blood. If using an electrical shaver, follow safety measures for electrical equipment (Chapter 8).

Rinse the safety razor often during the shaving procedure. Rinsing removes whiskers and lather. Then wipe the razor. Protect yourself from cuts by:

- Placing several thicknesses of tissues or paper towels on the overbed table. Do not hold them in your hand.
- Wiping the razor on the tissues or paper towels.

Follow Standard Precautions and the Bloodborne Pathogen Standard. Discard used razor blades and disposable shavers in the sharps container. Do not recap the razor.

Comfort

Some men have tender and sensitive skin. Usually the neck area below the jaw is tender and sensitive. Some electric shavers become very warm or hot while in use. Such heat can irritate the skin. Shave tender areas first while the shaver is cool. Then move to the other areas of the face.

Some people apply lotion or after-shave to the skin after shaving. Lotion softens the skin. After-shave closes skin pores. Heat is applied before shaving to soften the skin. It also opens pores.

SHAVING THE PERSON'S FACE WITH A SAFETY RAZOR

QUALITY OF LIFE

Remember to:
- Knock before entering the person's room.
- Address the person by name.
- Introduce yourself by name and title.

- Explain the procedure to the person before beginning and during the procedure.
- Protect the person's rights during the procedure.
- Handle the person gently during the procedure.

PRE-PROCEDURE

1 Follow *Delegation Guidelines: Shaving.*
See *Promoting Safety and Comfort: Shaving.*
2 Practice hand hygiene.
3 Collect the following:
- Wash basin
- Bath towel
- Hand towel
- Washcloth
- Safety razor
- Mirror
- Shaving cream, soap, or lotion
- Shaving brush

- After-shave or lotion
- Tissues or paper towels
- Paper towels
- Gloves

4 Arrange paper towels and supplies on the overbed table.
5 Identify the person. Check the ID bracelet against the assignment sheet. Also call the person by name.
6 Provide for privacy.
7 Raise the bed for body mechanics. Bed rails are up if used.

PROCEDURE

8 Fill the wash basin with warm water.
9 Place the basin on the overbed table.
10 Lower the bed rail near you if up.
11 Decontaminate your hands. Put on gloves.
12 Assist the person to semi-Fowler's position if allowed or to the supine position.
13 Adjust lighting to clearly see the person's face.
14 Place the bath towel over the person's chest and shoulders.
15 Adjust the overbed table for easy reach.
16 Tighten the razor blade to the shaver.
17 Wash the person's face. Do not dry.
18 Wet the washcloth or towel. Wring it out.
19 Apply the washcloth or towel to the face for a few minutes.

20 Apply shaving cream with your hands. Or use a shaving brush to apply lather.
21 Hold the skin taut with one hand.
22 Shave in the direction of hair growth. Use shorter strokes around the chin and lips (Fig. 16-5, p. 276).
23 Rinse the razor often. Wipe it with tissues or paper towels.
24 Apply direct pressure to any bleeding areas (Chapter 29).
25 Wash off any remaining shaving cream or soap. Pat dry with a towel.
26 Apply after-shave or lotion if requested. (If there are nicks or cuts, do not apply after-shave lotion.)
27 Remove the towel and gloves. Decontaminate your hands.

Continued

SHAVING THE PERSON'S FACE WITH A SAFETY RAZOR—cont'd

POST-PROCEDURE

28 Provide for comfort. (See the inside of the front book cover.)

29 Place the signal light within reach.

30 Lower the bed to its lowest position.

31 Raise or lower bed rails. Follow the care plan.

32 Clean and return equipment and supplies to their proper place. Discard a razor blade or a disposable razor into the sharps container. Discard other disposable items. Wear gloves.

33 Wipe off the overbed table with paper towels. Discard the paper towels.

34 Unscreen the person.

35 Complete a safety check of the room. (See the inside of the front book cover.)

36 Follow agency policy for dirty linen.

37 Remove the gloves. Decontaminate your hands.

38 Report nicks, cuts, irritation, or bleeding to the nurse at once. Also report and record other observations.

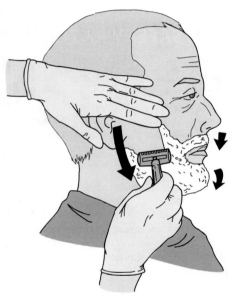

FIGURE 16-5 Shave in the direction of hair growth. Use longer strokes on the larger areas of the face. Use short strokes around the chin and lips.

❖ NAIL AND FOOT CARE

Nail and foot care prevents infection, injury, and odors. Hangnails, ingrown nails (nails that grow in at the side), and nails torn away from the skin cause skin breaks. Long or broken nails can scratch skin or snag clothing. Dirty feet, socks, or stockings harbor microbes and cause odors. Shoes and socks provide a warm, moist environment for the growth of microbes. Injuries occur from stubbing toes, stepping on sharp objects, or being stepped on. Shoes that fit poorly cause blisters.

Poor circulation prolongs healing. Diabetes and vascular diseases are common causes of poor circulation. Infections or foot injuries are very serious for older persons and persons with circulatory disorders. Trimming and clipping toenails can easily result in injuries.

Nails are easier to trim and clean right after soaking or bathing. Use nail clippers to cut fingernails. *Never use scissors.* Use extreme caution to prevent damage to nearby tissues.

Some agencies do not let nursing assistants cut or trim toenails. Follow agency policy.

See *Delegation Guidelines: Nail and Foot Care.*

See *Promoting Safety and Comfort: Nail and Foot Care.*

DELEGATION GUIDELINES
Nail and Foot Care

Before giving nail and foot care, you need this information from the nurse and the care plan:

- What water temperature to use
- How long to soak fingernails (usually 5 to 10 minutes)
- How long to soak feet (usually 15 to 20 minutes)
- What observations to report and record:
  - Reddened, irritated, or callused areas
  - Breaks in the skin
  - Very thick nails
  - Loose nails
- When to report observations
- What specific patient or resident concerns to report at once

PROMOTING SAFETY AND COMFORT
Nail and Foot Care

Safety

You do not cut or trim toenails if a person:
- Has diabetes
- Has poor circulation to the legs and feet
- Takes drugs that affect blood clotting
- Has very thick nails or ingrown toenails

The RN or podiatrist (foot *[pod]* doctor) cuts toenails and provides foot care for these persons.

Check between the toes for cracks and sores. These areas are often overlooked. If left untreated, a serious infection could occur.

The feet are easily burned. Persons with decreased sensation or circulatory problems may not feel hot temperatures.

After soaking, apply lotion or petroleum jelly to the feet. This can cause slippery feet. Help the person put on non-skid footwear before you transfer the person or let the person walk.

Breaks in the skin and bleeding can occur. Follow Standard Precautions and the Bloodborne Pathogen Standard.

Comfort

Sometimes just the fingernails are trimmed. Sometimes just foot care is given. Sometimes both are done. When both are done, the person sits at the overbed table (Fig. 16-6, p. 278). Make sure the person is warm and comfortable.

Promote your own comfort when giving nail and foot care. Sit in front of the overbed table when cleaning and trimming fingernails. When giving foot care, rest the person's lower leg and foot on your lap. Or you can kneel on the floor. Lay a towel across your lap or on the floor to protect your uniform. Remember to use good body mechanics. However you position yourself, you must support the person's foot and ankle when giving foot care.

GIVING NAIL AND FOOT CARE

QUALITY OF LIFE

Remember to:
- Knock before entering the person's room.
- Address the person by name.
- Introduce yourself by name and title.

- Explain the procedure to the person before beginning and during the procedure.
- Protect the person's rights during the procedure.
- Handle the person gently during the procedure.

PRE-PROCEDURE

1 Follow *Delegation Guidelines: Nail and Foot Care.* See *Promoting Safety and Comfort: Nail and Foot Care.*
2 Practice hand hygiene.
3 Collect the following:
   - Wash basin or whirlpool foot bath
   - Soap
   - Bath thermometer
   - Bath towel
   - Hand towel
   - Washcloth
   - Kidney basin
   - Nail clippers
   - Orangewood stick

   - Emery board or nail file
   - Lotion for the hands
   - Lotion or petroleum jelly for the feet
   - Paper towels
   - Bath mat
   - Gloves
4 Arrange paper towels and other items on the overbed table.
5 Identify the person. Check the ID bracelet against the assignment sheet. Also call the person by name.
6 Provide for privacy.
7 Assist the person to the bedside chair. Place the signal light within reach.

Continued

PROCEDURE

8 Place the bath mat under the feet.
9 Fill the wash basin or whirlpool foot bath two-thirds full with water. The nurse tells you what water temperature to use. (Measure water temperature with a bath thermometer. Or test it by dipping your elbow or inner wrist into the basin. Follow agency policy.) Also ask the person to check the water temperature. Adjust the water temperature as needed.
10 Place the basin or foot bath on the bath mat.
11 Put on gloves.
12 Help the person put the feet into the basin or foot bath. Make sure both feet are completely covered by water.
13 Adjust the overbed table in front of the person.
14 Fill the kidney basin two-thirds full with water. See step 9 for water temperature.
15 Place the kidney basin on the overbed table.
16 Place the person's fingers into the basin. Position the arms for comfort (see Fig. 16-6).
17 Let the fingers soak for 5 to 10 minutes. Let the feet soak for 15 to 20 minutes. Re-warm water as needed.
18 Remove the kidney basin.
19 Clean under the fingernails with the flat end of the orangewood stick. Use a towel to wipe the orangewood stick after each nail.

20 Dry the hands and between the fingers thoroughly.
21 Clip fingernails straight across with the nail clippers (Fig. 16-7).
22 Shape nails with an emery board or nail file. Nails are smooth with no rough edges. Check each nail for smoothness. File as needed.
23 Push cuticles back with the orangewood stick or a washcloth (Fig. 16-8).
24 Apply lotion to the hands. Warm lotion before applying it.
25 Move the overbed table to the side.
26 Lift a foot out of the water. Support the foot and ankle with one hand. With your other hand, wash the foot and between the toes with soap and a washcloth. Return the foot to the water for rinsing. Make sure you rinse between the toes.
27 Repeat step 26 for the other foot.
28 Remove the feet from the basin or foot bath. Dry thoroughly, especially between the toes.
29 Apply lotion or petroleum jelly to the tops and soles of the feet. Do not apply between the toes. Warm lotion or petroleum jelly before applying it. Remove excess lotion or petroleum jelly with a towel.
30 Remove and discard the gloves. Decontaminate your hands.
31 Help the person put on non-skid footwear.

POST-PROCEDURE

32 Provide for comfort. (See the inside of the front book cover.)
33 Place the signal light within reach.
34 Raise or lower bed rails. Follow the care plan.
35 Clean, dry, and return equipment and supplies to their proper place. Discard disposable items. Wear gloves for this step.

36 Unscreen the person.
37 Complete a safety check of the room. (See the inside of the front book cover.)
38 Follow agency policy for dirty linen.
39 Remove the gloves. Decontaminate your hands.
40 Report and record your observations.

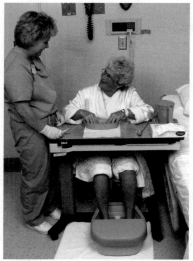

FIGURE 16-6 Nail and foot care. The feet soak in a whirlpool foot bath. The fingers soak in a kidney basin.

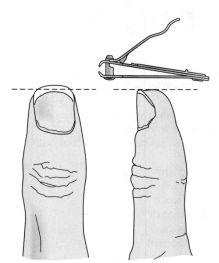

FIGURE 16-7 Clip fingernails straight across. Use a nail clipper.

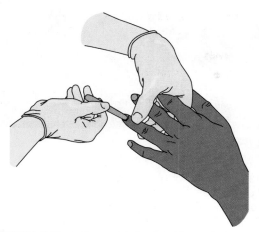

FIGURE 16-8 Push the cuticle back with an orangewood stick.

CHANGING CLOTHING AND HOSPITAL GOWNS

Gown or pajamas are changed after the bath and when wet or soiled. Some people wear street clothes during the day. Garments are changed whenever wet or soiled.

When changing clothes and hospital gowns, follow these rules:

- Provide for privacy. Do not expose the person.
- Encourage the person to do as much as possible.
- Let the person choose what to wear. Make sure the right undergarments are chosen.
- Remove clothing from the strong or "good" side first. This is often call the *unaffected side*.
- Put clothing on the weak side first. This is often called the *affected side*.
- Support the arm or leg when removing or putting on a garment.

Dressing and Undressing

Clothing changes are usually necessary on admission and discharge. Some people enter and leave the agency in a gown or pajamas. Most wear street clothes. Most nursing center residents wear street clothes during the day.

Some patients and residents dress and undress themselves. Others need help. Personal choice is a resident right. Let the person choose what to wear.

The rules listed above are followed for dressing and undressing.

See *Persons With Dementia: Dressing and Undressing.*
See *Focus on Communication: Dressing and Undressing.*
See *Delegation Guidelines: Dressing and Undressing.*

PERSONS WITH DEMENTIA
Dressing and Undressing

Persons with dementia may not want to change clothes. Or they may not know how. For example, a person may try to put slacks on over his or her head. The Alzheimer's Disease Education and Referral Center (ADEAR) suggests the following:

- Try to assist with dressing and undressing at the same time each day. The person will learn to expect these tasks as a part of his or her daily routine.
- Let the person dress himself or herself to the extent possible. Allow extra time for this task. Do not rush the person.
- Let the person choose what to wear from 2 or 3 outfits. If the person has a favorite outfit, the family may buy several of the same outfit. This makes dressing easier if the person insists on wearing the same outfit.
- Choose clothes that are comfortable to wear and easy to get on and off. Garments with elastic waistbands and Velcro closures are examples. The person does not have to handle zippers, buttons, hooks, snaps, or other closures.
- Stack clothes in the order that they will be put on. The person sees one item at a time. For example, underpants or undershorts are put on first. The item is on top of the stack.
- Give clear, simple, step-by-step directions.

FOCUS ON COMMUNICATION
Dressing and Undressing

Make sure you allow for personal choice and independence when assisting with dressing and undressing. You can ask:

- "What would you like to wear today?"
- "There's a concert today in the lounge. Do you want to wear something special?"
- "Can I help you with those buttons?"
- "Would you like me to help you with that zipper?"

DELEGATION GUIDELINES
Dressing and Undressing

Before assisting with dressing and undressing, you need this information from the nurse and the care plan:

- How much help the person needs
- Which side is the person's strong side
- If the person needs to wear certain garments
- What observations to report and record:
  - How much help was given
  - How the person tolerated the procedure
  - Any complaints by the person
  - Any changes in the person's behavior
- When to report observations
- What specific patient or resident concerns to report at once

UNDRESSING THE PERSON

QUALITY OF LIFE

Remember to:
- Knock before entering the person's room.
- Address the person by name.
- Introduce yourself by name and title.

- Explain the procedure to the person before beginning and during the procedure.
- Protect the person's rights during the procedure.
- Handle the person gently during the procedure.

PRE-PROCEDURE

1 Follow *Delegation Guidelines: Dressing and Undressing,* p. 279.
2 Practice hand hygiene.
3 Collect a bath blanket and clothing requested by the person.
4 Identify the person. Check the ID bracelet against the assignment sheet. Also call the person by name.

5 Provide for privacy.
6 Raise the bed for body mechanics. Bed rails are up if used.
7 Lower the bed rail on the person's weak side.
8 Position him or her supine.
9 Cover the person with a bath blanket. Fan-fold linens to the foot of the bed.

PROCEDURE

10 Remove garments that open in the back:
  a Raise the head and shoulders. Or turn him or her onto the side away from you.
  b Undo buttons, zippers, ties, or snaps.
  c Bring the sides of the garment to the sides of the person (Fig. 16-9). If he or she is in a side-lying position, tuck the far side under the person. Fold the near side onto the chest (Fig. 16-10).
  d Position the person supine.
  e Slide the garment off the shoulder on the strong side. Remove it from the arm (Fig. 16-11).
  f Remove the garment from the weak side.
11 Remove garments that open in the front:
  a Undo buttons, zippers, ties, or snaps.
  b Slide the garment off the shoulder and arm on the strong side.
  c Assist the person to sit up or raise the head and shoulders. Bring the garment over to the weak side (Fig. 16-12).
  d Lower the head and shoulders. Remove the garment from the weak side.
  e If you cannot raise the head and shoulders:
    (1) Turn the person toward you. Tuck the removed part under the person.
    (2) Turn him or her onto the side away from you.
    (3) Pull the side of the garment out from under the person. Make sure he or she will not lie on it when supine.
    (4) Return the person to the supine position.
    (5) Remove the garment from the weak side.

12 Remove pullover garments:
  a Undo buttons, zippers, ties, or snaps.
  b Remove the garment from the strong side.
  c Raise the head and shoulders. Or turn the person onto the side away from you. Bring the garment up to the person's neck (Fig. 16-13).
  d Remove the garment from the weak side.
  e Bring the garment over the person's head.
  f Position him or her in the supine position.
13 Remove pants or slacks:
  a Remove footwear and socks.
  b Position the person supine.
  c Undo buttons, zippers, ties, snaps, or buckles.
  d Remove the belt.
  e Ask the person to lift the buttocks off the bed. Slide the pants down over the hips and buttocks (Fig. 16-14). Have the person lower the hips and buttocks.
  f If the person cannot raise the hips off the bed:
    (1) Turn the person toward you.
    (2) Slide the pants off the hip and buttock on the strong side (Fig. 16-15, p. 282).
    (3) Turn the person away from you.
    (4) Slide the pants off the hip and buttock on the weak side (Fig. 16-16, p. 282).
  g Slide the pants down the legs and over the feet.
14 Dress the person. See procedure: *Dressing the Person,* p. 282.

POST-PROCEDURE

15 Provide for comfort. (See the inside of the front book cover.)
16 Place the signal light within reach.
17 Lower the bed to its lowest position.
18 Raise or lower bed rails. Follow the care plan.
19 Unscreen the person.

20 Complete a safety check of the room. (See the inside of the front book cover.)
21 Follow agency policy for soiled clothing.
22 Decontaminate your hands.
23 Report and record your observations.

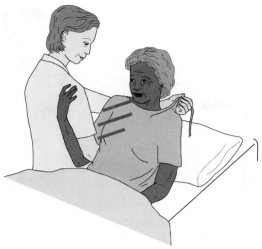

FIGURE 16-9 The sides of the garment are brought from the back to the sides of the person. (Note that the "weak" side is *indicated by slash marks.*)

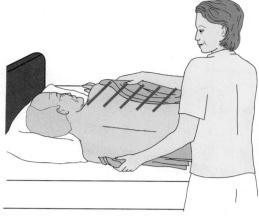

FIGURE 16-10 A garment that opens in the back is removed from the person in the side-lying position. The far side of the garment is tucked under the person. The near side is folded onto the person's chest. (Note that the "weak" side is *indicated by slash marks.*)

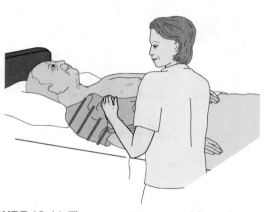

FIGURE 16-11 The garment is removed from the strong side first. (Note that the "weak" side is *indicated by slash marks.*)

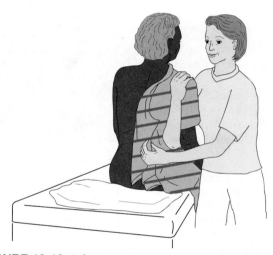

FIGURE 16-12 A front-opening garment is removed with the person's head and shoulders raised. The garment is removed from the strong side first. Then it is brought around the back to the weak side. (Note that the "weak" side is *indicated by slash marks.*)

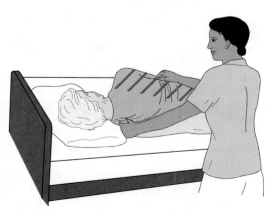

FIGURE 16-13 A pullover garment is removed from the strong side first. Then the garment is brought up to the person's neck so that it can be removed from the weak side. (Note that the "weak" side is *indicated by slash marks.*)

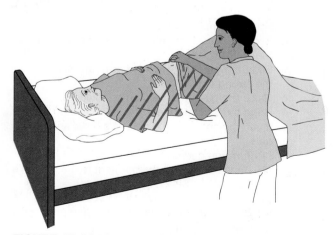

FIGURE 16-14 The person lifts the hips and buttocks for removing the pants. The pants are slid down over the hips and buttocks. (Note that the "weak" side is *indicated by slash marks.*)

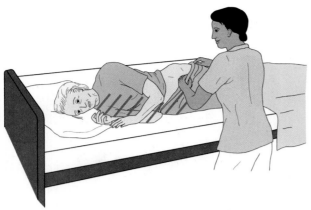

FIGURE 16-15 Pants are removed in the side-lying position. They are removed from the strong side first. They are slid over the hip and buttock. (Note that the "weak" side is *indicated by slash marks.*)

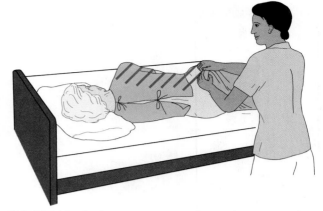

FIGURE 16-16 The person is turned onto the strong side. The pants are removed from the weak side. (Note that the "weak" side is *indicated by slash marks.*)

DRESSING THE PERSON

QUALITY OF LIFE

Remember to:
- Knock before entering the person's room.
- Address the person by name.
- Introduce yourself by name and title.
- Explain the procedure to the person before beginning and during the procedure.
- Protect the person's rights during the procedure.
- Handle the person gently during the procedure.

PRE-PROCEDURE

1 Follow *Delegation Guidelines: Dressing and Undressing,* p. 279.
2 Practice hand hygiene.
3 Ask the person what he or she would like to wear.
4 Get a bath blanket and clothing requested by the person.
5 Identify the person. Check the ID bracelet against the assignment sheet. Also call the person by name.
6 Provide for privacy.
7 Raise the bed for body mechanics. Bed rails are up if used.
8 Lower the bed rail (if up) on the person's strong side.
9 Position the person supine.
10 Cover the person with a bath blanket. Fan-fold linens to the foot of the bed.
11 Undress the person. (See procedure: *Undressing the Person,* p. 280.)

PROCEDURE

12 Put on garments that open in the back:
   a Slide the garment onto the arm and shoulder of the weak side.
   b Slide the garment onto the arm and shoulder of the strong side.
   c Raise the person's head and shoulders.
   d Bring the sides to the back.
   e If you cannot raise the person's head and shoulders:
     (1) Turn the person toward you.
     (2) Bring one side of the garment to the person's back (Fig. 16-17, *A*).
     (3) Turn the person away from you.
     (4) Bring the other side to the person's back (Fig. 16-17, *B*).
   f Fasten buttons, zippers, snaps, or other closures.
   g Position the person supine.

13 Put on garments that open in the front:
   a Slide the garment onto the arm and shoulder on the weak side.
   b Raise the head and shoulders. Bring the side of the garment around to the back. Lower the person down. Slide the garment onto the arm and shoulder of the strong arm.
   c If the person cannot raise the head and shoulders:
     (1) Turn the person away from you.
     (2) Tuck the garment under him or her.
     (3) Turn the person toward you.
     (4) Pull the garment out from under him or her.
     (5) Turn the person back to the supine position.
     (6) Slide the garment over the arm and shoulder of the strong arm.
   d Fasten buttons, zippers, ties, snaps, or other closures.

PROCEDURE—cont'd

14 Put on pullover garments:
  a Position the person supine.
  b Bring the neck of the garment over the head.
  c Slide the arm and shoulder of the garment onto the weak side.
  d Raise the person's head and shoulders.
  e Bring the garment down.
  f Slide the arm and shoulder of the garment onto the strong side.
  g If the person cannot assume a semi-sitting position:
    (1) Turn the person away from you.
    (2) Tuck the garment under the person.
    (3) Turn the person toward you.
    (4) Pull the garment out from under him or her.
    (5) Position the person supine.
    (6) Slide the arm and shoulder of the garment onto the strong side.
  h Fasten buttons, zippers, ties, snaps, or other closures.

15 Put on pants or slacks:
  a Slide the pants over the feet and up the legs.
  b Ask the person to raise the hips and buttocks off the bed.
  c Bring the pants up over the buttocks and hips.
  d Ask the person to lower the hips and buttocks.
  e If the person cannot raise the hips and buttocks:
    (1) Turn the person onto the strong side.
    (2) Pull the pants over the buttock and hip on the weak side.
    (3) Turn the person onto the weak side.
    (4) Pull the pants over the buttock and hip on the strong side.
    (5) Position the person supine.
  f Fasten buttons, zippers, ties, snaps, a belt buckle, or other closures.

16 Put socks and non-skid footwear on the person. Make sure socks are up all the way and smooth.

17 Help the person get out of bed. If the person will stay in bed, cover the person. Remove the bath blanket.

POST-PROCEDURE

18 Provide for comfort. (See the inside of the front book cover.)
19 Place the signal light within reach.
20 Lower the bed to its lowest position.
21 Raise or lower bed rails. Follow the care plan.
22 Unscreen the person.
23 Complete a safety check of the room. (See the inside of the front book cover.)
24 Follow agency policy for soiled clothing.
25 Decontaminate your hands.
26 Report and record your observations.

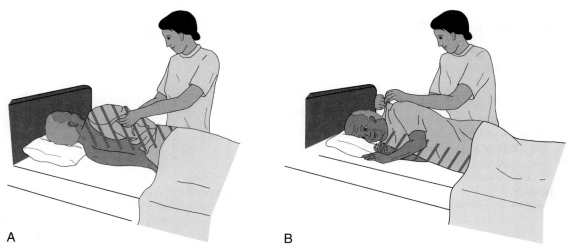

A   B

FIGURE 16-17 Dressing a person. **A,** The side-lying position can be used to put on garments that open in the back. Turn the person toward you after the garment is put on the arms. The side of the garment is brought to the person's back. **B,** Then turn the person away from you. The other side of the garment is brought to the back and fastened. (Note that the "weak" side is *indicated by slash marks.*)

❧ Changing Hospital Gowns

Many hospital patients wear gowns. So do some nursing center residents. Gowns are usually worn for IV (intravenous) therapy (Chapter 19). Some agencies have special gowns for IV therapy. They open along the sleeve and close with ties, snaps, or Velcro. Sometimes standard gowns are used.

If there is injury or paralysis, the gown is removed from the strong arm first. Support the weak arm while removing the gown. Put the clean gown on the weak arm first and then on the strong arm.

See *Delegation Guidelines: Changing Hospital Gowns.*

See *Promoting Safety and Comfort: Changing Hospital Gowns.*

DELEGATION GUIDELINES
Changing Hospital Gowns

Before changing a gown, you need this information from the nurse and the care plan:
- Which arm has the IV
- If the person has an IV pump (see *Promoting Safety and Comfort: Changing Hospital Gowns*)

PROMOTING SAFETY AND COMFORT
Changing Hospital Gowns

Safety

IV pumps control how fast fluid enters a vein. This is called the *flow rate* (Chapter 19). If the person has an IV pump and a standard gown, do not use the following procedure. The arm with the IV is not put through the sleeve.

If the person has an IV, changing the gown can cause the flow rate to change. Always ask the nurse to check the flow rate after you change a gown.

Do not disconnect or remove any part of the IV set-up.

Comfort

Some hospital gowns are secured with ties at the upper back. The back and buttocks are exposed when the person stands. Other gowns overlap in the back and tie at the side. These gowns provide more privacy. Because they tie at the side, uncomfortable bows and knots at the back are avoided.

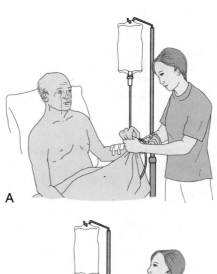

A

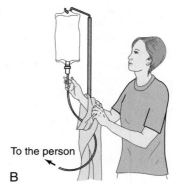

To the person

B

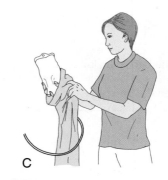

C

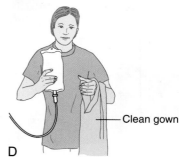

Clean gown

D

FIGURE 16-18 Changing a gown. **A,** The gown is removed from the arm with no IV. The sleeve on the arm with the IV is gathered up, slipped over the IV site and tubing, and removed from the arm and hand. **B,** The gathered sleeve is slipped along the IV tubing to the bag. **C,** The IV bag is removed from the pole and passed through the sleeve. **D,** The gathered sleeve of the clean gown is slipped over the IV bag at the shoulder part of the gown.

CHANGING THE GOWN OF THE PERSON WITH AN IV

QUALITY OF LIFE

Remember to:
- Knock before entering the person's room.
- Address the person by name.
- Introduce yourself by name and title.

- Explain the procedure to the person before beginning and during the procedure.
- Protect the person's rights during the procedure.
- Handle the person gently during the procedure.

PRE-PROCEDURE

1 Follow *Delegation Guidelines: Changing Hospital Gowns*.
See *Promoting Safety and Comfort: Changing Hospital Gowns*.
2 Practice hand hygiene.
3 Get a clean gown and a bath blanket.

4 Identify the person. Check the ID bracelet against the assignment sheet. Also call the person by name.
5 Provide for privacy.
6 Raise the bed for body mechanics. Bed rails are up if used.

PROCEDURE

7 Lower the bed rail near you (if up).
8 Cover the person with a bath blanket. Fan-fold linens to the foot of the bed.
9 Untie the gown. Free parts that the person is lying on.
10 Remove the gown from the arm with *no IV.*
11 Gather up the sleeve of the arm *with the IV.* Slide it over the IV site and tubing. Remove the arm and hand from the sleeve (Fig. 16-18, *A*).
12 Keep the sleeve gathered. Slide your arm along the tubing to the bag (Fig. 16-18, *B*).
13 Remove the bag from the pole. Slide the bag and tubing through the sleeve (Fig. 16-18, *C*). Do not pull on the tubing. Keep the bag above the person.

14 Hang the IV bag on the pole.
15 Gather the sleeve of the clean gown that will go on the arm with the IV infusion.
16 Remove the bag from the pole. Slip the sleeve over the bag at the shoulder part of the gown (Fig. 16-18, *D*). Hang the bag.
17 Slide the gathered sleeve over the tubing, hand, arm, and IV site. Then slide it onto the shoulder.
18 Put the other side of the gown on the person. Fasten the gown.
19 Cover the person. Remove the bath blanket.

POST-PROCEDURE

20 Provide for comfort. (See the inside of the front book cover.)
21 Place the signal light within reach.
22 Lower the bed to its lowest position.
23 Raise or lower bed rails. Follow the care plan.
24 Unscreen the person.

25 Complete a safety check of the room. (See the inside of the front book cover.)
26 Follow agency policy for dirty linen.
27 Decontaminate your hands.
28 Ask the nurse to check the flow rate.
29 Report and record your observations.

Focus on P R I D E
The Person, Family, and Yourself

Personal and Professional Responsibility—
Personal grooming measures are important. Self-esteem and body image improve when the person likes how he or she looks.

You may not like the person's hair style or clothing choices. Or you may not agree with the person's choice in personal care products. Do not judge the person by your own standards. Do not impose your choices or values on the person.

Always remain professional. Do not say things that make the person feel bad about his or her personal choices. Assist with grooming in a way that improves the person's self-esteem and pride.

Rights and Respect—People have different grooming preferences. Respect the person's right to choose. Ask the person what he or she prefers. For example, ask the person what he or she would like to wear. Or ask how the person wants his or her hair styled. Follow the person's grooming routines whenever possible.

Independence and Social Interaction—
Sometimes family members want to help with grooming. For example, they want to help style the person's hair. Or they want to apply lotion to the person's hands and feet.

With the person's permission, allow family members to assist with grooming measures as much as safely possible. This promotes social interaction. It also involves the family in the person's care.

Delegation and Teamwork—Working as a team involves considering the needs of co-workers. Some grooming equipment is shared among patients and residents. Shampoo trays, electric shavers, and whirlpool foot baths are examples. When finished using a shared item, clean and promptly return the item to its proper place. A co-worker should not have to clean or look for an item after you use it.

Ethics and Laws—OBRA requires courteous and dignified care. You need to:
- Groom hair and nails as the person wishes
- Assist with dressing in the right clothing for the time of day
- Assist with grooming measures for:
  - A neat and clean appearance
  - A clean, shaved face or a groomed beard
  - Clean and trimmed nails
  - Properly fastened clothing and shoes

REVIEW QUESTIONS

Circle the BEST answer.

1 A person has alopecia. This is
  a Excessive body hair
  b Dry, white flakes from the scalp
  c An infestation with lice
  d Hair loss

2 Which prevents hair from matting and tangling?
  a Bedrest
  b Daily brushing and combing
  c Daily shampooing
  d Cutting hair

3 A person's hair is not matted or tangled. When brushing hair, start at
  a The forehead and brush backward
  b The hair ends
  c The scalp
  d The back of the neck and brush forward

4 Brushing keeps the hair
  a Soft and shiny
  b Clean
  c Free of lice
  d Long

5 A person requests a shampoo. You should
  a Shampoo the hair during the person's shower
  b Shampoo hair at the sink
  c Shampoo the person in bed
  d Follow the care plan

6 When shaving a person's face, do the following except
  a Practice Standard Precautions
  b Follow the Bloodborne Pathogen Standard
  c Shave in the direction of hair growth
  d Shave when the skin is dry

7 A person is nicked during shaving. Your first action is to
  a Wash your hands
  b Apply direct pressure
  c Tell the nurse
  d Apply a bandage

8 Fingernails are cut with
  a An emery board
  b Scissors
  c A nail file
  d Nail clippers

9 A person has a loose toenail. You should
  a Tell the nurse
  b Cut the toenail
  c File the toenail
  d Remove the toenail

Circle T if the statement is *true*. Circle F if the statement is *false*.

10 T F Mr. Polk has a mustache and beard. To promote his comfort, you can shave his beard and mustache.

11 T F Clothing is removed from the strong side first.

12 T F The person chooses what to wear.

13 T F A person has poor circulation in the legs and feet. You can cut and trim the person's toenails.

14 T F You can cut matted hair.

Answers to these questions are on p. 527.

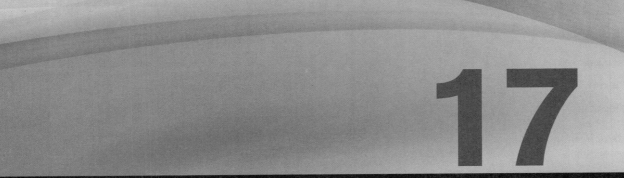

17

ASSISTING WITH URINARY ELIMINATION

PROCEDURES

- View Video! Video CLIP Giving the Bedpan
- View Video! Giving the Urinal
- View Video! Helping the Person to the Commode
- View Video! Video CLIP Giving Catheter Care
- View Video! Emptying a Urinary Drainage Bag
- View Video! Applying a Condom Catheter

OBJECTIVES

- Define the key terms and key abbreviations listed in this chapter.
- Describe normal urine.
- Describe the rules for normal urination.
- Describe urinary incontinence and the care required.
- Explain why catheters are used.
- Explain how to care for persons with catheters.
- Describe two methods of bladder training.
- Explain how to promote PRIDE in the person, the family, and yourself.
- Perform the procedures described in this chapter.

KEY TERMS

catheter A tube used to drain or inject fluid through a body opening

dysuria Painful or difficult (*dys*) urination (*uria*)

functional incontinence The person has bladder control but cannot use the toilet in time

hematuria Blood (*hemat*) in the urine (*uria*)

mixed incontinence Having more than one type of incontinence

nocturia Frequent urination (*uria*) at night (*noct*)

oliguria Scant amount (*olig*) of urine (*uria*); less than 500 mL in 24 hours

overflow incontinence Small amounts of urine leak from a bladder that is always full

polyuria Abnormally large amounts (*poly*) of urine (*uria*)

reflex incontinence The loss of urine at predictable intervals when the bladder is full

stress incontinence When urine leaks during exercise and certain movements that cause pressure on the bladder

urge incontinence The loss of urine in response to a sudden, urgent need to void; the person cannot get to a toilet in time

urinary frequency Voiding at frequent intervals

urinary incontinence The involuntary loss or leakage of urine

urinary urgency The need to void at once

urination The process of emptying urine from the bladder; voiding

voiding See "urination"

KEY ABBREVIATIONS

ID Identification

IV Intravenous

mL Milliliter

Eliminating waste is a physical need. The urinary system removes waste products from the blood. It also maintains the body's water balance.

NORMAL URINATION

The healthy adult produces about 1500 mL (milliliters) or 3 pints of urine a day. Many factors affect urine production. They include age, disease, the amount and kinds of fluid ingested, dietary salt, body temperature, perspiration, and drugs. Some substances increase urine production—coffee, tea, alcohol, and some drugs. A diet high in salt causes the body to retain water. When water is retained, less urine is produced.

Urination (voiding) means the process of emptying urine from the bladder. The amount of fluid intake, habits, and available toilet facilities affect frequency. So do activity, work, and illness. People usually void at bedtime, after sleep, and before meals. Some people void every 2 to 3 hours.

Some persons need help getting to the bathroom. Others use bedpans, urinals, or commodes. Follow the rules in Box 17-1 and the person's care plan.

See *Focus on Communication: Normal Urination.*

BOX 17-1 Rules for Normal Urination

- Practice medical asepsis.
- Follow Standard Precautions and the Bloodborne Pathogen Standard.
- Provide fluids as the nurse and care plan direct.
- Follow the person's voiding routines and habits. Check with the nurse and the care plan.
- Help the person to the bathroom when the request is made. Or provide the commode, bedpan, or urinal. The need to void may be urgent.
- Help the person assume a normal position for voiding if possible. Women sit or squat. Men stand.
- Warm the bedpan or urinal.
- Cover the person for warmth and privacy.
- Provide for privacy. Pull the curtain around the bed, close room and bathroom doors, and close window coverings. Leave the room if the person can be alone.
- Tell the person that running water, flushing the toilet, or playing music can mask voiding sounds. Voiding with others close by embarrasses some people.
- Stay nearby if the person is weak or unsteady.
- Place the signal light and toilet tissue within reach.
- Allow enough time. Do not rush the person.
- Promote relaxation. Some people like to read.
- Run water in a sink if the person cannot start the stream. Or place the person's fingers in warm water.
- Provide perineal care as needed (Chapter 15).
- Assist with hand washing after voiding. Provide a wash basin, soap, washcloth, and towel.
- Assist the person to the bathroom or offer the bedpan, urinal, or commode at regular times. Some people are embarrassed or are too weak to ask for help.

FOCUS ON COMMUNICATION
Normal Urination

Patients and residents may not use "voiding" or "urinating" terms. The person may not understand what you are saying. Instead, you can ask these questions:
- "Do you need to use the bathroom?"
- "Do you need to use the bedpan?"
- "Do you need to pass urine?"
- "Do you need to pee?"

Observations

Normal urine is pale yellow, straw-colored, or amber (Fig. 17-1). It is clear with no particles. A faint odor is normal. Observe urine for color, clarity, odor, amount, and particles.

Ask the nurse to observe urine that looks or smells abnormal. Report these problems:

- **Dysuria**—painful or difficult *(dys)* urination *(uria)*
- **Hematuria**—blood *(hemat)* in the urine *(uria)*
- **Nocturia**—frequent urination *(uria)* at night *(noct)*
- **Oliguria**—scant amount *(olig)* of urine *(uria)*; less than 500 mL in 24 hours
- **Polyuria**—abnormally large amounts *(poly)* of urine *(uria)*
- **Urinary frequency**—voiding at frequent intervals
- **Urinary incontinence**—the involuntary loss or leakage of urine
- **Urinary urgency**—the need to void at once

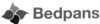 **Bedpans**

Bedpans are used by persons who cannot be out of bed. Women use bedpans for voiding and bowel movements. Men use them for bowel movements.

The *standard bedpan* is shown in Figure 17-2. A *fracture pan* has a thin rim. It is only about ½-inch deep at one end (see Fig. 17-2). The smaller end is placed under the buttocks (Fig. 17-3). Fracture pans are used:

- By persons with casts
- By persons in traction
- By persons with limited back motion
- After spinal cord injury or surgery
- After a hip fracture or hip replacement surgery
  See *Delegation Guidelines: Bedpans.*
  See *Promoting Safety and Comfort: Bedpans.*

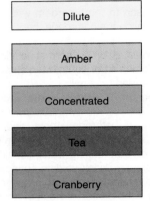

FIGURE 17-1 Color chart for urine. *(Redrawn from Welcon, Inc. Fort Worth, Texas.)*

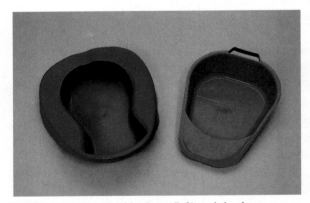

FIGURE 17-2 Standard bedpan *(left)* and the fracture pan *(right)*.

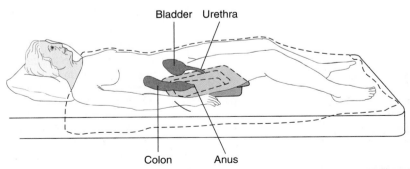

FIGURE 17-3 A person positioned on a fracture pan. The small end is under the buttocks.

<table>
<tr><td>

DELEGATION GUIDELINES
Bedpans

Before assisting with a bedpan, you need this information from the nurse and the care plan:

- What bedpan to use—standard bedpan or fracture pan
- Position or activity limits
- If you can leave the room or if you need to stay with the person
- If the nurse needs to observe the results before disposing of the contents
- What observations to report and record:
  - Urine color, clarity, and odor
  - Amount
  - Presence of particles
  - Complaints of urgency, burning, dysuria, or other problems
  - For bowel movements, see Chapter 18
- When to report observations
- What specific patient or resident concerns to report at once

</td><td>

PROMOTING SAFETY AND COMFORT
Bedpans

Safety

Urine and bowel movements may contain blood and microbes. Microbes can live and grow in dirty bedpans. Follow Standard Precautions and the Bloodborne Pathogen Standard when handling bedpans and their contents. Thoroughly clean and disinfect bedpans after use.

Remember to raise the bed as needed for good body mechanics. Lower the bed before leaving the room. Raise or lower the bed rails according to the care plan.

Comfort

Some older persons have fragile bones or painful joints. Fracture pans provide more comfort for them than standard bedpans.

The person must not sit on a bedpan for a long time. Bedpans are uncomfortable. And they can lead to pressure ulcers from prolonged pressure (Chapter 23).

</td></tr>
</table>

GIVING THE BEDPAN

QUALITY OF LIFE

Remember to:
- Knock before entering the person's room.
- Address the person by name.
- Introduce yourself by name and title.

- Explain the procedure to the person before beginning and during the procedure.
- Protect the person's rights during the procedure.
- Handle the person gently during the procedure.

PRE-PROCEDURE

1 Follow *Delegation Guidelines: Bedpans.*
  See *Promoting Safety and Comfort: Bedpans.*
2 Provide for privacy.
3 Practice hand hygiene.
4 Put on gloves.

5 Collect the following:
  - Bedpan
  - Bedpan cover
  - Toilet tissue
  - Waterproof pad (if required by the agency)
6 Arrange equipment on the chair or bed.

PROCEDURE

7 Lower the bed rail near you if up.
8 Position the person supine. Raise the head of the bed slightly.
9 Fold the top linens and gown out of the way. Keep the lower body covered.
10 Ask the person to flex the knees and raise the buttocks by pushing against the mattress with his or her feet.
11 Slide your hand under the lower back. Help raise the buttocks. If using a waterproof pad, place it under the person's buttocks.
12 Slide the bedpan under the person (Fig. 17-4, p. 292).

13 If the person cannot assist in getting on the bedpan:
  a Place the waterproof pad under the person's buttocks if using one.
  b Turn the person onto the side away from you.
  c Place the bedpan firmly against the buttocks (Fig. 17-5, *A*, p. 293).
  d Push the bedpan down and toward the person (Fig. 17-5, *B*, p. 293).
  e Hold the bedpan securely. Turn the person onto his or her back.
  f Make sure the bedpan is centered under the person.

Continued

GIVING THE BEDPAN—cont'd

PROCEDURE—cont'd

14 Cover the person.
15 Raise the head of the bed so the person is in a sitting position (Fowler's position) if the person uses a standard bedpan. (NOTE: Some state competency tests require that you remove gloves and wash your hands before raising the head of the bed.)
16 Make sure the person is correctly positioned on the bedpan (Fig. 17-6).
17 Raise the bed rail if used.
18 Place the toilet tissue and signal light within reach.
19 Ask the person to signal when done or when help is needed.
20 Remove the gloves. Practice hand hygiene.
21 Leave the room, and close the door.
22 Return when the person signals. Or check on the person every 5 minutes. Knock before entering.
23 Practice hand hygiene. Put on gloves.
24 Raise the bed for body mechanics. Lower the bed rail (if used) and lower the head of the bed.
25 Ask the person to raise the buttocks. Remove the bedpan. Or hold the bedpan and turn him or her onto the side away from you.

26 Clean the genital area if the person cannot do so. Clean from front (urethra) to back (anus) with toilet tissue. Use fresh tissue for each wipe. Provide perineal care if needed. Remove and discard the waterproof pad if using one.
27 Cover the bedpan. Take it to the bathroom. Raise the bed rail (if used) before leaving the bedside.
28 Note the color, amount, and character of urine or feces.
29 Empty the bedpan contents into the toilet and flush.
30 Rinse the bedpan. Pour the rinse into the toilet and flush.
31 Clean the bedpan with a disinfectant.
32 Remove soiled gloves. Practice hand hygiene, and put on clean gloves.
33 Return the bedpan and clean cover to the bedside stand.
34 Help the person with hand washing. (Wear gloves for this step.)
35 Remove the gloves. Practice hand hygiene.

POST-PROCEDURE

36 Provide for comfort. (See the inside of the front book cover.)
37 Place the signal light within reach.
38 Lower the bed to its lowest position.
39 Raise or lower bed rails. Follow the care plan.
40 Unscreen the person.

41 Complete a safety check of the room. (See the inside of the front book cover.)
42 Follow agency policy for soiled linen.
43 Practice hand hygiene.
44 Report and record your observations.

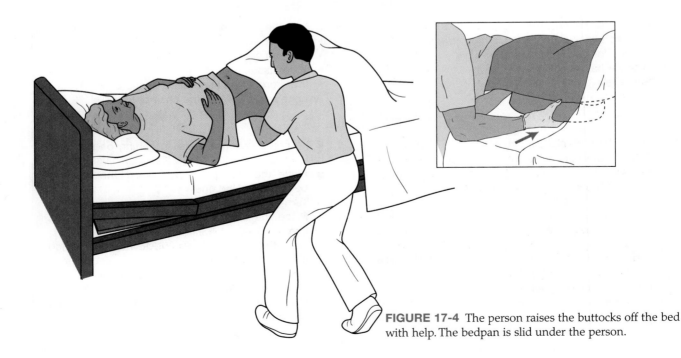

FIGURE 17-4 The person raises the buttocks off the bed with help. The bedpan is slid under the person.

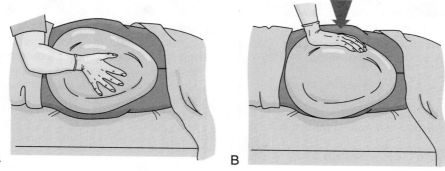

FIGURE 17-5 Giving a bedpan. **A,** Position the person on one side. Place the bedpan firmly against the buttocks. **B,** Push downward on the bedpan and toward the person.

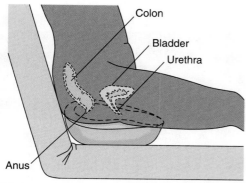

FIGURE 17-6 The person is positioned on the bedpan so the urethra and anus are directly over the opening.

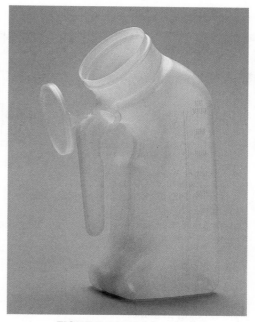

FIGURE 17-7 Male urinal.

 Urinals

Men use urinals to void (Fig. 17-7). Urinals have caps and hook-type handles. The urinal hooks to the bed rail within the man's reach. He stands to use the urinal if possible. Or he sits on the side of the bed or lies in bed to use it. Some men need support when standing. You may have to place and hold the urinal for some men.

After voiding, the urinal cap is closed. This prevents urine spills. Remind men to hang urinals on bed rails and to use the signal light after using them. Remind them not to place urinals on overbed tables and bedside stands. These surfaces must not be contaminated with urine.

Some beds may not have bed rails. Follow agency policy for where to place urinals.

See *Focus on Communication: Urinals.*
See *Delegation Guidelines: Urinals,* p. 294.
See *Promoting Safety and Comfort: Urinals,* p. 294.

FOCUS ON COMMUNICATION
Urinals

Some men are unable to use a urinal on their own. You may need to assist them. You may need to stay with the person. To make the person more comfortable, explain why you must help him. You can say:
- "Mr. Turner, I'll help you use your urinal. I need to stay with you to make sure you don't fall."
- "Mr. Gonzalez, I'll help you place and remove your urinal so it doesn't spill."

DELEGATION GUIDELINES
Urinals

Before assisting with urinals, you need this information from the nurse and the care plan:
- How the urinal is used—standing, sitting, or lying in bed
- If help is needed with placing or holding the urinal
- If the man needs support to stand (If yes, how many staff members are needed.)
- If you can leave the room or if you need to stay with the person
- If the nurse needs to observe the urine before its disposal
- What observations to report and record (see *Delegation Guidelines: Bedpans,* p. 291)
- When to report observations
- What specific patient or resident concerns to report at once

PROMOTING SAFETY AND COMFORT
Urinals

Safety

Follow Standard Precautions and the Bloodborne Pathogen Standard when handling urinals and their contents. Empty them promptly to prevent odors and the spread of microbes. A filled urinal spills easily, causing safety hazards. Also, it is an unpleasant sight and a source of odor. Urinals are cleaned and disinfected like bedpans.

Comfort

You may have to place the urinal for some men. This means that you have to place the penis in the urinal. This may embarrass both the person and you. Act in a professional manner at all times.

GIVING THE URINAL

QUALITY OF LIFE

Remember to:
- Knock before entering the person's room.
- Address the person by name.
- Introduce yourself by name and title.

- Explain the procedure to the person before beginning and during the procedure.
- Protect the person's rights during the procedure.
- Handle the person gently during the procedure.

PRE-PROCEDURE

1 Follow *Delegation Guidelines: Urinals.*
 See *Promoting Safety and Comfort: Urinals.*
2 Provide for privacy.
3 Determine if the man will stand, sit, or lie in bed.
4 Practice hand hygiene.

5 Put on gloves.
6 Collect the following:
 - Urinal
 - Non-skid footwear if the person will stand to void

PROCEDURE

7 Give him the urinal if he is in bed. Remind him to tilt the bottom down to prevent spills.
8 If he is going to stand:
 a Help him sit on the side of the bed.
 b Put non-skid footwear on him.
 c Help him stand. Provide support if he is unsteady.
 d Give him the urinal.
9 Position the urinal if necessary. Position his penis in the urinal if he cannot do so.
10 Place the signal light within reach. Ask him to signal when done or when he needs help.
11 Provide for privacy.
12 Remove the gloves. Practice hand hygiene.
13 Leave the room, and close the door.

14 Return when he signals for you. Or check on him every 5 minutes. Knock before entering.
15 Practice hand hygiene. Put on gloves.
16 Close the cap on the urinal. Take it to the bathroom.
17 Note the color, amount, and character of urine.
18 Empty the urinal into the toilet and flush.
19 Rinse the urinal with cold water. Pour rinse into the toilet and flush.
20 Clean the urinal with a disinfectant.
21 Return the urinal to its proper place.
22 Remove soiled gloves. Practice hand hygiene, and put on clean gloves.
23 Assist with hand washing.
24 Remove the gloves. Practice hand hygiene.

POST-PROCEDURE

25 Provide for comfort. (See the inside of the front book cover.)
26 Place the signal light within reach.
27 Raise or lower bed rails. Follow the care plan.
28 Unscreen him.

29 Complete a safety check of the room. (See the inside of the front book cover.)
30 Follow agency policy for soiled linen.
31 Practice hand hygiene.
32 Report and record your observations.

Commodes

A commode is a chair or wheelchair with an opening for a container (Fig. 17-8). Persons unable to walk to the bathroom often use commodes. The commode allows a normal position for elimination. The commode arms and back provide support and help prevent falls.

Some commodes are wheeled into bathrooms and placed over toilets. The container is removed if the commode is used with the toilet. Wheels are locked after the commode is positioned over the toilet.

See *Delegation Guidelines: Commodes.*
See *Promoting Safety and Comfort: Commodes.*

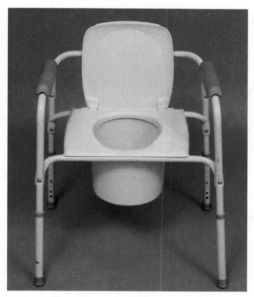

FIGURE 17-8 The commode has a toilet seat with a container. The container slides out from under the seat for emptying.

HELPING THE PERSON TO THE COMMODE

QUALITY OF LIFE

Remember to:
- Knock before entering the person's room.
- Address the person by name.
- Introduce yourself by name and title.
- Explain the procedure to the person before beginning and during the procedure.
- Protect the person's rights during the procedure.
- Handle the person gently during the procedure.

PRE-PROCEDURE

1 Follow *Delegation Guidelines: Commodes.*
   See *Promoting Safety and Comfort: Commodes.*
2 Provide for privacy.
3 Practice hand hygiene.
4 Put on gloves.

5 Collect the following:
   - Commode
   - Toilet tissue
   - Bath blanket
   - Transfer belt
   - Robe and non-skid footwear

Continued

PROCEDURE

6 Bring the commode next to the bed. Remove the chair seat and container lid.

7 Help the person sit on the side of the bed. Lower the bed rail if used.

8 Help him or her put on a robe and non-skid footwear.

9 Assist the person to the commode. Use the transfer belt.

10 Remove the transfer belt. Cover the person with a bath blanket for warmth.

11 Place the toilet tissue and signal light within reach.

12 Ask him or her to signal when done or when help is needed. (Stay with the person if necessary. Be respectful. Provide as much privacy as possible.)

13 Remove the gloves. Practice hand hygiene.

14 Leave the room. Close the door.

15 Return when the person signals. Or check on the person every 5 minutes. Knock before entering.

16 Decontaminate your hands. Put on the gloves.

17 Help the person clean the genital area as needed. Remove the gloves, and practice hand hygiene.

18 Apply the transfer belt. Help the person back to bed using the transfer belt. Remove the transfer belt, robe, and footwear. Raise the bed rail if used.

19 Put on clean gloves. Remove and cover the commode container. Clean the commode.

20 Take the container to the bathroom.

21 Observe urine and feces for color, amount, and character.

22 Empty the container contents into the toilet and flush.

23 Rinse the container. Pour the rinse into the toilet and flush.

24 Clean and disinfect the container.

25 Return the container to the commode. Return other supplies to their proper place.

26 Remove soiled gloves. Practice hand hygiene, and put on clean gloves.

27 Assist with hand washing.

28 Remove the gloves. Practice hand hygiene.

POST-PROCEDURE

29 Provide for comfort. (See the inside of the front book cover.)

30 Place the signal light within reach.

31 Raise or lower bed rails. Follow the care plan.

32 Unscreen the person.

33 Complete a safety check of the room. (See the inside of the front book cover.)

34 Follow agency policy for dirty linen.

35 Practice hand hygiene.

36 Report and record your observations.

URINARY INCONTINENCE

Urinary incontinence is the involuntary loss or leakage of urine. It may be temporary or permanent. The basic types of incontinence are:

- **Stress incontinence.** Urine leaks during exercise and certain movements that cause pressure on the bladder. Urine loss is small (less than 50 mL). Often called *dribbling*, it occurs with laughing, sneezing, coughing, lifting, or other activities.
- **Urge incontinence.** Urine is lost in response to a sudden, urgent need to void. The person cannot get to a toilet in time. Urinary frequency, urinary urgency, and night-time voidings are common.
- **Overflow incontinence.** Small amounts of urine leak from a bladder that is always full. The person feels like the bladder is not empty. The person only dribbles or has a weak urine stream.
- **Functional incontinence.** The person has bladder control but cannot use the toilet in time. Immobility, restraints, unanswered signal lights, no signal light within reach, and not knowing where to find the bathroom are causes. So is difficulty removing clothing. Confusion and disorientation are other causes.
- **Reflex incontinence.** Urine is lost at predictable intervals when the bladder is full. The person does not feel the need to void. Nervous system disorders and injuries are common causes.
- **Mixed incontinence.** A person can have more than one type of incontinence. Stress and urge incontinence often occur together.

Sometimes incontinence results from intestinal, rectal, and reproductive system surgeries. Incontinence may result from a physical illness. If incontinence is a new problem, tell the nurse at once.

Incontinence is embarrassing. Garments get wet, and odors develop. The person is uncomfortable. Skin irritation, infection, and pressure ulcers are risks. Falling is a risk when trying to get to the bathroom quickly. The person's pride, dignity, and self-esteem are affected. Social isolation, loss of independence, and depression are common. Quality of life suffers.

BOX 17-2   Nursing Measures for Persons With Urinary Incontinence

- Record the person's voidings. This includes incontinent times and successful use of the toilet, commode, bedpan, or urinal.
- Answer signal lights promptly. The need to void may be urgent.
- Promote normal urinary elimination (see Box 17-1).
- Promote normal bowel elimination (Chapter 18).
- Assist with elimination after sleep, before and after meals, and at bedtime.
- Follow the person's bladder training program (p. 306).
- Have the person wear easy-to-remove clothing. Incontinence can occur while trying to deal with buttons, zippers, other closures, and undergarments.
- Encourage the person to do pelvic muscle exercises as instructed by the nurse.
- Check the person to make sure he or she is clean and dry.
- Help prevent urinary tract infections:
  - Promote fluid intake as the nurse directs.
  - Have the person wear cotton underwear.
  - Keep the perineal area clean and dry.
- Decrease fluid intake at bedtime.
- Provide good skin care.

- Apply a barrier cream as directed by the nurse. The cream prevents irritation and skin damage.
- Provide dry garments and linens.
- Observe for signs of skin breakdown (Chapter 23).
- Use incontinence products as the nurse directs. Follow the manufacturer's instructions.
- Do not leave urinals in place to catch urine in men who are incontinent.
- Keep the perineal area clean and dry (Chapter 15). Remember to:
  - Use soap and water or a no-rinse incontinent cleanser (perineal rinse). Follow the care plan. If using soap and water, remember to use a safe and comfortable water temperature and rinse thoroughly.
  - Follow Standard Precautions and the Bloodborne Pathogen Standard.
  - Protect the person and dry garments and linen from the wet incontinence product.
  - Expose only the perineal area.
  - Dry the perineal area and buttocks.
  - Remove wet incontinence products, garments, and linen. Apply clean, dry ones.

The person's care plan may include some of the measures listed in Box 17-2. *Good skin care and dry garments and linens are essential.* Promoting normal urinary elimination prevents incontinence in some people (see Box 17-1). Others need bladder training (p. 306). Sometimes catheters are needed (p. 298).

Incontinence products help keep the person dry (Fig. 17-9). They have two layers and a waterproof back. Fluid passes through the first layer. It is absorbed by the lower layer. The nurse selects products that best meet the person's needs. Follow the manufacturer's instructions and agency procedures when using them.

Incontinence is beyond the person's control. It is not something the person chooses to do. The person may wet again right after skin care and changing wet garments and linens. Be patient. The person's needs are great. If you find yourself becoming short-tempered and impatient, talk to the nurse at once. The person has the right to be free from abuse, mistreatment, and neglect. Kindness, empathy, understanding, and patience are needed.

See *Persons With Dementia: Urinary Incontinence,* p. 298.

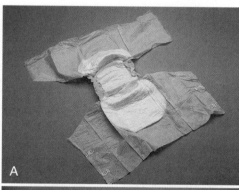
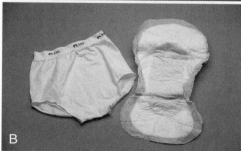

FIGURE 17-9 Disposable garment protectors. **A,** Complete incontinence brief. **B,** Pant liner and undergarment.

PERSONS WITH DEMENTIA
Urinary Incontinence

Persons with dementia may void in wrong places. Trash cans, planters, heating vents, and closets are examples. Some persons remove incontinence products and throw them on the floor or in the toilet. Other persons resist staff efforts to keep them clean and dry.

You must provide safe care for these persons. The care plan lists needed measures. The care plan may include these measures recommended by the Alzheimer's Disease Education and Referral Center (ADEAR):

- Follow the person's bathroom routine as closely as possible. For example, take the person to the bathroom every 3 hours during the day. Do not wait for the person to ask.
- Observe for signs that the person may need to void. Restlessness and pulling at clothes are examples. Respond quickly.
- Stay calm when the person is incontinent. Reassure the person if he or she becomes upset.
- Tell the nurse when the person is incontinent. Report the time, what the person was doing, and other observations. There may be a pattern to the person's incontinence. If so, measures can be taken to prevent the problem.
- Prevent episodes of incontinence during sleep. Limit the type and amount of fluids in the evening. Follow the care plan.
- Plan ahead if the person will leave the agency. Have the person wear clothing that is easy to remove. Pack an extra set of clothing. Know where to find restrooms.

You may need a co-worker's help to keep the person clean and dry. If you have questions, ask the nurse for help.

Remember, everyone has the right to safe care. They also have the right to be treated with dignity and privacy.

CATHETERS

A **catheter** is a tube used to drain or inject fluid through a body opening. Inserted through the urethra into the bladder, a urinary catheter drains urine. An *indwelling catheter (retention or Foley catheter)* is left in the bladder (Fig. 17-10). Urine drains constantly into a drainage bag. Tubing connects the catheter to the drainage bag.

Catheterization is the process of inserting a catheter. It is done by a doctor or nurse. With the proper education and supervision, some states and agencies let nursing assistants insert and remove catheters.

Some people are too weak or disabled to use the bedpan, urinal, commode, or toilet. For them, catheters can promote comfort and prevent incontinence. Catheters can protect wounds and pressure ulcers from contact with urine. They also allow hourly urinary output measurements. However, they are a last resort for incontinence. Catheters do not treat the cause of incontinence.

Persons with catheters are at high risk for infection. Follow the rules in Box 17-3.

See *Delegation Guidelines: Catheters, p. 300.*
See *Promoting Safety and Comfort: Catheters, p. 300.*
Text continued on p. 302

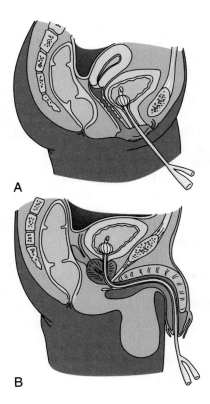

FIGURE 17-10 Indwelling catheter. **A,** Indwelling catheter in the female bladder. The inflated balloon at the tip prevents the catheter from slipping out through the urethra. **B,** Indwelling catheter with the balloon inflated in the male bladder.

BOX 17-3   Caring for Persons With Indwelling Catheters

- Follow the rules of medical asepsis.
- Follow Standard Precautions and the Bloodborne Pathogen Standard.
- Allow urine to flow freely through the catheter or tubing. Tubing should not have kinks. The person should not lie on the tubing.
- Keep the catheter connected to the drainage tubing. Follow the measures on p. 302 if the catheter and drainage tube are disconnected.
- Keep the drainage tube below the bladder. This prevents urine from flowing backward into the bladder.
- Move the bag to the other side of the bed when the person is turned and repositioned on his or her other side.
- Attach the drainage bag to the bed frame, back of the chair, or lower part of an IV (intravenous) pole. *Never attach the drainage bag to the bed rail.* Otherwise it is higher than the bladder when the bed rail is raised.
- Do not let the drainage bag rest on the floor. This can contaminate the system.
- Coil the drainage tubing on the bed. Secure it to the bottom linen (Fig. 17-11). Follow agency policy. Use a clip, bed sheet clamp, tape, safety pin with rubber band, or other device as directed by the nurse. Tubing must not loop below the drainage bag.
- Secure the catheter to the inner thigh (see Fig. 17-11). Or secure it to the man's abdomen. This prevents excess catheter movement and friction at the insertion site. Secure the catheter with a tube holder, tape, or other devices as the nurse directs.
- Check for leaks. Check the site where the catheter connects to the drainage bag. Report any leaks to the nurse at once.
- Provide catheter care daily, twice a day, after bowel movements, or when vaginal discharge is present. (See procedure: *Giving Catheter Care,* p. 301.) Some agencies consider perineal care to be sufficient. Follow the care plan.
- Provide perineal care daily or twice a day, after bowel movements, and when there is vaginal drainage. Follow the care plan.
- Empty the drainage bag at the end of the shift or as the nurse directs. Measure and record the amount of urine (see procedure: *Emptying a Urinary Drainage Bag,* p. 303). Report an increase or decrease in the amount of urine.
- Use a separate measuring container for each person. This prevents the spread of microbes from one person to another.
- Do not let the drain on the drainage bag touch any surface.
- Report complaints to the nurse at once—pain, burning, the need to void, or irritation. Also report the color, clarity, and odor of urine and the presence of particles.
- Encourage fluid intake as directed by the nurse and the care plan.

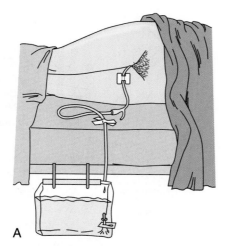 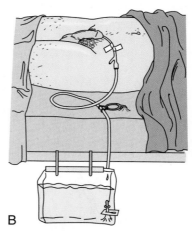

FIGURE 17-11 Securing catheters. **A,** The drainage tube is coiled on the bed and secured to the bottom linens. The catheter is secured to the inner thigh with tape. Drainage tubing is secured to bottom linens with tape. **B,** The catheter is secured to the man's abdomen with a tube holder. Drainage tubing is secured to bottom linens with a clamp.

DELEGATION GUIDELINES
Catheters

The nurse may delegate catheter care to you. If so, you need this information from the nurse and the care plan:

- When to give catheter care—daily, twice a day, after bowel movements, or when vaginal discharge is present
- Where to secure the catheter—thigh or abdomen
- How to secure the catheter—tube holder, tape, or other device
- How to secure drainage tubing—clip, bed sheet clamp, tape, safety pin with rubber band, or other device
- What observations to report and record:
  - Complaints of pain, burning, irritation, or the need to void (report at once)
  - Crusting, abnormal drainage, or secretions
  - The color, clarity, and odor of urine
  - Particles in the urine
  - Urine leaking at the insertion site
  - Drainage system leaks
- When to report observations
- What specific patient or resident concerns to report at once

PROMOTING SAFETY AND COMFORT
Catheters

Safety

Urine may contain microbes and blood. Follow Standard Precautions and the Bloodborne Pathogen Standard.

Be very careful when using a safety pin and rubber band to secure the drainage tubing to the bottom linens:

- The safety pin must work properly. It must not be stretched out of shape.
- The rubber band must be intact. It should not be frayed or over-stretched.
- Do not insert the pin through the catheter.
- Point the pin away from the person.

Comfort

The catheter must not pull at the insertion site. This causes discomfort and irritation. Hold the catheter securely during catheter care. Then properly secure the catheter. Make sure the tubing is not under the person. Besides obstructing urine flow, lying on the tubing is uncomfortable. It can also cause skin breakdown. To promote comfort, see Box 17-3.

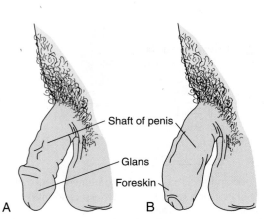

FIGURE 17-12 **A,** Circumcised male. **B,** Uncircumcised male.

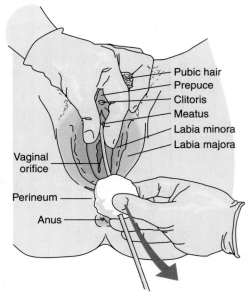

FIGURE 17-13 The catheter is cleaned starting at the meatus. About 4 inches of the catheter is cleaned.

GIVING CATHETER CARE

QUALITY OF LIFE

Remember to:
- Knock before entering the person's room.
- Address the person by name.
- Introduce yourself by name and title.

- Explain the procedure to the person before beginning and during the procedure.
- Protect the person's rights during the procedure.
- Handle the person gently during the procedure.

PRE-PROCEDURE

1   Follow *Delegation Guidelines:*
    a   *Perineal Care* (Chapter 15)
    b   *Catheters*
    See *Promoting Safety and Comfort:*
    a   *Perineal Care* (Chapter 15)
    b   *Catheters*
2   Practice hand hygiene.
3   Collect the following:
    - Items for perineal care (Chapter 15)
    - Gloves
    - Bath blanket
4   Cover the overbed table with paper towels. Arrange items on top of them.

5   Identify the person. Check the ID bracelet against the assignment sheet. Also call the person by name.
6   Provide for privacy.
7   Fill the wash basin. Water temperature is about 105° F (Fahrenheit) (40.5° C [centigrade]). Measure water temperature according to agency policy. Ask the person to check the water temperature. Adjust water temperature as needed.
8   Raise the bed for body mechanics. Bed rails are up if used.

PROCEDURE

9   Lower the bed rail near you if up.
10 Decontaminate your hands. Put on the gloves.
11 Cover the person with a bath blanket. Fan-fold top linens to the foot of the bed.
12 Drape the person for perineal care (Chapter 15).
13 Fold back the bath blanket to expose the genital area.
14 Place the waterproof pad under the buttocks. Ask the person to flex the knees and raise the buttocks off the bed.
15 Separate the labia (female). In an uncircumcised male, retract the foreskin (Fig. 17-12). Check for crusts, abnormal drainage, or secretions.
16 Give perineal care (Chapter 15).
17 Apply soap to a clean, wet washcloth.
18 Hold the catheter near the meatus.
19 Clean the catheter from the meatus down the catheter about 4 inches (Fig. 17-13). Clean downward, away from the meatus with 1 stroke. Do not tug or pull on the catheter. Repeat as needed with a clean area of the washcloth. Use a clean washcloth if needed.

20 Rinse the catheter with a clean washcloth. Rinse from the meatus down the catheter about 4 inches. Rinse downward, away from the meatus with 1 stroke. Do not tug or pull on the catheter. Repeat as needed with a clean area of the washcloth. Use a clean washcloth if needed.
21 Dry the catheter with a towel. Dry from the meatus down the catheter about 4 inches. Do not tug or pull on the catheter.
22 Pat dry the perineal area. Dry from front to back.
23 Return the foreskin to its natural position.
24 Secure the catheter. Coil and secure tubing (see Fig. 17-11).
25 Remove the waterproof pad.
26 Cover the person. Remove the bath blanket.
27 Remove the gloves. Practice hand hygiene.

POST-PROCEDURE

28 Provide for comfort. (See the inside of the front book cover.)
29 Place the signal light within reach.
30 Lower the bed to its lowest position.
31 Raise or lower bed rails. Follow the care plan.
32 Clean, dry, and return equipment to its proper place. Discard disposable items. (Wear gloves for this step.)

33 Unscreen the person.
34 Complete a safety check of the room. (See the inside of the front book cover.)
35 Follow agency policy for soiled linen.
36 Remove the gloves. Practice hand hygiene.
37 Report and record your observations.

Drainage Systems

A closed drainage system is used for indwelling catheters. Nothing can enter the system from the catheter to the drainage bag. The urinary system is sterile. Infection can occur if microbes enter the drainage system. The microbes travel up the tubing or catheter into the bladder and kidneys. A urinary tract infection can threaten health and life.

The drainage system has tubing and a drainage bag. Tubing attaches at one end to the catheter. At the other end, it attaches to the drainage bag.

The bag hangs from the bed frame, chair, or wheelchair. It must not touch the floor. The bag is always kept lower than the person's bladder (see Fig. 17-11).

Microbes can grow in urine. If the drainage bag is higher than the bladder, urine can flow back into the bladder. An infection can occur. *Therefore do not hang the drainage bag on a bed rail.* Otherwise when the bed rail is raised, the bag is higher than bladder level. When the person walks, the bag is held lower than the bladder.

Sometimes drainage systems are disconnected accidentally. If that happens, tell the nurse at once. Do not touch the ends of the catheter or tubing. Do the following:

- Practice hand hygiene. Put on gloves.
- Wipe the end of the tube with an antiseptic wipe.
- Wipe the end of the catheter with another antiseptic wipe.
- Do not put the ends down. Do not touch the ends after you clean them.
- Connect the tubing to the catheter.
- Discard the wipes into a biohazard bag.
- Remove the gloves. Practice hand hygiene.
  See *Delegation Guidelines: Drainage Systems.*
  See *Promoting Safety and Comfort: Drainage Systems.*

DELEGATION GUIDELINES
Drainage Systems

Your delegated tasks may involve urinary drainage systems. If so, you need this information from the nurse and the care plan:
- When to empty the drainage bag
- If the person uses a leg bag
- When to switch a drainage bag and leg bag
- If you should clean or discard the drainage bag
- What observations to report and record:
  - The amount of urine measured
  - The color, clarity, and odor of urine
  - Particles in the urine
  - Complaints of pain, burning, irritation, or the need to urinate
  - Drainage system leaks
- When to report observations
- What specific patient or resident concerns to report at once

---

PROMOTING SAFETY AND COMFORT
Drainage Systems

Safety
Urine may contain microbes and blood. Follow Standard Precautions and the Bloodborne Pathogen Standard.

A leg bag attaches to the thigh or calf (p. 304). Leg bags hold less than 1000 mL of urine. Most standard drainage bags hold at least 2000 mL of urine. Therefore leg bags fill faster than standard drainage bags. Check leg bags often. Empty the leg bag if it is becoming half full. Measure the contents.

Comfort
Having urine in a drainage bag embarrasses some people. Visitors can see the urine when they are with the person. To promote mental comfort, have visitors sit on the side away from the drainage bag. Sometimes you can empty the bag before visitors arrive. Make sure you measure, report, and record the amount of urine.

Some agencies provide drainage bag holders. The drainage bag is placed inside the holder. Urine cannot be seen.

EMPTYING A URINARY DRAINAGE BAG

QUALITY OF LIFE

Remember to:
- Knock before entering the person's room.
- Address the person by name.
- Introduce yourself by name and title.

- Explain the procedure to the person before beginning and during the procedure.
- Protect the person's rights during the procedure.
- Handle the person gently during the procedure.

PRE-PROCEDURE

1 Follow *Delegation Guidelines: Drainage Systems.* See *Promoting Safety and Comfort: Drainage Systems.*
2 Collect the following:
   - Graduate (measuring container)
   - Gloves
   - Paper towels

3 Practice hand hygiene.
4 Identify the person. Check the ID bracelet against the assignment sheet. Call the person by name.
5 Provide for privacy.

PROCEDURE

6 Put on the gloves.
7 Place a paper towel on the floor. Place the graduate on top of it.
8 Position the graduate under the collection bag.
9 Open the clamp on the drain.
10 Let all urine drain into the graduate. Do not let the drain touch the graduate (Fig. 17-14).
11 Close and position the clamp (see Fig. 17-11).
12 Measure urine.
13 Remove and discard the paper towel.

14 Empty the contents of the graduate into the toilet and flush.
15 Rinse the graduate. Empty the rinse into the toilet and flush.
16 Clean and disinfect the graduate.
17 Return the graduate to its proper place.
18 Remove the gloves. Practice hand hygiene.
19 Record the time and amount on the intake and output (I&O) record (Chapter 20).

POST-PROCEDURE

20 Provide for comfort. (See the inside of the front book cover.)
21 Place the signal light within reach.
22 Unscreen the person.

23 Complete a safety check of the room. (See the inside of the front book cover.)
24 Report and record the amount and other observations.

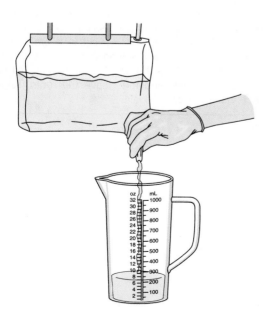

FIGURE 17-14 The clamp on the drainage bag is opened. The drain is directed into the graduate. The drain must not touch the inside of the graduate.

Condom Catheters

Condom catheters are often used for incontinent men. They also are called *external catheters*, *Texas catheters*, and *urinary sheaths*. A condom catheter is a soft sheath that slides over the penis. Tubing connects the condom catheter and the drainage bag. Many men prefer leg bags (Fig. 17-15).

Condom catheters are changed daily after perineal care. To apply a condom catheter, follow the manufacturer's instruction. Thoroughly wash the penis with soap and water. Then dry it before applying the catheter.

Some condom catheters are self-adhering. Adhesive inside the catheter adheres to the penis. Other catheters are secured in place with elastic tape. Use the elastic tape packaged with the catheter. Elastic tape expands when the penis changes size. This allows blood flow to the penis. *Never use adhesive tape to secure catheters. It does not expand. Blood flow to the penis is cut off, injuring the penis.*

See *Delegation Guidelines: Condom Catheters.*

See *Promoting Safety and Comfort: Condom Catheters.*

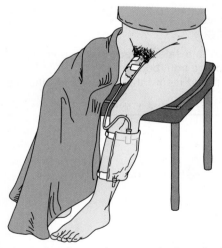

FIGURE 17-15 Condom catheter attached to a leg bag.

DELEGATION GUIDELINES
Condom Catheters

Before removing or applying a condom catheter, you need this information from the nurse and the care plan:
- What size to use—small, medium, or large
- When to remove the catheter and apply a new one
- If a leg bag or standard drainage system is used
- What observations to report and record:
  - Reddened or open areas on the penis
  - Swelling of the penis
  - Color, clarity, and odor of urine
  - Particles in the urine
- When to report observations
- What specific patient or resident concerns to report at once

---

PROMOTING SAFETY AND COMFORT
Condom Catheters

Safety

Do not apply a condom catheter if the penis is red, irritated, or shows signs of skin breakdown. Report your observations to the nurse at once.

If you do not know how to use the condom catheters used at your agency, ask the nurse to show you the correct application. Then ask the nurse to observe you applying the catheter.

Blood must flow to the penis. If tape is needed, use elastic tape packaged with the catheter. Apply it in a spiral.

Urine may contain microbes and blood. Follow Standard Precautions and the Bloodborne Pathogen Standard.

Comfort

To apply a condom catheter, you need to touch and handle the penis. This can embarrass the man. Some men become sexually aroused. Always act in a professional manner. If necessary, allow the man some privacy. Provide for his safety and place the urinal within reach. Tell him when you will return, and then leave the room. Knock before entering the room again.

APPLYING A CONDOM CATHETER

QUALITY OF LIFE

Remember to:
- Knock before entering the person's room.
- Address the person by name.
- Introduce yourself by name and title.
- Explain the procedure to the person before beginning and during the procedure.
- Protect the person's rights during the procedure.
- Handle the person gently during the procedure.

PRE-PROCEDURE

1 Follow *Delegation Guidelines:*
  a *Perineal Care* (Chapter 15)
  b *Condom Catheters*
  See *Promoting Safety and Comfort:*
  a *Perineal Care* (Chapter 15)
  b *Condom Catheters*
2 Practice hand hygiene.
3 Collect the following:
  - Condom catheter
  - Elastic tape
  - Drainage bag or leg bag
  - Cap for the drainage bag
  - Basin of warm water
  - Soap
  - Towel and washcloths
  - Bath blanket
  - Gloves
  - Waterproof pad
  - Paper towels
4 Arrange paper towels and equipment on the over-bed table.
5 Identify the person. Check the ID bracelet against the assignment sheet. Also call the person by name.
6 Provide for privacy.
7 Raise the bed for body mechanics. Bed rails are up if used.

PROCEDURE

8 Lower the bed rail near you if up.
9 Practice hand hygiene. Put on the gloves.
10 Cover the person with a bath blanket. Lower top linens to the knees.
11 Ask the person to raise his buttocks off the bed. Or turn him onto his side away from you.
12 Slide the waterproof pad under his buttocks.
13 Have the person lower his buttocks. Or turn him onto his back.
14 Secure the drainage bag to the bed frame. Or have a leg bag ready. Close the drain.
15 Expose the genital area.
16 Remove the condom catheter.
  a Remove the tape. Roll the sheath off the penis.
  b Disconnect the drainage tubing from the condom. Cap the drainage tube.
  c Discard the tape and condom.
17 Provide perineal care (Chapter 15). Observe the penis for reddened areas, skin breakdown, and irritation.
18 Remove the gloves, and practice hand hygiene. Put on clean gloves.

19 Remove the protective backing from the condom. This exposes the adhesive strip.
20 Hold the penis firmly. Roll the condom onto the penis. Leave a 1-inch space between the penis and the end of the catheter (Fig. 17-16).
21 Secure the condom.
  a For a self-adhering condom: press the condom to the penis.
  b For a condom secured with elastic tape: apply elastic tape in a spiral. See Figure 17-16. Do not apply tape completely around the penis.
22 Make sure the penis tip does not touch the condom. Make sure the condom is not twisted.
23 Connect the condom to the drainage tubing. Coil and secure excess tubing on the bed. Or attach a leg bag.
24 Remove the waterproof pad and gloves. Discard them. Practice hand hygiene.
25 Cover the person. Remove the bath blanket.

POST-PROCEDURE

26 Provide comfort. (See the inside of the front book cover.)
27 Place the signal light within reach.
28 Lower the bed to its lowest position.
29 Raise or lower bed rails. Follow the care plan.
30 Unscreen the person.
31 Practice hand hygiene. Put on clean gloves.
32 Measure and record the amount of urine in the bag. Clean or discard the collection bag.

33 Clean, dry, and return the wash basin and other equipment. Return items to their proper place.
34 Remove the gloves. Practice hand hygiene.
35 Complete a safety check of the room. (See the inside of the front book cover.)
36 Report and record your observations.

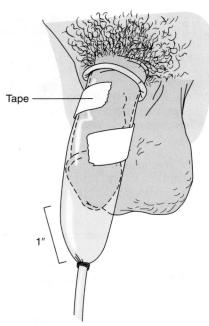

FIGURE 17-16 A condom catheter applied to the penis. A 1-inch space is between the penis and the end of the catheter. Elastic tape is applied in a spiral fashion to secure the condom catheter to the penis.

BLADDER TRAINING

Bladder training helps some persons with urinary incontinence. Some persons need bladder training after indwelling catheter removal. Control of urination is the goal. Bladder control promotes comfort and quality of life. It also increases self-esteem. You assist with bladder training as directed by the nurse and the care plan.

There are two basic methods for bladder training:

- The person uses the toilet, commode, bedpan, or urinal at certain times. The person is given 15 or 20 minutes to start voiding. The rules for normal elimination are followed. The normal position for urination is assumed if possible. Privacy is important.
- The person has a catheter. The catheter is clamped to prevent urine flow from the bladder (Fig. 17-17). It is usually clamped for 1 hour at first. Over time, it is clamped for 3 to 4 hours. Urine drains when the catheter is unclamped. When the catheter is removed, voiding is encouraged every 3 to 4 hours or as directed by the nurse and the care plan.

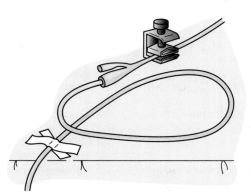

FIGURE 17-17 The clamped catheter prevents urine from draining out of the bladder. The clamp is applied directly to the catheter—not to the drainage tube.

Focus on P R I D E
The Person, Family, and Yourself

Personal and Professional Responsibility—You are responsible for reporting and recording what you have done and observed. When assisting with elimination, accurate reporting and recording are important. The nurse needs correct information about urine appearance, odor, and amount. Changes in urination may lead to changes in the person's care. Report urinary problems and abnormal urine to the nurse. If you are unsure what to report or record, ask the nurse.

Rights and Respect—People usually void in private. Illness, disease, and aging can affect this very private act. Respect the person's right to privacy. Allow as much privacy as safely possible. Follow the nurse's directions and the care plan.

Empty urinals, bedpans, and commodes promptly. Leaving urine-filled devices in the person's room does not respect the person's right to a neat and clean setting. It also may cause embarrassment. Do your best to promote comfort, dignity, and respect when assisting with elimination needs.

Independence and Social Interaction—Some persons can place bedpans and urinals themselves. Some can get on and off bedside commodes themselves. Other persons need some help but can be left alone to void. Allow persons to do as much as safely possible.

To safely promote independence, keep devices within reach for persons who use them without help. For persons who need some help, check on them often. Do not leave a person sitting on a bedpan or commode for a long time. Discomfort, odors, and skin breakdown are likely. Also, the person may think you forgot about him or her. The person may try to get off of the bedpan or commode alone. He or she may be harmed. Make sure the signal light is within reach. Respond promptly when a person calls for help.

Delegation and Teamwork—A person's need to void may be urgent. Waiting to urinate may cause incontinence. Then the person is wet and embarrassed. He or she is at risk for skin breakdown and infection. Also, you have extra work changing linens and garments.

Work as a team to help all persons with elimination needs as soon as possible. Answer signal lights promptly. Do so for co-workers as well. If a co-worker is busy, assist the person yourself. You may need to find out how much help the person needs. Some patients or residents can tell you themselves. Ask the nurse if you are unsure. You like help when you are busy. So do your co-workers.

Ethics and Laws—Each state has a nurse practice act. It regulates nursing practice in that state. The act is used to decide what nursing assistants can do in that state. The purpose is to protect the public's welfare and safety. Some states allow nursing assistants to insert a catheter into the bladder. If your state and agency allow you to insert urinary catheters:

- The procedure must be in your job description.
- You must have the necessary education and training.
- You must know how to use the agency's supplies and equipment.
- A nurse must be available to answer questions and supervise you.

REVIEW QUESTIONS

Circle the BEST answer.

1 Which is *false*?
   a Urine is normally clear and yellow or amber in color.
   b Urine normally has an ammonia odor.
   c Voiding usually occurs before going to bed and after sleep.
   d A person normally voids 1500 mL a day.

2 Which is *not* a rule for normal elimination?
   a Help the person assume a normal position for voiding.
   b Provide for privacy.
   c Help the person to the bathroom or commode. Or provide the bedpan or urinal as soon as requested.
   d Stay with the person who uses the bedpan.

3 The person using a standard bedpan is in
   a Fowler's position
   b The supine position
   c The prone position
   d The side-lying position

4 After using the urinal, the man should
   a Put it on the bedside stand
   b Use the signal light
   c Put it on the overbed table
   d Empty it

5 Urinary incontinence
   a Is always permanent
   b Requires good skin care
   c Is treated with a catheter
   d Requires bladder training

6 Which is *not* a cause of functional incontinence?
   a Unanswered signal light
   b No signal light within reach
   c Problems removing clothing
   d Urinary tract infection

7 A person has a catheter. Which is *not* correct?
   a Keep the drainage bag above the level of the bladder.
   b Keep drainage tubing free of kinks.
   c Coil the drainage tubing on the bed.
   d Secure the catheter according to agency policy.

8 A person has a catheter. Which is *not* correct?
   a Tape any leaks at the connection site.
   b Follow Standard Precautions and the Bloodborne Pathogen Standard.
   c Empty the drainage bag at the end of your shift.
   d Report complaints of pain, burning, the need to void, or irritation at once.

9 A person has a catheter. You are going to turn the person from the left side to the right side. What should you do with the drainage bag?
   a Move it to the right side.
   b Keep it on the left side.
   c Hang it from an IV pole.
   d Remove the catheter and the drainage bag.

10 When giving catheter care, you clean the catheter
   a From the meatus down the catheter about 4 inches
   b From the meatus down the entire catheter
   c From the drainage tube connection up the catheter to the meatus
   d From the drainage tube connection up the catheter about 4 inches

11 Mr. Cooper has a condom catheter. You apply elastic tape
   a Completely around the penis
   b To the inner thigh
   c To the abdomen
   d In a spiral fashion

12 The goal of bladder training is to
   a Remove the catheter
   b Allow the person to walk to the bathroom
   c Gain control of urination
   d Have the person void twice a day

Answers to these questions are on p. 528.

18

ASSISTING WITH BOWEL ELIMINATION

PROCEDURES

 Giving a Cleansing Enema
 Giving a Small-Volume Enema

OBJECTIVES

- Define the key terms and key abbreviations listed in this chapter.
- Describe normal defecation and the observations to report.
- Identify the factors that affect bowel elimination.
- Describe the common bowel elimination problems.
- Explain how to promote comfort and safety during defecation.
- Describe bowel training.
- Explain why enemas are given.
- Describe the common enema solutions.
- Describe the rules for giving enemas.
- Describe how to care for a person with an ostomy.
- Explain how to promote PRIDE in the person, the family, and yourself.
- Perform the procedures described in this chapter.

KEY TERMS

colostomy A surgically created opening (*stomy*) between the colon (*colo*) and abdominal wall

constipation The passage of a hard, dry stool

defecation The process of excreting feces from the rectum through the anus; a bowel movement

diarrhea The frequent passage of liquid stools

enema The introduction of fluid into the rectum and lower colon

fecal impaction The prolonged retention and buildup of feces in the rectum

fecal incontinence The inability to control the passage of feces and gas through the anus

feces The semi-solid mass of waste products in the colon that is expelled through the anus

flatulence The excessive formation of gas or air in the stomach and intestines

flatus Gas or air passed through the anus

ileostomy A surgically created opening (*stomy*) between the ileum (small intestine [*ileo*]) and the abdominal wall

ostomy A surgically created opening; see "colostomy" and "ileostomy"

stoma An opening; see "colostomy" and "ileostomy"

stool Excreted feces

suppository A cone-shaped, solid drug that is inserted into a body opening; it melts at body temperature

KEY ABBREVIATIONS

BM Bowel movement

C Centigrade

F Fahrenheit

ID Identification

IV Intravenous

mL Milliliter

oz Ounce

SSE Soapsuds enema

Bowel elimination is a basic physical need. Wastes are excreted from the gastro-intestinal system (Chapter 6). You assist patients and residents in meeting their elimination needs.

NORMAL BOWEL ELIMINATION

Some people have a bowel movement (BM) every day. Others have one every 2 to 3 days. Some people have 2 or 3 BMs a day. Many people have a BM after breakfast. Others do so in the evening.

To assist with bowel elimination, you need to know these terms:

- **Defecation**—the process of excreting feces from the rectum through the anus (bowel movement)
- **Feces**—the semi-solid mass of waste products in the colon that is expelled through the anus
- **Stool**—excreted feces

Observations

Stools are normally brown. Bleeding in the stomach and small intestine causes black or tarry stools. Bleeding in the lower colon and rectum causes red-colored stools. Diseases and infection can cause clay-colored or white, pale, orange-colored, or green-colored stools.

Stools are normally soft, formed, moist, and shaped like the rectum. They normally have an odor.

Carefully observe stools before disposing of them. Ask the nurse to observe abnormal stools. Observe and report the following to the nurse:

- Color
- Amount
- Consistency
- Presence of blood or mucus
- Odor
- Shape and size
- Frequency of defecation
- Complaints of pain or discomfort
  See *Focus on Communication: Observations.*

FOCUS ON COMMUNICATION
Observations

Many patients and residents tend to their own bowel elimination needs. However, information is still needed for the person's record and the nursing process. You may need to ask these questions:

- "Did you have a bowel movement today?"
- "Did you have more than one bowel movement today? If so, how many?"
- "What was the amount?"
- "Were the stools formed or loose?"
- "What was the color?"
- "Did you have any bleeding, pain, or problems having a bowel movement?"
- "Did you pass any gas?"
- "Do you feel that you need to pass more gas?"
- "Are you having any pain or discomfort now?"
- "Do you need help cleaning yourself?"

FACTORS AFFECTING BOWEL ELIMINATION

These factors affect stool frequency, consistency, color, and odor. The nurse considers them when using the nursing process to meet the person's elimination needs. Normal, regular elimination is the goal.

- *Privacy.* Lack of privacy can prevent a BM despite having the urge. Odors and sounds are embarrassing. Some people ignore the urge when others are present.
- *Habits.* Many people have a BM after breakfast. Some drink a hot beverage, read, or take a walk. These activities are relaxing. A BM is easier when a person is relaxed, not tense.
- *Diet—high-fiber foods.* High-fiber foods leave a residue for needed bulk and prevent constipation. Fruits, vegetables, and whole grain cereals and breads are high in fiber. Some people cannot chew these foods. They may not have teeth or dentures may fit poorly. In nursing centers, bran is added to cereal, prunes, or prune juice.
- *Diet—other foods.* Milk and milk products cause constipation or diarrhea. Chocolate and other foods cause similar reactions. Spicy foods can cause frequent stools or diarrhea. Gas-forming foods stimulate peristalsis, aiding defecation. Such foods include onions, beans, cabbage, cauliflower, radishes, and cucumbers.
- *Fluids.* Feces contain water. Stool consistency depends on the amount of water absorbed in the colon. Feces harden and dry when large amounts of water are absorbed or when fluid intake is poor. Hard, dry feces move slowly through the colon. Constipation can occur. Drinking 6 to 8 glasses of water daily promotes normal bowel elimination. Warm fluids—coffee, tea, hot cider, warm water—increase peristalsis.
- *Activity.* Exercise and activity maintain muscle tone and stimulate peristalsis.
- *Drugs.* Drugs can prevent constipation or control diarrhea. Other drugs have diarrhea or constipation as side effects.
- *Disability.* Some people cannot control BMs. They have a BM whenever feces enter the rectum. A bowel training program is needed (p. 313).
- *Aging.* Aging causes changes in the gastrointestinal tract. Feces pass through the intestines at a slower rate. Constipation is a risk. Some older persons lose bowel control (see "Fecal Incontinence," p. 312).

BOX 18-1   Safety and Comfort During Bowel Elimination

- Provide for privacy. Ask visitors to leave the room. Close doors and privacy curtains. Also close window coverings.
- Help the person to the toilet or commode. Or provide the bedpan as soon as requested.
- Wheel the person into the bathroom on the commode if possible. Place the commode over the toilet. This provides privacy. Remember to lock the commode wheels.
- Make sure the bedpan is warm.
- Position the person in a normal sitting or squatting position.
- Cover the person for warmth and privacy.
- Allow enough time for a BM.
- Place the signal light and toilet tissue within reach.
- Leave the room if the person can be alone. Check on the person every 5 minutes.
- Stay nearby if the person is weak or unsteady.
- Provide perineal care.
- Dispose of stools promptly. This reduces odors and prevents the spread of microbes.
- Assist the person with hand washing after elimination.
- Follow the care plan if the person has fecal incontinence. The care plan tells you when to assist with elimination.
- Follow Standard Precautions and the Bloodborne Pathogen Standard.

Safety and Comfort

The care plan includes measures to meet the person's elimination needs. It may involve diet, fluids, and exercise. Follow the measures in Box 18-1 to promote safety and comfort.

COMMON PROBLEMS

Common problems include constipation, fecal impaction, diarrhea, fecal incontinence, and flatulence.

Constipation

Constipation is the passage of a hard, dry stool. The person usually strains to have a bowel movement. Stools are large or marble-size. Large stools cause pain as they pass through the anus. Constipation occurs when feces move slowly through the bowel.

This allows more time for water absorption. Common causes of constipation include:
- A low-fiber diet
- Ignoring the urge to have a BM
- Decreased fluid intake
- Inactivity
- Drugs
- Aging
- Certain diseases

Diet changes, fluids, and activity prevent or relieve constipation. So do drugs and enemas.

Fecal Impaction

A **fecal impaction** is the prolonged retention and buildup of feces in the rectum. Feces are hard or putty-like. Fecal impaction results if constipation is not relieved. The person cannot have a BM. More water is absorbed from the already hard feces. Liquid feces pass around the hardened fecal mass in the rectum. The liquid feces seep from the anus.

The person tries many times to have a BM. Abdominal discomfort, abdominal distention (swelling), nausea, cramping, and rectal pain are common. Older persons may have poor appetite or confusion. Some persons may have a fever. Report these signs and symptoms to the nurse.

Diarrhea

Diarrhea is the frequent passage of liquid stools. Feces move through the intestines rapidly. This reduces the time for fluid absorption. The BM need is urgent. Some people cannot get to a bathroom in time. Abdominal cramping, nausea, and vomiting may occur.

Causes of diarrhea include infections, some drugs, irritating foods, and microbes in food and water. Diet and drugs are ordered to reduce peristalsis. You need to:
- Assist with elimination needs promptly.
- Dispose of stools promptly. This prevents odors and the spread of microbes.
- Give good skin care. Liquid stools irritate the skin. So does frequent wiping with toilet tissue. Skin breakdown and pressure ulcers are risks.
- Follow Standard Precautions and the Bloodborne Pathogen Standard when in contact with stools.

The amount of body water decreases with aging. Report signs of diarrhea at once. Ask the nurse to observe the stool.

See *Promoting Safety and Comfort: Diarrhea.*

PROMOTING SAFETY AND COMFORT
Diarrhea

Clostridium difficile (C. difficile) is a microbe that causes diarrhea and intestinal infections. It can cause death. Persons at risk include persons who are older, ill, or need the prolonged use of antibiotics. Signs and symptoms include:
- Watery diarrhea
- Fever
- Loss of appetite
- Nausea
- Abdominal pain or tenderness

The microbe is found in feces. A person becomes infected by touching items or surfaces contaminated with feces and then touching his or her mouth or mucous membranes. You can spread the microbe if your contaminated hands or gloves:
- Touch a person
- Contaminate surfaces

You must practice good hand hygiene. Also follow Standard Precautions.

PERSONS WITH DEMENTIA
Fecal Incontinence

Persons with dementia may not feel the urge to have a BM. Some are not aware of having a BM. They may smear stools on themselves, furniture, and walls. Some resist care. Follow the person's care plan. The measures for urinary incontinence (Chapter 17) may be part of the care plan. Be patient. Ask for help from co-workers. Talk to the nurse if you have problems keeping the person clean.

Fecal Incontinence

Fecal incontinence is the inability to control the passage of feces and gas through the anus. Causes include intestinal diseases and nervous system diseases and injuries. Fecal impaction, diarrhea, some drugs, and aging are other causes. So are unanswered signal lights.

Fecal incontinence affects the person emotionally. Frustration, embarrassment, anger, and humiliation are common. The person may need:
- Bowel training
- Help with elimination after meals and every 2 to 3 hours
- Incontinence products to keep garments and linens clean
- Good skin care

See *Persons With Dementia: Fecal Incontinence.*

Flatulence

Gas and air are normally in the stomach and intestines. They are expelled through the mouth (burping, belching, eructating) and anus. Gas or air passed through the anus is called **flatus**. **Flatulence** is the excessive formation of gas or air in the stomach and intestines. Causes include:

* Swallowing air while eating and drinking
* Bacterial action in the intestines
* Gas-forming foods (p. 311)
* Constipation
* Bowel and abdominal surgeries
* Drugs that decrease peristalsis

If flatus is not expelled, the intestines distend. That is, they swell or enlarge from the pressure of gases. Abdominal cramping or pain, shortness of breath, and a swollen abdomen occur. "Bloating" is a common complaint. Exercise, walking, moving in bed, and the left side-lying position often produce flatus. Doctors may order enemas and drugs to relieve flatulence.

BOWEL TRAINING

Bowel training has two goals:

* To gain control of bowel movements.
* To develop a regular pattern of elimination. Fecal impaction, constipation, and fecal incontinence are prevented.

Meals, especially breakfast, stimulate the urge for a BM. The person's usual time of day for a BM is noted on the care plan. So is toilet, commode, or bedpan use. Offer help with elimination at the times noted. Factors that promote elimination are part of the care plan and bowel training program.

The doctor may order a suppository to stimulate a BM. A **suppository** is a cone-shaped, solid drug that is inserted into a body opening. It melts at body temperature. A nurse inserts a rectal suppository into the rectum (Fig. 18-1). A BM occurs about 30 minutes later.

ENEMAS

An **enema** is the introduction of fluid into the rectum and lower colon. Doctors order enemas to remove feces and relieve constipation, fecal impaction, or flatulence. Sometimes enemas are given to clean the bowel of feces before certain surgeries and diagnostic procedures.

Safety and comfort measures for bowel elimination are practiced when giving an enema (see Box 18-1). So are the rules in Box 18-2, p. 314.

The doctor orders the enema solution. The solution depends on the enema's purpose:

* *Tap water enema*—obtained from a faucet.
* *Saline enema*—a solution of salt and water. For adults, add 1 to 2 teaspoons of table salt to 500 to 1000 mL (milliliters) of tap water.
* *Soapsuds enema (SSE)*—for adults, add 3 to 5 mL of castile soap to 500 to 1000 mL of tap water.
* *Small-volume enema*—the adult size contains about 120 mL (4 ounces [oz]) of solution.
* *Oil-retention enema*—mineral, olive, or cottonseed oil. The adult size contains about 120 mL (4 oz) of solution.

See *Delegation Guidelines: Enemas*, p. 314.
See *Promoting Safety and Comfort: Enemas*, p. 315.

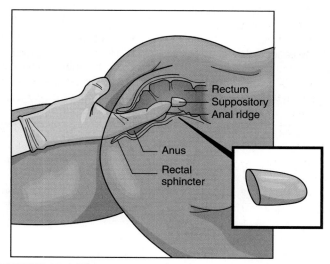

FIGURE 18-1 The suppository *(inset)* is inserted into the rectum.

BOX 18-2   Safety and Comfort Measures for Giving Enemas

- Have the person void first. This increases the person's comfort during the enema procedure.
- Measure solution temperature with a bath thermometer. See *Delegation Guidelines: Enemas.*
- Give the amount of solution ordered.
- Position the person as the nurse directs. The Sims' position or the left side-lying position is preferred.
- Ask the nurse and check the agency's procedure manual for how far to insert the enema tubing. It is usually inserted 2 to 4 inches in adults.
- Lubricate the enema tip before inserting it.
- Stop tube insertion if you feel resistance, the person complains of pain, or bleeding occurs.
- Ask the nurse how high to raise the enema bag. For adults, it is usually held 12 inches above the anus.

- Give the solution slowly. Usually it takes 10 to 15 minutes to give 750 to 1000 mL.
- Hold the enema tube in place while giving the solution.
- Ask the nurse how long the person should retain the solution. The length of time depends on the amount and type of solution.
- Make sure the bathroom will be vacant when the person needs to defecate. Make sure that another person will not use the bathroom. If the person uses the bedpan or commode, have the device ready.
- Ask the nurse to observe the enema results.

DELEGATION GUIDELINES
Enemas

Some states and agencies let nursing assistants give enemas. Others do not. Before giving an enema, make sure that:
- Your state allows you to perform the procedure.
- The procedure is in your job description.
- You have the necessary education and training.
- You review the procedure with the nurse.
- A nurse is available to answer questions and to supervise you.

If the above conditions are met, you need this information from the nurse:
- What type of enema to give—cleansing, small-volume (p. 317), or oil-retention (p. 318)
- What size enema tube to use
- When to give the enema
- How many times to repeat the enema
- The amount of solution ordered by the doctor—usually 500 to 1000 mL for a cleansing enema (for adults)
- How much castile soap to use for an SSE
- How much salt to use for a saline enema
- What the solution temperature should be—usually body temperature (98.6° F [Fahrenheit], 37° C [Centigrade]); sometimes warmer temperatures are used (105° F [40.5° C] for adults)

- How to position the person—Sims' or the left side-lying position
- How far to insert the enema tubing—usually 2 to 4 inches for adults
- How high to hold the solution container—usually 12 inches above the anus
- How fast to give the solution—750 to 1000 mL are usually given over 10 to 15 minutes
- How long the person should try to retain the solution
- What to report and record:
  - The amount of solution given
  - If you noted bleeding or resistance when inserting the tube
  - How long the person retained the enema solution
  - Color, amount, consistency, shape, and odor of stools
  - Complaints of cramping, pain, or discomfort
  - Complaints of nausea or weakness
  - How the person tolerated the procedure
- When to report observations
- What specific patient or resident concerns to report at once

PROMOTING SAFETY AND COMFORT
Enemas

Safety

Enemas are usually safe procedures. Many people give themselves enemas at home. However, enemas are dangerous for older persons and those with certain heart and kidney diseases.

Contact with stools is likely when giving enemas. They contain microbes and may contain blood. Follow Standard Precautions and the Bloodborne Pathogen Standard.

Comfort

Before starting the procedure, make sure that the bathroom is ready for the person's use. If the person will use the commode or bedpan, make sure the device is ready. Always keep a bedpan nearby in case the person starts to expel the enema solution and stools. Mental comfort is promoted when the person knows that the bathroom, commode, or bedpan is ready for his or her use.

Make sure the person is comfortable in the Sims' or left side-lying position. When comfortable, it is easier for the person to tolerate the procedure.

To prevent cramping:
- Use the correct water temperature. Cool water causes cramping.
- Give the solution slowly.

The Cleansing Enema

Cleansing enemas clean the bowel of feces and flatus. They relieve constipation and fecal impaction. They are needed before certain surgeries and diagnostic procedures. Cleansing enemas take effect in 10 to 20 minutes.

The doctor orders a tap water, saline, or soapsuds enema. The doctor may order *enemas until clear.* This means that enemas are given until the return solution is clear and free of stools. Ask the nurse how many enemas to give. Agency policy may allow repeating enemas 2 or 3 times.

View Video!

GIVING A CLEANSING ENEMA

QUALITY OF LIFE

Remember to:
- Knock before entering the person's room.
- Address the person by name.
- Introduce yourself by name and title.
- Explain the procedure to the person before beginning and during the procedure.
- Protect the person's rights during the procedure.
- Handle the person gently during the procedure.

PRE-PROCEDURE

1 Follow *Delegation Guidelines: Enemas.*
   See *Promoting Safety and Comfort: Enemas.*
2 Practice hand hygiene.
3 Collect the following before going to the person's room:
   - Disposable enema kit as directed by the nurse (enema bag, tube, clamp, and waterproof pad)
   - Bath thermometer
   - Waterproof pad (if not in the enema kit)
   - Water soluble lubricant
   - 3 to 5 mL (1 teaspoon) of castile soap or 1 to 2 teaspoons of salt
   - IV (intravenous) pole
   - Gloves
4 Arrange items in the person's room and bathroom.

5 Decontaminate your hands.
6 Identify the person. Check the ID (identification) bracelet against the assignment sheet. Also call the person by name.
7 Put on gloves.
8 Collect the following:
   - Commode or bedpan and cover
   - Toilet tissue
   - Bath blanket
   - Robe and non-skid footwear
   - Paper towels
9 Provide for privacy.
10 Raise the bed for body mechanics. Bed rails are up if used.

Continued

GIVING A CLEANSING ENEMA—cont'd

PROCEDURE

11 Lower the bed rail near you if up.

12 Remove the gloves, and decontaminate your hands. Put on clean gloves.

13 Cover the person with a bath blanket. Fan-fold top linens to the foot of the bed.

14 Position the IV pole so the enema bag is 12 inches above the anus. Or it is at the height directed by the nurse.

15 Raise the bed rail if used.

16 Prepare the enema:
  a Close the clamp on the tube.
  b Adjust water flow until it is lukewarm.
  c Fill the enema bag for the amount ordered.
  d Measure water temperature with the bath thermometer. The nurse tells you what temperature to use.
  e Prepare the solution as directed by the nurse:
   (1) Tap water: add nothing
   (2) Saline enema: add salt as directed
   (3) Soapsuds enema: add castile soap as directed
  f Stir the solution with the bath thermometer. Scoop off any suds (SSE).
  g Seal the bag.
  h Hang the bag on the IV pole.

17 Lower the bed rail near you if up.

18 Position the person in Sims' position or in a left side-lying position.

19 Place a waterproof pad under the buttocks.

20 Expose the anal area.

21 Place the bedpan behind the person.

22 Position the enema tube in the bedpan. Remove the cap from the tubing.

23 Open the clamp. Let solution flow through the tube to remove air. Clamp the tube.

24 Lubricate the tube 2 to 4 inches from the tip.

25 Separate the buttocks to see the anus.

26 Ask the person to take a deep breath through the mouth.

27 Insert the tube gently 2 to 4 inches into the adult's rectum (Fig. 18-2). Do this when the person is exhaling. Stop if the person complains of pain, you feel resistance, or bleeding occurs.

28 Check the amount of solution in the bag.

29 Unclamp the tube. Give the solution slowly (Fig. 18-3).

30 Ask the person to take slow deep breaths. This helps the person relax.

31 Clamp the tube if the person needs to defecate, has cramping, or starts to expel solution. Also clamp the tube if the person is sweating or complains of nausea or weakness. Unclamp when symptoms subside.

32 Give the amount of solution ordered. Stop if the person cannot tolerate the procedure.

33 Clamp the tube before it is empty. This prevents air from entering the bowel.

34 Hold toilet tissue around the tube and against the anus. Remove the tube.

35 Discard toilet tissue into the bedpan.

36 Wrap the tubing tip with paper towels. Place it inside the enema bag.

37 Assist the person to the bathroom or commode. The person wears a robe and non-skid footwear when up. The bed is in the lowest position. Or help the person onto the bedpan. Raise the head of the bed. Raise or lower bed rails according to the care plan.

38 Place the signal light and toilet tissue within reach. Remind the person not to flush the toilet.

39 Discard disposable items.

40 Remove the gloves. Practice hand hygiene.

41 Leave the room if the person can be left alone.

42 Return when the person signals. Or check on the person every 5 minutes. Knock before entering the room or bathroom.

43 Decontaminate your hands, and put on gloves. Lower the bed rail if up.

44 Observe enema results for amount, color, consistency, shape, and odor. Call the nurse to observe the results.

45 Provide perineal care as needed.

46 Remove the waterproof pad.

47 Empty, clean, and disinfect equipment. Flush the toilet after the nurse observes the results.

48 Return equipment to its proper place.

49 Remove the gloves, and practice hand hygiene.

50 Assist with hand washing. Wear gloves for this step.

51 Cover the person. Remove the bath blanket.

POST-PROCEDURE

52 Provide for comfort. (See the inside of the front book cover.)

53 Place the signal light within reach.

54 Lower the bed to its lowest position.

55 Raise or lower bed rails. Follow the care plan.

56 Unscreen the person.

57 Complete a safety check of the room. (See the inside of the front book cover.)

58 Follow agency policy for dirty linen and used supplies.

59 Practice hand hygiene.

60 Report and record your observations.

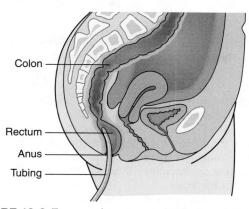

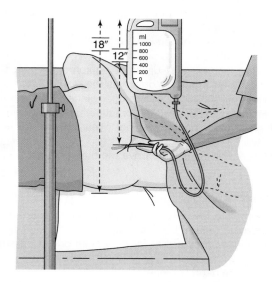

FIGURE 18-2 Enema tubing inserted into the adult rectum.

The Small-Volume Enema

Small-volume enemas irritate and distend the rectum. This causes a BM. They are often ordered for constipation or when the bowel does not need complete cleansing.

These enemas are ready to give. The solution is usually given at room temperature. To give the enema, squeeze and roll up the plastic bottle from the bottom. Do not release pressure on the bottle. Otherwise, solution is drawn from the rectum back into the bottle.

Urge the person to retain the solution until there is a need to have a BM. This usually takes about 5 to 10 minutes. Staying in the Sims' or left side-lying position helps retain the enema.

FIGURE 18-3 Giving an enema. The person is in Sims' position. The enema bag hangs from an IV pole. The bag is 12 inches above the anus and 18 inches above the mattress.

GIVING A SMALL-VOLUME ENEMA

QUALITY OF LIFE

Remember to:
- Knock before entering the person's room.
- Address the person by name.
- Introduce yourself by name and title.

- Explain the procedure to the person before beginning and during the procedure.
- Protect the person's rights during the procedure.
- Handle the person gently during the procedure.

PRE-PROCEDURE

1 Follow *Delegation Guidelines: Enemas*, p. 314. See *Promoting Safety and Comfort: Enemas*, p. 315.
2 Practice hand hygiene.
3 Collect the following before going to the person's room:
   - Small-volume enema
   - Waterproof pad
   - Gloves
4 Arrange items in the person's room.
5 Practice hand hygiene.
6 Identify the person. Check the ID bracelet against the assignment sheet. Also call the person by name.

7 Put on gloves.
8 Collect the following:
   - Commode or bedpan
   - Waterproof pad
   - Toilet tissue
   - Robe and non-skid footwear
   - Bath blanket
9 Provide for privacy.
10 Raise the bed for body mechanics. Bed rails are up if used.

Continued

PROCEDURE

11 Lower the bed rail near you if up.
12 Remove the gloves, and practice hand hygiene. Put on clean gloves.
13 Cover the person with a bath blanket. Fan-fold top linens to the foot of the bed.
14 Position the person in Sims' or a left side-lying position.
15 Place the waterproof pad under the buttocks.
16 Expose the anal area.
17 Position the bedpan near the person.
18 Remove the cap from the enema tip.
19 Separate the buttocks to see the anus.
20 Ask the person to take a deep breath through the mouth.
21 Insert the enema tip 2 inches into the adult's rectum (Fig. 18-4). Do this when the person is exhaling. Insert the tip gently. Stop if the person complains of pain, you feel resistance, or bleeding occurs.
22 Squeeze and roll the bottle gently. Release pressure on the bottle after you remove the tip from the rectum.
23 Put the bottle into the box, tip first.
24 Assist the person to the bathroom or commode when he or she has the urge to have a BM. The person wears a robe and non-skid footwear when up. The bed is in the lowest position. Or help the person onto the bedpan, and raise the head of the bed. Raise or lower bed rails according to the care plan.
25 Place the signal light and toilet tissue within reach. Remind the person not to flush the toilet.
26 Discard disposable items.
27 Remove the gloves. Practice hand hygiene.
28 Leave the room if the person can be left alone.
29 Return when the person signals. Or check on the person every 5 minutes. Knock before entering the room or bathroom.
30 Practice hand hygiene. Put on gloves.
31 Lower the bed rail if up.
32 Observe enema results for amount, color, consistency, shape, and odor. Call the nurse to observe the results.
33 Provide perineal care as needed.
34 Remove the waterproof pad.
35 Empty, clean, and disinfect equipment. Flush the toilet after the nurse observes the results.
36 Return equipment to its proper place.
37 Remove the gloves, and practice hand hygiene.
38 Assist with hand washing. Wear gloves for this step.
39 Cover the person. Remove the bath blanket.

POST-PROCEDURE

40 Provide for comfort. (See the inside of the front book cover.)
41 Place the signal light within reach.
42 Lower the bed to its lowest position.
43 Raise or lower bed rails. Follow the care plan.
44 Unscreen the person.
45 Complete a safety check of the room. (See the inside of the front book cover.)
46 Follow agency policy for dirty linen and used supplies.
47 Practice hand hygiene.
48 Report and record your observations.

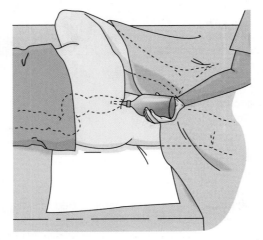

FIGURE 18-4 The small-volume enema tip is inserted 2 inches into the rectum.

The Oil-Retention Enema

Oil-retention enemas relieve constipation and fecal impactions. The oil is retained for 30 to 60 minutes or longer (1 to 3 hours). Retaining oil softens feces and lubricates the rectum. This lets feces pass with ease. Most oil-retention enemas are commercially prepared.

Giving an oil-retention enema is like giving a small-volume enema. After giving an oil-retention enema:

• Leave the person in the Sims' or left side-lying position. Cover the person for warmth.
• Urge the person to retain the enema for the time ordered.
• Place extra waterproof pads on the bed if needed.
• Check the person often while he or she retains the enema.

See *Promoting Safety and Comfort: The Oil-Retention Enema.*

PROMOTING SAFETY AND COMFORT
The Oil-Retention Enema

Safety

The oil-retention enema is retained for at least 30 to 60 minutes. You will leave the room after giving the enema. Make sure you check on the person often. After checking on the person, tell him or her when you will return. Remind the person to signal for you if he or she needs help.

THE PERSON WITH AN OSTOMY

Sometimes part of the intestines is removed surgically. Cancer, bowel disease, and trauma (stab or bullet wounds) are common reasons. An ostomy is sometimes necessary. An **ostomy** is a surgically created opening. The opening is called a **stoma.** The person wears a pouch over the stoma to collect stools and flatus.

Colostomy

A **colostomy** is a surgically created opening (*stomy*) between the colon (*colo*) and abdominal wall. Part of the colon is brought out onto the abdominal wall and a stoma is made. Feces and flatus pass through the stoma instead of through the anus.

With a permanent colostomy, the diseased part of the colon is removed. A temporary colostomy gives the diseased or injured bowel time to heal. After healing, surgery is done to reconnect the bowel.

The colostomy site depends on the site of disease or injury (Fig. 18-5). Stool consistency depends on the colostomy site. Consistency ranges from liquid to formed. The more colon remaining to absorb water, the more solid and formed the stool. If the colostomy is near the start of the colon, stools are liquid. A colostomy near the end of the colon results in formed stools.

Stools irritate the skin. Skin care prevents skin breakdown around the stoma. The skin is washed and dried. Then a skin barrier is applied around the stoma. It prevents stools from having contact with the skin. The skin barrier is part of the pouch or a separate device.

Ileostomy

An **ileostomy** is a surgically created opening (*stomy*) between the ileum (*small intestine [ileo]*) and the abdominal wall. Part of the ileum is brought out onto the abdominal wall, and a stoma is made. The entire colon is removed (Fig. 18-6, p. 320).

Liquid stools drain constantly from an ileostomy. Water is not absorbed because the colon was removed. Feces in the small intestine contain digestive

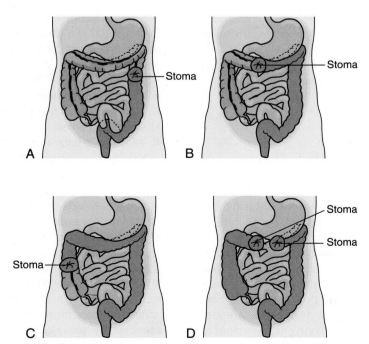

FIGURE 18-5 Colostomy sites. *Shading* shows the part of the bowel surgically removed. **A,** Sigmoid or descending colostomy. **B,** Transverse colostomy. **C,** Ascending colostomy. **D,** Double-barrel colostomy has two stomas. One allows for the excretion of feces. The other is for the introduction of drugs to help the bowel heal. This type of colostomy is usually temporary.

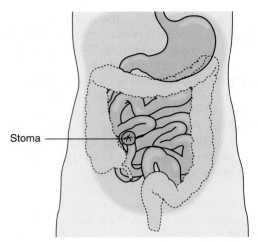

FIGURE 18-6 An ileostomy. The entire large intestine is surgically removed.

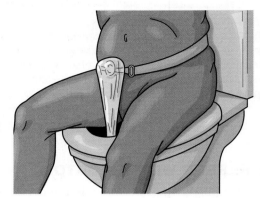

FIGURE 18-7 The ostomy pouch is secured to an ostomy belt. The pouch is emptied by directing it into the toilet and opening the end.

juices that are very irritating to the skin. The ileostomy pouch must fit well. Stools must not touch the skin. Good skin care is required.

Ostomy Pouches

The pouch has an adhesive backing that is applied to the skin. Sometimes pouches are secured to ostomy belts (Fig. 18-7).

Many pouches have a drain at the bottom that closes with a clip, clamp, or wire closure. The drain is opened to empty the pouch. The pouch is emptied when stools are present. It is opened when it balloons or bulges with flatus. The drain is wiped with toilet tissue before it is closed.

The pouch is changed every 3 to 7 days and when it leaks. Frequent changes can damage the skin.

Odors are prevented by:
- Good hygiene.
- Emptying the pouch.
- Avoiding gas-forming foods.
- Putting deodorants into the pouch. The nurse tells you what to use.

The person can wear normal clothes. However, tight garments can prevent feces from entering the pouch. Also, bulging from stools and flatus can be seen with tight clothes.

Peristalsis increases after eating and drinking. Therefore stomas are usually quiet after sleep. That is, expelling feces is less likely at this time. If the person showers or bathes with the pouch off, it is best done before breakfast. Showers and baths are delayed for 1 to 2 hours after applying a new pouch. This gives the adhesive time to seal to the skin.

Do not flush pouches down the toilet. Follow agency policy for disposing of them.

Focus on P R I D E
The Person, Family, and Yourself

Personal and Professional Responsibility—Odors and sounds often occur with bowel elimination. You must control your verbal and non-verbal responses. Act in a professional manner at all times. Do not laugh at or make fun of another person. Such reactions are unprofessional. They lessen the person's dignity and self-esteem.

Rights and Respect—Bowel elimination is typically done in private. Illness, disease, surgery, and aging can affect this private act. Some persons may feel embarrassed to have a BM in a strange environment. You can help the person feel more comfortable by respecting his or her privacy. To promote comfort and privacy:
- Ask others to leave the room.
- Close doors, curtains, and window coverings.
- Turn on water or music to mask sounds.
- Cover the person.
- Allow the person enough time. Place the signal light nearby and instruct the person to call if help is needed.
- Knock before entering the room. Tell the person who you are. Ask the person if you may enter before opening the door completely.
- Use a spray for odors that is provided by the agency.

Independence and Social Interaction—Persons with ostomies manage their own care if able. Some have had ostomies for a long time. They may have special routines or care measures. Do not react to things that seem odd to you. Follow their choices in ostomy care. Allow the person to do as much as is safely possible. Doing so promotes independence.

D elegation and Teamwork—The nurse may delegate a task to you that you have not done before. For example, a nurse asks you to give an enema or empty a colostomy bag. Never attempt a task that you are not comfortable doing alone. Make sure the task is in your job description. Also, make sure your state allows you to perform the procedure. If those conditions are met, politely tell the nurse. You can say: "I'm sorry, but I have never done that task before. I do not feel comfortable doing it on my own. Would you please show me how it is done?" Take pride in making the right choice to tell the nurse about your delegation concern.

E thics and Laws—Leaving a person sitting or lying in his or her urine or feces is neglect. It is a form of physical abuse. Federal and state laws require the reporting and investigating of abuse. If found guilty of abuse, neglect, or mistreatment of a patient or resident, you will lose your job. The offense is noted on your registry information. You cannot work in a nursing center or on a skilled care nursing unit in a hospital. Protect yourself from being accused of neglect. Check on your patients or residents often. Do not allow them to be left sitting or lying in urine or feces.

REVIEW QUESTIONS

Circle the BEST answer.

1 Which is *false?*
 a A person must have a bowel movement every day.
 b Stools are normally brown, soft, and formed.
 c Diarrhea occurs when feces move rapidly through the bowels.
 d Constipation results when feces move slowly through the colon.
2 The prolonged retention and accumulation of feces in the rectum is called
 a Constipation
 b Fecal impaction
 c Diarrhea
 d Fecal incontinence
3 Which does *not* promote comfort and safety for bowel elimination?
 a Asking visitors to leave the room
 b Helping the person to a sitting position
 c Offering the bedpan after meals
 d Telling the person that you will return very soon
4 Bowel training is aimed at
 a Bowel control and regular elimination
 b Ostomy control
 c Preventing fecal impaction, constipation, and fecal incontinence
 d Preventing bleeding
5 Which is *not* used for a cleansing enema?
 a Castile soap
 b Salt
 c Oil
 d Tap water

6 These statements are about enemas. Which is *false?*
 a The solution should be cool.
 b The Sims' position is used.
 c The enema bag is held 12 inches above the anus.
 d The solution is given slowly.
7 In adults, the enema tube is inserted
 a 2 to 4 inches
 b 4 to 6 inches
 c 6 to 8 inches
 d 8 to 10 inches
8 The oil-retention enema is retained for at least
 a 10 to 15 minutes
 b 15 to 30 minutes
 c 30 to 60 minutes
 d 60 to 90 minutes
9 These statements are about ostomies. Which is *false?*
 a Good skin care around the stoma is needed.
 b Deodorants can control odors.
 c The person wears a pouch.
 d Stools are liquid.
10 An ostomy pouch is usually emptied
 a Every 4 to 6 hours
 b Every shift
 c Every 3 to 7 days
 d When stools are present

Answers to these questions are on p. 528.

19

ASSISTING WITH NUTRITION AND FLUIDS

PROCEDURES

- Preparing the Person for a Meal
- Serving Meal Trays
- Feeding the Person
- Providing Drinking Water

OBJECTIVES

- Define the key terms and key abbreviations listed in this chapter.
- Explain the purpose and use of the MyPyramid food guidance system.
- Describe the functions of nutrients.
- Describe the factors that affect eating and nutrition.
- Describe the OBRA requirements for serving food.
- Describe the special diets and between-meal snacks.
- Identify the signs, symptoms, and precautions for aspiration and regurgitation.
- Describe fluid requirements and the causes of dehydration.
- Explain what to do when the person has special fluid orders.
- Explain how to assist with food and fluid needs.
- Explain how to assist with enteral nutrition and IV therapy.
- Explain how to promote PRIDE in the person, the family, and yourself.
- Perform the procedures described in this chapter.

KEY TERMS

anorexia The loss of appetite

aspiration Breathing fluid, food, vomitus, or an object into the lungs

calorie The amount of energy produced when the body burns food

dehydration A decrease in the amount of water in body tissues

dysphagia Difficulty (*dys*) swallowing (*phagia*)

edema The swelling of body tissues with water

enteral nutrition Giving nutrients into the gastro-intestinal (GI) tract (*enteral*) through a feeding tube

flow rate The number of drops per minute

gavage The process of giving a tube feeding

intravenous (IV) therapy Giving fluids through a needle or catheter inserted into a vein; IV and IV infusion

nutrition The processes involved in the ingestion, digestion, absorption, and use of foods and fluids by the body

regurgitation The backward flow of stomach contents into the mouth

KEY ABBREVIATIONS

GI Gastro-intestinal

ID Identification

IV Intravenous

mg Milligram

mL Milliliter

NG Naso-gastric

NPO Non per os; nothing by mouth

OBRA Omnibus Budget Reconciliation Act of 1987

oz Ounce

Food and water are physical needs. They are necessary for life. The person's diet affects physical and mental well-being. A poor diet and poor eating habits:

- Increase the risk for diseases and infection
- Cause healing problems
- Affect physical and mental function, increasing the risk for accidents and injuries

BASIC NUTRITION

Nutrition is the processes involved in the ingestion, digestion, absorption, and use of foods and fluids by the body. Good nutrition is needed for growth, healing, and body functions. A *nutrient* is a substance that is ingested, digested, absorbed, and used by the body. Nutrients are grouped into fats, proteins, carbohydrates, vitamins, minerals, and water.

Fats, proteins, and carbohydrates give the body fuel for energy. A **calorie** is the amount of energy produced when the body burns food:

- 1 gram of fat—9 calories
- 1 gram of protein—4 calories
- 1 gram of carbohydrate—4 calories

MyPlate

The MyPlate symbol (Fig. 19-1) encourages healthy eating from 5 food groups. MyPlate, issued by the United States Department of Agriculture (USDA), helps you make wise food choices by:

- Balancing calories
  - Eating less
  - Avoiding over-sized portions
- Increasing certain foods
  - Making half of your plate fruits and vegetables
  - Making at least half of your grains whole grains
  - Drinking fat-free or low-fat (1%) milk
- Reducing certain foods
  - Choosing low-sodium foods
  - Drinking water instead of sugary drinks

The amount needed from each food group depends on age, sex, and physical activity (Table 19-1). Activity should be moderate or vigorous (Box 19-1). The USDA recommends that adults do at least one of the following:

- 2 hours and 30 minutes each week of moderate physical activity
- 1 hour and 15 minutes each week of vigorous physical activity

Physical activity at least 3 days a week is best. Each activity should be for at least 10 minutes at a time. Adults should also do strengthening activities at least 2 days a week. Push-ups, sit-ups, and weight-lifting are examples.

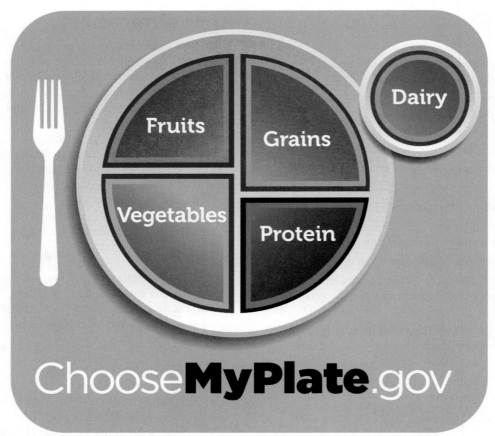

FIGURE 19-1 The MyPlate Symbol. *(Courtesy U.S. Department of Agriculture, Washington, DC., 2011.)*

BOX 19-1 Moderate and Vigorous Physical Activities

Moderate Physical Activities

- Walking briskly (about 3½ miles per hour)
- Bicycling (less than 10 miles per hour)
- Gardening (raking, trimming bushes)
- Dancing
- Golf (walking and carrying clubs)
- Water aerobics
- Canoeing
- Tennis (doubles)

Vigorous Physical Activities

- Running and jogging (5 miles per hour)
- Walking very fast (4½ miles per hour)
- Bicycling (more than 10 miles per hour)
- Heavy yard work (chopping wood)
- Swimming (freestyle laps)
- Aerobics
- Basketball (competitive)
- Tennis (singles)

From *What is Physical Activity?*, *U.S. Department of Agriculture, June 4, 2011.*

Grains Group. Foods made from wheat, rice, oats, cornmeal, barley, or other cereal grain are grain products. Bread, pasta, oatmeal, breakfast cereals, tortillas, and grits are examples. The two types of grains are:

- *Whole grains* have the entire grain kernel. Whole-wheat flour, bulgur (cracked wheat), oatmeal, whole cornmeal, and brown rice are examples.
- *Refined grains* were processed to remove the grain kernel. These grains have a fine texture. White flour, white bread, and white rice are examples. They have less dietary fiber than whole grains.

Grains, especially whole grains, have these health benefits:

- Reduce the risk of heart disease.
- May prevent constipation.
- May help with weight management.
- May prevent certain birth defects.
- Contain these nutrients—dietary fiber, several B vitamins (thiamin, riboflavin, niacin, folate), and minerals (iron, magnesium, and selenium).

TABLE 19-1 MyPlate Serving Sizes

Group	Daily Servings	Serving Sizes
Grains	• Adult women: 5 to 6 oz; at least 3 oz from whole grains • Adult men: 6 to 8 oz; at least 3 to 4 oz from whole grains	1 oz = 1 slice of bread 1 oz = 1 cup of breakfast cereal 1 oz = ½ cup of cooked rice, cereal, or pasta
Vegetables	• Adult women: 2 to 2½ cups • Adult men: 2½ to 3 cups	1 cup = 1 cup of raw or cooked vegetables or vegetable juice 1 cup = 2 cups of raw leafy greens
Fruits	• Adult women: 1½ to 2 cups • Adult men: 2 cups	1 cup = 1 cup of fruit 1 cup = 1 cup of fruit juice 1 cup = ½ cup of dried fruit
Dairy	• Adult women: 3 cups • Adult men: 3 cups	1 cup = 1 cup milk or yogurt 1 cup = 1½ oz natural cheese 1 cup = 2 oz processed cheese

Modified from MyPlate, U.S. Department of Agriculture, June 2011.

Continued

TABLE 19-1	MyPlate Serving Sizes—cont'd	
Group	**Daily Servings**	**Serving Sizes**
Protein foods	• Adult women: 5 to 5½ oz • Adult men: 5 ½ to 6½ oz	1 oz = 1 oz of lean meat, poultry, or fish 1 oz = 1 egg 1 oz = 1 tablespoon peanut butter 1 oz = ¼ cup cooked dry beans 1 oz = ½ oz of nuts or seeds

Vegetable Group. Vegetables can be eaten raw or cooked. They may be fresh, frozen, canned, dried, or juice. You can eat them whole, cut-up, or mashed. The 5 vegetable subgroups are:

* *Dark green vegetables*—bok choy, broccoli, collard greens, dark green leafy lettuce, kale, mesclun, mustard greens, romaine lettuce, spinach, turnips, watercress
* *Red and orange vegetables*—acorn, butternut, and hubbard squashes; carrots; pumpkin; red peppers; sweet potatoes; tomatoes; tomato juice
* *Beans and peas*—black beans, black-eyed peas, garbanzo beans (chickpeas), kidney beans, lentils, navy beans, pinto beans, soy beans, split peas, and white beans
* *Starchy vegetables*—corn, green bananas, green peas, green lima beans, plantains, potatoes, taro, water chestnuts
* *Other vegetables*—artichokes, asparagus, avocado, bean sprouts, beets, Brussels sprouts, cabbage, cauliflower, celery, cucumbers, eggplant, green beans, green peppers, iceberg (head) lettuce, mushrooms, okra, onions, parsnips, turnips, wax beans, zucchini

Vegetables have these health benefits:
* May reduce the risk for stroke, heart disease, high blood pressure, cardiovascular diseases, obesity, type 2 diabetes.
* May protect against certain cancers. Cancers of the mouth, stomach, and colon-rectum are examples.
* May reduce the risk of developing kidney stones.
* May reduce the risk of bone loss.
* May help prevent constipation.
* May help lower calorie intake. Most vegetables are low in fat and calories.
* Contain no cholesterol. (**Cholesterol** is a soft, waxy substance. It is found in the bloodstream and all body cells. Dietary sources are from animal foods—egg yolks, meat, poultry, shellfish, milk, and milk products.)
* May prevent certain birth defects.

* Contain these nutrients—potassium, dietary fiber, folate (folic acid), vitamins A and C.

Fruit Group. Any fruit or 100% fruit juice counts as part of the fruit group. Fruits may be fresh, frozen, canned, or dried. They may be eaten whole, cut-up, or pureed. Avoid fruits canned in syrup. Syrup contains added sugar. Choose fruits canned in 100% fruit juice or water.

Fruits have these health benefits:
* May reduce the risk for stroke, heart disease, high blood pressure, cardiovascular diseases, obesity, and type 2 diabetes.
* May protect against certain cancers. Cancers of the mouth, stomach, and colon-rectum are examples.
* May reduce the risk of developing kidney stones.
* May reduce the risk of bone loss.
* May help prevent constipation.
* May help lower calorie intake. Most fruits are low in fat and calories.
* Contain no cholesterol.
* Are low in sodium.
* May prevent certain birth defects.
* Contain these nutrients—potassium, dietary fiber, vitamin C, and folate (folic acid).

Dairy Group. All fluid milk products are part of the dairy group. So are many foods made from milk. Low-fat or fat-free choices are best. The milk group includes all fluid milk, yogurt, and cheese. (Cream, cream cheese, and butter are not in this group.)

Milk has these health benefits:
* Helps build and maintain bone mass throughout life. This may reduce the risk of osteoporosis.
* May reduce the risk of cardiovascular disease, type 2 diabetes, and high blood pressure.
* Contains these nutrients—calcium, potassium, and vitamin D.

Protein Foods Group. This group includes all foods made from meat, poultry, seafood, beans and peas, eggs, processed soy products, nuts, and seeds.

When selecting foods from this group, remember:

- To choose lean or low-fat meat and poultry. Higher fat choices include regular ground beef (75 to 80% lean) and chicken with skin.
- Using fat for cooking increases the calories. Fried chicken and eggs fried in butter are examples.
- Salmon, trout, and herring are rich in substances that may reduce the risk of heart disease.
- Liver and other organ meats are high in cholesterol.
- Egg yolks are high in cholesterol. Egg whites are cholesterol-free.
- Processed meats have added sodium (salt). They include ham, sausage, frankfurters, and luncheon and deli meats.

Many protein foods are high in fat and cholesterol. Heart disease is a major risk. However, this group provides nutrients needed for health and body maintenance:

- Protein
- B vitamins (niacin, thiamin, riboflavin, and B$_6$) and vitamin E
- Iron, zinc, and magnesium

Oils. Oils are fats that are liquid at room temperature. Vegetable oils for cooking are examples. They include canola oil, corn oil, and olive oil. Oils come from plants and fish. Because they have nutrients, the USDA includes oils in food patterns. However, *oils are not a food group.*

Adult women are allowed 5 to 6 teaspoons of oils daily. Adult men are allowed 6 to 7 teaspoons daily. Some foods are high in oil—nuts, olives, some fish, and avocados. When making oil choices, remember:

- Oils are high in calories.
- The best oil choices come from fish, nuts, and vegetable oils.

- Some foods are mainly oil. Mayonnaise, certain salad dressings, and soft margarine (tub or squeeze) are examples.
- Oils from plant sources do not contain cholesterol.
- *Solid fats* are solid at room temperature. Common solid fats include butter, milk fat, beef fat (tallow, suet), chicken fat, pork fat (lard), stick margarine, and shortening.
- Oils and solid fats have about 120 calories in each tablespoon.
- Enough oil is usually consumed daily from nuts, fish, cooking oil, and salad dressings.

Nutrients

No food or food group has every essential nutrient. A well-balanced diet assures an adequate intake of essential nutrients.

- *Protein* is the most important nutrient. It is needed for tissue growth and repair. Sources include meat, fish, poultry, eggs, milk and milk products, cereals, beans, peas, and nuts.
- *Carbohydrates* provide energy and fiber for bowel elimination. They are found in fruits, vegetables, breads, cereals, and sugar. Fiber is not digested. It provides the bulky part of chyme for elimination.
- *Fats* provide energy. They add flavor to food and help the body use certain vitamins. Sources include meats, lard, butter, shortening, oils, milk, cheese, egg yolks, and nuts. Dietary fat not needed by the body is stored as body fat (*adipose tissue*).
- *Vitamins* are needed for certain body functions. They do not provide calories. The body stores vitamins A, D, E, and K. Vitamin C and the B complex vitamins are not stored. They must be ingested daily. The lack of a certain vitamin can cause illness.
- *Minerals* are needed for bone and tooth formation, nerve and muscle function, fluid balance, and other body processes.
- *Water* is needed for all body processes (p. 334).

FACTORS AFFECTING EATING AND NUTRITION

Many factors affect nutrition and eating habits. Some begin during infancy and continue throughout life. Others develop later.

* *Age.* Many changes occur in the digestive system with aging. See Chapter 7.
* *Culture.* Culture influences dietary practices, food choices, and food preparation. Frying, baking, smoking, or roasting food and eating raw food are cultural practices. So is the use of sauces, herbs, and spices. See *Caring About Culture: Food Practices.*
* *Religion.* Selecting, preparing, and eating food often involve religious practices. A person may follow all, some, or none of the dietary practices of his or her faith. You must respect the person's religious practices.
* *Appetite.* Appetite relates to the desire for food. A hungry person seeks food and eats until satisfied. However, loss of appetite **(anorexia)** can occur. Causes include illness, drugs, anxiety, pain, and depression. Unpleasant sights, thoughts, and smells are other causes. Older persons may have loss of appetite from decreased senses of taste and smell.
* *Personal choice.* Food likes and dislikes are influenced by foods served in the home. Usually food likes expand with age and social experiences.
* *Body reactions.* People usually avoid foods that cause allergic reactions. They also avoid foods that cause nausea, vomiting, diarrhea, indigestion, gas, or headaches.

* *Illness.* Appetite usually decreases during illness and recovery from injuries. However, nutrition needs are increased. The body must fight infection, heal tissue, and replace lost blood cells. Nutrients lost through vomiting and diarrhea need replacement. Some diseases and drugs cause a sore mouth. This makes eating painful.
* *Disability.* Disease or injury can affect the hands, wrists, and arms. Assistive devices let the person eat independently (Fig. 19-2).

OBRA DIETARY REQUIREMENTS

The Omnibus Budget Reconciliation Act of 1987 (OBRA) has requirements for food served in nursing centers:

* Each person's nutritional and dietary needs are met.
* The person's diet is well-balanced. It is nourishing and tastes good. Food is well-seasoned. It is not too salty or too sweet.
* Food is appetizing. It has an appealing aroma and is attractive.
* The foods served vary in color and texture.
* Hot food is served hot. Cold food is served cold.
* Food is served promptly. Hot food must stay hot. Cold food must stay cold.
* Food is prepared to meet each person's needs. Some people need food cut, ground, or chopped. Others have special diets ordered by the doctor.
* Other foods are offered if the person refused the food served. Substituted food must have a similar nutritional value to the first foods served.
* Each person receives at least 3 meals a day. A bedtime snack is offered.
* The center provides needed assistive devices and utensils (see Fig. 19-2). Such devices promote independence in eating. Make sure the person has needed equipment.

SPECIAL DIETS

Doctors may order special diets for a nutritional deficiency or a disease. They also order them for weight control or to remove or decrease certain substances in the diet.

Regular diet, general diet, and *house diet* mean no dietary limits or restrictions. Table 19-2 describes common diets.

The sodium-controlled diet is often ordered. So is a diabetes meal plan. Persons with difficulty swallowing may need a dysphagia diet.

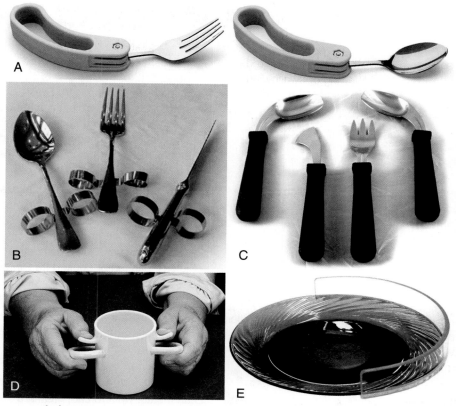

FIGURE 19-2 Eating utensils for persons with special needs. **A,** The fork and spoon are angled. Fingers are inserted through the opening or wrapped around the handle. **B,** The utensils can be adjusted for the person's grip strength. **C,** Eating utensils have tapered and angled handles. The knife cuts with slicing and rocking motions. **D,** The thumb grips on the cup help prevent spilling. **E,** The plate guard helps keep food on the plate. (*Courtesy ElderStore, Alpharetta, Georgia.*)

TABLE 19-2 Special Diets		
Diet	**Use**	**Foods Allowed**
Clear-liquid—foods liquid at body temperature and that leave small amounts of residue; non-irritating and non-gasforming	Post-operatively, acute illness, infection, nausea and vomiting, and to prepare for gastro-intestinal (GI) exams	Water, tea, and coffee (without milk or cream); carbonated drinks; gelatin; clear fruit juices (apple, grape, cranberry); fat-free clear broth; hard candy, sugar, and Popsicles
Full-liquid—foods liquid at room temperature or melt at body temperature	Advance from clear-liquid diet post-operatively; for stomach irritation, fever, nausea, and vomiting; for persons unable to chew, swallow, or digest solid foods	Foods on the clear-liquid diet; custard; eggnog; strained soups; strained fruit and vegetable juices; milk and milk shakes; strained, cooked cereals; plain ice cream and sherbet; pudding; yogurt

Continued

TABLE 19-2 Special Diets—cont'd

Diet	Use	Foods Allowed
Mechanical soft—semi-solid foods that are easily digested	Advance from full-liquid diet, chewing or swallowing problems, GI disorders, and infections	All liquids; eggs (not fried); broiled, baked, or roasted meat, fish, or poultry that is chopped or shredded; mild cheeses (American, Swiss, cheddar, cream, cottage); strained fruit juices; refined bread (no crust) and crackers; cooked cereal; cooked or pureed vegetables; cooked or canned fruit without skin or seeds; pudding; plain cakes and soft cookies without fruit or nuts
Fiber- and residue-restricted—food that leaves a small amount of residue in the colon	Diseases of the colon and diarrhea	Coffee, tea, milk, carbonated drinks, strained fruit juices; refined bread and crackers; creamed and refined cereal; rice; cottage and cream cheese; eggs (not fried); plain puddings and cakes; gelatin; custard; sherbet and ice cream; strained vegetable juices; canned or cooked fruit without skin or seeds; potatoes (not fried); strained cooked vegetables; plain pasta; no raw fruits or vegetables
High-fiber—foods that increase the amount of residue and fiber in the colon to stimulate peristalsis	Constipation and GI disorders	All fruits and vegetables; whole-wheat bread; whole-grain cereals; fried foods; whole-grain rice; milk, cream, butter, and cheese; meats
Bland—foods that are mechanically and chemically non-irritating and low in roughage; foods served at moderate temperatures; no strong spices or condiments	Ulcers, gallbladder disorders, and some intestinal disorders; after abdominal surgery	Lean meats; white bread; creamed and refined cereals; cream or cottage cheese; gelatin; plain puddings, cakes, and cookies; eggs (not fried); butter and cream; canned fruits and vegetables without skin and seeds; strained fruit juices; potatoes (not fried); pastas and rice; strained or soft cooked carrots, peas, beets, spinach, squash, and asparagus tips; creamed soups from allowed vegetables; no fried foods
High-calorie—calorie intake is increased to about 3000 to 4000 daily; includes 3 full meals and between-meal snacks	Weight gain and some thyroid imbalances	Dietary increases in all foods; large portions of regular diet with 3 between-meal snacks
Calorie-controlled—provides adequate nutrients while controlling calories to promote weight loss and reduce body fat	Weight reduction	Foods low in fats and carbohydrates and lean meats; avoid butter, cream, rice, gravies, salad oils, noodles, cakes, pastries, carbonated and alcoholic drinks, candy, potato chips, and similar foods
High-iron—foods that are high in iron	Anemia, following blood loss, for women during the reproductive years	Liver and other organ meats, lean meats, egg yolks, shellfish, dried fruits, dried beans, green leafy vegetables, lima beans, peanut butter, enriched breads and cereals

TABLE 19-2   Special Diets—cont'd

Diet	Use	Foods Allowed
Fat-controlled (low cholesterol)—foods low in fat and prepared without adding fat	Heart disease, gallbladder disease, disorders of fat digestion, liver disease, diseases of the pancreas	Skim milk (fat free) or buttermilk; cottage cheese (no other cheeses allowed); gelatin; sherbet; fruit; lean meat, poultry, and fish (baked, broiled, or roasted); fat-free broth; soups made with skim milk (fat free); margarine; rice, pasta, breads, and cereals; vegetables; potatoes
High-protein—aids and promotes tissue healing	For burns, high fever, infection, and some liver diseases	Meat, milk, eggs, cheese, fish, poultry; breads and cereals; green leafy vegetables
Sodium-controlled—a certain amount of sodium is allowed	Heart disease, fluid retention, liver disease, and some kidney diseases	Fruits and vegetables and unsalted butter are allowed; adding salt at the table is not allowed; highly salted foods and foods high in sodium are not allowed; the use of salt during cooking may be restricted
Diabetes meal plan—the same amounts of carbohydrates, protein, and fat are eaten at the same time each day	Diabetes	Determined by nutritional and energy requirements

The Sodium-Controlled Diet

The average amount of sodium in the daily diet is 3000 to 5000 milligrams (mg). The body needs no more than 2400 mg a day. Healthy people excrete excess sodium in the urine.

Heart, liver, and kidney diseases and certain drugs cause the body to retain extra sodium. Sodium causes the body to retain water. With too much sodium, the body retains more water. Tissues swell with water. There is excess fluid in the blood vessels. The heart has to work harder. Sodium control decreases the amount of sodium in the body. The body retains less water. Less water in the tissues and blood vessels reduces the heart's workload.

The doctor orders the amount of sodium allowed. Sodium-controlled diets involve:

- Omitting high-sodium foods (Box 19-2, p. 332)
- Not adding salt when eating
- Limiting the amount of salt used in cooking

Diabetes Meal Planning

Diabetes is a chronic illness in which the body cannot produce or use insulin properly (Chapter 26). The pancreas produces and secretes insulin. Insulin lets the body use sugar. Without enough insulin, sugar builds up in the bloodstream. It is not used by cells for energy. Diabetes is usually treated with insulin or other drugs, diet, and exercise.

The dietitian and person develop a meal plan for healthy eating. Consistency is key. It involves:

- Food preferences (likes, eating habits, meal times, culture, and life-style). Food amounts and preparation may be restricted.
- Calories needed. The same amounts of carbohydrates, protein, and fat are eaten each day.
- Eating meals and snacks at regular times. The person should eat at the same time every day. Doing so maintains a certain blood sugar level.

Serve the person's meals and snacks on time. Always check the tray to see what the person ate. Tell the nurse what the person did and did not eat. A between-meal snack makes up for food the person did not eat. The nurse tells you what to give the person.

BOX 19-2 High-Sodium Foods

Grains (Orange Band)
- Baked goods—biscuits, muffins, cakes, cookies, pies, pastries, sweet rolls, donuts, and so on
- Breads and rolls
- Cereals—cold, instant hot
- Noodle mixes
- Pancakes
- Salted snack foods—pretzels, corn chips, popcorn, crackers, chips, and so on
- Stuffing mixes
- Waffles

Vegetables (Green Band)
- Canned vegetables
- Olives
- Pickles and other pickled vegetables
- Relish
- Sauerkraut
- Tomato sauce or paste
- Vegetable juices—tomato, V-8, bloody Mary mixes
- Vegetables with sauces, creams, or seasonings

Fruits (Red Band)
- None—fruits are not high in sodium

Milk (Blue Band)
- Buttermilk
- Cheese
- Commercial dips made with sour cream

Meat and Beans (Purple Band)
- Bacon
- Canadian bacon
- Canned meats and fish—chicken, tuna, salmon, anchovies, sardines
- Caviar
- Chipped and corned beef
- Dried beef and other meats
- Dried fish
- Ham
- Herring
- Hot dogs (frankfurters)
- Liverwurst
- Lox
- Luncheon meats—turkey, ham, bologna, salami
- Mackerel
- Pastrami
- Pepperoni
- Salt pork
- Sausages
- Scrapple
- Shellfish—shrimp, crab, clams, oysters, scallops, lobster
- Smoked salmon

Oils (Yellow Band)
- Mayonnaise
- Salad dressings

Other
- Asian foods—Chinese, Japanese, East Indian, Thai, Vietnamese
- Baking soda and baking powder
- Catsup (ketchup)
- Cocoa mixes
- Commercially prepared dinners—frozen, canned, boxed, and so on
- Mexican foods
- Mustard
- Pasta dishes—lasagna, manicotti, ravioli
- Peanut butter
- Pizzas
- Pot pies
- Salted nuts or seeds
- Sauces—soy, teriyaki, Worcestershire, steak, barbecue, pasta, chili, cocktail
- Seasoning salts—garlic, onion, celery, meat tenderizers, monosodium glutamate (MSG), and so on
- Soups—canned, packaged, instant, dried, bouillon

BOX 19-3 Dysphagia Diet

CONSISTENCY	DESCRIPTION
Thickened liquid	No lumps. Pureed with milk, gravy, or broth to thickness of baby food. Thickener is added to some pureed foods as needed. Does not mound on a plate. May be called creamy or a sauce. Stir before serving if the food settles. Use a spoon.
Medium thick	The thickness of nectar or V-8 juice (does not hold its shape). Stir right before serving.
Extra thick	Thick like honey. Mounds a bit on a spoon. Drinkable from a cup. Stir before serving.
Yogurt-like	Thick like yogurt or pudding. Holds its shape. Served with a spoon.
Puree	No lumps; mounds on a plate. May be thick like mashed potatoes.

BOX 19-4 Signs and Symptoms of Dysphagia

- The person avoids food that needs chewing.
- The person avoids food with certain textures and temperatures.
- The person tires during a meal.
- Food spills out of the person's mouth while eating.
- Food "pockets" or is "squirreled" in the person's cheeks.
- The person eats slowly, especially solid foods.
- The person complains that food will not go down or that the food is stuck.
- The person frequently coughs or chokes before, during, or after swallowing.
- The person regurgitates food after eating (p. 343).
- The person spits out food suddenly and almost violently.
- Food comes up through the person's nose.
- The person is hoarse—especially after eating.
- After swallowing, the person makes gargling sounds while talking or breathing.
- The person has a runny nose, sneezes, or has excessive drooling of saliva.
- The person complains of frequent heartburn.
- Appetite is decreased.

The Dysphagia Diet

Dysphagia means difficulty *(dys)* swallowing *(phagia)*. A *slow swallow* means the person has difficulty getting enough food and fluids for good nutrition and fluid balance. An *unsafe swallow* means that food enters the airway (aspiration). **Aspiration** is breathing fluid, food, vomitus, or an object into the lungs.

Food thickness is changed to meet the person's needs (Box 19-3). You may need to feed a person with dysphagia. To promote safety and comfort, you must:

- Know the signs and symptoms of dysphagia (Box 19-4).
- Feed the person according to the care plan.
- Follow aspiration precautions (Box 19-5).
- Report changes in how the person eats.
- Observe for signs and symptoms of aspiration: choking, coughing, difficulty breathing during or after meals, and abnormal breathing or respiratory sounds. Report these observations at once.

BOX 19-5 Aspiration Precautions

- Help the person with meals and snacks. Follow the care plan.
- Position the person in Fowler's position or upright in a chair for meals and snacks.
- Support the upper back, shoulders, and neck with a pillow. Follow the care plan.
- Observe for signs and symptoms of aspiration during meals and snacks.
- Check the person's mouth after eating for pocketing. Check inside the cheeks, under the tongue, and on the roof of the mouth. Remove any food.
- Position the person in a chair or in semi-Fowler's position after eating. The person maintains this position for at least 1 hour after eating. Follow the care plan.
- Provide mouth care after eating.
- Report and record your observations.

FLUID BALANCE

Water is needed to live. Death can result from too much or too little water. Water is ingested through fluids and foods. It is lost through urine, feces, vomit, the skin (perspiration), and the lungs (expiration).

Fluid balance is needed for health. The amount of fluid taken in (*intake*) and the amount of fluid lost (*output*) must be equal. If fluid intake exceeds fluid output, body tissues swell with water. This is called **edema.** Edema is common in people with heart and kidney diseases. **Dehydration** is a decrease in the amount of water in body tissues. Fluid output exceeds intake. Common causes are poor fluid intake, vomiting, diarrhea, bleeding, excess sweating, and increased urine production.

Normal Fluid Requirements

An adult needs 1500 milliliters (mL) of water daily to survive. About 2000 to 2500 mL are needed for normal fluid balance. Water requirements increase with hot weather, exercise, fever, illness, and excess fluid losses.

Body water decreases with age. So does the thirst sensation. Older people may not feel thirsty even when their bodies need water. Offer fluids according to the care plan.

Special Fluid Orders

The doctor may order the amount of fluid a person can have in 24-hours. This is done to maintain fluid balance. Intake records are kept (Chapter 20). Found in the care plan and Kardex, common orders are:

- *Encourage fluids.* The person drinks an increased amount of fluid. The order states the amount to ingest. A variety of fluids are offered and kept within the person's reach. Serve them at the correct temperature. Offer fluids often to persons who cannot feed themselves.
- *Restrict fluids.* Fluids are limited to a certain amount. They are offered in small amounts and in small containers. The water pitcher is removed from the room or kept out of sight. Frequent oral hygiene keeps the mouth moist.

- *Nothing by mouth.* The person cannot eat or drink anything. *NPO* stands for *non per os.* It means nothing (*non*) by (*per*) mouth (*os*). NPO is ordered before and after surgery, before some diagnostic tests, and to treat certain illnesses. An NPO sign is posted above the bed. The water pitcher and glass are removed. Frequent oral hygiene is needed, but the person must not swallow any fluid. The person is NPO for at least 6 to 8 hours before surgery and before some diagnostic tests. Follow agency policy.
- *Thickened liquids.* All fluids are thickened, including water. Thickness depends on the person's ability to swallow (see Box 19-3). Thickener is added before fluids are served. Or commercial fluids are used. They are already thickened.

MEETING FOOD AND FLUID NEEDS

Weakness, illness, and confusion can affect appetite and ability to eat. So can unpleasant odors, sights, and sounds. An uncomfortable position, the need for oral hygiene, the need to eliminate, and pain also affect appetite.

See *Focus on Communication: Meeting Food and Fluid Needs.*

FOCUS ON COMMUNICATION
Meeting Food and Fluid Needs

The person may not eat or drink all the food and fluids served. You need to find out why and tell the nurse. You can politely ask these questions:
- "Did your food taste okay?"
- "Weren't you hungry?"
- "Was your food too hot or too cold?"
- "Is there a reason why you didn't eat everything?"
- "Was there something you didn't like?"
- "Would you like something else?"

Preparing for Meals

Preparing patients and residents for meals promotes comfort. When they are ready to eat, you can serve meal trays faster. Foods stay at the correct temperature.

See *Delegation Guidelines: Preparing for Meals.*

See *Promoting Safety and Comfort: Preparing for Meals.*

PROMOTING SAFETY AND COMFORT
Preparing for Meals

Safety
Before meals, the person needs to eliminate and have oral hygiene. Follow Standard Precautions and the Bloodborne Pathogen Standard. Also follow them when cleaning equipment and the room.

Comfort
The meal setting must be free of unpleasant sights, sounds, and odors. Remove unpleasant equipment from the room.

DELEGATION GUIDELINES
Preparing for Meals

To prepare a person for a meal, you need this information from the nurse and the care plan:
- How much help the person needs
- Where the person will eat—room or dining room
- What the person uses for elimination—bathroom, commode, bedpan, urinal, or specimen pan
- What type of oral hygiene the person needs
- If the person wears dentures
- How to position the person—in bed, a chair, or a wheelchair
- If the person wears eyeglasses or hearing aids
- How the person gets to the dining room—by self or with help
- If the person uses a wheelchair, walker, or cane

PREPARING THE PERSON FOR A MEAL

QUALITY OF LIFE

Remember to:
- Knock before entering the person's room.
- Address the person by name.
- Introduce yourself by name and title.

- Explain the procedure to the person before beginning and during the procedure.
- Protect the person's rights during the procedure.
- Handle the person gently during the procedure.

PRE-PROCEDURE

1 Follow *Delegation Guidelines: Preparing for Meals.* See *Promoting Safety and Comfort: Preparing for Meals.*
2 Practice hand hygiene.
3 Collect the following:
- Equipment for oral hygiene
- Bedpan and cover, urinal, commode, or specimen pan

- Toilet tissue
- Wash basin
- Soap
- Washcloth
- Towel
- Gloves

4 Provide for privacy.

Continued

PREPARING THE PERSON FOR A MEAL—cont'd

PROCEDURE

5 Make sure eyeglasses and hearing aids are in place.
6 Assist with oral hygiene. Make sure dentures are in place. Wear gloves, and decontaminate your hands after removing them.
7 Assist with elimination. Make sure the incontinent person is clean and dry. Wear gloves, and practice hand hygiene after removing them.
8 Assist with hand washing. Wear gloves, and practice hand hygiene after removing them.
9 Do the following if the person will eat in bed:
  a Raise the head of the bed to a comfortable position. Fowler's position is preferred.
  b Remove items from the overbed table. Clean the overbed table.
  c Adjust the overbed table in front of the person.
10 Do the following if the person will sit in a chair:
  a Position the person in a chair or wheelchair.
  b Remove items from the overbed table. Clean the table.
  c Adjust the overbed table in front of the person.
11 Assist the person to the dining area. (This step is for the person who eats in a dining area.)

POST-PROCEDURE

12 Provide for comfort. (See the inside of the front book cover.)
13 Place the signal light within reach.
14 Empty, clean, and disinfect equipment. Return equipment to its proper place. Wear gloves, and practice hand hygiene after removing them.
15 Straighten the room. Eliminate unpleasant noise, odors, or equipment.
16 Unscreen the person.
17 Complete a safety check of the room. (See the inside of the front book cover.)
18 Decontaminate your hands.

Dining Programs

The needs of nursing center residents vary. Some are alert, others are confused. Some cannot feed themselves. The following dining programs are common in nursing centers:

- *Social dining.* A dining room table seats 4 to 6 residents. Food is served as in a restaurant. Residents are oriented and can feed themselves.
- *Family dining.* Food is served in bowls and on platters like at home. Residents serve and feed themselves.
- *Assistive dining.* Horse-shoe shaped tables are in the dining room. You sit at the center of the table and feed up to 4 people (Fig. 19-3).
- *Low-stimulation dining.* Mealtime distractions are prevented. The health team decides on the best place for each person to sit.
- *Restaurant-style menus.* The person selects food from a menu. This program allows more food choices. The person is served as in a restaurant.
- *Open-dining.* A buffet is open for several hours. Breakfast is an example. Residents can eat any time while the buffet is open.

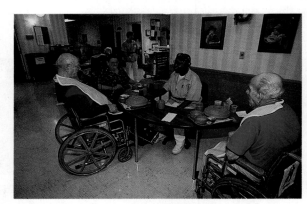

FIGURE 19-3 A horse-shoe shaped table is used for assistive dining. The nursing assistant feeds three residents at one time. Residents are in the company of others.

Serving Meal Trays

Food is served in containers that keep foods at the correct temperature. Hot food is kept hot. Cold food is kept cold.

You serve meal trays after preparing patients and residents for meals. You can serve trays promptly if they are ready to eat. Prompt serving keeps food at the correct temperature.

If food is not served within 15 minutes, re-check food temperatures. Follow agency policy. If not at the correct temperature, get a fresh tray. Some agencies allow re-heating in microwave ovens.

See *Delegation Guidelines: Serving Meal Trays.*

See *Promoting Safety and Comfort: Serving Meal Trays.*

DELEGATION GUIDELINES
Serving Meal Trays

Before serving meal trays, you need this information from the nurse and the care plan:
- What assistive devices the person uses
- How much help the person needs opening cartons, cutting food, buttering bread, and so on
- If the person's intake is measured (Chapter 20)
- If calorie counts are done (p. 340)

PROMOTING SAFETY AND COMFORT
Serving Meal Trays

Safety

Always check food temperature after re-heating. Food that is too hot can burn the person.

Comfort

Check the person's position when serving meal trays. The position may have changed after the person was prepared to eat. Provide other comfort measures as needed. See the inside of the front book cover for comfort measures.

View Video!

SERVING MEAL TRAYS

QUALITY OF LIFE

Remember to:
- Knock before entering the person's room.
- Address the person by name.
- Introduce yourself by name and title.

- Explain the procedure to the person before beginning and during the procedure.
- Protect the person's rights during the procedure.
- Handle the person gently during the procedure.

PRE-PROCEDURE

1 Follow *Delegation Guidelines: Serving Meal Trays.* See *Promoting Safety and Comfort: Serving Meal Trays.*

2 Practice hand hygiene.

PROCEDURE

3 Make sure the tray is complete. Check items on the tray with the dietary card. Make sure assistive devices are included.

4 Identify the person. Check the ID (identification) bracelet against the dietary card. Also call the person by name.

5 Place the tray within the person's reach. Adjust the overbed table as needed.

6 Remove food covers. Open cartons, cut food into bite-size pieces, butter bread, and so on as needed. Season food as the person prefers and is allowed on the care plan.

7 Place the napkin, clothes protector, assistive devices, and eating utensils within reach.

8 Place the signal light within reach.

9 Do the following when the person is done eating:
 a Measure and record intake if ordered (Chapter 20).
 b Note the amount and type of foods eaten. (See "Calorie Counts" on p. 340.)
 c Check for and remove any food in the mouth (pocketing). Wear gloves. Decontaminate your hands after removing them.
 d Remove the tray.
 e Clean spills. Change soiled linen and clothing.
 f Help the person return to bed if needed.
 g Assist with oral hygiene and hand washing. Wear gloves. Decontaminate your hands after removing the gloves.

Continued

SERVING MEAL TRAYS—cont'd

POST-PROCEDURE

10 Provide for comfort. (See the inside of the front book cover.)
11 Place the signal light within reach.
12 Raise or lower bed rails. Follow the care plan.
13 Complete a safety check of the room. (See the inside of the front book cover.)

14 Follow agency policy for soiled linen.
15 Decontaminate your hands.
16 Report and record your observations.

 ### Feeding the Person

You need to feed some people. Weakness, paralysis, casts, confusion, and other limits may make self-feeding impossible.

Serve food and fluids in the order the person prefers. Offer fluids during the meal. Fluids help the person chew and swallow.

Use teaspoons. They are less likely to cause injury than forks. A teaspoon portion one-third full is chewed and swallowed easily. Some people need smaller portions. Follow the care plan.

Persons who need to be fed are often angry, humiliated, and embarrassed. Some refuse to eat. Let them do as much as possible. Some can manage "finger foods" (bread, cookies, crackers). If strong enough, let them hold milk or juice glasses (never hot drinks). Follow activity limits ordered by the doctor. Provide support. Encourage them to try, even if food is spilled.

Visually impaired persons are often very aware of food aromas. They may know the food served. Always tell the person what is on the tray. When feeding visually impaired persons, describe what you are offering. For persons who feed themselves, describe foods and fluids and their place on the tray. Use the numbers on a clock for the location of foods (Fig. 19-4).

Many people pray before eating. Allow time and privacy for prayer. This shows respect and caring.

Meals provide social contact with others. Engage the person in pleasant conversation. However, allow time for chewing and swallowing. Also, sit facing the person. Sitting is more relaxing. It shows that you have time for the person. By facing the person, you can see how well the person is eating. You can also see swallowing problems.

See *Persons With Dementia: Feeding the Person.*
See *Delegation Guidelines: Feeding the Person.*
See *Promoting Safety and Comfort: Feeding the Person.*

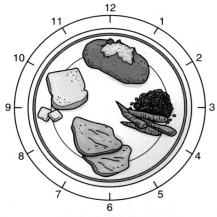

FIGURE 19-4 The numbers on a clock are used to help a visually impaired person locate food.

PERSONS WITH DEMENTIA
Feeding the Person

Persons with dementia may become distracted during meals. Some cannot sit long enough for a meal. Others forget how to use eating utensils. Some persons resist your efforts to help them eat. A confused person may throw or spit food.

The Alzheimer's Disease Education and Referral Center (ADEAR) recommends the following. The measures may be part of the person's care plan.

- Provide a calm, quiet setting for eating. Limit noise and other distractions. This helps the person focus on the meal.
- Limit the number of food choices.
- Offer several small meals throughout the day instead of larger ones.
- Use straws or cups with lids. These make drinking easier.
- Provide finger foods if the person has problems with utensils. A bowl may be easier to use than a plate.
- Provide healthy snacks. Keep snacks where the person can see them.

Be patient. Talk to the nurse if you feel upset or impatient. Remember, the person has the right to be treated with dignity and respect.

DELEGATION GUIDELINES
Feeding the Person

Before feeding a person, you need this information from the nurse and the care plan:
- Why the person needs help
- How much help the person needs
- If the person can manage finger foods
- What the person's activity limits are
- What the person's dietary restrictions are
- What size portion to feed the person—⅓ teaspoonful or less
- What safety measures are needed if the person has dysphagia
- If the person can use a straw
- What observations to report and record:
  - The amount and kind of food eaten
  - Complaints of nausea or dysphagia
  - Signs and symptoms of dysphagia
  - Signs and symptoms of aspiration
- When to report observations
- What specific patient or resident concerns to report at once

PROMOTING SAFETY AND COMFORT
Feeding the Person

Safety

Check food temperature. Very hot foods can burn the person.

Prevent aspiration. Check the person's mouth before offering more food or fluids. The person's mouth must be empty between bites and swallows.

Comfort

The person will eat better if not rushed. Sit to show the person that you have time for him or her. Standing communicates that you are in a hurry.

Wipe the person's hands, face, and mouth as needed during the meal. Use the napkin. If necessary, use a wet washcloth. Then dry the person with a towel.

FEEDING THE PERSON

QUALITY OF LIFE

Remember to:
- Knock before entering the person's room.
- Address the person by name.
- Introduce yourself by name and title.

- Explain the procedure to the person before beginning and during the procedure.
- Protect the person's rights during the procedure.
- Handle the person gently during the procedure.

PRE-PROCEDURE

1 Follow *Delegation Guidelines: Feeding the Person.* See *Promoting Safety and Comfort: Feeding the Person.*
2 Practice hand hygiene.

3 Position the person in a comfortable position for eating—usually sitting or Fowler's.
4 Get the tray. Place it on the overbed table or dining table.

PROCEDURE

5 Identify the person. Check the ID bracelet against the dietary card. Also call the person by name.
6 Drape a napkin across the person's chest and underneath the chin.
7 Tell the person what foods and fluids are on the tray.
8 Prepare food for eating. Cut food into bite-size pieces. Season foods as the person prefers and is allowed on the care plan.
9 Place the chair where you can sit comfortably. Sit facing the person.

10 Serve foods in the order the person prefers. Identify foods as you serve them. Alternate between solid and liquid foods. Use a spoon for safety (Fig. 19-5, p. 340). Allow enough time for chewing and swallowing. Do not rush the person. Also offer water, coffee, tea, or other beverage on the tray.
11 Check the person's mouth before offering more food or fluids. Make sure the person's mouth is empty between bites and swallows.
12 Use straws for liquids if the person cannot drink out of a glass or cup. Have one straw for each liquid. Provide short straws for weak persons.

Continued

FEEDING THE PERSON—cont'd

PROCEDURE—cont'd

13 Wipe the person's hands, face, and mouth as needed during the meal. Use the napkin.
14 Follow the care plan if the person has dysphagia. (Some persons with dysphagia do not use straws.) Give thickened liquid with a spoon.
15 Converse with the person in a pleasant manner.
16 Encourage him or her to eat as much as possible.
17 Wipe the person's mouth with a napkin. Discard the napkin.

18 Note how much and which foods were eaten. See "Calorie Counts".
19 Measure and record intake if ordered (Chapter 20).
20 Remove the tray.
21 Take the person back to his or her room (if in a dining area).
22 Assist with oral hygiene and hand washing. Provide for privacy, and put on gloves. Decontaminate your hands after removing the gloves.

POST-PROCEDURE

23 Provide for comfort. (See the inside of the front book cover.)
24 Place the signal light within reach.
25 Raise or lower bed rails. Follow the care plan.
26 Complete a safety check of the room. (See the inside of the front book cover.)

27 Return the food tray to the food cart.
28 Decontaminate your hands.
29 Report and record your observations.

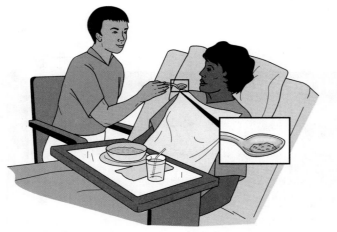

FIGURE 19-5 A spoon is used to feed the person. The spoon is one-third full.

Between-Meal Snacks

Many special diets involve between-meal snacks. Common snacks are crackers, milk, juice, a milkshake, cake, wafers, a sandwich, gelatin, and custard.

Snacks are served upon arrival on the nursing unit. Provide needed utensils, a straw, and a napkin. Follow the same considerations and procedures for serving meal trays and feeding persons.

Calorie Counts

The nurse tells you which persons need calorie counts. On a flow sheet, note what the person ate and how much. For example, a chicken breast, rice, beans, a roll, pudding, and two pats of butter were served. The person ate all the chicken, half the rice, and the roll. One pat of butter was used. The beans and pudding were not eaten. Note these on the flow sheet. A nurse or dietitian converts these portions into calories.

❧ Providing Drinking Water

Patients and residents need fresh drinking water each shift. They also need water whenever the pitcher is empty.

Some agencies do not use the procedure that follows. Each person's water pitcher is filled as needed. The pitcher is taken to an ice and water dispenser. If so, fill the water pitcher with ice first. Then add water to the pitcher.

See *Delegation Guidelines: Providing Drinking Water.*
See *Promoting Safety and Comfort: Providing Drinking Water.*

DELEGATION GUIDELINES
Providing Drinking Water

Before providing water, you need this information from the nurse and the care plan:
- The person's fluid orders
- If the person can have ice
- If the person uses a straw

PROMOTING SAFETY AND COMFORT
Providing Drinking Water

Safety

Water glasses and pitchers can spread microbes. To prevent the spread of microbes:

- Make sure the water pitcher is labeled with the person's name and room and bed number.
- Do not touch the rim or inside of the water cup or pitcher.
- Do not let the ice scoop touch the rim or inside of the water cup or pitcher.
- Do not put the ice scoop in the ice container or dispenser. Place it in the scoop holder or on a towel for the scoop.
- Make sure the person's water pitcher and cup are clean. Also check for cracks and chips. Provide a new water pitcher or cup as needed.

PROVIDING DRINKING WATER

QUALITY OF LIFE

Remember to:
- Knock before entering the person's room.
- Address the person by name.
- Introduce yourself by name and title.

- Explain the procedure to the person before beginning and during the procedure.
- Protect the person's rights during the procedure.
- Handle the person gently during the procedure.

PRE-PROCEDURE

1. Follow *Delegation Guidelines: Providing Drinking Water.*
   See *Promoting Safety and Comfort: Providing Drinking Water.*
2. Obtain a list of persons who have special fluid orders from the nurse. Or use your assignment sheet.
3. Practice hand hygiene.
4. Collect the following:
   - Cart
   - Ice chest filled with ice

   - Cover for the ice chest
   - Scoop
   - Disposable cups
   - Straws
   - Paper towels
   - Water pitchers for patient and resident use
   - Large water pitcher filled with cold water (optional, depending on agency procedure)
   - Towel for the scoop
5. Cover the cart with paper towels. Arrange equipment on top of the paper towels.

PROCEDURE

6. Take the cart to the person's room door. Do not take the cart into the room.
7. Check the person's fluid orders. Use the list from the nurse.
8. Identify the person. Check the ID bracelet against the fluid orders sheet or your assignment sheet. Also call the person by name.
9. Take the pitcher from the person's overbed table. Empty it into the bathroom sink.
10. Determine if a new water pitcher is needed.
11. Use the scoop to fill the pitcher with ice (Fig. 19-6, p. 342). Do not let the scoop touch the rim or inside of the pitcher.

12. Place the ice scoop on the towel.
13. Fill the water pitcher with water. Get water from the bathroom or use the larger water pitcher on the cart.
14. Place the pitcher, disposable cup, and straw (if used) on the overbed table. Fill the cup with water. Do not let the water pitcher touch the rim or inside of the cup.
15. Make sure the water pitcher, cup, and straw (if used) are within the person's reach.

POST-PROCEDURE

16. Provide for comfort. (See the inside of the front book cover.)
17. Place the signal light within reach.

18. Complete a safety check of the room. (See the inside of the front book cover.)
19. Decontaminate your hands.
20. Repeat steps 6 through 19 for each person.

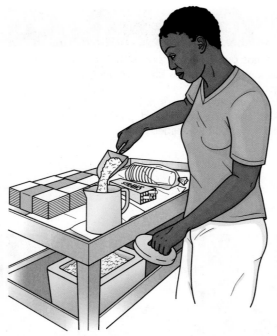

FIGURE 19-6 Providing drinking water.

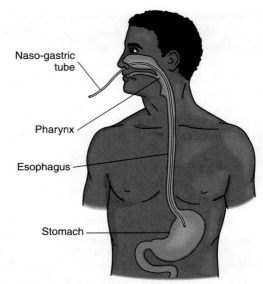

FIGURE 19-8 A naso-gastric (NG) tube inserted through the nose and esophagus and into the stomach.

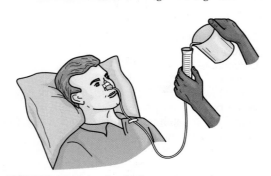

FIGURE 19-7 A tube feeding given with a syringe.

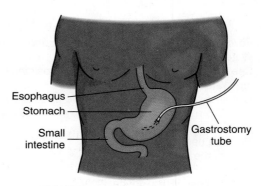

FIGURE 19-9 A gastrostomy tube.

ASSISTING WITH SPECIAL NEEDS

Many persons cannot eat or drink because of illness, surgery, or injury. The doctor may order nutritional support or IV (intravenous) therapy to meet food and fluid needs.

Enteral Nutrition

Some persons cannot or will not ingest, chew, or swallow food. Or food cannot pass from the mouth into the esophagus and into the stomach or small intestine. They may require enteral nutrition. **Enteral nutrition** is giving nutrients into the gastro-intestinal (GI) tract *(enteral)* through a feeding tube. **Gavage** is the process of giving a tube feeding (Fig. 19-7).

- A *naso-gastric (NG) tube* is inserted through the nose *(naso)* into the stomach *(gastro)* (Fig. 19-8).
- A *gastrostomy tube* *(stomach tube)* is inserted into the stomach *(gastro)*. It involves a surgically created opening *(stomy)* (Fig. 19-9).

Observations Diarrhea, constipation, delayed stomach emptying, and aspiration (p. 333) are risks. Report the following at once:

- Nausea
- Discomfort during the feeding
- Vomiting
- Distended (enlarged and swollen) abdomen
- Coughing
- Complaints of indigestion or heartburn
- Redness, swelling, drainage, odor, or pain at the ostomy site
- Fever
- Signs and symptoms of respiratory distress (Chapter 24)
- Increased pulse rate
- Complaints of flatulence (Chapter 18)
- Diarrhea (Chapter 18)

Preventing Aspiration Aspiration is a major risk from tube feedings. It can cause pneumonia and death. Aspiration can occur:

* *During insertion.* An NG tube can slip into the airway. An x-ray is taken after insertion to check tube placement.
* *From tube movement out of place.* Coughing, sneezing, vomiting, suctioning, and poor positioning are common causes. A tube can move from the stomach or intestines into the esophagus and then into the airway. *The RN checks tube placement before a tube feeding. You are never responsible for checking feeding tube placement.*
* *From regurgitation.* **Regurgitation** is the backward flow of stomach contents into the mouth. Delayed stomach emptying and over-feeding are common causes.

To assist the nurse in preventing regurgitation and aspiration:

* Position the person in Fowler's or semi-Fowler's position before the feeding. Follow the care plan and the nurse's directions.
* Maintain Fowler's or semi-Fowler's position for 1 to 2 hours after the feeding or at all times. The position allows formula to move through the GI tract. Follow the care plan and the nurse's directions.
* Avoid the left side-lying position. It prevents the stomach from emptying.

Comfort Measures Persons with feeding tubes usually are NPO. Dry mouth, dry lips, and sore throat cause discomfort. Sometimes hard candy or gum is allowed. These measures are common:

* Oral hygiene every 2 hours while the person is awake.
* Lubricant for the lips every 2 hours while the person is awake.
* Mouth rinses every 2 hours while the person is awake.
* Cleaning the nose and nostrils every 4 to 8 hours. NG tubes can irritate and cause pressure on the nose. They can change nostril shape or cause pressure ulcers. To prevent these problems:
* Secure the tube to the nose (Fig. 19-10). Use tape or a tube holder. Tube holders have foam cushions that prevent pressure on the nose. Re-taping is not needed. Re-taping irritates the nose.
* Secure the tube to the person's garment at the shoulder area (see Fig. 19-7). Taping the tube to the garment is common. Follow agency policy.

Intravenous Therapy

Intravenous (IV) therapy is giving fluids through a needle or catheter inserted into a vein. *IV* and

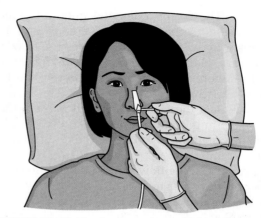

FIGURE 19-10 The feeding tube is secured to the nose.

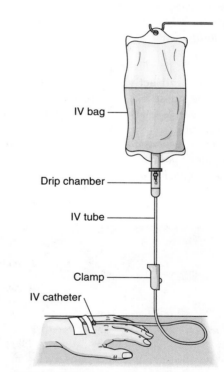

IV bag

Drip chamber

IV tube

Clamp

IV catheter

FIGURE 19-11 Equipment for IV therapy.

IV infusion also refer to IV therapy. See Figure 19-11 for the basic equipment used.

* The solution container is a plastic bag. It is called the *IV bag.*
* A *catheter* or *needle* is inserted into a vein.
* The *IV tube* or *infusion tubing* connects the IV bag to the catheter or needle.
* Fluid drips from the bag into the *drip chamber.*
* The *clamp* is used to regulate the flow rate.
* The IV bag hangs from an IV pole or ceiling hook. *IV standard* is another name for an IV pole.

Flow rate The doctor orders the amount of fluid to give (infuse) and the amount of time to give it in. With this information, the RN figures the flow rate. The **flow rate** is the number of drops per minute (*gtt/min*). The abbreviation *gtt* means drops. The Latin word *guttae* means drops.

The RN sets the clamp for the flow rate. Or an electronic pump controls the flow rate. An alarm sounds if something is wrong. Tell the nurse at once if you hear an alarm.

You can check the flow rate. The RN tells you the number of drops per minute. To check the flow rate, count the number of drops in 1 minute (Fig. 19-12). Tell the RN at once if:

- No fluid is dripping.
- The rate is too fast.
- The rate is too slow.
- The bag is empty or close to being empty.
  See *Promoting Safety and Comfort: Flow Rate.*

Assisting With IV Therapy You help meet the safety, hygiene, and activity needs of persons with IVs. Follow the nurse's direction, the care plan, and the safety measures in Box 19-6. Report any of the signs and symptoms listed in Box 19-7 at once.

You are never responsible for starting or maintaining IV therapy. Nor do you regulate the flow rate or change IV bags. You never give blood or IV drugs.

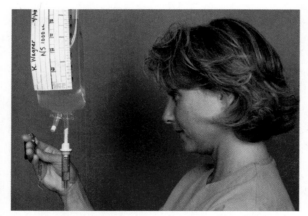

FIGURE 19-12 The flow rate is checked by counting the number of drops per minute.

PROMOTING SAFETY AND COMFORT
Flow Rate

Safety

The person can suffer serious harm if the flow rate is too fast or too slow. The flow rate can change from position changes. Kinked tubes and lying on the tube also affect the flow rate.

Never change the position of the clamp or adjust any controls on infusion pumps. Tell the nurse at once if there is a problem with the flow rate.

BOX 19-6 | Safety Measures for IV Therapy

- Follow Standard Precautions and the Bloodborne Pathogen Standard.
- Do not move the needle or catheter. Needle or catheter position must be maintained. If the needle or catheter is moved, it may come out of the vein. Then fluid flows into tissues (infiltration). Or the flow stops.
- Protect the IV bag, tubing, and needle or catheter when the person walks. Portable IV standards are rolled along next to the person.
- Assist the person with turning and repositioning. Move the IV bag to the side of the bed on which the person is lying. Always allow enough slack in the tubing. The needle or catheter can move from pressure on the tube.
- Tell the nurse at once if bleeding occurs from the insertion site. Follow Standard Precautions and the Bloodborne Pathogen Standard.
- Tell the nurse at once of any signs and symptoms listed in Box 19-7.

BOX 19-7   Signs and Symptoms of IV Therapy Complications

Local—At the IV Site
- Bleeding
- Puffiness, swelling, or leaking fluid
- Pale or reddened skin
- Complaints of pain at or above the IV site
- Hot or cold skin near the site

Systemic—Involving the Whole Body
- Fever
- Itching
- Drop in blood pressure
- Pulse rate greater than 100 beats per minute
- Irregular pulse
- Cyanosis (bluish color)
- Confusion or changes in mental function
- Loss of consciousness
- Difficulty breathing
- Shortness of breath
- Decreasing or no urine output
- Chest pain
- Nausea

Focus on PRIDE
The Person, Family, and Yourself

Personal and Professional Responsibility—Many hospitals are serving food in new ways. The purpose is to allow freedom and personal choice. For example, some hospitals offer:

- *24-hour catering.* Meals and snacks are provided 24 hours a day. This is for persons who cannot or do not want to eat at the usual mealtimes. The person can order food directly from the food service department. The person orders the foods he or she wants within the person's ordered diet.
- *Mobile food carts.* Food service staff bring a food cart to the nursing unit. The patient selects food and a tray is prepared.

With such systems, you may have new responsibilities. For example, you may need to watch for the arrival of food trays more often. Or you may need to assist persons with reading or filling out menus. Know your agency's food ordering and delivery system and your role in that system. Take pride in helping others meet their nutritional needs.

Rights and Respect—Persons have different food preferences. Cultural, social, religious, medical, and personal factors affect a person's food choices. Persons commonly express their food likes and dislikes. You may hear a person say the food is too cold. Or it is too bland. Or the food tastes bad.

Persons have the right to express their preferences. Do not become angry or upset. The person should not feel as if he or she is complaining or being picky. Learning the person's likes and dislikes can improve nutrition. It also shows interest and concern for the person. Respect the person's right to express personal food choices.

Independence and Social Interaction—Meals can provide a time for social contact with others. A friendly, social setting is important. Some nursing centers have areas where residents can dine with a partner, family, or friends. They can enjoy holidays, birthdays, anniversaries, and other special events together. The dietary department provides the meal. Or the meal is brought by the family.

Delegation and Teamwork—In some agencies, meal trays arrive on the nursing unit in a meal cart. Each tray is in a slot. Trays are served in the order that they appear in the cart. The entire nursing team serves trays. You may serve trays to patients or residents of other staff members. They do the same for you. The team works together to serve food promptly and at the correct temperature.

Ethics and Laws—OBRA requires that patients and residents receive proper nutrition. Survey teams make sure that:

- Needed help is provided
- Assistive devices are provided
- Medical asepsis is practiced when serving food and fluids
- Meals and snacks are served promptly
- Other food is offered if the person refuses the food served

REVIEW QUESTIONS

Circle the BEST answer.

1 The MyPyramid food guidance system encourages the following *except*
   a The same diet for everyone
   b Smart food choices
   c Physical activity
   d Small steps to improve diet and life-style

2 On a 2000 calorie a day diet, what is the amount of grains needed?
   a 6 ounces
   b 4 to 5 ounces
   c 3 to 4 ounces
   d 2 ounces

3 On a 2000 calorie a day diet, what is the amount of meat and beans needed?
   a 2½ ounces
   b 3 to 4 ounces
   c 4 to 5 ounces
   d 5½ ounces

4 Which food group contains the *most* fat?
   a Grains
   b Vegetables
   c Milk
   d Meat and beans

5 These statements are about oils. Which is *false?*
   a Oils are high in calories.
   b The best oil choices come from fish, nuts, and vegetable oils.
   c Oils from plant sources contain cholesterol.
   d Mayonnaise, some salad dressings, and soft margarine are mainly oil.

6 Protein is needed for
   a Tissue growth and repair
   b The fiber for bowel elimination
   c Body heat and to protect organs from injury
   d Improving the taste of food

7 Which foods provide the *most* protein?
   a Butter and cream
   b Tomatoes and potatoes
   c Meats and fish
   d Corn and lettuce

8 The sodium-controlled diet involves
   a Omitting high-sodium foods
   b Adding salt to food at the table
   c Using 2400 mg of salt in cooking
   d A sodium-intake flow sheet

9 Diabetes meal planning involves the following *except*
   a Food the person likes
   b Eating the same amount of carbohydrates, protein, and fat each day
   c Eating at regular times
   d Sodium control

10 OBRA requires
   a 2 regular meals
   b Between-meal snacks
   c 3 regular meals and a bedtime snack
   d Meals every 6 hours

11 Which is *not* a sign of a swallowing problem?
   a Drooling
   b Coughing while eating
   c Pocketing
   d Edema

12 Adult fluid requirements for normal fluid balance are about
   a 1000 to 1500 mL daily
   b 1500 to 2000 mL daily
   c 2000 to 2500 mL daily
   d 2500 to 3000 mL daily

13 A person is NPO. You should
   a Provide a variety of fluids
   b Offer fluids in small amounts and in small containers
   c Remove the water pitcher and cup from the room
   d Remove oral hygiene equipment from the room

14 You are feeding a person. Which action is *not correct?*
   a Ask if he or she wants to pray before eating.
   b Use a fork to feed the person.
   c Ask the person the order in which to serve food and fluids.
   d Engage the person in a pleasant conversation.

15 Before providing fresh drinking water, you need to know the person's
   a Intake
   b Diet
   c Fluid orders
   d Preferred beverages

16 Which position prevents regurgitation after a tube feeding?
   a Fowler's or semi-Fowler's position
   b The supine position
   c The left or right side-lying position
   d The prone position

17 A person with a feeding tube is NPO. You should do the following *except*
   a Give the person hard candy or gum
   b Provide oral hygiene
   c Provide mouth rinses
   d Apply lubricant to the lips

18 A person has an NG tube. The care plan includes the following measures to prevent nasal irritation. Which measure should you question?
   a Clean the nose and nostrils every 4 hours.
   b Tape the tube to the nose.
   c Remove the tube every 4 hours.
   d Secure the tube to the person's gown.

19 A nurse asks you to check an IV flow rate. What should you do?
   a Count the drops in 30 seconds; multiply the number by 2.
   b Count the drops for 1 minute.
   c Check if the fluid is dripping too fast or slow.
   d Measure the amount of fluid.

20 You note bleeding from an IV insertion site. What should you do?
   a Tell the nurse.
   b Move the needle or catheter.
   c Discontinue the IV.
   d Clamp the IV tubing.

Answers to these questions are on p. 528.

20

ASSISTING WITH ASSESSMENT

PROCEDURES

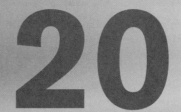

- Taking a Temperature With a Glass Thermometer
- Taking a Temperature With an Electronic Thermometer
- Taking a Radial Pulse
- Taking an Apical Pulse
- Counting Res0irations
- Measuring Blood Pressure
- Measuring Intake and Output
- Measuring Weight and Height

OBJECTIVES

- Define the key terms and key abbreviations listed in this chapter.
- Explain why vital signs are measured.
- List the factors affecting vital signs.
- Identify the normal ranges for each temperature site.
- Explain when to use each temperature site.
- Identify the pulse sites.
- Describe normal respirations.
- Describe the practices to follow when measuring blood pressure.
- Explain why intake and output are measured.
- Identify the fluids counted as intake and the fluids counted as output.
- Explain how to prepare the person for weight and height measurements.
- Explain how to assist with assessment.
- Explain how to promote PRIDE in the person, the family, and yourself.
- Perform the procedures described in this chapter.

KEY TERMS

blood pressure The amount of force exerted against the walls of an artery by the blood

body temperature The amount of heat in the body that is a balance between the amount of heat produced and the amount lost by the body

diastolic pressure The pressure in the arteries when the heart is at rest

fever Elevated body temperature

hypertension Blood pressure measurements that remain above (hyper) a systolic pressure of 140 mm Hg or a diastolic pressure above 90 mm Hg

hypotension When the systolic blood pressure is below (hypo) 90 mm Hg and the diastolic pressure is below 60 mm Hg

intake The amount of fluid taken in

output The amount of fluid lost

pulse The beat of the heart felt at an artery as a wave of blood passes through the artery

pulse rate The number of heartbeats or pulses felt in 1 minute

respiration Breathing air into (inhalation) and out of (exhalation) the lungs

systolic pressure The pressure in the arteries when the heart contracts

vital signs Temperature, pulse, respirations, and blood pressure

KEY ABBREVIATIONS

C Centigrade; Celsius

F Fahrenheit

Hg Mercury

ID Identification

I&O Intake and output

IV Intravenous

mL Milliliter

mm Millimeter

mm Hg Millimeters of mercury

You assist the nurse with the assessment step of the nursing process. Some observations involve measurements:

- **Vital signs**—temperature, pulse, respirations (TPR), blood pressure (BP). Some agencies consider "pain" to be a vital sign (p. 366).
- Intake and output.
- Weight and height.

VITAL SIGNS

Vital signs reflect three body processes: regulation of body temperature, breathing, and heart function. A person's vital signs vary within certain limits. They are affected by sleep, activity, eating, weather, noise, exercise, drugs, anger, fear, anxiety, pain, and illness.

Vital signs show even minor changes in the person's condition. They tell about responses to treatment. They often signal life-threatening events.

Accuracy is essential when you measure, record, and report vital signs. If unsure of your measurements, promptly ask the nurse to take them again. Unless otherwise ordered, take vital signs with the person at rest lying or sitting. Report the following at once:

- Any vital sign that is changed from a prior measurement
- Vital signs above or below the normal range
  See *Persons With Dementia: Vital Signs.*
  See *Focus on Communication: Vital Signs.*

PERSONS WITH DEMENTIA
Vital Signs

Measuring vital signs on persons with dementia may be difficult. The person may move about, hit at you, and grab equipment. This is not safe for the person or for you. Two workers may be needed. One uses touch and a soothing voice to calm and distract the person. The other measures the vital signs.

You may need to try the procedure when the person is calmer. Or take the pulse and respirations at one time. Then take the temperature and blood pressure at another time.

Always approach the person calmly. Use a soothing voice. Tell the person what you are going to do. Do not rush the person. Follow the care plan. If you cannot measure vital signs, tell the nurse right away.

FOCUS ON COMMUNICATION
Vital Signs

When measuring vital signs, you may not be able to feel a pulse or hear a blood pressure. Or a measurement may be abnormal. Do not alarm the person. You can say:

- "I'm not sure that I counted your pulse correctly. I want the nurse to check it too."
- "I'm not sure that I heard your blood pressure correctly. I'll ask the nurse to take it again."
- "Your pulse is a little slow (or fast). I'll ask the nurse to check it."
- "Your temperature is higher than normal. I'm going to try another thermometer. I'll also ask the nurse to check you."

BOX 20-1 Temperature Sites

Oral Site

Oral temperatures are *not* taken if the person:
- Is under 4 or 5 years of age
- Is unconscious
- Has had surgery or an injury to the face, neck, nose, or mouth
- Is receiving oxygen
- Breathes through the mouth
- Has a naso-gastric tube
- Is delirious, restless, confused, or disoriented
- Is paralyzed on one side of the body
- Has a sore mouth
- Has a convulsive (seizure) disorder

Rectal Site

The rectal site is used for infants and children under 3 years old. Rectal temperatures are taken when the oral site cannot be used. Rectal temperatures are *not* taken if the person:
- Has diarrhea
- Has a rectal disorder or injury
- Has heart disease
- Had rectal surgery
- Is confused or agitated

Tympanic Membrane Site

The site has fewer microbes than the mouth or rectum. Therefore, the risk of spreading infection is reduced. This site is *not* used if the person has:
- An ear disorder
- Ear drainage

Temporal Artery Site

Measures body temperature at the temporal artery in the forehead. The site is non-invasive.

Axillary Site

Less reliable than the other sites. It is used when the other sites cannot be used.

TABLE 20-1 Normal Body Temperatures

Site	Baseline	Normal Range
Oral	98.6° F (37° C)	97.6° to 99.6° F (36.5° to 37.5° C)
Rectal	99.6° F (37.5° C)	98.6° to 100.6° F (37.0° to 38.1° C)
Axillary	97.6° F (36.5° C)	96.6° to 98.6° F (35.9° to 37.0° C)
Tympanic membrane	98.6° F (37° C)	98.6° F (37° C)
Temporal artery	99.6° F (37.5° C)	99.6° F (37.5° C)

Body Temperature

Body temperature is the amount of heat in the body. It is a balance between the amount of heat produced and the amount lost by the body. Heat is produced as cells use food for energy. It is lost through the skin, breathing, urine, and feces. Body temperature stays fairly stable. It is lower in the morning and higher in the afternoon and evening. See "Vital Signs" for the factors affecting body temperature.

Thermometers are used to measure temperature. It is measured using the Fahrenheit (F) and centigrade or Celsius (C) scales. Temperature sites are the mouth, rectum, axilla (underarm), tympanic membrane (ear), and temporal artery (forehead) (Box 20-1). Each site has a normal range (Table 20-1).

Older persons have lower body temperatures than younger persons. An oral temperature of 98.6° F may signal **fever** (elevated body temperature) in an older person.

See *Promoting Safety and Comfort: Body Temperature.*

Glass Thermometers The glass thermometer is a hollow glass tube (Fig. 20-1) with a bulb (tip) at the end. The device is filled with a substance—mercury-free mixture or mercury. When heated, the substance expands and rises in the tube. When cooled, the substance contracts and moves down the tube.

PROMOTING SAFETY AND COMFORT
Body Temperature

Safety
Rectal temperatures are dangerous for persons with heart disease. The thermometer can stimulate the vagus nerve in the rectum. This nerve also affects the heart. Stimulation of the vagus nerve slows the heart rate. The heart rate can slow to dangerous levels in some persons.

PROMOTING SAFETY AND COMFORT
Glass Thermometers

Safety
If a mercury-glass thermometer breaks, tell the nurse at once. Mercury is a hazardous substance. Do not touch the mercury. Do not let the person do so. The agency must follow special procedures for handling all hazardous materials. See Chapter 8.

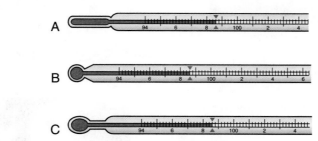

FIGURE 20-1 Types of glass thermometers. **A,** The long or slender tip. **B,** The stubby tip (rectal thermometer). **C,** The pear-shaped tip.

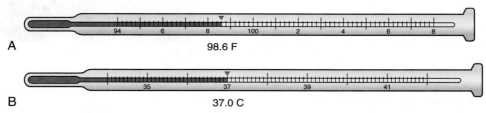

FIGURE 20-2 **A,** A Fahrenheit thermometer. The temperature measurement is 98.6° F. **B,** Centigrade thermometer. The temperature measurement is 37.0° C.

Long- or slender-tip thermometers are used for oral and axillary temperatures. So are thermometers with stubby and pear-shaped tips. Rectal thermometers have stubby tips. Thermometers are color-coded:

- Blue—oral and axillary thermometers
- Red—rectal thermometers

Glass thermometers are re-usable. However, the following are problems:

- They take a long time to register—3 to 10 minutes depending on the site (p. 352).
- They break easily. Broken thermometers can injure the rectum and colon.
- The person may bite down and break an oral thermometer. Cuts in the mouth are risks. Swallowed mercury can cause mercury poisoning.

See *Promoting Safety and Comfort: Glass Thermometers.*

Reading a Glass Thermometer Fahrenheit thermometers have long and short lines. Every other long line is an even degree from 94° to 108° F. The short lines mean 0.2 (two-tenths) of a degree (Fig. 20-2, *A*).

On a centigrade thermometer, each long line means 1 degree. Degrees range from 34° to 42° C. Each short line means 0.1 (one-tenth) of a degree (Fig. 20-2, *B*).

To read a glass thermometer:

- Hold it at the stem (Fig. 20-3, p. 352). Bring it to eye level.
- Turn it until you can see the numbers and the long and short lines.
- Turn it back and forth slowly until you can see the silver or red line.
- Read the nearest degree (long line).
- Read the nearest tenth of a degree (short line)—an even number on a Fahrenheit thermometer.

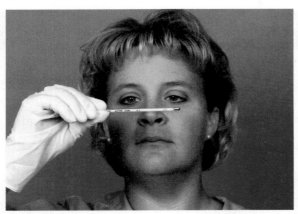

FIGURE 20-3 The thermometer is held at the stem. It is read at eye level.

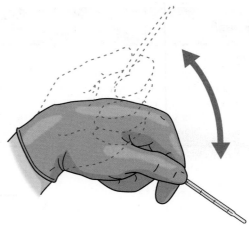

FIGURE 20-4 The wrist is snapped to shake down the thermometer.

Using a Glass Thermometer Do the following to prevent infection, promote safety, and obtain an accurate measurement:

- Use the person's thermometer.
- Use a rectal thermometer only for rectal temperatures.
- Rinse the thermometer under cold, running water if it was soaking in a disinfectant. Dry it from the stem to the bulb end with tissues.
- Check the thermometer for breaks, cracks, and chips. Discard it following agency policy if it is broken, cracked, or chipped.
- Shake down the thermometer to move the substance down in the tube. Hold it at the stem; stand away from walls, tables, or other hard surfaces. Flex and snap your wrist until the substance is below 94° F or 34° C. See Figure 20-4.
- Use plastic covers following agency policy (Fig. 20-5). To take a temperature, insert the thermometer into a cover. Remove the cover to read the thermometer. Discard the cover after use.
- Clean and store the thermometer following agency policy. Wipe it with tissues first to remove mucus, feces, or sweat. Do not use hot water. It causes the mercury or mercury-free mixture to expand so much that the thermometer could break. After cleaning, rinse the thermometer under cold, running water. Then store it in a container with a disinfectant solution.
- Practice medical asepsis. Follow Standard Precautions and the Bloodborne Pathogen Standard.

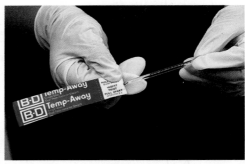

FIGURE 20-5 The thermometer is inserted into a plastic cover.

Taking Temperatures Glass thermometers are used for oral, rectal, and axillary temperatures. Special measures are needed for each site.

- *The oral site.* The glass thermometer remains in place 2 to 3 minutes or as required by agency policy.
- *The rectal site.* Lubricate the bulb end of the rectal thermometer for easy insertion and to prevent tissue injury. Hold the thermometer in place so it is not lost into the rectum or broken. A glass thermometer remains in the rectum for 2 minutes or as required by agency policy. Privacy is important. The buttocks and anus are exposed. The procedure embarrasses many people.
- *The axillary site.* The axilla (underarm) must be dry. Do not use this site right after bathing. The glass thermometer stays in place for 5 to 10 minutes or as required by agency policy.

See *Focus on Communication: Taking Temperatures.*
See *Delegation Guidelines: Taking Temperatures.*
See *Promoting Safety and Comfort: Taking Temperatures.*

FOCUS ON COMMUNICATION
Taking Temperatures

Checking a rectal temperature can be embarrassing and uncomfortable. Be professional. Tell the person what you are going to do. Explain why you must check the person's temperature using the rectal route. You can say: "Mr. Presney, I need to check your temperature. I must check a rectal temperature because your oxygen changes the temperature in your mouth. The thermometer has to stay in place for 2 minutes. Please tell me if you feel pain."

When using a glass thermometer, the thermometer remains in the rectum for at least 2 minutes. This can cause discomfort. To promote comfort, talk the person through the procedure. You can say: "I'm almost done. There's about 1 minute left. Are you doing okay?"

DELEGATION GUIDELINES
Taking Temperatures

Before taking temperatures, you need this information from the nurse and the care plan:
- What thermometer to use for each person—glass, electronic, or other type
- What site to use for each person—oral, rectal, axillary, tympanic membrane, or temporal artery
- How long to leave a glass thermometer in place
- When to take temperatures
- Which persons are at risk for elevated temperatures
- What observations to report and record:
  - A temperature that is changed from a prior measurement
  - A temperature above or below the normal range for the site used
- When to report observations
- What specific patient or resident concerns to report at once

PROMOTING SAFETY AND COMFORT
Taking Temperatures

Safety

Thermometers are inserted into the mouth, rectum, axilla, and ear. Each area has many microbes. The area may contain blood. Therefore each person has his or her own glass thermometer. This prevents the spread of microbes and infection. Follow Standard Precautions and the Bloodborne Pathogen Standard when taking temperatures.

When taking a rectal temperature, your gloved hands may come in contact with feces. If so, remove the gloves and decontaminate your hands. Then note the temperature on your notepad or assignment sheet. Put on clean gloves to complete the procedure.

Comfort

Remove the thermometer in a timely manner. Do not leave it in place longer than needed. This affects the person's comfort. For example, an oral glass thermometer is left in place for 2 to 3 minutes. Do not leave it in place longer than that.

 # TAKING A TEMPERATURE WITH A GLASS THERMOMETER

QUALITY OF LIFE

Remember to:
- Knock before entering the person's room.
- Address the person by name.
- Introduce yourself by name and title.

- Explain the procedure to the person before beginning and during the procedure.
- Protect the person's rights during the procedure.
- Handle the person gently during the procedure.

PRE-PROCEDURE

1. Follow *Delegation Guidelines: Taking Temperatures.* See *Promoting Safety and Comfort:*
   a *Glass Thermometers,* p. 351
   b *Taking Temperatures*
2. For an *oral temperature,* ask the person not to eat, drink, smoke, or chew gum for at least 15 to 20 minutes before the measurement or as required by agency policy.
3. Practice hand hygiene.
4. Collect the following:
   - Oral or rectal thermometer and holder
   - Tissues

- Plastic covers if used
- Gloves
- Toilet tissue (rectal temperature)
- Water-soluble lubricant (rectal temperature)
- Towel (axillary temperature)
5. Decontaminate your hands.
6. Identify the person. Check the ID (identification) bracelet against the assignment sheet. Also call the person by name.
7. Provide for privacy.

Continued

PROCEDURE

8 Put on the gloves.
9 Rinse the thermometer in cold water if it was soaking in a disinfectant. Dry it with tissues.
10 Check for breaks, cracks, or chips.
11 Shake down the thermometer below the lowest number. Hold the thermometer by the stem.
12 Insert it into a plastic cover if used.
13 For an *oral temperature:*
   a Ask the person to moisten his or her lips.
   b Place the bulb end of the thermometer under the tongue and to one side (Fig. 20-6).
   c Ask the person to close the lips around the thermometer to hold it in place.
   d Ask the person not to talk. Remind the person not to bite down on the thermometer.
   e Leave it in place for 2 to 3 minutes or as required by agency policy.
14 For a *rectal temperature:*
   a Position the person in Sims' position.
   b Put a small amount of lubricant on a tissue.
   c Lubricate the bulb end of the thermometer.
   d Fold back top linens to expose the anal area.
   e Raise the upper buttock to expose the anus (Fig. 20-7).
   f Insert the thermometer 1 inch into the rectum. Do not force the thermometer. Remember, glass thermometers can break.
   g Hold the thermometer in place for 2 minutes or as required by agency policy. Do not let go of it while it is in the rectum.
15 For an *axillary temperature:*
   a Help the person remove an arm from the gown. Do not expose the person.

b Dry the axilla with the towel.
c Place the bulb end of the thermometer in the center of the axilla.
d Ask the person to place the arm over the chest to hold the thermometer in place (Fig. 20-8). Hold it and the arm in place if he or she cannot help.
e Leave the thermometer in place for 5 to 10 minutes or as required by agency policy.
16 Remove the thermometer.
17 Use tissues to remove the plastic cover. Discard the cover and tissues. Wipe the thermometer with a tissue if no cover was used. Wipe from the stem to the bulb end. Discard the tissue.
18 Read the thermometer.
19 Note the person's name and temperature on your notepad or assignment sheet. Write *R* for a rectal temperature. Write *A* for an axillary temperature.
20 For a *rectal temperature:*
   a Place used toilet tissue on several thicknesses of clean toilet tissue.
   b Place the thermometer on clean toilet tissue.
   c Wipe the anal area to remove excess lubricant and any feces.
   d Cover the person.
21 For an *axillary temperature:* Help the person put the gown back on.
22 Shake down the thermometer.
23 Clean the thermometer according to agency policy. Return it to the holder.
24 Discard tissues and dispose of toilet tissue.
25 Remove the gloves. Decontaminate your hands.

POST-PROCEDURE

26 Provide for comfort. (See the inside of the front book cover.)
27 Place the signal light within reach.
28 Unscreen the person.
29 Complete a safety check of the room. (See the inside of the front book cover.)

30 Decontaminate your hands.
31 Report and record the temperature. Note the temperature site when reporting and recording. Report an abnormal temperature at once.

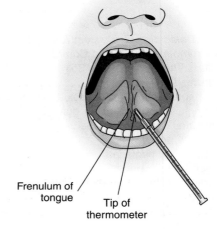

FIGURE 20-6 The thermometer is placed at the base of the tongue and to one side.

Frenulum of tongue

Tip of thermometer

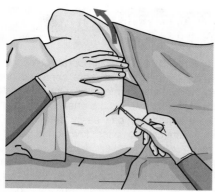

FIGURE 20-7 The rectal temperature is taken with the person in Sims' position. The buttock is raised to expose the anus.

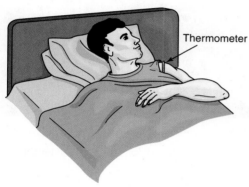

FIGURE 20-8 The thermometer is held in place in the axilla by bringing the person's arm over the chest.

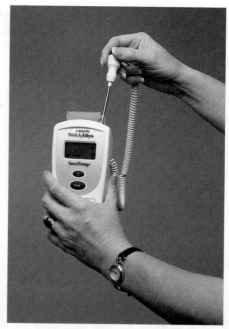

FIGURE 20-9 Electronic thermometer.

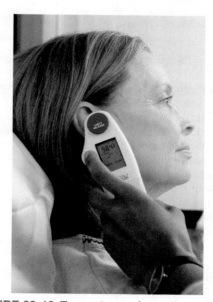

FIGURE 20-10 Tympanic membrane thermometer.

✿ Electronic Thermometers Electronic thermometers are battery-operated (Fig. 20-9). They measure temperature in a few seconds. The temperature is shown on the front of the device. Some contain batteries. Others are kept in battery chargers when not in use.

Some electronic thermometers have oral and rectal probes. A disposable cover (sheath) protects the probe. The probe cover is discarded after use. This helps prevent the spread of infection.

Tympanic Membrane Thermometers Tympanic membrane thermometers measure temperature at the tympanic membrane in the ear (Fig. 20-10). The covered probe is gently inserted into the ear. The temperature is measured in 1 to 3 seconds.

Temporal Artery Thermometers Body temperature is measured at the temporal artery in the forehead (Fig. 20-11, p. 356). The device is gently stroked across the forehead and across the temporal artery. It measures the temperature of the blood in the temporal artery—the same temperature of the blood coming from the heart.

These thermometers measure body temperature in 3 to 4 seconds. They are non-invasive. Nothing is inserted into the mouth, ear, or rectum. Follow the manufacturer's instructions for using, cleaning, and storing the device.

See *Persons With Dementia: Electronic Thermometers,* p. 356.

FIGURE 20-11 Temporal artery thermometer.

PERSONS WITH DEMENTIA
Electronic Thermometers

Tympanic membrane and temporal artery thermometers are used for persons who are confused and resist care. They are fast and comfortable. Oral and rectal glass and electronic thermometers are unsafe because:

- A glass thermometer can easily break if the person moves, resists care, or bites down on it. Serious injury can occur.
- An electronic thermometer can injure the mouth and teeth if the person bites down on it. It also can cause injury if the person moves quickly and without warning.

TAKING A TEMPERATURE WITH AN ELECTRONIC THERMOMETER

QUALITY OF LIFE

Remember to:
- Knock before entering the person's room.
- Address the person by name.
- Introduce yourself by name and title.

- Explain the procedure to the person before beginning and during the procedure.
- Protect the person's rights during the procedure.
- Handle the person gently during the procedure.

PRE-PROCEDURE

1 Follow *Delegation Guidelines: Taking Temperatures,* p. 353.
  See *Promoting Safety and Comfort: Taking Temperatures,* p. 353.
2 For an oral temperature, ask the person not to eat, drink, smoke, or chew gum for at least 15 to 20 minutes before the measurement or as required by agency policy.
3 Practice hand hygiene.
4 Collect the following:
  - Thermometer—electronic, tympanic membrane, temporal artery

- Probe (Blue for an oral or axillary temperature. Red for a rectal temperature.)
- Probe covers
- Toilet tissue (rectal temperature)
- Water-soluble lubricant (rectal temperature)
- Gloves
- Towel (axillary temperature)
5 Plug the probe into the thermometer. (This is not done for a tympanic membrane or temporal artery thermometer.)
6 Decontaminate your hands.
7 Identify the person. Check the ID bracelet against the assignment sheet. Also call the person by name.

PROCEDURE

8 Provide for privacy. Position the person for an oral, rectal, axillary, or tympanic membrane temperature.
9 Put on gloves if contact with blood, body fluids, secretions, or excretions is likely.
10 Insert the probe into a probe cover.
11 For an *oral temperature:*
  a Ask the person to open the mouth and raise the tongue.
  b Place the covered probe at the base of the tongue and to one side (see Fig. 20-6).
  c Ask the person to lower the tongue and close the mouth.

12 For a *rectal temperature:*
  a Place some lubricant on toilet tissue.
  b Lubricate the end of the covered probe.
  c Expose the anal area.
  d Raise the upper buttock.
  e Insert the probe ½ inch into the rectum.
  f Hold the probe in place.
13 For an *axillary temperature:*
  a Help the person remove an arm from the gown. Do not expose the person.
  b Dry the axilla with the towel.
  c Place the covered probe in the center of the axilla.
  d Place the person's arm over the chest.
  e Hold the probe in place.

PROCEDURE—cont'd

14 For a *tympanic membrane temperature:*
  a Ask the person to turn his or her head so the ear is in front of you.
  b Pull up and back on the adult's ear to straighten the ear canal (Fig. 20-12).
  c Insert the covered probe gently.
15 Start the thermometer.
16 Hold the probe in place until you hear a tone or see a flashing or steady light.
17 Read the temperature on the display.
18 Remove the probe. Press the eject button to discard the cover.

19 Note the person's name and temperature on your notepad or assignment sheet. Note the temperature site. Write *R* for a rectal temperature. Write *A* for an axillary temperature.
20 Return the probe to the holder.
21 Help the person put the gown back on (axillary temperature). For a rectal temperature:
  a Wipe the anal area with toilet tissue to remove lubricant.
  b Cover the person.
  c Dispose of used toilet tissue.
  d Remove the gloves. Decontaminate your hands.

POST-PROCEDURE

22 Provide for comfort. (See the inside of the front book cover.)
23 Place the signal light within reach.
24 Unscreen the person.
25 Complete a safety check of the room. (See the inside of the front book cover.)

26 Return the thermometer to the charging unit.
27 Decontaminate your hands.
28 Report and record the temperature. Note the temperature site when reporting and recording. Report an abnormal temperature at once.

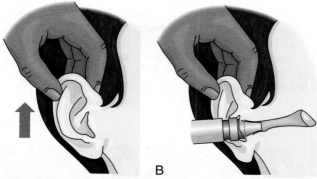

FIGURE 20-12 Using a tympanic membrane thermometer. **A,** The ear is pulled up and back. **B,** The probe is inserted into the ear canal.

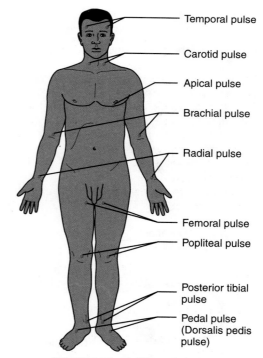

FIGURE 20-13 The pulse sites.

Pulse

The **pulse** is the beat of the heart felt at an artery as a wave of blood passes through the artery. A pulse is felt every time the heart beats.

The temporal, carotid, brachial, radial, femoral, popliteal, posterior tibial, and dorsalis pedis (pedal) pulses are on each side of the body (Fig. 20-13). The radial pulse is used most often. It is easy to reach and find. You can take a radial pulse without disturbing or exposing the person.

The apical pulse is felt over the heart. The apex *(apical)* of the heart is at the tip of the heart, just below the left nipple (p. 359). This pulse is taken with a stethoscope.

Using a Stethoscope A *stethoscope* is an instrument used to listen to the sounds produced by the heart, lungs, and other body organs (Fig. 20-14). It is used to take apical pulses and blood pressures. To use a stethoscope:

- Wipe the earpieces and diaphragm with antiseptic wipes before and after use.
- Place the earpiece tips in your ears. The bend of the tips points forward. Earpieces should fit snugly to block out noises. They should not cause pain or ear discomfort.
- Tap the diaphragm gently. You should hear the tapping. If not, turn the chest piece at the tubing. Gently tap the diaphragm again. Proceed if you hear the tapping sound. Check with the nurse if you do not hear the tapping.
- Place the diaphragm over the artery. Hold it in place as in Figure 20-15.
- Prevent noise. Do not let anything touch the tubing. Ask the person to be silent.

  See *Focus on Communication: Using a Stethoscope.*

  See *Promoting Safety and Comfort: Using a Stethoscope.*

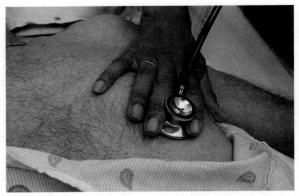

FIGURE 20-15 The stethoscope is held in place with the fingertips of the index and middle fingers.

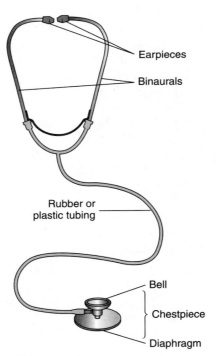

FIGURE 20-14 Parts of a stethoscope.

Earpieces

Binaurals

Rubber or plastic tubing

Bell

Chestpiece

Diaphragm

FOCUS ON COMMUNICATION
Using a Stethoscope

Hearing through the stethoscope is hard if the person is talking. You must ask the person to be silent. Be polite. Explain the procedure. Tell the person when and for how long he or she must remain silent. You can say: "Mr. Bradley, I am going to check your pulse using my stethoscope. It is hard for me to hear your heart beat when you talk. Please do not talk when my stethoscope is on your chest. It will take about 1 minute."

Sometimes persons forget and begin talking. You can politely say: "I am almost finished. Please stay quiet for just a little longer." Thank the person when you are done.

PROMOTING SAFETY AND COMFORT
Using a Stethoscope

Safety

Stethoscopes are in contact with many persons and staff. Therefore you must prevent infection. Wipe the earpieces and diaphragm with antiseptic wipes before and after use.

Comfort

Stethoscope diaphragms tend to be cold. Warm the diaphragm in your hand before applying it to the person (Fig. 20-16). Cold diaphragms can startle the person.

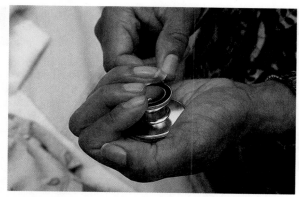

FIGURE 20-16 The diaphragm of the stethoscope is warmed in the palm of the hand.

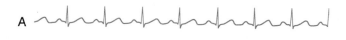

A

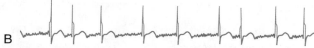

B

FIGURE 20-17 **A,** The electrocardiogram shows a regular pulse. The beats occur at regular intervals. **B,** These beats are at irregular intervals.

Pulse Rate The **pulse rate** is the number of heartbeats or pulses felt in 1 minute. The factors affecting "Vital Signs" (p. 349) cause the heart rate to change. Some drugs also increase the pulse rate. Other drugs slow down the pulse.

The adult pulse rate is between 60 and 100 beats per minute. A rate of less than 60 or more than 100 is considered abnormal. Report abnormal pulses to the nurse at once.

Rhythm and Force of the Pulse The *rhythm* of the pulse should be regular. That is, pulses are felt in a pattern. The same time interval occurs between beats. An irregular pulse occurs when the beats are not evenly spaced or beats are skipped (Fig. 20-17).

Force relates to pulse strength. A forceful pulse is easy to feel. It is described as *strong, full,* or *bounding.* Hard-to-feel pulses are described as *weak, thready,* or *feeble.*

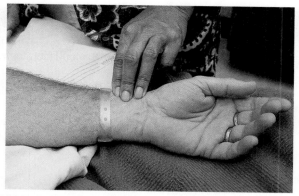

FIGURE 20-18 The middle three fingertips are used to take the radial pulse.

Taking Pulses You take radial and apical pulses.
- The radial pulse is used for routine vital signs. Place the first 2 or 3 fingertips of one hand against the radial artery. The radial artery is on the thumb side of the wrist (Fig. 20-18). Count the pulse for 30 seconds. Then multiply the number by 2. This gives the number of beats per minute. If the pulse is irregular, count it for 1 minute. In some agencies, all radial pulses are taken for 1 minute.
- The apical pulse is on the left side of the chest slightly below the nipple (Fig. 20-19). It is taken with a stethoscope. Count the apical pulse for 1 minute. The heartbeat normally sounds like a *lub-dub.* Count each *lub-dub* as one beat. Do not count the *lub* as one beat and the *dub* as another. Apical pulses are taken on:
  - Persons who have heart disease
  - Persons who have irregular heart rhythms
  - Persons who take drugs that affect the heart

See *Delegation Guidelines: Taking Pulses,* p. 360.
See *Promoting Safety and Comfort: Taking Pulses,* p. 360.

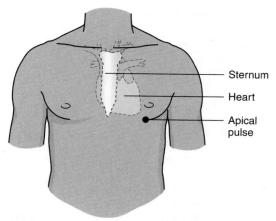

Sternum

Heart

Apical pulse

FIGURE 20-19 The apical pulse is located 2 to 3 inches to the left of the sternum (breastbone) and below the left nipple.

TAKING A RADIAL PULSE

NNAAP™

QUALITY OF LIFE

Remember to:
- Knock before entering the person's room.
- Address the person by name.
- Introduce yourself by name and title.

- Explain the procedure to the person before beginning and during the procedure.
- Protect the person's rights during the procedure.
- Handle the person gently during the procedure.

PRE-PROCEDURE

1 Follow *Delegation Guidelines: Taking Pulses.* See *Promoting Safety and Comfort: Taking Pulses.*
2 Practice hand hygiene.
3 Identify the person. Check the ID bracelet against the assignment sheet. Also call the person by name.
4 Provide for privacy.

PROCEDURE

5 Have the person sit or lie down.
6 Locate the radial pulse on the thumb side of the person's wrist. Use your first 2 or 3 middle fingertips (see Fig. 20-18).
7 Note if the pulse is strong or weak, and regular or irregular.

8 Count the pulse for 30 seconds. Multiply the number of beats by 2. Or count the pulse for 1 minute if:
 a Directed by the nurse and care plan.
 b Required by agency policy.
 c The pulse was irregular.
 d Required for your state competency test.
9 Note the person's name and pulse on your notepad or assignment sheet. Note the strength of the pulse. Note if it was regular or irregular.

POST-PROCEDURE

10 Provide for comfort. (See the inside of the front book cover.)
11 Place the signal light within reach.
12 Unscreen the person.
13 Complete a safety check of the room. (See the inside of the front book cover.)

14 Decontaminate your hands.
15 Report and record the pulse rate and your observations. Report an abnormal pulse at once.

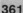

TAKING AN APICAL PULSE

QUALITY OF LIFE

Remember to:
- Knock before entering the person's room.
- Address the person by name.
- Introduce yourself by name and title.

- Explain the procedure to the person before beginning and during the procedure.
- Protect the person's rights during the procedure.
- Handle the person gently during the procedure.

PRE-PROCEDURE

1 Follow *Delegation Guidelines: Taking Pulses*. See *Promoting Safety and Comfort: Using a Stethoscope*, p. 358.
2 Practice hand hygiene.
3 Collect a stethoscope and antiseptic wipes.

4 Decontaminate your hands.
5 Identify the person. Check the ID bracelet against the assignment sheet. Also call the person by name.
6 Provide for privacy.

PROCEDURE

7 Clean the earpieces and diaphragm with the wipes.
8 Have the person sit or lie down.
9 Expose the nipple area of the left chest. Limit exposure of a woman's breasts to the extent necessary.
10 Warm the diaphragm in your palm.
11 Place the earpieces in your ears.

12 Find the apical pulse. Place the diaphragm 2 to 3 inches to the left of the breastbone and below the left nipple (see Fig. 20-19).
13 Count the pulse for 1 minute. Note if it was regular or irregular.
14 Cover the person. Remove the earpieces.
15 Note the person's name and pulse on your notepad or assignment sheet. Note if the pulse was regular or irregular.

POST-PROCEDURE

16 Provide for comfort. (See the inside of the front book cover.)
17 Place the signal light within reach.
18 Unscreen the person.
19 Complete a safety check of the room. (See the inside of the front book cover.)
20 Clean the earpieces and diaphragm with the wipes.

21 Return the stethoscope to its proper place.
22 Decontaminate your hands.
23 Report and record your observations. Record the pulse rate with *Ap* for apical. Report an abnormal pulse rate at once.

 Respirations

Respiration means breathing air into *(inhalation)* and out of *(exhalation)* the lungs. Each respiration involves 1 inhalation and 1 exhalation. Respirations are normally quiet, effortless, and regular. Both sides of the chest rise (inhalation) and fall (exhalation) equally.

The healthy adult has 12 to 20 respirations per minute. See "Vital Signs" (p. 349) for the factors affecting respirations. Heart and respiratory diseases usually increase the respiratory rate.

People tend to change their breathing patterns when they know their respirations are being counted. Therefore the person should not know that you are counting them.

Count respirations right after taking a pulse. Keep your fingers or stethoscope over the pulse site. (The person assumes you are taking the pulse.) To count respirations, watch the chest rise and fall. Count them for 30 seconds. Multiply the number by 2 for the number of respirations in 1 minute. If an abnormal pattern is noted, count the respirations for 1 minute.

In some agencies, respirations are counted for 1 minute. Follow agency policy.

See *Delegation Guidelines: Respirations,* p. 362.

DELEGATION GUIDELINES
Respirations

Before counting respirations, you need this information from the nurse and the care plan:
- How long to count respirations for each person—30 seconds or 1 minute
- When to count respirations
- If the nurse has concerns about certain patients or residents
- What other vital signs to measure

- What observations to report and record:
  - The respiratory rate
  - Equality and depth of respirations
  - If the respirations were regular or irregular
  - If the person has pain or difficulty breathing
  - Any respiratory noises
  - An abnormal respiratory pattern (Chapter 24)
- When to report observations
- What specific patient or resident concerns to report at once

COUNTING RESPIRATIONS

PROCEDURE

1 Follow *Delegation Guidelines: Respirations.*
2 Keep your fingers or stethoscope over the pulse site.
3 Do not tell the person you are counting respirations.
4 Begin counting when the chest rises. Count each rise and fall of the chest as 1 respiration.
5 Note the following:
  a If respirations are regular
  b If both sides of the chest rise equally
  c The depth of respirations
  d If the person has any pain or difficulty breathing
  e An abnormal respiratory pattern

6 Count respirations for 30 seconds. Multiply the number by 2. Count respirations for 1 minute if:
  a Directed by the nurse and care plan.
  b Required by agency policy.
  c They are abnormal or irregular.
  d Required for your state competency test.
7 Note the person's name, respiratory rate, and other observations on your notepad or assignment sheet.

POST-PROCEDURE

8 Provide for comfort. (See the inside of the front book cover.)
9 Place the signal light within reach.
10 Unscreen the person.
11 Complete a safety check of the room. (See the inside of the front book cover.)

12 Decontaminate your hands.
13 Report and record the respiratory rate and your observations. Report abnormal respirations at once.

Blood Pressure

Blood pressure is the amount of force exerted against the walls of an artery by the blood. The period of heart muscle contraction is called *systole.* The period of heart muscle relaxation is called *diastole.*

Systolic and diastolic pressures are measured. The **systolic pressure** is the pressure in the arteries when the heart contracts. It is the higher pressure.

The **diastolic pressure** is the pressure in the arteries when the heart is at rest. It is the lower pressure.

Blood pressure is measured in millimeters (mm) of mercury (Hg). The systolic pressure is recorded over the diastolic pressure. A systolic pressure of 120 mm Hg (millimeters of mercury) and a diastolic pressure of 80 mm Hg is written as 120/80 mm Hg.

Normal and Abnormal Blood Pressures Blood pressure can change from minute to minute. Because it can vary so easily, blood pressure has normal ranges:

*   *Systolic pressure*—less than 120 mm Hg
*   *Diastolic pressure*—less than 80 mm Hg
    Treatment is indicated for:
*   **Hypertension**—blood pressure measurements that remain above *(hyper)* a systolic pressure of 140 mm Hg or a diastolic pressure above 90 mm Hg. Report any systolic measurement at or above 120 mm Hg. Also report a diastolic pressure at or above 80 mm Hg.
*   **Hypotension**—when the systolic blood pressure is below *(hypo)* 90 mm Hg and the diastolic pressure is below 60 mm Hg. Report a systolic pressure below 90 mm Hg. Also report a diastolic pressure below 60 mm Hg.

Equipment A stethoscope and a sphygmomanometer are used to measure blood pressure. The *sphygmomanometer* has a cuff and a measuring device.

*   The *aneroid type* has a round dial and a needle that points to the numbers (Fig. 20-20, *A*).
*   The *mercury type* has a column of mercury within a calibrated tube (Fig. 20-20, *B*).
*   The *electronic type* shows the systolic and diastolic blood pressures on the front of the device (Fig. 20-20, *C*). It also shows the pulse rate. To use the device, follow the manufacturer's instructions.

The blood pressure cuff is wrapped around the upper arm. Tubing connects the cuff to the manometer. Another tube connects the cuff to a small, hand-held bulb. A valve on the bulb is turned clockwise to close the valve so the cuff inflates as the bulb is squeezed. The inflated cuff causes pressure over the brachial artery. The valve is turned counterclockwise to open the valve to deflate the cuff. Blood pressure is measured as the cuff is deflated.

Sounds are produced as the blood flows through the arteries. The stethoscope is used to listen to the sounds in the brachial artery as the cuff is deflated. Stethoscopes are not needed with electronic manometers.

See *Promoting Safety and Comfort: Equipment.*

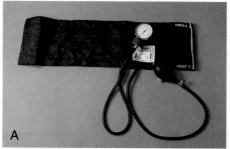
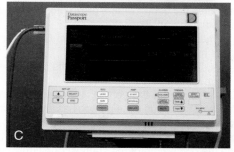
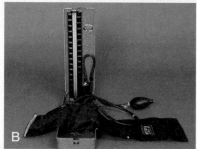

FIGURE 20-20 Blood pressure equipment. **A,** Aneroid manometer and cuff. **B,** Mercury manometer and cuff. **C,** Electronic sphygmomanometer.

PROMOTING SAFETY AND COMFORT
Equipment

Safety

Mercury is a hazardous substance. Mercury manometers are being phased out of health care. Some agencies may still use them. Handle mercury manometers carefully. If one breaks, call for the nurse at once. Do not touch the mercury. Do not let the person touch it. The agency must follow special procedures for handling all hazardous substances. See Chapter 8.

Comfort

Inflate the cuff only to the extent necessary (see procedure: *Measuring Blood Pressure*, p. 365). The inflated cuff causes discomfort. The higher the inflation, the greater the discomfort.

🌸 **Measuring Blood Pressure** Blood pressure is normally measured in the brachial artery. Box 20-2 lists the guidelines for measuring blood pressure.

See *Delegation Guidelines: Measuring Blood Pressure.*

BOX 20-2   Guidelines for Measuring Blood Pressure

- Do not take blood pressure on an arm with an IV (intravenous) infusion, a cast, or a dialysis access site. If a person had breast surgery, do not take blood pressure on that side. Avoid taking blood pressure on an injured arm.
- Let the person rest for 10 to 20 minutes before measuring blood pressure.
- Measure blood pressure with the person sitting or lying. Sometimes the doctor orders blood pressure measured in the standing position.
- Apply the cuff to the bare upper arm. Clothing can affect the measurement.
- Make sure the cuff is snug. Loose cuffs can cause inaccurate readings.
- Use a larger cuff if the person is obese or has a large arm. Use a small cuff if the person has a very small arm. Ask the nurse what size to use. Also check the care plan.
- Place the diaphragm of the stethoscope firmly over the brachial artery. The entire diaphragm must have contact with the skin.
- Make sure the room is quiet. Talking, TV, radio, and sounds from the hallway can affect an accurate measurement.
- Have the sphygmomanometer where you can clearly see it.
- Measure the systolic and diastolic pressures.
  - Expect to hear the first blood pressure sound at the point where you last felt the radial or brachial pulse. The first sound is the systolic pressure.
  - The point where the sound disappears is the diastolic pressure.
- Take the blood pressure again if you are not sure of an accurate measurement. Wait 30 to 60 seconds before repeating the measurement. Ask the nurse to take the blood pressure if you are unsure of the measurement.
- Tell the nurse at once if you cannot hear the blood pressure.

DELEGATION GUIDELINES
Measuring Blood Pressure

Before measuring blood pressure, you need this information from the nurse and the care plan:
- When to measure blood pressure
- What arm to use
- The person's normal blood pressure range
- If the nurse has concerns about certain patients or residents
- If the person needs to be lying down, sitting, or standing
- What size cuff to use—regular, child-size, or extra large
- What observations to report and record
- When to report the blood pressure measurement
- What specific patient or resident concerns to report at once

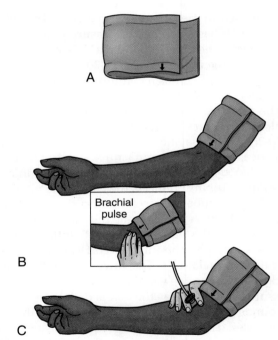

FIGURE 20-21 Measuring blood pressure. **A,** The arrow is used for correct cuff alignment. **B,** The cuff is placed so the arrow is aligned with brachial artery. **C,** The diaphragm of the stethoscope is over the brachial artery.

MEASURING BLOOD PRESSURE

QUALITY OF LIFE

Remember to:
- Knock before entering the person's room.
- Address the person by name.
- Introduce yourself by name and title.

- Explain the procedure to the person before beginning and during the procedure.
- Protect the person's rights during the procedure.
- Handle the person gently during the procedure.

PRE-PROCEDURE

1 Follow *Delegation Guidelines: Measuring Blood Pressure.*
  See *Promoting Safety and Comfort:*
  a *Using a Stethoscope,* p. 358
  b *Equipment,* p. 363
2 Practice hand hygiene.
3 Collect the following:
  - Sphygmomanometer
  - Stethoscope
  - Antiseptic wipes
4 Decontaminate your hands.
5 Identify the person. Check the ID bracelet against the assignment sheet. Also call the person by name.
6 Provide for privacy.

PROCEDURE

7 Wipe the stethoscope earpieces and diaphragm with the wipes. Warm the diaphragm in your palm.
8 Have the person sit or lie down.
9 Position the person's arm level with the heart. The palm is up.
10 Stand no more than 3 feet away from the manometer. The mercury type is vertical, on a flat surface, and at eye level. The aneroid type is directly in front of you.
11 Expose the upper arm.
12 Squeeze the cuff to expel any remaining air. Close the valve on the bulb.
13 Find the brachial artery at the inner aspect of the elbow. (The brachial artery is on the little finger side of the arm.) Use your fingertips.
14 Locate the arrow on the cuff (Fig. 20-21, *A*). Place the arrow over the brachial artery (Fig. 20-21, *B*). Wrap the cuff around the upper arm at least 1 inch above the elbow. It is even and snug.
15 Place the stethoscope earpieces in your ears.
16 Find the radial or brachial pulse.
17 *Method one:*
  a Inflate the cuff until you can no longer feel the pulse. Note this point.
  b Inflate the cuff 30 mm Hg beyond the point where you last felt the pulse.

18 *Method two:*
  a Inflate the cuff until you can no longer feel the pulse. Note this point.
  b Inflate the cuff 30 mm Hg beyond the point where you last felt the pulse.
  c Deflate the cuff slowly. Note the point when you feel the pulse.
  d Wait 30 seconds.
  e Inflate the cuff again, 30 mm Hg beyond the point where you felt the pulse return.
19 Place the diaphragm of the stethoscope over the brachial artery (Fig. 20-21, *C*). Do not place it under the cuff.
20 Deflate the cuff at an even rate of 2 to 4 millimeters per second. Turn the valve counter-clockwise to deflate the cuff.
21 Note the point where you hear the first sound. This is the systolic reading. It is near the point where the radial pulse disappeared.
22 Continue to deflate the cuff. Note the point where the sound disappears. This is the diastolic reading.
23 Deflate the cuff completely. Remove it from the person's arm. Remove the stethoscope earpieces from your ears.
24 Note the person's name and blood pressure on your notepad or assignment sheet.
25 Return the cuff to the case or wall holder.

POST-PROCEDURE

26 Provide for comfort. (See the inside of the front book cover.)
27 Place the signal light within reach.
28 Unscreen the person.
29 Complete a safety check of the room. (See the inside of the front book cover.)

30 Clean the earpieces and diaphragm with the wipes.
31 Return the equipment to its proper place.
32 Decontaminate your hands.
33 Report and record the blood pressure. Note which arm was used. Report an abnormal blood pressure at once.

PAIN

Pain means to ache, hurt, or be sore (Chapter 14). Pain is a warning from the body. It means there is tissue damage. Pain often causes the person to seek health care.

Pain is personal. It differs for each person. What *hurts* to one person may *ache* to another. What one person calls *sore*, another may call *aching*. If a person complains of pain or discomfort, the person *has* pain or discomfort. You must believe the person.

There are different types of pain.

- *Acute pain* is felt suddenly from injury, disease, trauma, or surgery. There is tissue damage. Acute pain lasts a short time, usually less than 6 months. It lessens with healing.
- *Chronic pain (persistent pain)* lasts for a long time (months or years) or occurs off and on. There is no longer tissue damage. Chronic pain remains long after healing. Arthritis and cancer are common causes.
- *Radiating pain* is felt at the site of tissue damage and in nearby areas. Pain from a heart attack is often felt in the left chest, left jaw, left shoulder, and left arm. Gallbladder disease can cause pain in the right upper abdomen, the back, and the right shoulder (Fig. 20-22).
- *Phantom pain* is felt in a body part that is no longer there. A person with an amputated leg may still sense leg pain.

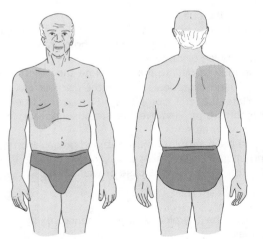

FIGURE 20-22 Gallbladder pain radiates to the right upper abdomen, the back, and the right shoulder.

Signs and Symptoms

You cannot see, hear, feel, or smell the person's pain. You must rely on what the person tells you. Promptly report any information you collect about pain. Write down what the person says. Use the person's exact words when reporting and recording. The nurse needs this information:

- *Location.* Where is the pain? Ask the person to point to the area of pain. Pain can radiate. Ask the person if the pain is anywhere else and to point to those areas.
- *Onset and duration.* When did the pain start? How long has it lasted?
- *Intensity.* Does the person complain of mild, moderate, or severe pain? Ask the person to rate the pain on a scale of 1 to 10, with 10 as the most severe (Fig. 20-23). Or use the Wong-Baker Faces Pain Rating Scale (Fig. 20-24). Designed for children, the scale is useful for persons of all ages. To use the scale, tell the person that each face shows how a person is feeling. Read the description for each face. Then ask the person to choose the face that best describes how he or she feels.
- *Description.* Ask the person to describe the pain.
- *Factors causing pain.* These are called *precipitating* factors. To precipitate means to cause. Such factors include moving or turning in bed, coughing or deep breathing, and exercise. Ask what the person was doing before the pain started and when it started.
- *Factors affecting pain.* Ask the person what makes the pain better. Also ask what makes it worse.
- *Vital signs.* Measure the person's pulse, respirations, and blood pressure. Increases in these vital signs often occur with acute pain. Vital signs may be normal with chronic pain.
- *Other signs and symptoms.* Does the person have other symptoms—dizziness, nausea, vomiting, weakness, numbness or tingling, or others? Box 20-3 lists the signs and symptoms that often occur with pain.

See *Focus on Communication: Signs and Symptoms.*

PAIN: Ask person to rate pain on scale of 0-10										
No pain										Worst pain imaginable
0	1	2	3	4	5	6	7	8	9	10

FIGURE 20-23 Pain rating scale. *(Modified from deWit SC: Fundamental concepts and skills for nursing, ed 3, St Louis, 2009, Saunders.)*

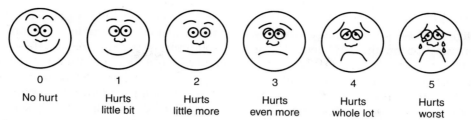

FIGURE 20-24 Wong-Baker Faces Pain Rating Scale. *(From Hockenberry MJ, Wilson D: Wong's nursing care of infants and children, ed 8, St Louis, 2007, Mosby.)*

0	1	2	3	4	5
No hurt	Hurts little bit	Hurts little more	Hurts even more	Hurts whole lot	Hurts worst

BOX 20-3   Signs and Symptoms of Pain

Body Responses
- Appetite: changes in
- Dizziness
- Nausea
- Numbness
- Pulse, respirations, and blood pressure: increased
- Skin: pale (pallor)
- Sleep: difficulty with
- Sweating (diaphoresis)
- Tingling
- Vomiting
- Weakness

Behaviors
- Crying
- Gasping
- Grimacing
- Groaning
- Grunting
- Holding the affected body part (splinting; guarding)
- Irritability
- Moaning
- Mood: changes in
- Positioning: maintaining one position; refusing to move
- Quietness
- Restlessness
- Rubbing
- Screaming
- Speech: slow or rapid; loud or quiet

FOCUS ON COMMUNICATION
Signs and Symptoms

A person may use the word "hurt" instead of "pain." Some persons say they are uncomfortable. Others describe what they feel but deny pain. For example, a person may say: "I'm not having pain. It's just pressure." Use words that the person uses.

Some persons are unable to tell you they are in pain. You must look for nonverbal signs and symptoms. The person's behavior and body responses can suggest pain. See Box 20-3. Tell the nurse if you suspect the person is in pain.

Some persons find it hard to describe pain. You may need to give the person some options. Some common words to describe pain are:
- Aching
- Burning
- Cramping
- Dull
- Pressure
- Sharp
- Stabbing
- Sore
- Throbbing

INTAKE AND OUTPUT

The doctor or nurse may order intake and output (I&O) measurements.
- **Intake** is the amount of fluid taken in.
- **Output** is the amount of fluid lost.

I&O records are kept. They are used to evaluate fluid balance and kidney function. They also are kept when the person has special fluid orders (Chapter 19).

All fluids taken by mouth are measured and recorded—water, milk, coffee, tea, juices, soups, and soft drinks. So are foods that melt at room temperature—ice cream, sherbet, custard, pudding, gelatin, and Popsicles. The nurse measures and records IV fluids and tube feedings (Chapter 19). Output includes urine, vomitus, diarrhea, and wound drainage.

Measuring Intake and Output

Intake and output are measured in milliliters (mL). You need to know these amounts:
- 1 ounce equals 30 mL
- 1 pint is about 500 mL
- 1 quart is about 1000 mL

You also need to know the serving sizes of bowls, dishes, cups, pitchers, glasses, and other containers. This information may be on the I&O record (Fig. 20-25).

A measuring container for fluid is called a *graduate*. It is used to measure left-over fluids, urine, vomitus, and drainage from suction. Like a measuring cup, the graduate is marked in ounces and milliliters (Fig. 20-26). Plastic urinals and kidney basins also have amounts marked. The measuring device is held at eye level to read the amount.

An I&O record is kept at the bedside. When I&O are measured, the amount is recorded in the correct column (see Fig. 20-25). Amounts are totaled at the end of the shift and recorded in the person's chart.

The urinal, commode, bedpan, or specimen pan is used for voiding. Remind the person not to void in the toilet. Also remind the person not to put toilet tissue into the receptacle.

See *Delegation Guidelines: Intake and Output.*
See *Promoting Safety and Comfort: Intake and Output.*

OSF
ST. JOSEPH MEDICAL CENTER
Bloomington, Illinois

DATE __6/15__

FLUID BALANCE CHART

Water Glass	250mL		Ice Cream	120mL
Styrofoam Cup	180mL		Ice Chips	1/2 amt. of mL's in cup
Cup (coffee)	250mL			
Milk Carton	240mL		Pitcher	
Pop (1 can)	360mL		(Yellow)	1000mL
Broth-Soup	175mL			
Juice Carton	120mL			
Juice Glass	120mL			
Jello	120mL			

TIME	ORAL	Parenteral	Amt. mL Absbd.	URINE Method Collected	URINE Amt. (mL)	OTHER Method Collected	OTHER Amt. (mL)	CONT. IRRIGATION In	CONT. IRRIGATION Out
2400-0100		mL from previous shift		V	150				
0100-0200						Vom.	150		
0200-0300									
0300-0400									
0400-0500									
0500-0600	125			V	200				
0600-0700									
0700-0800									
	125	8 - hour Sub-total		8-hr T	350	8-hr T	150		
0800-0900	400	mL from previous shift		V	250				
0900-1000	100								
1000-1100									
1100-1200									
1200-1300	400			V	250				
1300-1400									
1400-1500	200								
1500-1600									
	1100	8 - hour Sub-total		8-hr T	500	8-hr T			
1600-1700		mL from previous shift		V	270				
1700-1800	350								
1800-1900	50								
1900-2000	200								
2000-2100				V	400				
2100-2200									
2200-2300									
2300-2400									
	600	8 - hour Sub-total		8-hr T	670	8-hr T			
	1825	24 - hour Sub-total		24-hr T	1520	24-hr T	150		

310' Marie Mills

Source Key:
URINE
V - Voided
C - Catheter
INC - Incontinent
U.C. - Ureteral Catheter

Source Key:
OTHER
G.I.T. - Gastric Intestinal Tube
T.T. - T. Tube
Vom. - Vomitus
Liq S. - Liquid Stool
H.V. - Hemovac

Form No. MF36722 (Rev. 5/97) **MFI**

FIGURE 20-25 An intake and output record. (*Modified from OSF St. Joseph Medical Center, Bloomington, Ill.*)

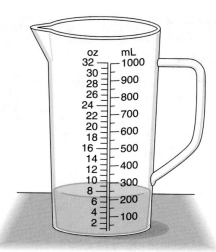

FIGURE 20-26 A graduate marked in ounces and milliliters.

When measuring I&O, you need this information from the nurse and the care plan:
- Does the person have a special fluid order—encourage fluids, restrict fluids, NPO (nothing by mouth), or thickened fluids
- When to report measurements—hourly or end-of-shift
- What the person uses for voiding—urinal, bedpan, commode, or specimen pan (Chapter 21)
- If the person has a catheter
- What specific patient or resident concerns to report at once

PROMOTING SAFETY AND COMFORT
Intake and Output

Safety

Urine may contain microbes or blood. Microbes can grow in urinals, commodes, bedpans, specimen pans, and drainage systems. Follow Standard Precautions and the Bloodborne Pathogen Standard when handling such equipment. Thoroughly clean the item after it is used. Use a disinfectant for cleaning.

Comfort

Promptly measure the contents of urinals, bedpans, commodes, and specimen pans. This helps prevent or reduce odors. Odors can disturb the person.

MEASURING INTAKE AND OUTPUT

QUALITY OF LIFE

Remember to:
- Knock before entering the person's room.
- Address the person by name.
- Introduce yourself by name and title.

- Explain the procedure to the person before beginning and during the procedure.
- Protect the person's rights during the procedure.
- Handle the person gently during the procedure.

PRE-PROCEDURE

1 Follow *Delegation Guidelines: Intake and Output.* See *Promoting Safety and Comfort: Intake and Output.*
2 Practice hand hygiene.

3 Collect the following:
- I&O record
- Graduates
- Gloves

PROCEDURE

4 Put on gloves.
5 Measure intake as follows:
  a Pour liquid remaining in the container into the graduate.
  b Measure the amount at eye level or on a flat surface. Keep the container level.
  c Check the serving amount on the I&O record.

  d Subtract the remaining amount from the full serving amount. Note the amount.
  e Pour fluid in the graduate back into the container.
  f Repeat steps 5a through 5e for each liquid.
  g Add the amounts from each liquid together.
  h Record the time and amount on the I&O record.

Continued

MEASURING INTAKE AND OUTPUT—cont'd

PROCEDURE—cont'd

6 Measure output as follows:
   a Pour the fluid into the graduate used to measure output.
   b Measure the amount at eye level or on a flat surface. Keep the container level.
   c Dispose of fluid in the toilet. Avoid splashes.
7 Clean and rinse the graduates. Dispose of rinse into the toilet. Return the graduates to their proper place.

8 Clean and rinse the bedpan, urinal, commode container, specimen pan, kidney basin, or other drainage container. Dispose of the rinse into the toilet. Return the item to its proper place.
9 Remove the gloves. Practice hand hygiene.
10 Record the output amount on the I&O record.

POST-PROCEDURE

11 Provide for comfort. (See the inside of the front book cover.)
12 Make sure the signal light is within reach.

13 Complete a safety check of the room. (See the inside of the front book cover.)
14 Report and record your observations.

❖ WEIGHT AND HEIGHT

Weight and height are measured on admission to the agency. Then the person is weighed daily, weekly, or monthly. This is done to measure weight gain or loss.

Standing, chair, bed, and lift scales are used. Chair, bed, and lift scales are used for persons who cannot stand. Follow the manufacturer's instructions and agency procedures.

When measuring weight and height, follow these guidelines:

* The person only wears a gown or pajamas. Clothes add weight. No footwear is worn. Footwear adds to the weight and height measurements.
* The person voids before being weighed. A full bladder adds weight.
* Weigh the person at the same time of day. Before breakfast is the best time. Food and fluids add weight.
* Use the same scale for daily, weekly, and monthly weights. Scales weigh differently.
* Balance the scale at zero (0) before weighing the person. For balance scales, move the weights to zero. A digital scale should read at zero.
  See *Delegation Guidelines: Weight and Height.*
  See *Promoting Safety and Comfort: Weight and Height.*

DELEGATION GUIDELINES
Weight and Height

Before measuring weight and height, you need this information from the nurse and the care plan:
* When to measure weight and height
* What scale to use
* When to report the measurements
* What specific patient and resident concerns to report at once

PROMOTING SAFETY AND COMFORT
Weight and Height

Safety
Follow the manufacturer's instructions when using chair, bed, or lift scales. Also follow the agency's procedures. Practice safety measures to prevent falls.

Comfort
The person wears only a gown or pajamas for the weight measurement. Prevent chilling and drafts (Chapter 14).

MEASURING WEIGHT AND HEIGHT

QUALITY OF LIFE

Remember to:
- Knock before entering the person's room.
- Address the person by name.
- Introduce yourself by name and title.

- Explain the procedure to the person before beginning and during the procedure.
- Protect the person's rights during the procedure.
- Handle the person gently during the procedure.

PRE-PROCEDURE

1 Follow *Delegation Guidelines: Weight and Height.* See *Promoting Safety and Comfort: Weight and Height.*
2 Ask the person to void.
3 Practice hand hygiene.
4 Bring the scale and paper towels (for a standing scale) to the person's room.

5 Decontaminate your hands.
6 Identify the person. Check the ID bracelet against the assignment sheet. Also call the person by name.
7 Provide for privacy.

PROCEDURE

8 Place the paper towels on the scale platform.
9 Raise the height rod.
10 Move the weights to zero (0). The pointer is in the middle.
11 Have the person remove the robe and footwear. Assist as needed.
12 Help the person stand on the scale. The person stands in the center of the scale. Arms are at the sides.
13 Move the weights until the balance pointer is in the middle (Fig. 20-27).
14 Note the weight on your notepad or assignment sheet.

15 Ask the person to stand very straight.
16 Lower the height rod until it rests on the person's head (Fig. 20-28, p. 372).
17 Note the height on your notepad or assignment sheet.
18 Raise the height rod. Help the person step off of the scale.
19 Help the person put on a robe and non-skid footwear if he or she will be up. Or help the person back to bed.
20 Lower the height rod. Adjust the weights to zero (0) if this is your agency's policy.

POST-PROCEDURE

21 Provide for comfort. (See the inside of the front book cover.)
22 Place the signal light within reach.
23 Raise or lower bed rails. Follow the care plan.
24 Unscreen the person.

25 Complete a safety check of the room. (See the inside of the front book cover.)
26 Discard the paper towels.
27 Return the scale to its proper place.
28 Decontaminate your hands.
29 Report and record the measurements.

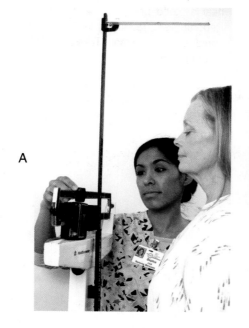

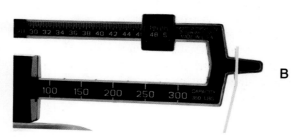

FIGURE 20-27 A, The person is weighed. **B,** The weight is read when the balance pointer is in the middle.

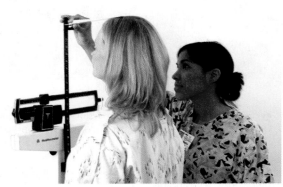

FIGURE 20-28 Height is measured.

Focus on P R I D E
The Person, Family, and Yourself

Personal and Professional Responsibility—Measurements and observations about the person are important for the nursing process. They help the nurse plan for and evaluate the person's care. You are responsible for knowing normal measurements and observations. For example, you must know normal vital sign ranges. The person is at risk if you do not.

Report abnormal measurements and observations to the nurse. If you are unsure, tell the nurse. Take pride in safely assisting the nurse with assessment.

Rights and Respect—Often patients and residents like to know their vital signs and other measurements. If agency policy allows, you can tell the person the measurements. Remember, this information is private and confidential. Respect the person's right to privacy. Roommates and visitors must not hear what you are saying.

Independence and Social Interaction—Personal choices promote independence. The person may prefer that you use the right or left arm for pulses and blood pressures. If safe to do so, use the arm the person prefers.

Delegation and Teamwork—Equipment is often shared with the nursing team. Electronic and tympanic membrane thermometers, scales, and electronic sphygmomanometers are examples. When using these devices, tell your co-workers what equipment you have. Work quickly, but carefully. Return the device to the charging unit or storage area as soon as possible. Do not have your co-workers wait or look for equipment. Take pride in being a courteous team member by using equipment responsibly.

Ethics and Laws—Your measurements must be accurate. Tell the nurse if you are unsure of any measurement. For example, you cannot feel a pulse or hear a blood pressure. Never make up a measurement. Reporting and recording false measurements is wrong. It could harm the person. Take pride in doing the right thing by honest reporting and recording.

REVIEW QUESTIONS

Circle the BEST answer.

1 Which should you report at once?
  a An oral temperature of 98.4° F
  b A rectal temperature of 101.6° F
  c An axillary temperature of 97.6° F
  d An oral temperature of 99.0° F

2 A rectal temperature is taken when the person
  a Is unconscious
  b Has heart disease
  c Is confused
  d Has diarrhea

3 Which is usually used to take an adult's pulse?
  a The radial pulse
  b The apical pulse
  c The carotid pulse
  d The brachial pulse

4 Which is reported to the nurse at once?
  a An adult has a pulse of 124 beats per minute.
  b An adult has a pulse of 90 beats per minute.
  c An adult has a pulse of 86 beats per minute.
  d An adult has a pulse of 64 beats per minute.

5 In an adult, normal respirations are
  a 10 to 18 per minute
  b 12 to 20 per minute
  c Less than 20 per minute
  d More than 20 per minute

6 Respirations are usually counted
  a After taking the temperature
  b After taking the pulse
  c Before taking the pulse
  d After taking the blood pressure

7 Which blood pressure is normal for an adult?
  a 88/54 mm Hg
  b 140/90 mm Hg
  c 100/58 mm Hg
  d 112/78 mm Hg

8 When measuring blood pressure, you should do the following except
  a Use the arm with an IV infusion
  b Apply the cuff to a bare upper arm
  c Turn off the TV
  d Locate the brachial artery

9 The systolic pressure is the point
  a Where the pulse is no longer felt
  b Where the first sound is heard
  c Where the last sound is heard
  d 30 mm Hg above where the pulse was felt

10 A person has pain in the left chest, the left jaw, and the left shoulder and arm. This is
  a Acute pain
  b Chronic pain
  c Radiating pain
  d Phantom pain

11 A person complains of pain. You should ask the person to do the following except
  a Point to where the pain is felt
  b Tell you when the pain started
  c Describe the pain
  d Let you look at the pain

12 Which are not counted as liquid foods?
  a Coffee, tea, juices, and soft drinks
  b Butter, sauces, and melted cheese
  c Ice cream, sherbet, custard, pudding
  d Jell-O, Popsicles, and creamed cereals

13 Which is not measured as output?
  a Urine
  b Vomitus
  c Perspiration
  d Wound drainage

14 For an accurate weight measurement, the person
  a Wears footwear
  b Wears a robe and gown
  c Voids first
  d Chooses what scale to use

Answers to these questions are on p. 528.

21

ASSISTING WITH SPECIMENS

PROCEDURES

- Collecting a Random Urine Specimen
- 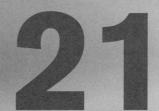 Collecting a Midstream Specimen
- Collecting a Double-Voided Specimen
- Testing Urine With Reagent Strips
- Collecting a Stool Specimen
- Collecting a Sputum Specimen

OBJECTIVES

- Define the key terms and key abbreviations listed in this chapter.
- Explain why specimens are collected.
- Explain the rules for collecting specimens.
- Describe the different types of specimens.
- Explain how to promote PRIDE in the person, the family, and yourself.
- Perform the procedures described in this chapter.

KEY TERMS

acetone A substance that appears in urine from the rapid breakdown of fat for energy; ketone body or ketone

glucosuria Sugar *(glucos)* in the urine *(uria)*; glycosuria

glycosuria Sugar *(glycos)* in the urine *(uria)*; glucosuria

hematuria Blood *(hemat)* in the urine *(uria)*

hemoptysis Bloody *(hemo)* sputum *(ptysis means to spit)*

ketone See "acetone"

ketone body See "acetone"

sputum Mucus from the respiratory system that is expectorated *(expelled)* through the mouth

KEY ABBREVIATIONS

ID Identification

I&O Intake and output

mL Milliliter

oz Ounce

TB Tuberculosis

Specimens *(samples)* are collected and tested to prevent, detect, and treat disease. The doctor orders what specimen to collect and the test needed. Most specimens are tested in the laboratory. All specimens sent to the laboratory require requisition slips. The slip has the person's identifying information and the test ordered. And the specimen container is labeled according to agency policy. Some tests are done at the bedside. When collecting specimens, follow the rules in Box 21-1.

URINE SPECIMENS

Urine specimens are collected for urine tests. Follow the rules in Box 21-1.

See *Delegation Guidelines: Urine Specimens.*

See *Promoting Safety and Comfort: Urine Specimens,* p. 376.

BOX 21-1   Rules for Collecting Specimens

- Follow the rules of medical asepsis.
- Follow Standard Precautions and the Bloodborne Pathogen Standard.
- Use a clean container for each specimen.
- Use the correct container.
- Do not touch the inside of the container or lid.
- Identify the person. Check the ID bracelet against the laboratory requisition slip or assignment sheet. Compare *all* information.
- Label the container in the person's presence. Provide accurate information.
- Collect the specimen at the correct time.
- Ask the person not to have a bowel movement when collecting a urine specimen. The specimen must not contain stools.
- Ask the person to void before collecting a stool specimen. The specimen must not contain urine.
- Ask the person to put toilet tissue in the toilet or wastebasket. Urine and stool specimens must not contain tissue.
- Place the specimen container in a labeled BIOHAZARD plastic bag. Do not let the container touch the outside of the bag. Seal the bag.
- Deliver the specimen and requisition slip to the laboratory. Or take it to the storage area. Follow agency policy.

DELEGATION GUIDELINES
Urine Specimens

Before collecting a urine specimen, you need this information from the nurse and the care plan:

- If the person uses the toilet, bedpan, urinal, or commode for voiding
- The type of specimen needed
- What time to collect the specimen
- What special measures are needed
- If you need to test the specimen (p. 380)
- If measuring intake and output (I&O) is ordered
- What observations to report and record:
  - Problems obtaining the specimen
  - Color, clarity, and odor of urine
  - Particles in the urine
  - Complaints of pain, burning, urgency, dysuria, or other problems
- When to report observations
- What specific patient or resident concerns to report at once

PROMOTING SAFETY AND COMFORT
Urine Specimens

Safety
Microbes can grow in urine. Urine also may contain blood. Follow Standard Precautions and the Bloodborne Pathogen Standard.

Comfort
Urine specimens may embarrass some people. They do not like clear specimen containers that show urine. Placing the urine specimen container in a paper bag is often helpful.

 ## The Random Urine Specimen

The random urine specimen is collected for a routine urinalysis. It is collected any time during a 24-hour period. Many people can collect the specimen themselves. Weak and very ill persons need help.

COLLECTING A RANDOM URINE SPECIMEN

QUALITY OF LIFE

Remember to:
- Knock before entering the person's room.
- Address the person by name.
- Introduce yourself by name and title.

- Explain the procedure to the person before beginning and during the procedure.
- Protect the person's rights during the procedure.
- Handle the person gently during the procedure.

PRE-PROCEDURE

1 Follow *Delegation Guidelines: Urine Specimens,* p. 375. See *Promoting Safety and Comfort: Urine Specimens.*
2 Practice hand hygiene.
3 Collect the following before going to the person's room:
   - Laboratory requisition slip
   - Specimen container and lid
   - Specimen label
   - Plastic bag
   - BIOHAZARD label (if needed)
   - Gloves
4 Arrange collected items in the person's bathroom.
5 Decontaminate your hands.

6 Identify the person. Check the ID (identification) bracelet against the requisition slip. Also call the person by name.
7 Label the container in the person's presence.
8 Put on gloves.
9 Collect the following:
   - Voiding receptacle—bedpan and cover, urinal, commode, or specimen pan (Fig. 21-1)
   - Graduate to measure output
10 Provide for privacy.

PROCEDURE

11 Ask the person to void into the receptacle. Remind him or her to put toilet tissue into the wastebasket or toilet. Toilet tissue is not put in the bedpan or specimen pan.
12 Take the receptacle to the bathroom.
13 Pour about 120 mL (milliliters) (4 ounces [oz]) into the specimen container.
14 Place the lid on the specimen container. Put the container in the plastic bag. Do not let the container touch the outside of the bag. Apply a BIOHAZARD label according to agency policy.

15 Measure urine if I&O are ordered. Include the amount in the specimen container.
16 Empty, clean, and disinfect equipment. Return equipment to its proper place.
17 Remove the gloves, and practice hand hygiene. Put on clean gloves.
18 Assist with hand washing.
19 Remove the gloves. Practice hand hygiene.

POST-PROCEDURE

20 Provide for comfort. (See the inside of the front book cover.)
21 Place the signal light within reach.
22 Raise or lower bed rails. Follow the care plan.
23 Unscreen the person.
24 Complete a safety check of the room. (See the inside of the front book cover.)

25 Decontaminate your hands.
26 Deliver the specimen and the requisition slip to the laboratory or storage area. Follow agency policy. Wear gloves.
27 Report and record your observations.

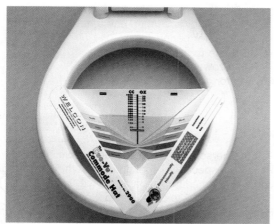

FIGURE 21-1 The specimen pan is placed at the front of the toilet on the toilet rim. This pan has a color chart for urine. *(Courtesy Welcon, Inc., Forth Worth, Tex.)*

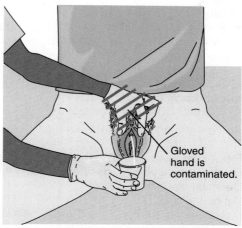

Gloved hand is contaminated.

FIGURE 21-2 The labia are separated to collect a midstream specimen.

❖ The Midstream Specimen

The midstream specimen is also called a *clean-voided specimen* or *clean-catch specimen*. The perineal area is cleaned before collecting the specimen. This reduces the number of microbes in the urethral area. The person starts to void into a receptacle. Then the person stops the stream of urine, and a sterile specimen container is positioned. The person voids into the container until the specimen is obtained.

Stopping the stream of urine is hard for many people. You may need to position and hold the specimen container in place after the person starts to void (Fig. 21-2).

See *Focus on Communication: The Midstream Specimen.*

COLLECTING A MIDSTREAM SPECIMEN

PRE-PROCEDURE

1 Follow *Delegation Guidelines: Urine Specimens,* p. 375. See *Promoting Safety and Comfort: Urine Specimens,* p. 376.
2 Practice hand hygiene.
3 Collect the following before going to the person's room:
   - Laboratory requisition slip
   - Midstream specimen kit—includes specimen container, label, and towelettes; may include sterile gloves
   - Plastic bag
   - Sterile gloves (if not part of the kit)
   - Disposable gloves
   - BIOHAZARD label (if needed)

4 Arrange your work area.
5 Decontaminate your hands.
6 Identify the person. Check the ID bracelet against the requisition slip. Also call the person by name.
7 Put on disposable gloves.
8 Collect the following:
   - Voiding receptacle—bedpan and cover, urinal, commode, or specimen pan if needed
   - Supplies for perineal care
   - Graduate to measure output
   - Paper towel
9 Provide for privacy.

PROCEDURE

10 Provide perineal care. (Wear gloves for this step. Decontaminate your hands after removing them.)
11 Open the sterile kit.
12 Put on the sterile gloves.
13 Open the packet of towelettes inside the kit.
14 Open the sterile specimen container. Do not touch the inside of the container or lid. Set the lid down so the inside is up.
15 *For a female*—clean the perineal area with the towelettes.
   a Spread the labia with your thumb and index finger. Use your non-dominant hand. (This hand is now contaminated. It must not touch anything sterile.)
   b Clean down the urethral area from front to back. Use a clean towelette for each stroke.
   c Keep the labia separated to collect the urine specimen (steps 17 through 20).
16 *For a male*—clean the penis with the towelettes.
   a Hold the penis with your non-dominant hand. (This hand is now contaminated. It must not touch anything sterile.)
   b Clean the penis starting at the meatus. Clean in a circular motion. Start at the center and work outward.
   c Keep holding the penis until the specimen is collected (steps 17 through 20).

17 Ask the person to void into a receptacle.
18 Pass the specimen container into the stream of urine. Keep the labia separated (see Fig. 21-2).
19 Collect about 30 to 60 mL (1 to 2 oz) of urine.
20 Remove the specimen container before the person stops voiding.
21 Release the labia or penis. Let the person finish voiding into the receptacle.
22 Put the lid on the specimen container. Touch only the outside of the container and lid. Wipe the outside of the container. Set the container on a paper towel.
23 Provide toilet tissue after the person is done voiding.
24 Take the receptacle to the bathroom.
25 Measure urine if I&O are ordered. Include the amount in the specimen container.
26 Empty, clean, and disinfect equipment. Return equipment to its proper place.
27 Remove the gloves, and practice hand hygiene. Put on clean disposable gloves.
28 Label the specimen container in the person's presence. Place the container in the plastic bag. Do not let the container touch the outside of the bag. Apply a BIOHAZARD label according to agency policy.
29 Assist with hand washing.
30 Remove the gloves. Practice hand hygiene.

POST-PROCEDURE

31 Provide for comfort. (See the inside of the front book cover.)
32 Place the signal light within reach.
33 Raise or lower bed rails. Follow the care plan.
34 Unscreen the person.
35 Complete a safety check of the room. (See the inside of the front book cover.)

36 Decontaminate your hands.
37 Deliver the specimen and the requisition slip to the laboratory or storage area. Follow agency policy. Wear gloves.
38 Report and record your observations.

The Double-Voided Specimen

Fresh-fractional urine specimen is another term for double-voided specimen. The person voids twice. The first time the bladder is emptied of "stale" urine. "Fresh" urine collects in the bladder after the first voiding. In 30 minutes the person voids again. The second voiding is usually a small or "fractional" amount of urine.

Fresh-fractional urine specimens are used to test urine for glucose and ketones (p. 380). Specimen containers and urine testing equipment are usually kept in the person's bathroom.

COLLECTING A DOUBLE-VOIDED SPECIMEN

QUALITY OF LIFE

Remember to:
- Knock before entering the person's room.
- Address the person by name.
- Introduce yourself by name and title.

- Explain the procedure to the person before beginning and during the procedure.
- Protect the person's rights during the procedure.
- Handle the person gently during the procedure.

PRE-PROCEDURE

1 Follow *Delegation Guidelines: Urine Specimens,* p. 375. See *Promoting Safety and Comfort: Urine Specimens,* p. 376.
2 Practice hand hygiene. Put on gloves.
3 Collect the following:
   - Voiding receptacle—bedpan and cover, urinal, commode, or specimen pan
   - Two specimen containers

- Urine testing equipment
- Graduate to measure output
- Gloves

4 Remove the gloves. Decontaminate your hands.
5 Identify the person. Check the ID bracelet against the assignment sheet. Also call the person by name.
6 Provide for privacy.

PROCEDURE

7 Put on gloves.
8 Ask the person to void into the receptacle. Remind the person not to put toilet tissue in the receptacle.
9 Take the receptacle to the bathroom.
10 Measure urine if I&O are ordered.
11 Pour some urine into a specimen container.
12 Test the specimen in case the person cannot provide a second specimen (p. 380). Discard the urine. Note the result on your assignment sheet.
13 Empty, clean, and disinfect equipment. Return equipment to its proper place.
14 Remove the gloves, and practice hand hygiene. Put on clean gloves.
15 Assist with hand washing.
16 Remove the gloves. Practice hand hygiene.

17 Ask the person to drink an 8-ounce glass of water.
18 Do the following before leaving the room:
   a Provide for comfort. (See the inside of the front book cover.)
   b Place the signal light within reach.
   c Raise or lower the bed rails. Follow the care plan.
   d Unscreen the person.
   e Complete a safety check of the room. (See the inside of the front book cover.)
   f Decontaminate your hands.
19 Return to the room in 20 to 30 minutes. Decontaminate your hands.
20 Repeat steps 2 through 16.

POST-PROCEDURE

21 Provide for comfort. (See the inside of the front book cover.)
22 Place the signal light within reach.
23 Raise or lower the bed rails. Follow the care plan.
24 Unscreen the person.

25 Complete a safety check of the room. (See the inside of the front book cover.)
26 Decontaminate your hands.
27 Report and record the results of the second test and any other observations.

Testing Urine

The nurse may ask you to do simple urine tests. You can test for pH, glucose, and blood using reagent strips. The doctor orders the type and frequency of urine tests.

- *Testing for pH*—Urine pH measures if urine is acidic or alkaline. Changes in normal pH (4.6 to 8.0) occur from illness, food, and drugs. A routine urine specimen is needed.
- *Testing for glucose and ketones*—In diabetes, the pancreas does not secrete enough insulin (Chapter 26). The body needs insulin to use sugar for energy. If not used, sugar builds up in the blood. Some sugar appears in the urine. **Glucosuria** or **glycosuria** means sugar *(glucos, glycos)* in the urine *(uria)*. The diabetic person may also have **acetone (ketone bodies, ketones)** in the urine. These substances appear in urine from the rapid breakdown of fat for energy. The body uses fat for energy if it cannot use sugar. Urine is also tested for ketones. These tests are usually done four times a day—30 minutes before each meal and at bedtime. The doctor uses the test to make drug and diet decisions. Double-voided specimens are best for these tests.
- *Testing for blood*—Injury and disease can cause **hematuria.** It means blood *(hemat)* in the urine *(uria)*. Sometimes blood is seen in the urine. At other times it is unseen *(occult)*. A routine urine specimen is needed.

See *Delegation Guidelines: Testing Urine.*

See *Promoting Safety and Comfort: Testing Urine.*

DELEGATION GUIDELINES
Testing Urine

When testing urine is delegated to you, you need this information from the nurse and the care plan:
- What test is needed
- What urine specimen to collect
- What equipment to use
- When to test urine
- Instructions for the test ordered
- If the nurse wants to observe the results of each test
- What observations to report and record:
  - The time you collected and tested the specimen
  - Test results
  - Problems obtaining the specimen
  - Color, clarity, and odor of urine
  - Particles in the urine
  - Complaints of pain, burning, urgency, difficulty voiding, or other problems
- When to report test results and observations
- What specific patient or resident concerns to report at once

---

PROMOTING SAFETY AND COMFORT
Testing Urine

Safety

You must be accurate when testing urine. Promptly report the results to the nurse. Ordered drugs may depend on the results.

Urine may contain microbes and blood. Follow Standard Precautions and the Bloodborne Pathogen Standard.

Comfort

The person may want to know the test results. If allowed by agency policy, you can tell the person the results. Remember, this information is private and confidential. Make sure only the person hears what you are saying.

Using Reagent Strips Reagent strips have sections that change color when they react with urine. To use a reagent strip:
- Do not touch the test area on the strip.
- Dip the strip into urine.
- Compare the strip with the color chart on the bottle (Fig. 21-3).

See *Promoting Safety and Comfort: Using Reagent Strips.*

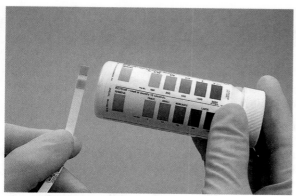

FIGURE 21-3 Reagent strip for sugar and ketones.

TESTING URINE WITH REAGENT STRIPS

QUALITY OF LIFE

Remember to:
- Knock before entering the person's room.
- Address the person by name.
- Introduce yourself by name and title.

- Explain the procedure to the person before beginning and during the procedure.
- Protect the person's rights during the procedure.
- Handle the person gently during the procedure.

PRE-PROCEDURE

1 Follow *Delegation Guidelines: Testing Urine.* See *Promoting Safety and Comfort:*
   a *Testing Urine*
   b *Using Reagent Strips*
2 Practice hand hygiene.
3 Collect gloves and the reagent strips ordered.
4 Decontaminate your hands.
5 Identify the person. Check the ID bracelet against the assignment sheet. Also call the person by name.
6 Put on gloves.
7 Collect equipment for collecting the urine specimen needed. (See procedure: *Collecting a Random Urine Specimen,* p. 376, or *Collecting a Double-Voided Specimen*, p. 379.)
8 Provide for privacy.

PROCEDURE

9 Collect the urine specimen. (See procedure: *Collecting a Random Urine Specimen,* p. 376, or *Collecting a Double-Voided Specimen,* p. 379.)
10 Remove the strip from the bottle. Put the cap on the bottle at once. It must be on tight.
11 Dip the strip test areas into the urine.
12 Remove the strip after the correct amount of time. See the manufacturer's instructions.
13 Tap the strip gently against the container. This removes excess urine.
14 Wait the required amount of time. See the manufacturer's instructions.
15 Compare the strip with the color chart on the bottle (see Fig. 21-3). Read the results.
16 Discard disposable items and the specimen.
17 Empty, clean, and disinfect equipment. Return equipment to its proper place.
18 Remove the gloves. Practice hand hygiene.

POST-PROCEDURE

19 Provide for comfort. (See the inside of the front book cover.)
20 Place the signal light within reach.
21 Raise or lower bed rails. Follow the care plan.
22 Unscreen the person.
23 Complete a safety check of the room. (See the inside of the front book cover.)
24 Decontaminate your hands.
25 Report and record the test results and other observations.

STOOL SPECIMENS

When internal bleeding is suspected, stools are checked for blood. Stools also are studied for fat, microbes, worms, and other abnormal contents.

The stool specimen must not be contaminated with urine. The person uses one receptacle for voiding and another for a bowel movement. Some tests require a warm stool. The specimen is taken at once to the laboratory or to the storage area for transport to the laboratory. Follow the rules in Box 21-1.

See *Focus on Communication: Stool Specimens.*
See *Delegation Guidelines: Stool Specimens.*
See *Promoting Safety and Comfort: Stool Specimens.*

FOCUS ON COMMUNICATION
Stool Specimens

Always explain the procedure before you begin. Explain what the person needs to do and what you will do. Also show what equipment and supplies you will use. For example:

"The doctor wants your stools tested. Meaning, we need a specimen from a bowel movement. I'm going to place this specimen pan (show the specimen pan) at the back of the toilet seat. You will urinate into the toilet. Your bowel movement will collect in the specimen pan rather than in the toilet. Please put toilet tissue in the toilet, not in the specimen pan. After you have a bowel movement, put your signal light on right away. I'll use a tongue blade (show the tongue blade) to take some stool from the specimen pan to put in this specimen container (show the specimen container)."

After explaining the procedure, ask the person if he or she has any questions. If you do not know the answer, refer questions to the nurse.

Also make sure the person understands what to do. You can say: "Mrs. Clark, please help me make sure that you understand what I said. To collect a stool specimen, please tell me what you're going to do."

DELEGATION GUIDELINES
Stool Specimens

Before collecting a stool specimen, you need this information from the nurse:
- What time to collect the specimen
- What special measures are needed
- What observations to report and record:
  - Problems obtaining the specimen
  - Color, amount, consistency, and odor of stools
  - Complaints of pain or discomfort
  - The time when the specimen was collected
- When to report observations
- What specific patient or resident concerns to report at once

---

PROMOTING SAFETY AND COMFORT
Stool Specimens

Safety

Stools contain microbes. And they may contain blood. Follow Standard Precautions and the Bloodborne Pathogen Standard.

Comfort

Stools normally have an odor. A person may be embarrassed that you need to collect a specimen. Complete the task quickly and carefully. Also act in a professional manner.

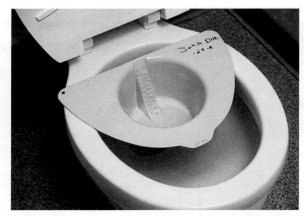

FIGURE 21-4 The specimen pan is placed at the back of the toilet for a stool specimen.

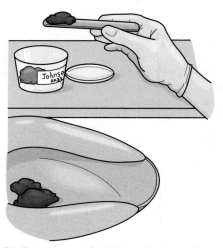

FIGURE 21-5 A tongue blade is used to transfer a small amount of stool from the bedpan to the specimen container.

COLLECTING A STOOL SPECIMEN

QUALITY OF LIFE

Remember to:
- Knock before entering the person's room.
- Address the person by name.
- Introduce yourself by name and title.

- Explain the procedure to the person before beginning and during the procedure.
- Protect the person's rights during the procedure.
- Handle the person gently during the procedure.

PRE-PROCEDURE

1 Follow *Delegation Guidelines: Stool Specimens.* See *Promoting Safety and Comfort: Stool Specimens.*
2 Practice hand hygiene.
3 Collect the following before going to the person's room:
   - Laboratory requisition slip
   - Specimen pan for the toilet
   - Specimen container and lid
   - Specimen label
   - Tongue blade
   - Disposable bag
   - Plastic bag
   - BIOHAZARD label (if needed)
   - Gloves

4 Arrange collected items in the person's bathroom.
5 Decontaminate your hands.
6 Identify the person. Check the ID bracelet against the requisition slip. Also call the person by name.
7 Label the specimen container in the person's presence.
8 Put on gloves.
9 Collect the following:
   - Receptacle for voiding—bedpan and cover, urinal, commode, or specimen pan
   - Toilet tissue
10 Provide for privacy.

PROCEDURE

11 Ask the person to void. Provide the receptacle for voiding if the person does not use the bathroom. Empty, clean, and disinfect the device. Return it to its proper place.
12 Put the specimen pan on the toilet if the person will use the bathroom. Place it at the back of the toilet (Fig. 21-4). Or provide a bedpan or commode.
13 Ask the person not to put toilet tissue into the bedpan, commode, or specimen pan. Provide a bag for toilet tissue.
14 Place the signal light and toilet tissue within reach. Raise or lower bed rails. Follow the care plan.
15 Remove the gloves. Decontaminate your hands. Leave the room.
16 Return when the person signals. Or check on the person every 5 minutes. Knock before entering.
17 Decontaminate your hands. Put on clean gloves.
18 Lower the bed rail near you if up.
19 Remove the bedpan. Note the color, amount, consistency, and odor of stools.
20 Provide perineal care if needed.

21 Collect the specimen:
   a Use a tongue blade to take about 2 tablespoons of formed or liquid stool to the specimen container (Fig. 21-5). Take the sample from the middle of a formed stool.
   b Include pus, mucus, or blood present in the stool.
   c Take stool from 2 different places in the bowel movement if required by agency policy.
   d Put the lid on the specimen container.
   e Place the container in the plastic bag. Do not let the container touch the outside of the bag. Apply a BIOHAZARD label according to agency policy.
22 Wrap the tongue blade in toilet tissue. Discard it into the disposable bag.
23 Empty, clean, and disinfect equipment. Return equipment to its proper place.
24 Remove the gloves, and practice hand hygiene. Put on clean gloves.
25 Assist with hand washing.
26 Remove the gloves. Practice hand hygiene.

POST-PROCEDURE

27 Provide for comfort. (See the inside of the front book cover.)
28 Place the signal light within reach.
29 Raise or lower bed rails. Follow the care plan.
30 Unscreen the person.

31 Complete a safety check of the room. (See the inside of the front book cover.)
32 Deliver the specimen and requisition slip to the laboratory or storage area. Follow agency policy. Wear gloves.
33 Report and record your observations.

❖ SPUTUM SPECIMENS

Respiratory disorders cause the lungs, bronchi, and trachea to secrete mucus. Mucus from the respiratory system is called **sputum** when expectorated *(expelled)* through the mouth. Sputum specimens are studied for blood, microbes, and abnormal cells.

The person coughs up sputum from the bronchi and trachea. This is often painful and hard to do. It is easier to collect a specimen in the morning. Secretions collect in the trachea and bronchi during sleep. They are coughed up on awakening.

To collect a specimen, follow the rules in Box 21-1. Also have the person rinse the mouth with water. Rinsing decreases saliva and removes food particles. Mouthwash is not used. It destroys some of the microbes in the mouth.

See *Delegation Guidelines: Sputum Specimens.*
See *Promoting Safety and Comfort: Sputum Specimens.*

PROMOTING SAFETY AND COMFORT
Sputum Specimens

Safety

Follow Standard Precautions and the Bloodborne Pathogen Standard to prevent contact with mucus. It may contain blood or microbes.

The doctor may order Isolation Precautions if the person has or may have tuberculosis (TB) (Chapter 26). Protect yourself by wearing a TB respirator (Chapter 11).

Comfort

The procedure can embarrass the person. Coughing and expectorating sounds can disturb those nearby. Also, sputum is not pleasant to look at. For these reasons, privacy is important. Cover the specimen container and place it in a bag. Some sputum specimen containers are cloudy in color to hide the contents.

DELEGATION GUIDELINES
Sputum Specimens

Before collecting a sputum specimen, you need this information from the nurse:
- When to collect the specimen
- How much sputum is needed—usually 1 to 2 teaspoons
- If the person uses the bathroom
- If the person can hold the specimen container
- What observations to report and record:
  - The time the specimen was collected
  - The amount of sputum collected
  - How easily the person raised the sputum
  - Sputum color—clear, white, yellow, green, brown, or red
  - Sputum odor—none or foul odor
  - Sputum consistency—thick, watery, or frothy (with bubbles or foam)
  - **Hemoptysis**—bloody *(hemo)* sputum *(ptysis,* meaning *to spit)*
  - If the person was not able to produce sputum
  - Any other observations
- When to report observations
- What specific patient or resident concerns to report at once

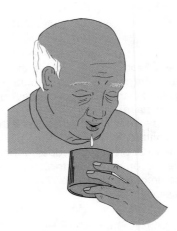

FIGURE 21-6 The person expectorates into the center of the specimen container.

COLLECTING A SPUTUM SPECIMEN

QUALITY OF LIFE

Remember to:
- Knock before entering the person's room.
- Address the person by name.
- Introduce yourself by name and title.
- Explain the procedure to the person before beginning and during the procedure.
- Protect the person's rights during the procedure.
- Handle the person gently during the procedure.

PRE-PROCEDURE

1 Follow *Delegation Guidelines: Sputum Specimens.* See *Promoting Safety and Comfort: Sputum Specimens.*
2 Practice hand hygiene.
3 Collect the following before going to the person's room:
   - Laboratory requisition slip
   - Sputum specimen container and lid
   - Specimen label
   - Plastic bag
   - BIOHAZARD label (if needed)
4 Arrange collected items in the person's bathroom.
5 Decontaminate your hands.
6 Identify the person. Check the ID bracelet against the requisition slip. Also call the person by name.
7 Label the specimen container in the person's presence.
8 Collect gloves and tissues.
9 Provide for privacy. If able, the person uses the bathroom for the procedure.

PROCEDURE

10 Put on gloves.
11 Ask the person to rinse the mouth out with clear water.
12 Have the person hold the container. Only the outside is touched.
13 Ask the person to cover the mouth and nose with tissues when coughing. Follow agency policy for used tissues.
14 Ask him or her to take 2 or 3 deep breaths and cough up the sputum.
15 Have the person expectorate directly into the container (Fig. 21-6). Sputum should not touch the outside of the container.
16 Collect 1 to 2 teaspoons of sputum unless told to collect more.
17 Put the lid on the container.
18 Place the container in the plastic bag. Do not let the container touch the outside of the bag. Apply a BIOHAZARD label according to agency policy.
19 Remove the gloves, and decontaminate your hands. Put on clean gloves.
20 Assist with hand washing.
21 Remove the gloves. Decontaminate your hands.

POST-PROCEDURE

22 Provide for comfort. (See the inside of the front book cover.)
23 Place the signal light within reach.
24 Raise or lower bed rails. Follow the care plan.
25 Unscreen the person.
26 Complete a safety check of the room. (See the inside of the front book cover.)
27 Decontaminate your hands.
28 Deliver the specimen and the requisition slip to the laboratory or storage area. Follow agency policy. Wear gloves.
29 Report and record your observations.

Focus on P R I D E
The Person, Family, and Yourself

Personal and Professional Responsibility—When collecting specimens, you are responsible for correctly identifying the person. You must collect and test specimens on the right person. Otherwise one or both persons could suffer harm. Before collecting or testing a specimen, carefully identify the person. Check the ID bracelet against the laboratory requisition slip or assignment sheet. Compare all information, not just the person's name.

Some agencies require placing collection information on the specimen container. Collection date, collection time, and the collector's name or initials are examples. Follow agency policy for labeling specimens. Take pride in promoting safety by labeling specimens properly.

Rights and Respect—Specimen collection embarrasses many people. Respect the person's right to privacy when collecting specimens. To promote comfort and privacy:
- Politely ask visitors to leave the room.
- Close doors, privacy curtains, and window coverings.
- Leave the room if it is safe to do so. If you cannot leave, explain this to the person.
- Place the specimen container in a paper bag or wrap it in a paper towel or washcloth so others do not see the specimen.
- Always act professionally. Do not make statements that may embarrass the person.

Independence and Social Interaction—Some persons can collect their own urine and sputum specimens. Doing so promotes independence. It also helps reduce embarrassment.

Explain the procedure to the person. This helps the person know how to correctly collect the specimen. Show the person the specimen container and how it is used. Also, ask the person where you should place the container. When ready to collect the specimen, the person knows where to find the container.

Delegation and Teamwork—You may need to take a specimen to the laboratory. Before you go, tell the nurse and your co-workers that you are leaving the area. Also, ask if other staff need specimens taken to the laboratory. Doing so saves staff time. This also prevents having too many staff members off the unit at the same time. Return from the laboratory promptly.

Ethics and Laws—Ethics is concerned with right and wrong behavior. If you did not collect a specimen correctly, do not send it to the laboratory. Tell the nurse what happened. Then collect the specimen at the next opportunity. Test results must be accurate for correct diagnosis and treatment. Take pride in honestly reporting mistakes.

REVIEW QUESTIONS

Circle the BEST answer.

1   A random urine specimen is collected
   a   Upon awakening
   b   Before meals
   c   After meals
   d   Any time

2   Perineal care is given before collecting a
   a   Random specimen
   b   Midstream specimen
   c   Stool specimen
   d   Double-voided specimen

3   Urine is tested for sugar and ketones
   a   At bedtime
   b   30 minutes after meals and at bedtime
   c   30 minutes before meals and at bedtime
   d   Before breakfast

4   Which specimen is best for sugar and ketone testing?
   a   A random specimen
   b   A clean-voided specimen
   c   A reagent specimen
   d   A double-voided specimen

5   A stool specimen must be kept warm. After collecting the specimen
   a   Put it in an oven
   b   Put it in a paper bag
   c   Cover it with a towel
   d   Take it to the laboratory

6   The best time to collect a sputum specimen is
   a   On awakening
   b   After meals
   c   At bedtime
   d   After oral hygiene

7   A sputum specimen is needed. You should ask the person to
   a   Use mouthwash
   b   Rinse the mouth with clear water
   c   Brush the teeth
   d   Remove dentures

Answers to these questions are on p. 528.

22

ASSISTING WITH EXERCISE AND ACTIVITY

PROCEDURES

- Performing Range-of-Motion Exercises
- Helping the Person Walk

OBJECTIVES

- Define the key terms and key abbreviations listed in this chapter.
- Describe bedrest and how to prevent related complications.
- Describe the devices used to support and maintain body alignment.
- Describe range-of-motion exercises.
- Describe four walking aids.
- Explain how to promote PRIDE in the person, the family, and yourself.
- Perform the procedures described in this chapter.

KEY TERMS

abduction Moving a body part away from the midline of the body

adduction Moving a body part toward the midline of the body

ambulation The act of walking

atrophy The decrease in size or the wasting away of tissue

contracture The lack of joint mobility caused by abnormal shortening of a muscle

dorsiflexion Bending the toes and foot up at the ankle

extension Straightening a body part

external rotation Turning the joint outward

flexion Bending a body part

footdrop The foot falls down at the ankle; permanent plantar flexion

hyperextension Excessive straightening of a body part

internal rotation Turning the joint inward

orthostatic hypotension Abnormally low *(hypo)* blood pressure when the person suddenly stands up *(ortho* and *static)*; postural hypotension

plantar flexion The foot *(plantar)* is bent *(flexion)*; bending the foot down at the ankle

postural hypotension See "orthostatic hypotension"

pronation Turning the joint downward

range of motion (ROM) The movement of a joint to the extent possible without causing pain

rotation Turning the joint

supination Turning the joint upward

KEY ABBREVIATIONS

ADL Activities of daily living

ID Identification

ROM Range of motion

Illness, surgery, injury, pain, and aging can limit activity. Inactivity, whether mild or severe, affects every body system. It also affects mental well-being.

You assist the nurse in promoting exercise and activity in all persons to the extent possible. The care plan and your assignment sheet include the person's activity level and needed exercises.

See *Persons With Dementia: Assisting With Exercise and Activity.*

PERSONS WITH DEMENTIA
Assisting With Exercise and Activity

Persons with dementia may resist exercise and activity. They do not understand what is happening and may fear harm. They may become agitated and combative. Some cry out for help. Do not force the person to exercise or take part in activities. Stay calm, and ask the nurse for help. Follow the care plan.

BEDREST

The doctor orders bedrest to treat a health problem. Sometimes it is a nursing measure if the person's condition changes. Bedrest is ordered to:
* Reduce physical activity
* Reduce pain
* Encourage rest
* Regain strength
* Promote healing
  These types of bedrest are common:
* *Strict bedrest.* Everything is done for the person. No activities of daily living (ADL) are allowed.
* *Bedrest.* Some ADL are allowed. Self-feeding, oral hygiene, bathing, shaving, and hair care are often allowed.
* *Bedrest with commode privileges.* The person uses the commode for elimination.
* *Bedrest with bathroom privileges (bedrest with BRP).* The person uses the bathroom for elimination.

Complications of Bedrest

Bedrest and lack of exercise and activity can cause serious complications. Pressure ulcers, constipation, and fecal impaction can result. Urinary tract infections and renal calculi (kidney stones) can occur. So can blood clots (thrombi) and pneumonia (inflammation and infection of the lung).

The musculoskeletal system is affected by lack of exercise and activity. These complications must be prevented to maintain normal movement:
* A **contracture** is the lack of joint mobility caused by abnormal shortening of a muscle. The contracted muscle is fixed into position, is deformed, and cannot stretch (Fig. 22-1, p. 390). Common sites are the fingers, wrists, elbows, toes, ankles, knees, and hips. They can also occur in the neck and spine. The person is permanently deformed and disabled.
* **Atrophy** is the decrease in size or the wasting away of tissue. Tissues shrink in size. Muscle atrophy is a decrease in size or a wasting away of muscle (Fig. 22-2, p. 390).

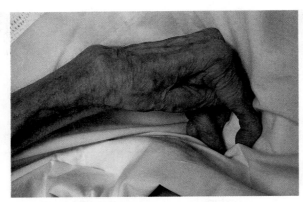

FIGURE 22-1 A contracture.

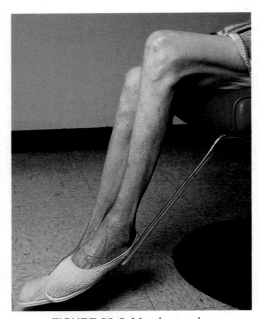

FIGURE 22-2 Muscle atrophy.

Orthostatic hypotension is abnormally low *(hypo)* blood pressure when the person suddenly stands up *(ortho* and *static)*. It is also called **postural hypotension.** *(Postural* relates to posture or standing.) When a person moves from lying or sitting to a standing position, blood pressure drops. The person is dizzy and weak and has spots before the eyes. Fainting can occur. Slowly changing positions is key to preventing orthostatic hypotension.

Good nursing care prevents complications from bedrest. Good alignment, range-of-motion exercises, and frequent position changes are important measures. These are part of the care plan.

See *Focus on Communication: Complications of Bedrest.*

Positioning

Body alignment and positioning were discussed in Chapter 12. Supportive devices are often used to support and maintain the person in a certain position:

- *Bedboards*—are placed under the mattress to prevent it from sagging (Fig. 22-3).
- *Footboards*—prevent plantar flexion that can lead to footdrop. In **plantar flexion,** the foot *(plantar)* is bent *(flexion)*. **Footdrop** is when the foot falls down at the ankle (permanent plantar flexion). The footboard is placed so the soles of the feet are flush against it (Fig. 22-4). Footboards also keep top linens off the feet and toes.
- *Trochanter rolls*—prevent the hips and legs from turning outward (external rotation) (Fig. 22-5). A bath blanket is folded to the desired length and rolled up. The loose end is placed under the person from the hip to the knee. Then the roll is tucked alongside the body.
- *Hip abduction wedges*—keep the hips abducted (Fig. 22-6). The wedge is placed between the person's legs. These are common after hip replacement surgery.
- *Handrolls or handgrips*—prevent contractures of the thumb, fingers, and wrist (Fig. 22-7). Foam rubber sponges, rubber balls, and finger cushions (Fig. 22-8) also are used.
- *Splints*—keep the elbows, wrists, thumbs, fingers, ankles, and knees in normal position (Fig. 22-9, p. 392).
- *Bed cradles*—keep the weight of top linens off the feet and toes (Fig. 22-10, p. 392). The weight of top linens can cause footdrop and pressure ulcers.

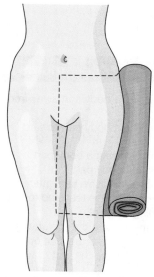

FIGURE 22-3 Bedboards. **A,** Mattress sagging without bedboards. **B,** Bedboards are under the mattress. No sagging occurs.

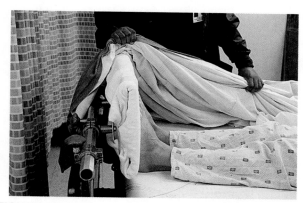

FIGURE 22-4 A footboard. Feet are flush with the board to keep them in normal alignment.

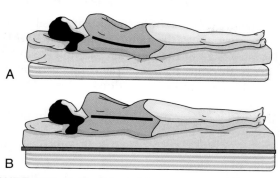

FIGURE 22-5 A trochanter roll is made from a bath blanket. It extends from the hip to the knee.

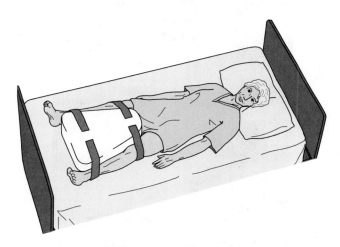

FIGURE 22-6 Hip abduction wedge.

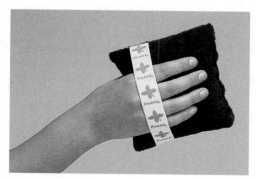

FIGURE 22-7 Handgrip. (*Image courtesy J. T. Posey Co., Arcadia, Calif.*)

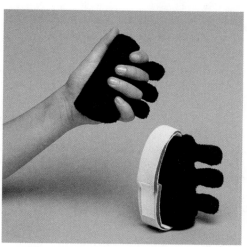

FIGURE 22-8 Finger cushion. (*Image courtesy J. T. Posey Co., Arcadia, Calif.*)

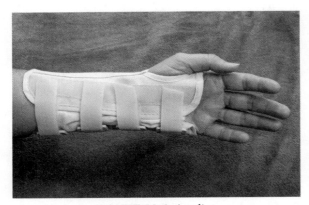

FIGURE 22-9 A splint.

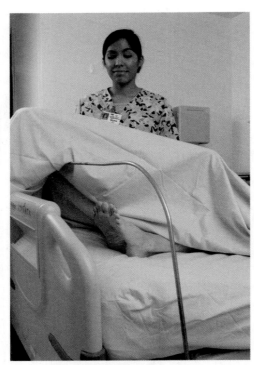

FIGURE 22-10 A bed cradle.

 RANGE-OF-MOTION EXERCISES

The movement of a joint to the extent possible without causing pain is the **range of motion (ROM)** of that joint. Range-of-motion exercises involve moving the joints through their complete range of motion (Box 22-1). They are usually done at least 2 times a day.

- *Active* ROM—are done by the person himself or herself.
- *Passive* ROM—you move the joints through their range of motion.
- *Active-assistive* ROM—the person does the exercises with some help.

See *Focus on Communication: Range-of-Motion Exercises.*

See *Delegation Guidelines: Range-of-Motion Exercises.*

See *Promoting Safety and Comfort: Range-of-Motion Exercises.*

Text continued on p. 398

BOX 22-1 Joint Movements

Abduction—moving a body part away from the midline of the body
Adduction—moving a body part toward the midline of the body
Extension—straightening a body part
Flexion—bending a body part
Hyperextension—excessive straightening of a body part
Dorsiflexion—bending the toes and foot up at the ankle
Rotation—turning the joint
Internal rotation—turning the joint inward
External rotation—turning the joint outward
Plantar flexion—bending the foot down at the ankle
Pronation—turning the joint downward
Supination—turning the joint upward

FOCUS ON COMMUNICATION
Range-of-Motion Exercises

You must not force a joint beyond its present range of motion or to the point of pain. Ask the person to tell you if he or she:
- Feels that the joint cannot move any farther
- Feels pain or discomfort in the joint

DELEGATION GUIDELINES
Range-of-Motion Exercises

When delegated ROM exercises, you need this information from the nurse and the care plan:

- The kind of ROM ordered—active, passive, active-assistive
- Which joints to exercise
- How often the exercises are done
- How many times to repeat each exercise
- What observations to report and record:
  - The time the exercises were performed
  - The joints exercised
  - The number of times the exercises were performed on each joint
  - Complaints of pain or signs of stiffness or spasm
  - The degree to which the person took part in the exercises
- When to report observations
- What specific patient or resident concerns to report at once

PROMOTING SAFETY AND COMFORT
Range-of-Motion Exercises

Safety

Range-of-motion exercises can cause injury if not done properly. Muscle strain, joint injury, and pain are possible. Practice the rules in Box 22-2 when performing or assisting with ROM exercises.

ROM exercises to the neck can cause serious injury if not done properly. Some agencies require that nursing assistants have special training before doing such exercises. Other agencies do not let nursing assistants do them. Know your agency's policy. *Perform ROM exercises to the neck only if allowed by your agency and if the nurse instructs you to do so.*

Comfort

To promote physical comfort during ROM exercises, follow the rules in Box 22-2. Also cover the person with a bath blanket. Expose only the part being exercised. Providing for privacy promotes physical and mental comfort.

BOX 22-2   Performing Range-of-Motion Exercises

- Exercise only the joints the nurse tells you to exercise.
- Expose only the body part being exercised.
- Use good body mechanics.
- Support the part being exercised.
- Move the joint slowly, smoothly, and gently.
- Do not force a joint beyond its present range of motion.
- Do not force a joint to the point of pain.
- Ask the person if he or she has pain or discomfort.
- *Perform range-of-motion exercises to the neck only if allowed by agency policy.* In some agencies, only physical or occupational therapists do neck exercises. This is because of the danger of neck injuries.

PERFORMING RANGE-OF-MOTION EXERCISES

QUALITY OF LIFE

Remember to:
- Knock before entering the person's room.
- Address the person by name.
- Introduce yourself by name and title.

- Explain the procedure to the person before beginning and during the procedure.
- Protect the person's rights during the procedure.
- Handle the person gently during the procedure.

PRE-PROCEDURE

1. Follow *Delegation Guidelines: Range-of-Motion Exercises.* See *Promoting Safety and Comfort: Range-of-Motion Exercises.*
2. Practice hand hygiene.
3. Identify the person. Check the ID (identification) bracelet against the assignment sheet. Also call the person by name.
4. Obtain a bath blanket.
5. Provide for privacy.
6. Raise the bed for body mechanics. Bed rails are up if used.

Continued

PERFORMING RANGE-OF-MOTION EXERCISES—cont'd

PROCEDURE

7 Lower the bed rail near you if up.

8 Position the person supine.

9 Cover the person with a bath blanket. Fan-fold top linens to the foot of the bed.

10 Exercise the neck *if allowed by your agency and if the RN instructs you to do so* (Fig. 22-11):

   a Place your hands over the person's ears to support the head. Support the jaws with your fingers.

   b Flexion—bring the head forward. The chin touches the chest.

   c Extension—straighten the head.

   d Hyperextension—bring the head backward until the chin points up.

   e Rotation—turn the head from side to side.

   f Lateral flexion—move the head to the right and to the left.

   g Repeat flexion, extension, hyperextension, rotation, and lateral flexion 5 times—or the number of times stated on the care plan.

11 Exercise the shoulder (Fig. 22-12):

   a Grasp the wrist with one hand. Grasp the elbow with the other hand.

   b Flexion—raise the arm straight in front and over the head.

   c Extension—bring the arm down to the side.

   d Hyperextension—move the arm behind the body. (Do this if the person sits in a straight-backed chair or is standing.)

   e Abduction—move the straight arm away from the side of the body.

   f Adduction—move the straight arm to the side of the body.

   g Internal rotation—bend the elbow. Place it at the same level as the shoulder. Move the forearm down toward the body.

   h External rotation—move the forearm toward the head.

   i Repeat flexion, extension, hyperextension, abduction, adduction, and internal and external rotation 5 times—or the number of times stated on the care plan.

12 Exercise the elbow (Fig. 22-13, p. 396):

   a Grasp the person's wrist with one hand. Grasp the elbow with your other hand.

   b Flexion—bend the arm so the same-side shoulder is touched.

   c Extension—straighten the arm.

   d Repeat flexion and extension 5 times—or the number of times stated on the care plan.

13 Exercise the forearm (Fig. 22-14, p. 396):

   a Continue to support the wrist and elbow.

   b Pronation—turn the hand so the palm is down.

   c Supination—turn the hand so the palm is up.

   d Repeat pronation and supination 5 times—or the number of times stated on the care plan.

14 Exercise the wrist (Fig. 22-15, p. 396):

   a Hold the wrist with both of your hands.

   b Flexion—bend the hand down.

   c Extension—straighten the hand.

   d Hyperextension—bend the hand back.

   e Radial flexion—turn the hand toward the thumb.

   f Ulnar flexion—turn the hand toward the little finger.

   g Repeat flexion, extension, hyperextension, and radial flexion and ulnar flexion 5 times—or the number of times stated on the care plan.

15 Exercise the thumb (Fig. 22-16, p. 396):

   a Hold the person's hand with one hand. Hold the thumb with your other hand.

   b Abduction—move the thumb out from the inner part of the index finger.

   c Adduction—move the thumb back next to the index finger.

   d Opposition—touch each fingertip with the thumb.

   e Flexion—bend the thumb into the hand.

   f Extension—move the thumb out to the side of the fingers.

   g Repeat abduction, adduction, opposition, flexion, and extension 5 times—or the number of times stated on the care plan.

16 Exercise the fingers (Fig. 22-17, p. 396):

   a Abduction—spread the fingers and the thumb apart.

   b Adduction—bring the fingers and thumb together.

   c Flexion—make a fist.

   d Extension—straighten the fingers so the fingers, hand, and arm are straight.

   e Repeat abduction, adduction, flexion, and extension 5 times—or the number of times stated on the care plan.

PROCEDURE—cont'd

17 Exercise the hip (Fig. 22-18, p. 397):
  a Support the leg. Place one hand under the knee. Place your other hand under the ankle.
  b Flexion—raise the leg.
  c Extension—straighten the leg.
  d Abduction—move the leg away from the body.
  e Adduction—move the leg toward the other leg.
  f Internal rotation—turn the leg inward.
  g External rotation—turn the leg outward.
  h Repeat flexion, extension, abduction, adduction, and internal and external rotation 5 times—or the number of times stated on the care plan.

18 Exercise the knee (Fig. 22-19, p. 397):
  a Support the knee. Place one hand under the knee. Place your other hand under the ankle.
  b Flexion—bend the knee.
  c Extension—straighten the knee.
  d Repeat flexion and extension of the knee 5 times—or the number of times stated on the care plan.

19 Exercise the ankle (Fig. 22-20, p. 397):
  a Support the foot and ankle. Place one hand under the foot. Place your other hand under the ankle.
  b Dorsiflexion—pull the foot forward. Push down on the heel at the same time.

  c Plantar flexion—turn the foot down. Or point the toes.
  d Repeat dorsiflexion and plantar flexion 5 times—or the number of times stated on the care plan.

20 Exercise the foot (Fig. 22-21, p. 397):
  a Continue to support the foot and ankle.
  b Pronation—turn the outside of the foot up and the inside down.
  c Supination—turn the inside of the foot up and the outside down.
  d Repeat pronation and supination 5 times—or the number of times stated on the care plan.

21 Exercise the toes (Fig. 22-22, p. 397):
  a Flexion—curl the toes.
  b Extension—straighten the toes.
  c Abduction—spread the toes apart.
  d Adduction—pull the toes together.
  e Repeat flexion, extension, abduction, and adduction 5 times—or the number of times stated on the care plan.

22 Cover the leg. Raise the bed rail if used.
23 Go to the other side. Lower the bed rail near you if up.
24 Repeat steps 11 through 21.

POST-PROCEDURE

25 Provide for comfort. (See the inside of the front book cover.)
26 Remove the bath blanket.
27 Place the signal light within reach.
28 Lower the bed to its lowest level.
29 Raise or lower bed rails. Follow the care plan.

30 Fold and return the bath blanket to its proper place.
31 Unscreen the person.
32 Complete a safety check of the room. (See the inside of the front book cover.)
33 Decontaminate your hands.
34 Report and record your observations.

Flexion   Extension   Hyperextension   Rotation   Lateral flexion

FIGURE 22-11 *Range-of-motion exercises for the neck.*

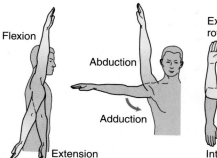   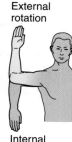

FIGURE 22-12 *Range-of-motion exercises for the shoulder.*

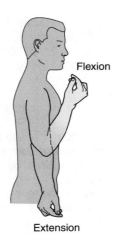

Flexion

Extension

FIGURE 22-13 Range-of-motion exercises for the elbow.

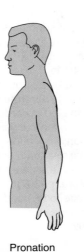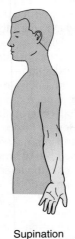

Pronation   Supination

FIGURE 22-14 Range-of-motion exercises for the forearm.

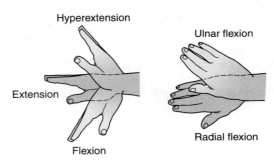

Hyperextension

Ulnar flexion

Extension

Flexion

Radial flexion

FIGURE 22-15 Range-of-motion exercises for the wrist.

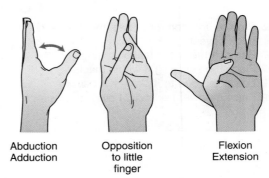

Abduction   Opposition   Flexion
Adduction   to little   Extension
             finger

FIGURE 22-16 Range-of-motion exercises for the thumb.

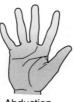

Abduction   Adduction   Flexion   Extension

FIGURE 22-17 Range-of-motion exercises for the fingers.

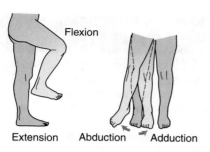

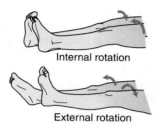

FIGURE 22-18 Range-of-motion exercises for the hip.

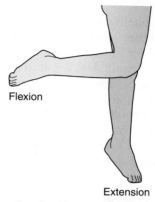

FIGURE 22-19 Range-of-motion exercises for the knee.

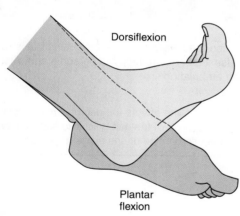

FIGURE 22-20 Range-of-motion exercises for the ankle.

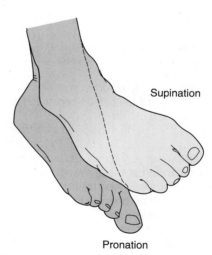

FIGURE 22-21 Range-of-motion exercises for the foot.

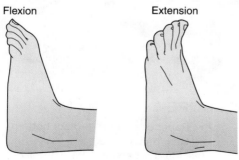

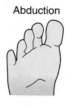

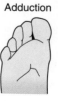

FIGURE 22-22 Range-of-motion exercises for the toes.

✦ AMBULATION

Ambulation is the act of walking. After bedrest, activity increases slowly and in steps. First the person dangles (sits on the side of the bed). Sitting in a bedside chair follows. Next the person walks in the room and then in the hallway.

Some people are weak and unsteady from bedrest, illness, surgery, or injury. Follow the care plan when helping a person walk. Use a gait (transfer) belt if the person is weak or unsteady. The person also uses hand rails along the wall. Always check the person for orthostatic hypotension (p. 390).

See *Focus on Communication: Ambulation*
See *Delegation Guidelines: Ambulation.*
See *Promoting Safety and Comfort: Ambulation.*

FOCUS ON COMMUNICATION
Ambulation

Before ambulating, talk with the person about the activity. Doing so promotes comfort and reduces fear. Explain to the person:
- The distance to walk
- What assistive devices will be used
- How you will assist
- What the person is to report to you
- How you will help if the person begins to fall
  For example, you can say:
  "Mr. Owens, I am going to help you walk from your bed to the doorway and back. This belt is to help support you while you walk. I will stay by your side and keep hold of the belt at all times. Let me know right away if you feel unsteady, dizzy, or weak. Also tell me if you feel any pain or discomfort. If you do begin to fall, I will use the belt to pull you close to me and gently lower you to the ground. Do you have any questions?"

DELEGATION GUIDELINES
Ambulation

Before helping with ambulation, you need this information from the nurse and the care plan:
- How much help the person needs
- If the person uses a cane, walker, crutches, or a brace
- Areas of weakness—right arm or leg, left arm or leg
- How far to walk the person
- What observations to report and record:
  - How well the person tolerated the activity
  - Shuffling, sliding, limping, or walking on tip-toes
  - Complaints of pain or discomfort
  - Complaints of orthostatic hypotension—weakness, dizziness, spots before the eyes, feeling faint
  - The distance walked
- When to report observations
- What specific patient or resident concerns to report at once

PROMOTING SAFETY AND COMFORT
Ambulation

Safety
Practice the safety measures to prevent falls (Chapter 9). Use a gait belt to help the person stand. Also use it during ambulation.

Comfort
The fear of falling affects the person's mental comfort. Explain the purpose of the gait belt. Also explain how you will help the person if he or she starts to fall (Chapter 9).

HELPING THE PERSON WALK

QUALITY OF LIFE

Remember to:
- Knock before entering the person's room.
- Address the person by name.
- Introduce yourself by name and title.

- Explain the procedure to the person before beginning and during the procedure.
- Protect the person's rights during the procedure.
- Handle the person gently during the procedure.

PRE-PROCEDURE

1 Follow *Delegation Guidelines: Ambulation.*
   See *Promoting Safety and Comfort: Ambulation.*
2 Practice hand hygiene.
3 Collect the following:
   - Robe and non-skid shoes

- Paper or sheet to protect bottom linens
- Gait (transfer) belt
4 Identify the person. Check the ID bracelet against the assignment sheet. Also call the person by name.
5 Provide for privacy.

PROCEDURE

6 Lower the bed to its lowest position. Lock the bed wheels. Lower the bed rail if up.

7 Fan-fold top linens to the foot of the bed.

8 Place the paper or sheet under the person's feet. Put the shoes on the person. Fasten the shoes.

9 Help the person sit on the side of the bed. (See procedure: *Sitting on the Side of the Bed [Dangling]*, Chapter 13.)

10 Help the person put on the robe.

11 Make sure the person's feet are flat on the floor.

12 Apply the gait belt. (See procedure: *Applying a Transfer/Gait Belt*, Chapter 9.)

13 Help the person stand. (See procedure: *Transferring the Person to a Chair or Wheelchair*, Chapter 13.) Grasp the gait belt at each side. If not using a gait belt, place your arms under the person's arms around to the shoulder blades.

14 Stand at the person's weak side while he or she gains balance. Hold the belt at the side and back. If not using a gait belt, have one arm around the back and the other at the elbow to support the person.

15 Encourage the person to stand erect with the head up and back straight.

16 Help the person walk. Walk to the side and slightly behind the person on the person's weak side. Provide support with the gait belt (Fig. 22-23). If not using a gait belt, have one arm around the back and the other at the elbow to support the person. Encourage the person to use the hand rail on his or her strong side.

17 Encourage the person to walk normally. The heel strikes the floor first. Discourage shuffling, sliding, or walking on tip-toes.

18 Walk the required distance if the person tolerates the activity. Do not rush the person.

19 Help the person return to bed. Remove the gait belt. (See procedure: *Transferring the Person From a Chair or Wheelchair to a Bed*, Chapter 13.)

20 Lower the head of the bed. Help the person to the center of the bed.

21 Remove the shoes. Remove and discard the paper or sheet over the bottom sheet.

POST-PROCEDURE

22 Provide for comfort. (See the inside of the front book cover.)

23 Place the signal light within reach.

24 Raise or lower bed rails. Follow the care plan.

25 Return the robe and shoes to their proper place.

26 Unscreen the person.

27 Complete a safety check of the room. (See the inside of the front book cover.)

28 Decontaminate your hands.

29 Report and record your observations.

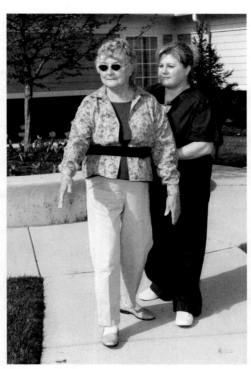

FIGURE 22-23 The nursing assistant walks at the person's side and slightly behind her.

Walking Aids

Walking aids support the body. The physical therapist or nurse measures and teaches the person to use the device.

Crutches. Crutches are used when the person cannot use one leg or when one or both legs need to gain strength. Some persons with permanent leg weakness can use crutches. Falls are a risk. Follow these safety measures:

- Check the crutch tips. They must not be worn down, torn, or wet. Replace worn or torn crutch tips. Dry wet tips with a towel or paper towels.
- Check crutches for flaws. Check wooden crutches for cracks and metal crutches for bends.
- Tighten all bolts.
- Street shoes are worn. They must be flat and have non-skid soles.
- Clothes must fit well. Loose clothes may get caught between the crutches and underarms. Loose clothes and long skirts can hang forward and block the person's view of the feet and crutch tips.
- Practice safety rules to prevent falls (Chapter 9).
- Keep crutches within the person's reach. Put them by the person's chair or against a wall.

Canes. Canes are used for weakness on one side of the body. They help provide balance and support (Fig. 22-24).

A cane is held on the *strong side* of the body. (If the left leg is weak, the cane is held in the right hand.) The cane tip is about 6 to 10 inches to the side of the foot. It is about 6 to 10 inches in front of the foot on the strong side. The grip is level with the hip. The person walks as follows:

- *Step A:* The cane is moved forward 6 to 10 inches (Fig. 22-25, *A*).
- *Step B:* The weak leg (opposite the cane) is moved forward even with the cane (Fig. 22-25, *B*).
- *Step C:* The strong leg is moved forward and ahead of the cane and the weak leg (Fig. 22-25, *C*).

Walkers. A walker gives more support than a cane. Wheeled walkers are common (Fig. 22-26). They have wheels on the front legs and rubber tips on the back legs. The person pushes the walker about 6 to 8 inches in front of his or her feet. Rubber tips on the back legs prevent the walker from moving while the person is walking or standing. Some have a braking action when weight is applied to the walker's back legs.

Baskets, pouches, and trays attach to the walker. They are used for needed items. This allows more independence. They also free the hands to grip the walker.

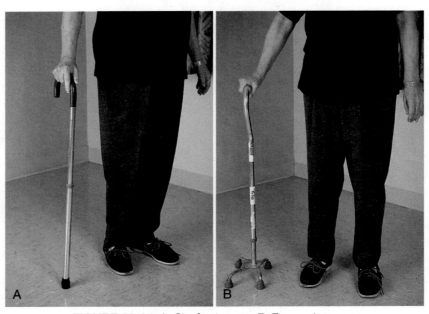

FIGURE 22-24 A, Single-tip cane. **B,** Four-point cane.

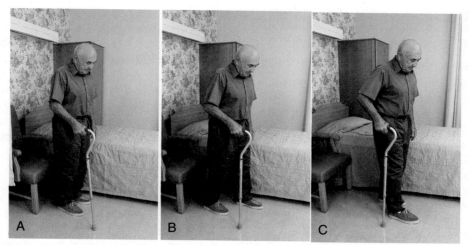

FIGURE 22-25 Walking with a cane. **A,** The cane is moved forward about 6 to 10 inches. **B,** The leg opposite the cane (weak leg) is brought forward even with the cane. **C,** The leg on the cane side (strong side) is moved ahead of the cane and the weak leg.

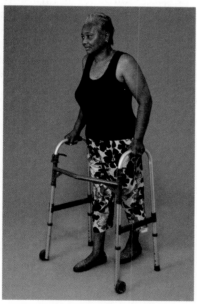

FIGURE 22-26 Wheeled walker.

Braces. Braces support weak body parts. They also prevent or correct deformities or prevent joint movement. Metal, plastic, or leather is used for braces. A brace is applied over the ankle, knee, or back (Fig. 22-27).

Skin and bony points under braces are kept clean and dry. This prevents skin breakdown. Report redness or signs of skin breakdown at once. Also report complaints of pain or discomfort. The nurse assesses the skin under braces every shift. The care plan tells you when to apply and remove a brace.

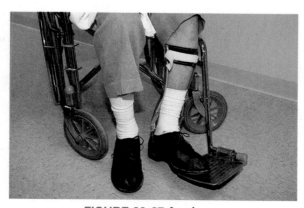

FIGURE 22-27 Leg brace.

Focus on P R I D E
The Person, Family, and Yourself

Personal and Professional Responsibility—
Exercise and activity help maintain normal joint and muscle function. They also promote normal function of all body systems. Good conditioning has long-term effects. The more active a person is in the present, the more likely that he or she will remain active in the future.

Every person has a responsibility to do his or her best to be active. Disease, injury, pain, and aging affect a person's ability to do daily activities. Even with such limits, you can promote activity, exercise, and well-being. You can:

- Encourage the person to be as active as possible.
- Resist the urge to do things for the person that he or she can safely do alone or with some assistance.
- Focus on the person's abilities.
- Tell the person when you notice he or she is doing well or making progress.
- Tell the person you are proud of what he or she did or tried to do.

Rights and Respect—Make sure the person's garments provide needed privacy during exercise and activity. When ambulating, the person must not walk in the room or hallway with a gown open in the back. During range-of-motion exercises, cover the person with a bath blanket. Expose only the body part being exercised. Protect the person's right to privacy. Privacy promotes dignity and mental comfort.

Independence and Social Interaction—Recreational activities are social events and are mentally stimulating. A good activity program improves a person's quality of life. Allow personal choice in selecting activities. Independence and well-being are promoted when the person attends activities that he or she chooses. Do not force the person to take part in activities that do not interest him or her.

Delegation and Teamwork—When delegated a task, you must know the person's activity limits. The person's care plan and your assignment sheet tell you the activities allowed. Always ask the nurse what bedrest means for each person. Also, follow the delegation guidelines in this chapter. Check with the nurse if you have questions about a person's activity limits. Take pride in providing safe care by knowing and following the person's activity level.

Ethics and Laws—The Omnibus Budget Reconciliation Act of 1987 requires activity programs for nursing center residents. The programs are important for physical and mental well-being. Activities must meet the interests and physical, mental, and social needs of each resident. Bingo, movies, dances, exercise groups, shopping and museum trips, concerts, and guest speakers are often arranged. Some centers have gardening activities.

Encourage residents to be involved in activities. Ask the resident and family about activities the person enjoys. Listen and suggest options that the person may like. The resident and family may not be aware of the activities offered. Take pride in being a good resource. Inform residents and families about your nursing center's activity programs.

REVIEW QUESTIONS

Circle the BEST answer.

1 The purpose of bedrest is to
   a Prevent orthostatic hypotension
   b Reduce pain and promote healing
   c Prevent pressure ulcers, constipation, and blood clots
   d Cause contractures and muscle atrophy

2 Which helps prevent plantar flexion?
   a Bedboards
   b A footboard
   c A trochanter roll
   d Handrolls

3 Which prevents the hip from turning outward?
   a Bedboards
   b A footboard
   c Trochanter roll
   d A leg brace

4 A contracture is
   a The loss of muscle strength from inactivity
   b The lack of joint mobility from shortening of a muscle
   c A decrease in the size of a muscle
   d A blood clot in the muscle

5 Passive range-of-motion exercises are performed by
   a The person
   b Someone else
   c The person with the help of another
   d The person with the use of handgrips

6 ROM exercises are ordered. You do the following *except*
   a Support the part being exercised
   b Move the joint slowly, smoothly, and gently
   c Force the joint through its full range of motion
   d Exercise only the joints indicated by the nurse

7 Flexion involves
   a Bending the body part
   b Straightening the body part
   c Moving the body part toward the body
   d Moving the body part away from the body

8 When ambulating a person
   a A gait belt is used if the person is weak or unsteady
   b The person can shuffle or slide when walking after bedrest
   c Walking aids are needed
   d You walk on the person's strong side

9 You are getting a person ready to crutch walk. You should do the following *except*
   a Check the crutch tips
   b Have the person wear non-skid shoes
   c Get a pair of crutches from physical therapy
   d Tighten the bolts on the crutches

10 A single-tip cane is used
   a At waist level
   b On the strong side
   c On the weak side
   d On either side

Circle T if the statement is *true*. Circle F if the statement is *false*.

11 T F A walker and a four-point cane give the same support.

12 T F When using a cane, the feet are moved first.

13 T F When using a walker, the feet are moved first.

14 T F A person has a brace. Bony areas need protection from skin breakdown.

Answers to these questions are on p. 528.

23

ASSISTING WITH WOUND CARE

PROCEDURES

- Applying Elastic Stockings
- Applying Elastic Bandages
- Applying a Dry, Non-Sterile Dressing
- Applying Heat and Cold Applications

OBJECTIVES

- Define the key terms and key abbreviations listed in this chapter.
- Describe pressure ulcers, skin tears, circulatory ulcers, and diabetic foot ulcers and how to prevent them.
- Identify the pressure points in each body position.
- Describe what to observe about wounds.
- Explain how to secure dressings.
- Explain the rules for applying dressings.
- Explain the purpose, effects, and complications of heat and cold applications.
- Describe the rules for applying heat and cold.
- Explain how to promote PRIDE in the person, the family, and yourself.
- Perform the procedures described in this chapter.

KEY TERMS

constrict To narrow

dilate To expand or open wider

pressure ulcer A localized injury to the skin and/or underlying tissue usually over a bony prominence; the result of pressure or pressure in combination with shear and/or friction

skin tear A break or rip in the skin; the epidermis (top skin layer) separates from the underlying tissues

ulcer A shallow or deep crater-like sore of the skin or a mucous membrane

wound A break in the skin or mucous membrane

KEY ABBREVIATIONS

C Centigrade

F Fahrenheit

ID Identification

TJC The Joint Commission

A **wound** is a break in the skin or mucous membrane. Common causes are:

- Surgery
- *Trauma*—an accident or violent act that injures the skin, mucous membranes, bones, and organs
- Pressure ulcers from unrelieved pressure
- Decreased blood flow through the arteries or veins
- Nerve damage

The wound is a portal of entry for microbes. Infection is a major threat. Wound care involves preventing infection and further injury to the wound and nearby tissues.

PRESSURE ULCERS

The National Pressure Ulcer Advisory Panel defines a **pressure ulcer** as a localized injury to the skin and/or underlying tissue usually over a bony prominence. It is the result of pressure or pressure in combination with shear and/or friction. *Decubitus ulcer, bed sore,* or *pressure sore* are other terms for pressure ulcer.

A pressure ulcer usually occurs over a bony prominence. *Prominence* means to stick out. A *bony prominence* is an area where the bone sticks out or projects from the flat surface of the body. The back of the head, shoulder blades, elbows, hips, spine, sacrum, knees, ankles, heels, and toes are bony prominences (Fig. 23-1, p. 406).

Causes and Risk Factors

Pressure, shearing, and friction are causes of skin breakdown and pressure ulcers. Risk factors include breaks in the skin, poor circulation to an area, moisture, dry skin, and irritation by urine and feces. Older and disabled persons are at great risk for pressure ulcers. Their skin is easily injured. Causes include age-related skin changes, chronic disease, and general debility.

Pressure occurs when the skin over a bony area is squeezed between hard surfaces (Fig. 23-2, p. 407). The bone is one hard surface. The other is usually the mattress or chair seat. Squeezing or pressure prevents blood flow to the skin and underlying tissues. Lack of blood flow means oxygen and nutrients cannot get to the cells. Therefore involved skin and tissues die (Fig. 23-3, p. 407).

Friction scrapes the skin, causing an open area. The open area needs to heal. A good blood supply is needed. A poor blood supply or an infection can lead to a pressure ulcer.

Shearing is when the skin sticks to a surface (usually the bed or chair) while deeper tissues move downward. This occurs when the person slides down in the bed or chair. Blood vessels and tissues are damaged. Blood flow to the area is reduced.

Persons at Risk

Persons at risk for pressure ulcers are those who:

- Are *bedfast* (confined to a bed) or *chairfast* (confined to a chair)
- Need some or total help in moving
- Are agitated or have involuntary muscle movements
- Have loss of bowel or bladder control
- Are exposed to moisture
- Have poor nutrition or poor fluid balance
- Have lowered mental awareness
- Have problems sensing pain or pressure
- Have circulatory problems
- Are older, obese, or very thin

Pressure Ulcer Stages

In persons with light skin, a reddened bony area is the first sign of a pressure ulcer. In persons with dark skin, skin color may differ from surrounding areas. The color change remains after the pressure is relieved. The area may feel warm or cool. The person may complain of pain, burning, tingling, or itching in the area. Some persons do not feel anything unusual. Figure 23-4, p. 407 shows pressure ulcer stages.

See *Focus on Communication: Pressure Ulcer Stages*, p. 408.

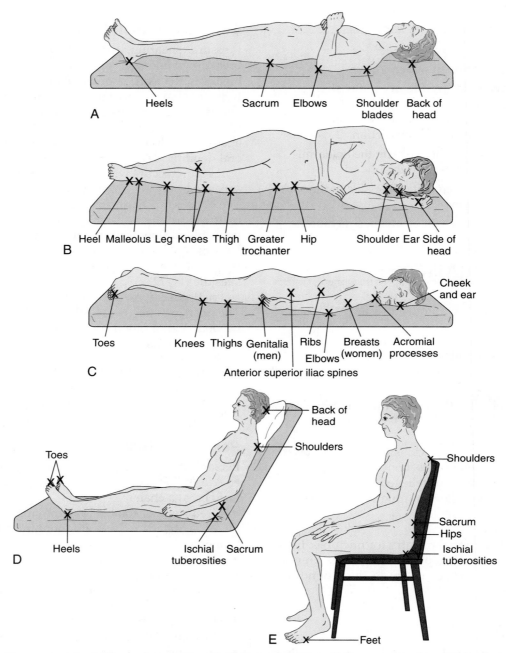

FIGURE 23-1 Pressure points. **A,** The supine position. **B,** The lateral position. **C,** The prone position. **D,** Fowler's position. **E,** Sitting position.

Sites

Pressure ulcers usually occur over bony areas. The bony areas are called *pressure points*. This is because they bear the weight of the body in a certain position (see Fig. 23-1). Pressure from body weight can reduce the blood supply to the area.

The ears also are sites for pressure ulcers. This is from pressure of the ear on the mattress when in the side-lying position. Eyeglasses and oxygen tubing (Chapter 24) also can cause pressure on the ears.

In obese people, pressure ulcers can occur in areas where skin has contact with skin. Common sites are between abdominal folds, the legs, the buttocks, the thighs, and under the breasts. Friction occurs in these areas.

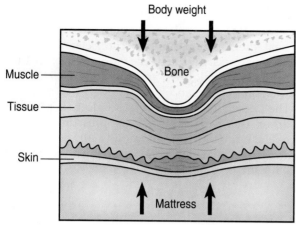

FIGURE 23-2 Tissue under pressure. The skin is squeezed between two hard surfaces: the bone and the mattress. *(Redrawn from* Understanding your body: what are pressure ulcers? *US Department of Health & Human Services, Agency for Healthcare Research and Quality, September 2009.)*

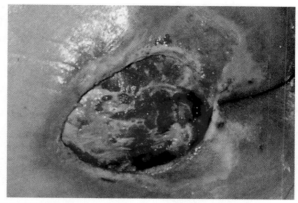

FIGURE 23-3 A pressure ulcer. *(From "Proceedings from the November National V.A.C.®,"* Ostomy Wound Management, Feb 2005, Vol. 51, Issue 2A[suppl], p. 75, HMP Communication.)

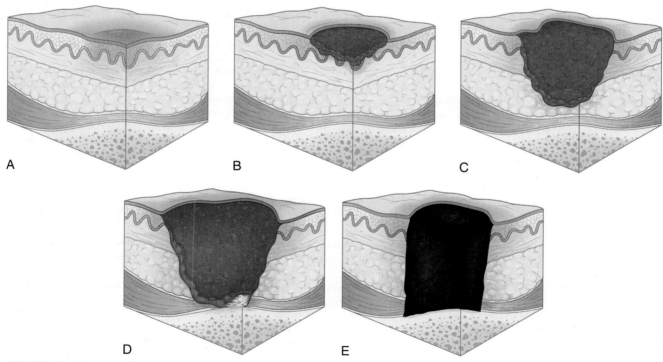

FIGURE 23-4 Stages of pressure ulcers. **A,** Stage 1—the skin is intact. There is usually redness over a bony prominence. The color does not return to normal when the skin is relieved of pressure. In persons with dark skin, skin color may differ from surrounding areas. **B,** Stage 2—partial-thickness skin loss. The wound may involve a blister or shallow ulcer. An ulcer may appear to be reddish-pink. A blister may be intact or open. **C,** Stage 3—full-thickness tissue loss. The skin is gone. Subcutaneous fat may be exposed. Tissue shedding *(slough)* may be present. **D,** Stage 4—full-thickness tissue loss with muscle, tendon, and bone exposure. Slough (tissue shedding) or *eschar* (a scab or dry crust) may be present. **E,** Unstageable—full-thickness tissue loss with the ulcer covered by slough and/or eschar. Slough is yellow, tan, gray, green, or brown. Eschar is tan, brown, or black. *(Redrawn from National Pressure Ulcer Advisory Panel, 2007.)*

Tell the nurse if you notice areas of redness, skin color changes, blisters, or skin or tissue loss. Describe what you saw as best as you can. Tell the nurse the location. The nurse needs to assess the area. For example, you can say to the nurse:

- "I noticed a reddened area on Mr. Drake's left heel. It was about the size of a quarter. The skin looked intact. Would you please take a look at it?"
- "I just gave Ms. Richards a bath. I noticed a reddened area with a blister on her left buttock. I didn't see any drainage. Would you please take a look at it? I can help you turn her."

Prevention and Treatment

Preventing pressure ulcers is much easier than trying to heal them. Good nursing care, cleanliness, and skin care are essential. The measures in Box 23-1 help prevent skin breakdown and pressure ulcers. Follow the person's care plan.

The person at risk for pressure ulcers is placed on a surface that reduces or relieves pressure. Such surfaces include foam, air, alternating air, gel, or water mattresses. The health team decides on the best surface for the person.

BOX 23-1 | **Measures to Prevent Pressure Ulcers**

Handling, Moving, and Positioning

- Follow the repositioning schedule in the person's care plan. Reposition bedfast persons at least every 1 to 2 hours. Reposition chairfast persons every hour. Some persons are repositioned every 15 minutes.
- Position the person according to the care plan. Use pillows for support as instructed by the nurse. The 30-degree lateral position is recommended (Fig. 23-5).
- Prevent shearing and friction during handling, moving, and transfer procedures. Use assist devices as directed by the nurse and the care plan.
- Prevent friction in bed. Powder sheets lightly to prevent friction. Follow the care plan.
- Prevent shearing. Do not raise the head of the bed more than 30 degrees. Follow the care plan. The care plan tells you:
  - When to raise the head of the bed
  - How far to raise the head of the bed
  - How long (in minutes) to raise the head of the bed
- Use pillows, foam wedges, or other devices to prevent bony areas from contact with bony areas. The knees and ankles are examples. Follow the care plan.
- Keep the heels and ankles off the bed. Use pillows or other devices as the nurse directs. Place the pillows or devices under the lower legs from mid-calf to the ankles.
- Use protective devices as the nurse and care plan direct.
- Remind persons sitting in chairs to shift their positions every 15 minutes. This decreases pressure on bony points.

Skin Care

- Do not use hot water to bathe or clean the skin. Hot water can irritate the skin.
- Use a cleansing agent as directed by the nurse and the care plan. Soap can dry and irritate the skin.
- Provide good skin care. The skin is clean and dry after bathing. The skin is free of moisture from urine, stools, perspiration, and wound drainage.
- Follow the care plan to prevent incontinence.
- Prevent skin exposure to moisture. Check persons who are incontinent of urine or feces often. Provide good skin care at once and change linens and garments as needed. Use incontinence products as directed by the nurse and the care plan.
- Check persons often who perspire heavily or have wound drainage. Change linens and garments as needed. Provide good skin care.
- Apply moisturizer to dry areas—hands, elbows, legs, ankles, heels, and so on. The nurse tells you what to use and what areas need attention.
- Give a back massage when repositioning the person. *Do not massage bony areas.*
- Do not massage over pressure points. *Never rub or massage reddened areas.*
- Keep linens clean, dry, and wrinkle-free.
- Apply cornstarch where skin touches skin. Apply it in a thin layer.
- Do not irritate the skin. Avoid scrubbing or vigorous rubbing when bathing or drying the person.
- Use pillows and blankets to prevent skin from being in contact with skin. They also reduce moisture and friction.
- Make sure socks and shoes are in good repair. Socks should not have wrinkles or creases. Make sure there is nothing in the shoes before the person puts them on.

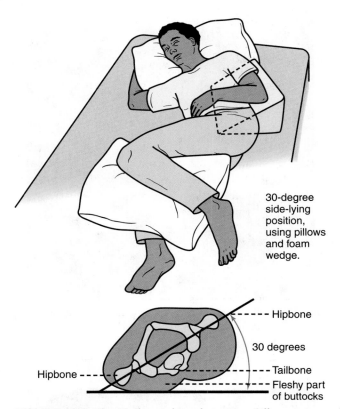

FIGURE 23-5 The 30-degree lateral position. Pillows are placed under the head, shoulder, and leg. This position inclines (lifts up) the hip to avoid pressure on the hip. The person does not lie on the hip as in the side-lying position.

The doctor orders wound care products, drugs, treatments, and special equipment to promote healing. The nurse and care plan tell you what to do. Protective devices are often used to prevent and treat pressure ulcers and skin breakdown. These devices are common:

- *Bed cradle*—A bed cradle is a metal frame placed on the bed and over the person (Chapter 22). Top linens are brought over the cradle to prevent pressure on the legs, feet, and toes.
- *Heel and elbow protectors*—These devices are made of foam padding, pressure-relieving gel, sheepskin, and other cushion materials. They fit the shape of heels and elbows (Fig. 23-6).
- *Heel and foot elevators*—These raise the heels and feet off of the bed (Fig. 23-7, p. 410). They prevent pressure. Some also prevent footdrop (Chapter 22). Many are secured in place with Velcro straps.
- *Gel or fluid-filled pads and cushions*—These devices involve a pressure-relieving gel or fluid (Fig. 23-8, p. 410). They are used for chairs and wheelchairs to prevent pressure. The outer case is vinyl. The pad or cushion is placed in a fabric cover to protect the person's skin.
- *Eggcrate-type pads*—These devices are placed on beds or in chairs or wheelchairs (Fig. 23-9, p. 410). The foam pad looks like an egg carton. Peaks in the pad distribute the person's weight more evenly. The pad is put in a special cover. The cover protects against heat, moisture, and soiling. Only a bottom sheet is used over the eggcrate-type pad and cover. No other bottom linens are used.
- *Special beds*—Some beds have air flowing through the mattresses (Fig. 23-10, p. 410). The person *floats* on the mattress. Body weight is distributed evenly. There is little pressure on body parts. Some beds allow repositioning without moving the person. The person is turned to the prone or supine position or the bed is tilted various degrees. Alignment does not change. Pressure points change as the position changes. There is little friction. Some beds constantly rotate from side to side. They are useful for persons with spinal cord injuries.
- *Other equipment*—Pillows, trochanter rolls, footboards, and other positioning devices are used (Chapter 22). They help keep the person in good alignment.

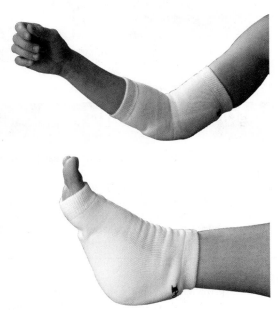

FIGURE 23-6 Heel and elbow protector. *(Image courtesy J. T. Posey Co., Arcadia, Calif.)*

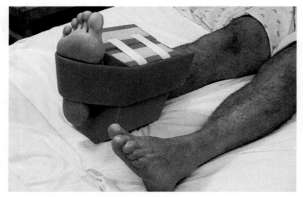

FIGURE 23-7 Heel elevator.

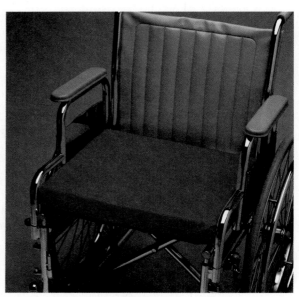

FIGURE 23-8 Gel and foam cushion. (*Image courtesy J. T. Posey Co., Arcadia, Calif.*)

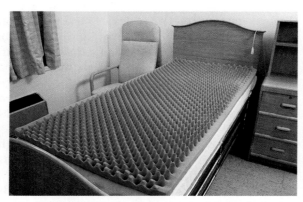

FIGURE 23-9 Eggcrate-type pad on the bed.

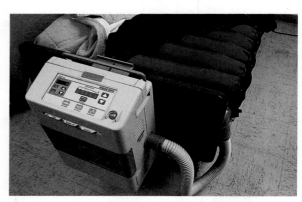

FIGURE 23-10 Air flotation bed.

SKIN TEARS

A **skin tear** is a break or rip in the skin. The epidermis (top skin layer) separates from the underlying tissues. Skin tears are caused by friction, shearing (Chapter 13), pulling, or pressure on the skin.

Bumping a hand, arm, or leg on any hard surface can cause a skin tear. Beds, bed rails, chairs, wheelchair footplates, and tables are dangers. So is holding the person's arm or leg too tight.

Skin tears are painful. They are portals of entry for microbes. Wound complications can develop. Tell the nurse at once if you cause or find a skin tear. To prevent skin tears, follow the care plan and the measures in Box 23-2.

See *Persons With Dementia: Skin Tears.*

PERSONS WITH DEMENTIA
Skin Tears

Some persons are confused and may resist care. They often move quickly and without warning. Or they pull away from you during care. Some try to hit or kick. These sudden movements can cause skin tears.

Never force care on a person. Chapter 28 describes how to care for persons who are confused and resist care. Always follow the care plan.

- Keep your fingernails short and smoothly filed.
- Keep the person's fingernails short and smoothly filed. Report long and tough toenails.
- Do not wear rings with large or raised stones. Do not wear bracelets.
- Be patient and calm when the person is confused or agitated or resists care.
- Follow the care plan and safety rules to handle, move, turn, position, or transfer the person.
  - Prevent shearing and friction.
  - Use an assist device to move and turn the person in bed.
  - Use pillows to support arms and legs. Follow the care plan.
- Pad bed rails and wheelchair arms, footplates, and leg supports. Follow the care plan.
- Follow the care plan and safety rules to bathe the person.
- Dress and undress the person carefully.
- Dress the person in soft clothes with long sleeves and long pants.
- Provide good lighting so the person can see. The person needs to avoid bumping into furniture, walls, and equipment.
- Provide a safe area for wandering (Chapter 28).
- Keep the skin moisturized. Apply lotion according to the care plan.
- Offer fluids. Follow the care plan.

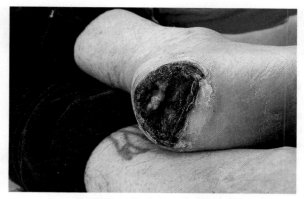

FIGURE 23-11 Venous ulcer.

- *Venous ulcers (stasis ulcers)* are open sores on the lower legs or feet. They are caused by poor blood flow through the veins (Fig. 23-11). The heels and inner aspect of the ankles are common sites. They can occur from skin injury. Scratching is an example. Or they can occur without trauma.
- *Arterial ulcers* are open wounds on the lower legs or feet caused by poor arterial blood flow. They are found between the toes, on top of the toes, and on the outer side of the ankle.
- A *diabetic foot ulcer* is an open wound on the foot caused by complications from diabetes. Diabetes (Chapter 26) can affect the nerves and blood vessels. When nerves are affected, the person can lose complete or partial sensation in a foot or leg. The person may not feel pain, heat, or cold. Therefore the person may not feel a cut, blister, burn, or other trauma to the foot. Infection and a large sore can develop. When blood vessels are affected, blood flow decreases. Tissues and cells do not get needed oxygen and nutrients. A sore does not heal properly. Tissue death (gangrene) can occur. Sometimes amputation of the affected part is needed to prevent the spread of gangrene.

CIRCULATORY ULCERS

Some diseases affect blood flow to and from the legs and feet. Such poor circulation can lead to pain, open wounds, and edema (swelling of tissues). Infection and gangrene can result from the open wound and poor circulation. *Gangrene* is a condition in which there is death of tissue.

An **ulcer** is a shallow or deep crater-like sore of the skin or a mucous membrane. *Circulatory ulcers (vascular ulcers)* are open sores on the lower legs or feet. They are caused by decreased blood flow through the arteries or veins. Persons with diseases affecting the blood vessels are at risk. These wounds are painful and hard to heal.

Prevention and Treatment

The doctor orders drugs and treatments as needed. You must help prevent skin breakdown on the legs and feet (Box 23-3, p. 412). Check the person's feet and legs every day. Report any sign of a problem to the nurse at once. Follow the care plan to prevent and treat circulatory ulcers.

BOX 23-3 Measures to Prevent Circulatory Ulcers

- Remind the person not to sit with the legs crossed.
- Reposition the person according to the care plan. The person is repositioned at least every 2 hours.
- Do not use elastic or rubber band-type garters to hold socks or hose in place.
- Do not dress the person in tight clothes.
- Provide good skin care daily. Keep the feet clean and dry. Clean and dry between the toes.
- Do not scrub or rub the skin during bathing and drying.
- Keep linens clean, dry, and wrinkle-free.
- Avoid injury to the legs and feet.
- Make sure shoes fit well.
- Keep pressure off the heels and other bony areas. Use pillows or other devices as the nurse and care plan direct.
- Check the person's legs and feet. Report skin breaks or changes in skin color.
- Do not massage over pressure points. *Never rub or massage reddened areas.*
- Use protective devices as the nurse directs. Follow the care plan.
- Follow the care plan for walking and exercise.

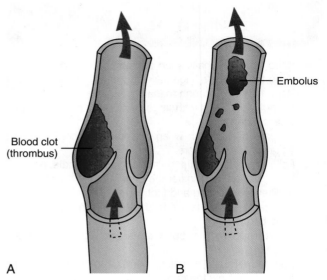

FIGURE 23-12 A, A blood clot is attached to the wall of a vein. The arrow shows the direction of blood flow. **B,** Part of the thrombus breaks off and becomes an embolus. The embolus travels in the bloodstream until it lodges in a distant vessel.

Elastic Stockings Elastic stockings exert pressure on the veins. The pressure promotes venous blood return to the heart. By doing so, the stockings help prevent blood clots *(thrombi).* A blood clot is called a *thrombus.*

If blood flow is sluggish, blood clots may form. They can form in the deep leg veins in the lower leg or thigh (Fig. 23-12, *A*). A blood clot can break loose and travel through the bloodstream. It then becomes an embolus. An *embolus* is a blood clot that travels through the vascular system until it lodges in a vessel (Fig. 23-12, *B*). An embolus from a vein lodges in the lungs *(pulmonary embolism).* A pulmonary embolus can cause severe respiratory problems and death. Report chest pain or shortness of breath at once.

Elastic stockings also are called AE stockings (AE means *anti-embolism* or *anti-embolic*). They also are called TED hose (TED means *thrombo-embolic disease*). Persons at risk for thrombi include those who:

- Have heart and circulatory disorders
- Are on bedrest
- Have had surgery
- Are older
- Are pregnant

DELEGATION GUIDELINES
Elastic Stockings

Before applying elastic stockings, you need this information from the nurse and the care plan:
- What size to use—small, medium, or large
- What length to use—thigh-high or knee-high
- When to remove them and for how long—usually every 8 hours for 30 minutes
- What observations to report and record:
  - The size and length of stockings applied
  - When you applied the stockings
  - Skin color and temperature
  - Leg and foot swelling
  - Skin tears, wounds, or signs of skin breakdown
  - Complaints of pain, tingling, or numbness
  - When you removed the stockings and for how long
  - When you re-applied the stockings
  - When you washed the stockings
- When to report observations
- What specific patient or resident concerns to report at once

The person usually has two pairs of stockings. One pair is washed while the other pair is worn. Wash the stockings by hand with a mild soap. Hang them to dry.

See *Delegation Guidelines: Elastic Stockings.*

See *Promoting Safety and Comfort: Elastic Stockings.*

PROMOTING SAFETY AND COMFORT
Elastic Stockings

Safety

Apply the stocking so the opening in the toe area is over the top of the toes. The opening is used to check circulation to the toes.

Stockings should not have twists, creases, or wrinkles after you apply them. Twists can affect circulation. Creases and wrinkles can cause skin breakdown.

Loose stockings do not promote venous blood return to the heart. Stockings that are too tight can affect circulation. Tell the nurse if stockings are loose or too tight.

Comfort

Stockings are applied before the person gets out of bed. Otherwise the person's legs can swell from sitting or standing. Stockings are hard to put on when the legs are swollen. The person lies in bed while they are off. This prevents the legs from swelling.

Gently handle and move the person's foot and leg. Do not force the joints (toes, foot, ankle, knee, and hip) beyond their range of motion or to the point of pain.

APPLYING ELASTIC STOCKINGS

QUALITY OF LIFE

Remember to:
- Knock before entering the person's room.
- Address the person by name.
- Introduce yourself by name and title.

- Explain the procedure to the person before beginning and during the procedure.
- Protect the person's rights during the procedure.
- Handle the person gently during the procedure.

PRE-PROCEDURE

1 Follow *Delegation Guidelines: Elastic Stockings.* See *Promoting Safety and Comfort: Elastic Stockings.*
2 Practice hand hygiene.
3 Obtain elastic stockings in the correct size and length.

4 Identify the person. Check the ID (identification) bracelet against the assignment sheet. Also call the person by name.
5 Provide for privacy.
6 Raise the bed for body mechanics. Bed rails are up if used.

PROCEDURE

7 Lower the bed rail near you if up.
8 Position the person supine.
9 Expose the legs. Fan-fold top linens toward the thighs.
10 Turn the stocking inside out down to the heel.
11 Slip the foot of the stocking over the toes, foot, and heel (Fig. 23-13, *A,* p. 414). Make sure the stocking heel is properly positioned on the person's heel.

12 Grasp the stocking top. Pull the stocking up the leg. It turns right side out as it is pulled up. The stocking is even and snug (Fig. 23-13, *B ,* p. 414).
13 Remove twists, creases, or wrinkles.
14 Repeat steps 10 through 13 for the other leg.

POST-PROCEDURE

15 Cover the person.
16 Provide for comfort. (See the inside of the front book cover.)
17 Place the signal light within reach.
18 Lower the bed to its lowest position.
19 Raise or lower bed rails. Follow the care plan.

20 Unscreen the person.
21 Complete a safety check of the room. (See the inside of the front book cover.)
22 Decontaminate your hands.
23 Report and record your observations.

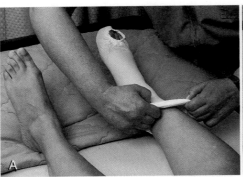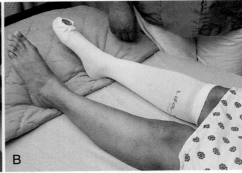

FIGURE 23-13 Applying elastic stockings. **A,** The stocking is slipped over the toes, foot, and heel. **B,** The stocking turns right side out as it is pulled up over the leg.

Elastic Bandages Elastic bandages have the same purposes as elastic stockings. They also provide support and reduce swelling from injuries. Sometimes they are used to hold dressings in place. They are applied to arms and legs. When applying bandages:

- Use the correct size. Use the proper length and width to bandage the extremity.
- Position the person in good alignment.
- Face the person during the procedure.
- Start at the lower (*distal*) part of the extremity. Work upward to the top (*proximal*) part.
- Expose fingers or toes if possible. This allows circulation checks.
- Apply the bandage with firm, even pressure.
- Check the color and temperature of the extremity every hour.
- Re-apply a loose or wrinkled bandage.
- Replace a moist or soiled bandage.
  See *Focus on Communication: Elastic Bandages.*
  See *Delegation Guidelines: Elastic Bandages.*
  See *Promoting Safety and Comfort: Elastic Bandages.*

DELEGATION GUIDELINES
Elastic Bandages

Before applying elastic bandages, you need this information from the nurse and the care plan:
- Where to apply the bandage
- What width and length to use
- When to remove the bandage and for how long—usually every 8 hours for 30 minutes
- What to do if the bandage is wet or soiled
- What observations to report and record:
  - The width and length applied
  - When you applied the bandage
  - Skin color and temperature
  - Swelling of the part
  - Skin tears, wounds, or signs of skin breakdown
  - Complaints of pain, itching, tingling, or numbness
  - When you removed the bandage and for how long
  - When you re-applied the bandage
- When to report observations
- What specific patient and resident concerns to report at once

---

FOCUS ON COMMUNICATION
Elastic Bandages

Elastic bandages should promote comfort. To check for comfort, you can ask:
- "Does the bandage feel too tight?"
- "Do you feel pain, itching, tingling, or numbness?" If yes: "What do you feel?" "Where do you feel it?"

PROMOTING SAFETY AND COMFORT
Elastic Bandages

Safety

Elastic bandages must be firm and snug but not tight. A tight bandage can affect circulation.

Elastic bandages are secured in place with clips, tape, or Velcro. Clips are made of metal or plastic. Clips can injure the skin if they become loose, fall off, or cause pressure. Use clips only if the nurse tells you to. Check the bandage often to make sure the clips are correctly in place.

Some agencies do not let nursing assistants apply elastic bandages. Know your agency's policy.

Comfort

A tight bandage can cause pain and discomfort. Apply it with firm, even pressure. If the person complains of pain, tingling, or numbness, remove the bandage and tell the nurse at once.

APPLYING ELASTIC BANDAGES

QUALITY OF LIFE

Remember to:
- Knock before entering the person's room.
- Address the person by name.
- Introduce yourself by name and title.

- Explain the procedure to the person before beginning and during the procedure.
- Protect the person's rights during the procedure.
- Handle the person gently during the procedure.

PRE-PROCEDURE

1 Follow *Delegation Guidelines: Elastic Bandages.* See *Promoting Safety and Comfort: Elastic Bandages.*
2 Practice hand hygiene.
3 Collect the following:
- Elastic bandage as directed by the nurse
- Tape or clips (unless the bandage has Velcro)

4 Identify the person. Check the ID bracelet against the assignment sheet. Also call the person by name.
5 Provide for privacy.
6 Raise the bed for body mechanics. Bed rails are up if used.

PROCEDURE

7 Lower the bed rail near you if up.
8 Help the person to a comfortable position. Expose the part you will bandage.
9 Make sure the area is clean and dry.
10 Hold the bandage so the roll is up. The loose end is on the bottom (Fig. 23-14, *A*).
11 Apply the bandage to the smallest part of the wrist, foot, ankle, or knee.
12 Make two circular turns around the part (Fig. 23-14, *B*).

13 Make overlapping spiral turns in an upward direction. Each turn overlaps about ½ to ⅔ of the previous turn (Fig. 23-14, *C*). Make sure each overlap is equal.
14 Apply the bandage smoothly with firm, even pressure. It is not tight.
15 End the bandage with two circular turns.
16 Secure the bandage in place with Velcro, tape, or clips. The clips are not under the body part.
17 Check the fingers or toes for coldness or cyanosis (bluish color). Ask about pain, itching, numbness, or tingling. Remove the bandage if any are noted. Report your observations to the nurse.

POST-PROCEDURE

18 Provide for comfort. (See the inside of the front book cover.)
19 Place the signal light within reach.
20 Lower the bed to its lowest position.
21 Raise or lower bed rails. Follow the care plan.

22 Unscreen the person.
23 Complete a safety check of the room. (See the inside of the front book cover.)
24 Decontaminate your hands.
25 Report and record your observations.

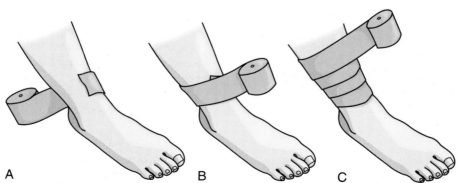

FIGURE 23-14 Applying an elastic bandage. **A,** The roll of the bandage is up. The loose end is at the bottom. **B,** The bandage is applied to the smallest part with two circular turns. **C,** The bandage is applied with spiral turns in an upward direction.

DRESSINGS

Wound dressings have many functions. They:
- Protect wounds from injury and microbes.
- Absorb drainage.
- Remove dead tissue.
- Promote comfort.
- Cover unsightly wounds.
- Provide a moist environment for wound healing.
- Apply pressure (pressure dressings) to help control bleeding.

Securing Dressings

Dressings must be secured over wounds. Microbes can enter the wound, and drainage can escape if the dressing is dislodged. Tape and Montgomery ties are used to secure dressings. Binders hold dressings in place.

Tape. Adhesive, paper, plastic, cloth, and elastic tapes are common. Adhesive tape sticks well to the skin. Any adhesive remaining on the skin is hard to remove. It can irritate the skin. Allergies to adhesive tape are common. Paper, plastic, and cloth tapes usually do not cause allergic reactions. Elastic tape allows movement of the body part.

Tape is applied to the top, middle, and bottom parts of the dressing. The tape extends several inches beyond each side of the dressing (Fig. 23-15). *Tape is not applied to circle the entire body part. If swelling occurs, circulation to the part is impaired.*

See *Focus on Communication: Tape.*

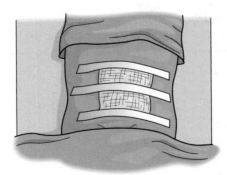

FIGURE 23-15 Tape is applied at the top, middle, and bottom of the dressing. The tape extends several inches beyond both sides of the dressing.

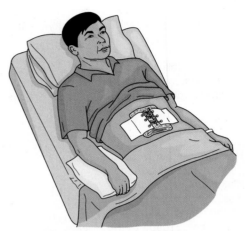

FIGURE 23-16 Montgomery ties.

Montgomery Ties. Montgomery ties (Fig. 23-16) are used for large dressings and frequent dressing changes. A Montgomery tie has an adhesive strip and a cloth tie. When the dressing is in place, the adhesive strips are placed on both sides of the dressing. Then the cloth ties are secured over the dressing. Two or three Montgomery ties may be needed on each side. The ties are undone for the dressing change. The adhesive strips stay in place. They are not removed unless soiled.

Applying Dressings

Some agencies let you apply simple, dry, non-sterile dressings to simple wounds. Box 23-4 lists the rules for applying dressings.

See *Focus on Communication: Applying Dressings.*
See *Delegation Guidelines: Applying Dressings.*
See *Promoting Safety and Comfort: Applying Dressings.*

BOX 23-4   Rules for Applying Dressings

- Allow pain drugs time to take effect, usually 30 minutes. The dressing change may cause discomfort. The nurse gives the drug and tells you how long to wait.
- Meet the person's fluid and elimination needs before you begin.
- Collect needed equipment and supplies before you begin.
- Do not bend or reach over your work area.
- Control your non-verbal communication. Wound odors, appearance, and drainage may be unpleasant. Do not communicate your thoughts or reactions to the person.
- Remove soiled dressings so the person cannot see the soiled side. The drainage and its odor may upset the person.
- Do not force the person to look at the wound. A wound can affect body image and self-esteem. The nurse helps the person deal with the wound.
- Remove tape by pulling it toward the wound.
- Remove dressings gently. They may stick to the wound, drain, or surrounding skin. If the dry dressing sticks, the nurse may have you wet the dressing with a saline solution. A wet dressing is easier to remove.
- Touch only the outer edges of old and new dressings.
- Report and record your observations. See *Delegation Guidelines: Applying Dressings.*

FOCUS ON COMMUNICATION
Applying Dressings

The person may not report discomfort from a dressing. You should ask:
- "Is the dressing comfortable?"
- "Does the tape cause pain or itching?"

PROMOTING SAFETY AND COMFORT
Applying Dressings

Safety

Contact with blood, body fluids, secretions, or excretions is likely. Follow Standard Precautions and the Bloodborne Pathogen Standard. Wear personal protective equipment as needed.

Do not apply tape to irritated, injured, or non-intact skin. Tape can further damage the skin.

Comfort

Wounds and dressing changes can cause discomfort or pain. If so, the nurse gives a pain-relief drug before the dressing change. Allow time for the drug to take effect. Be gentle when applying and removing tape and dressings.

DELEGATION GUIDELINES
Applying Dressings

When applying a dressing is delegated to you, make sure that:
- Your state allows you to perform the procedure
- The procedure is in your job description
- You have the necessary training
- You are familiar with the equipment
- You review the procedure with the nurse
- A nurse is available to answer questions and to supervise you

If the above conditions are met, you need this information from the nurse:
- When to change the dressing
- When the person received a pain-relief drug; when it will take effect
- What to do if the dressing sticks to the wound
- How to clean the wound
- What dressings to use
- How to secure the dressing—tape or Montgomery ties
- What kind of tape to use—adhesive, paper, plastic, cloth, or elastic
- What size tape to use—½-, ¾-, 1-, 2-, or 3-inch width
- What observations to report and record:
  - What you used to dress the wound and secure the dressing
  - A red or swollen wound
  - An area around the wound that is warm to touch
  - If wound edges are closed or separated
  - A wound that has broken open
  - Drainage appearance—clear, bloody, or watery and blood-tinged; thick and green, yellow, or brown
  - The amount of drainage
  - Wound or drainage odor
  - Intactness and color of surrounding tissues
  - Swelling of surrounding tissues
  - Possible dressing contamination—urine, feces; other body fluids, secretions, or excretions; dislodged dressing
  - Pain
  - Fever
- When to report observations
- What specific patient and resident concerns to report at once

View Video!

APPLYING A DRY, NON-STERILE DRESSING

QUALITY OF LIFE

Remember to:
- Knock before entering the person's room.
- Address the person by name.
- Introduce yourself by name and title.

- Explain the procedure to the person before beginning and during the procedure.
- Protect the person's rights during the procedure.
- Handle the person gently during the procedure.

PRE-PROCEDURE

1 Follow *Delegation Guidelines: Applying Dressings,* p. 417. See *Promoting Safety and Comfort: Applying Dressings,* p. 417.
2 Practice hand hygiene.
3 Collect the following:
- Gloves
- Personal protective equipment as needed
- Tape or Montgomery ties
- Dressings as directed by the nurse
- Saline solution as directed by the nurse
- Cleansing solution as directed by the nurse
- Adhesive remover

- Dressing set with scissors and forceps
- Plastic bag
- Bath blanket
4 Decontaminate your hands.
5 Identify the person. Check the ID bracelet against the assignment sheet. Also call the person by name.
6 Provide for privacy.
7 Arrange your work area. You should not have to reach over or turn your back on your work area.
8 Raise the bed for body mechanics. Bed rails are up if used.

PROCEDURE

9 Lower the bed rail near you if up.
10 Help the person to a comfortable position.
11 Cover the person with a bath blanket. Fan-fold top linens to the foot of the bed.
12 Expose the affected body part.
13 Make a cuff on the plastic bag. Place it within reach.
14 Decontaminate your hands.
15 Put on needed personal protective equipment. Put on gloves.
16 Remove tape or undo Montgomery ties.
   a *Tape:* hold the skin down. Gently pull the tape toward the wound.
   b *Montgomery ties:* fold ties away from the wound.
17 Remove any adhesive from the skin. Wet a 4 × 4 gauze dressing with adhesive remover. Clean away from the wound.
18 Remove gauze dressings. Start with the top dressing, and remove each layer. Keep the soiled side of each dressing away from the person's sight. Put

dressings in the plastic bag. They must not touch the outside of the bag.
19 Remove the dressing over the wound very gently. It may stick to the wound or drain site. Moisten the dressing with saline if it sticks to the wound.
20 Observe the wound, drain site, and wound drainage.
21 Remove the gloves, and put them in the plastic bag. Decontaminate your hands.
22 Open the new dressings.
23 Cut the length of tape needed.
24 Put on clean gloves.
25 Clean the wound with saline as directed by the nurse. See Figure 23-17.
26 Apply dressings as directed by the nurse.
27 Secure the dressings in place. Use tape or Montgomery ties.
28 Remove the gloves. Put them in the bag.
29 Remove and discard personal protective equipment.
30 Decontaminate your hands.
31 Cover the person. Remove the bath blanket.

POST-PROCEDURE

32 Provide for comfort. (See the inside of the front book cover.)
33 Place the signal light within reach.
34 Lower the bed to its lowest position.
35 Raise or lower bed rails. Follow the care plan.
36 Return equipment and supplies to the proper place. Leave extra dressings and tape in the room.
37 Discard used supplies into the bag. Tie the bag closed. Discard the bag following agency policy. (Wear gloves for this step.)

38 Clean your work area. Follow the Bloodborne Pathogen Standard.
39 Unscreen the person.
40 Complete a safety check of the room. (See the inside of the front book cover.)
41 Decontaminate your hands.
42 Report and record your observations.

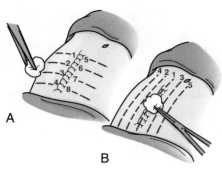

FIGURE 23-17 Cleaning a wound. **A,** Clean starting at the wound and stroking out to the surrounding skin. Use new gauze for each stroke. **B,** Clean the wound from the top to bottom. Start at the wound. Then clean the surrounding areas. Use new gauze for each stroke. *(Redrawn from Potter PA, Perry AG:* Fundamentals of nursing, *ed 7, St Louis, 2009, Mosby.)*

BOX 23-5   Rules for Applying Binders

- Follow the manufacturer's instructions.
- Apply the binder so there is firm, even pressure over the area.
- Apply the binder so it is snug. It must not interfere with breathing or circulation.
- Position the person in good alignment.
- Re-apply the binder if it is loose or wrinkled.
- Re-apply the binder if it is out of position or causes discomfort.
- Secure safety pins so they point away from the wound.
- Change binders that are moist or soiled. This prevents the growth of microbes.
- Tell the nurse at once if there is a change in the person's breathing.
- Check the person's skin under and around the binder. Tell the nurse at once if there is redness, irritation, or other signs of a skin problem.

BINDERS

Binders are wide bands of elastic fabric. They are applied to the abdomen, chest, or perineal areas. Binders promote healing because they support wounds and hold dressings in place. They also prevent or reduce swelling, promote comfort, and prevent injury.

Box 23-5 lists the rules for applying these binders:

- *Abdominal binder*—provides abdominal support and holds dressings in place (Fig. 23-18). The top part is at the person's waist. The lower part is over the hips. Binders are secured in place with Velcro or with hook and loop closures.

- *Breast binder*—supports the breasts after surgery (Fig. 23-19, p. 420). It also applies pressure to the breasts after childbirth in the non-breastfeeding mother. Pressure from the binder helps dry up the milk in the breasts. The binder also promotes comfort and supports swollen breasts after childbirth. Breast binders are secured in place with Velcro or padded zippers.

- *T-binders*—secure dressings in place after rectal and perineal surgeries. The single T-binder is for women (Fig. 23-20, *A,* p. 420). The double T-binder is for men (Fig. 23-20, *B,* p. 420). If perineal dressings are large, women many need double T-binders. The waistbands are brought around the waist and pinned at the front. The tails are brought between the legs and up to the waistband. They are pinned in place at the waistband.

See *Focus on Communication: Binders,* p. 420.
See *Promoting Safety and Comfort: Binders,* p. 420.

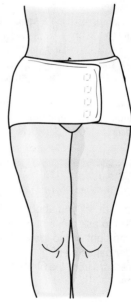

FIGURE 23-18 Abdominal binder.

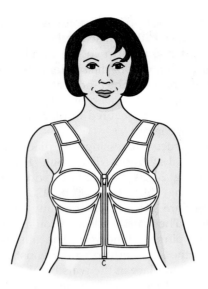

FIGURE 23-19 Breast binder.

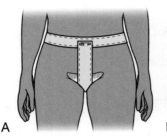
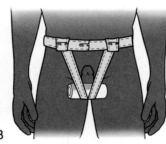

FIGURE 23-20 **A,** Single T-binder. **B,** Double T-binder. *(From deWit SC:* Fundamental concepts and skills for nursing, *ed 2, Philadelphia, 2005, Saunders.)*

FOCUS ON COMMUNICATION
Binders

The person may not tell you about pain or discomfort. Therefore, you need to ask these questions:
- "Is the binder too tight or too loose?"
- "Does the binder cause pain?"
- "Do you feel pressure from the binder?" If yes: "Where? Please show me."

PROMOTING SAFETY AND COMFORT
Binders

Safety
Binders must be applied properly. Otherwise, severe discomfort, skin irritation, and circulatory and respiratory problems can occur. Correct application is needed for the person's safety and for the binder to work effectively.

Comfort
A binder should promote comfort. Re-apply the binder if it causes pain or discomfort.

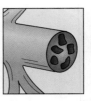

A Normal   B Dilated   C Constricted

FIGURE 23-21 **A,** Blood vessel under normal conditions. **B,** Dilated blood vessel. **C,** Constricted blood vessel.

HEAT AND COLD APPLICATIONS

Heat and cold applications promote healing and comfort. They also reduce tissue swelling. Heat and cold have opposite effects on body function.

Heat Applications

Heat applications are often used for musculoskeletal injuries or problems (arthritis). They relieve pain, relax muscles, and decrease joint stiffness. They also promote healing and reduce tissue swelling.

When heat is applied to the skin, blood vessels in the area dilate. **Dilate** means to expand or open wider (Fig. 23-21). Blood flow increases. Tissues have more oxygen and nutrients for healing. Excess fluid is removed from the area faster. The skin is red and warm.

Complications. High temperatures can cause burns. Report pain, excessive redness, and blisters at once.

Also observe for pale skin. When heat is applied too long, blood vessels **constrict** (narrow) (see Fig. 23-21). Blood flow decreases. Tissues receive less blood. Tissue damage occurs, and the skin is pale.

Older and fair-skinned persons have fragile skin that is easily burned. Persons with problems sensing heat and pain are also at risk. Nervous system damage, loss of consciousness, and circulatory disorders affect sensation. So do confusion and some drugs.

Metal implants pose risks. Metal conducts heat. Deep tissues can be burned. Pacemakers (cardiac devices) and joint replacements are made of metal. Do not apply heat to an implant area.

See *Persons With Dementia: Complications (Heat Applications).*

PERSONS WITH DEMENTIA
Complications (Heat Applications)

Confused persons and those with dementia may not recognize pain. Look for changes in the person's behavior. Behavior changes can signal pain.

Moist and Dry Heat Applications. With a *moist heat application,* water is in contact with the skin. Water conducts heat. Moist heat has greater and faster effects than dry heat. Heat penetrates deeper with a moist application. To prevent injury, moist heat applications have lower (cooler) temperatures than dry heat applications. Moist heat applications include:

- *Hot compresses* (Fig. 23-22, *A*)—a *compress* is a soft pad applied over a body area. It is usually made of cloth.
- *Hot soaks* (Fig. 23-22, *B*)—a body part is put into water.

- *Sitz baths* (Fig. 23-22, *C*)—the perineal and rectal areas are immersed in warm or hot water. (*Sitz* means *seat* in German.)
- *Hot packs* (Fig. 23-22, *D*)—a *pack* involves wrapping a body part.

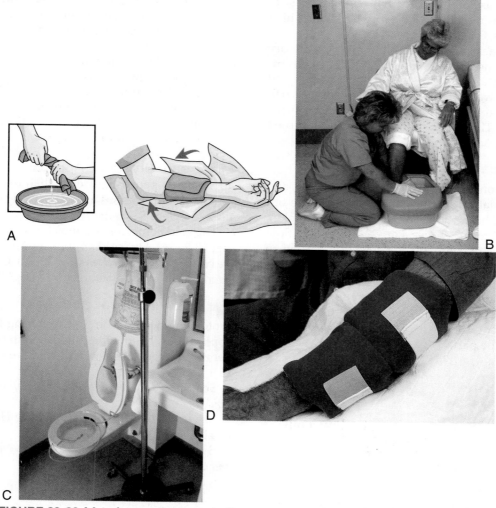

FIGURE 23-22 Moist heat applications. **A,** Compress. **B,** Hot soak. **C,** Disposable sitz bath. **D,** Hot pack.

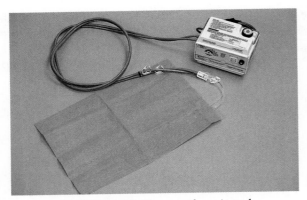

FIGURE 23-23 The aquathermia pad.

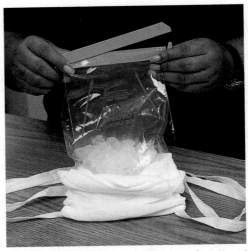

FIGURE 23-24 The ice bag is filled ½ to ⅔ full with ice.

With *dry heat applications,* water is not in contact with the skin. A dry heat application stays at the desired temperature longer. Dry heat does not penetrate as deeply as moist heat. Because water is not used, dry heat needs higher (hotter) temperatures to achieve the desired effect. Therefore burns are still a risk.

Some hot packs and the aquathermia pad are dry heat applications. The aquathermia pad is an electrical device (Fig. 23-23). Tubes inside the pad are filled with distilled water. Heated water flows to the pad through a hose. Another hose returns water to the heating unit. The water is reheated and returned back into the pad.

Cold Applications

Cold applications reduce pain, prevent swelling, and decrease circulation and bleeding. Cold has the opposite effect of heat. When cold is applied to the skin, blood vessels constrict (see Fig. 23-21). Blood flow decreases. Less oxygen and nutrients are carried to the tissues.

Cold applications are useful right after an injury. Decreased blood flow reduces the amount of bleeding. Less fluid collects in the tissues. Cold has a numbing effect on the skin. This helps reduce or relieve pain in the part.

Complications. Complications include pain, burns, blisters, and poor circulation. Burns and blisters occur from intense cold. They also occur when dry cold is in direct contact with the skin.

When cold is applied for a long time, blood vessels dilate. Blood flow increases. The prolonged application of cold has the same effect as heat applications.

Older and fair-skinned persons have fragile skin. They are at great risk for complications. So are persons with sensory impairments.

Moist and Dry Cold Applications. Moist cold applications penetrate deeper than dry ones. Therefore moist applications are not as cold as dry applications.

The cold compress is a moist cold application (see Fig. 23-22, *A*). Dry cold applications include ice bags, ice collars, and ice gloves (Fig. 23-24). Cold packs can be moist or dry applications (see Fig. 23-22, *D*).

Applying Heat and Cold

Protect the person from injury during heat and cold applications. Follow the rules listed in Box 23-6. Temperature ranges for heat and cold are listed in Table 23-1.

See *Focus on Communication: Applying Heat and Cold.*

See *Delegation Guidelines: Applying Heat and Cold,* p. 424.

See *Promoting Safety and Comfort: Applying Heat and Cold,* p. 424.

BOX 23-6   Rules for Applying Heat and Cold

- Know how to use the equipment. Follow the manufacturer's instructions for commercial devices.
- Measure the temperature of moist applications. Use a bath thermometer. Or follow agency policy for measuring temperature.
- Follow agency policies for safe temperature ranges. See Table 23-1.
- Do not apply *very hot* (above 106° F [Fahrenheit] or 46.1° C [centigrade]) applications. Tissue damage can occur. A nurse applies *very hot* applications.
- Ask the nurse what the temperature of the application should be.
  - Heat—cooler temperatures are needed for persons at risk.
  - Cold—warmer temperatures are needed for persons at risk.
- Know the exact site of the application. Ask the nurse to show you the site.
- Cover dry heat or cold applications before applying them. Use a flannel cover, towel, or other cover as directed by the nurse.
- Provide for privacy. Properly screen and drape the person. Expose only the body part involved. Avoid unnecessary exposure.
- Maintain comfort and body alignment during the procedure.
- Observe the skin every 5 minutes for signs of complications. See *Delegation Guidelines: Applying Heat and Cold*, p. 424.
- Do not let the person change the temperature of the application.
- Know how long to leave the application in place. See *Delegation Guidelines: Applying Heat and Cold*, p. 424. Carefully watch the time. Heat and cold are applied no longer than 15 to 20 minutes.
- Follow the rules of electrical safety when using electrical appliances to apply heat.
- Place the signal light within the person's reach.
- Complete a safety check before leaving the room. (See the inside of the front book cover.)

TABLE 23-1   Heat and Cold Temperature Ranges

Temperature	Fahrenheit Range	Centigrade Range
Hot	98° to 106° F	36.6° to 41.1° C
Warm	93° to 98° F	33.8° to 36.6° C
Tepid	80° to 93° F	26.6° to 33.8° C
Cool	65° to 80° F	18.3° to 26.6° C
Cold	50° to 65° F	10.0° to 18.3° C

Modified from Perry AG, Potter PA: *Clinical nursing skills and techniques*, ed 7, St Louis, 2010, Mosby.

FOCUS ON COMMUNICATION
Applying Heat and Cold

The person may not tell you about pain or discomfort. The person may not know what symptoms to report. For heat and cold applications, you need to ask:
- "Does the application feel too hot or too cold?"
- "Do you feel any pain, numbness, or burning?"
- "Are you warm enough?"
- "Do you feel weak, faint, or drowsy?" If yes: "Tell me how you feel."

DELEGATION GUIDELINES
Applying Heat and Cold

Before applying heat or cold, you need this information from the nurse and the care plan:

- The type of application—hot compress or pack, commercial compress, hot soak, sitz bath, aquathermia pad; ice bag, ice collar, ice glove, cold pack, or cold compress
- How to cover the application
- What temperature to use (see Table 23-1)
- The application site
- How long to leave the application in place
- What observations to report and record:
  - Complaints of pain or discomfort, numbness, or burning
  - Excessive redness
  - Blisters
  - Pale, white, or gray skin
  - *Cyanosis* (bluish color)
  - Shivering
  - Rapid pulse, weakness, faintness, and drowsiness (sitz bath)
  - Time, site, and length of application
- When to report observations
- What specific patient or resident concerns to report at once

PROMOTING SAFETY AND COMFORT
Applying Heat and Cold

Safety

Check the person every 5 minutes. Also follow these safety measures:

- *Sitz bath.* Blood flow increases to the perineum and rectum. Therefore less blood flows to other body parts. The person may become weak or feel faint. Drowsiness can occur from the bath's relaxing effect. Observe for signs of weakness, fainting, or fatigue. Also protect the person from injury. Check the person often. Keep the signal light within reach, and prevent chills and burns.
- *Commercial hot and cold packs.* Read warning labels and follow the manufacturer's instructions.
- *Aquathermia pad:*
  - Follow electrical safety precautions (Chapter 8).
  - Check the device for damage or flaws.
  - Follow the manufacturer's instructions.
  - Place the heating unit on an even, uncluttered surface. This prevents it from being knocked over or knocked off of the surface.
  - Use a flannel cover to insulate the pad. It absorbs perspiration at the application site. (Some agencies use towels or pillowcases.)
  - Secure the pad in place with ties, tape, or rolled gauze. Do not use pins. They can puncture the pad and cause leaks.
  - Do not place the pad under the person or under a body part. This prevents the escape of heat. Burns can result if heat cannot escape.

Some persons have medicated patches or ointments applied to the skin. Do not apply heat over such areas.

Comfort

Cold applications can cause chilling and shivering. Provide for warmth. Use bath blankets or other blankets as needed.

APPLYING HEAT AND COLD APPLICATIONS

QUALITY OF LIFE

Remember to:
- Knock before entering the person's room.
- Address the person by name.
- Introduce yourself by name and title.

- Explain the procedure to the person before beginning and during the procedure.
- Protect the person's rights during the procedure.
- Handle the person gently during the procedure.

PRE-PROCEDURE

1 Follow *Delegation Guidelines: Applying Heat and Cold*. See *Promoting Safety and Comfort: Applying Heat and Cold*.
2 Practice hand hygiene.
3 Collect needed equipment.
  a For a *hot compress:*
    • Basin
    • Bath thermometer
    • Small towel, washcloth, or gauze squares
    • Plastic wrap or aquathermia pad
    • Ties, tape, or rolled gauze
    • Bath towel
    • Waterproof pad
  b For a *hot soak:*
    • Water basin or arm or foot bath
    • Bath thermometer
    • Waterproof pad
    • Bath blanket
    • Towel
  c For a *sitz bath:*
    • Disposable sitz bath
    • Bath thermometer
    • Two bath blankets, bath towels, and a clean gown

  d For a *hot or cold pack:*
    • Commercial pack
    • Pack cover
    • Ties, tape, or rolled gauze (if needed)
    • Waterproof pad
  e For an *aquathermia pad:*
    • Aquathermia pad and heating unit
    • Distilled water
    • Flannel cover or other cover as directed by the nurse
    • Ties, tape, or rolled gauze
  f For an *ice bag, ice collar, ice glove,* or *dry cold pack:*
    • Ice bag, collar, or glove or cold pack
    • Crushed ice (except for a cold pack)
    • Flannel cover or other cover as directed by the nurse
    • Paper towels
  g For a *cold compress:*
    • Large basin with ice
    • Small basin with cold water
    • Gauze squares, washcloths, or small towels
    • Waterproof pad
4 Identify the person. Check the ID bracelet against the assignment sheet. Also call the person by name.
5 Provide for privacy.

PROCEDURE

6 Position the person for the procedure.
7 Place the waterproof pad (if needed) under the body part.
8 For a *hot compress:*
  a Fill the basin ½ to ⅔ full with hot water as directed by the nurse. Measure water temperature.
  b Place the compress in the water.
  c Wring out the compress.
  d Apply the compress over the area. Note the time.
  e Cover the compress quickly. Use one of the following as directed by the nurse:
    (1) Apply plastic wrap and then a bath towel. Secure the towel in place with ties, tape, or rolled gauze.
    (2) Apply an aquathermia pad.

9 For a *hot soak:*
  a Fill the container ½ full with hot water as directed by the nurse. Measure water temperature.
  b Place the part into the water. Pad the edge of the container with a towel. Note the time.
  c Cover the person with a bath blanket for warmth.
10 For a *sitz bath:*
  a Place the disposable sitz bath on the toilet seat.
  b Fill the sitz bath ⅔ full with water as directed by the nurse. Measure water temperature.
  c Secure the gown above the waist.
  d Help the person sit on the sitz bath. Note the time.
  e Provide for warmth. Place a bath blanket around the shoulders. Place another over the legs.
  f Stay with the person if he or she is weak or unsteady.

Continued

APPLYING HEAT AND COLD APPLICATIONS—cont'd

PROCEDURE—cont'd

11 For a *hot or cold pack:*
   a Squeeze, knead, or strike the pack as directed by the manufacturer.
   b Place the pack in the cover.
   c Apply the pack. Note the time.
   d Secure the pack in place with ties, tape, or rolled gauze. Some packs are secured with Velcro straps.

12 For an *aquathermia pad:*
   a Fill the heating unit to the fill line with distilled water.
   b Remove the bubbles. Place the pad and tubing below the heating unit. Tilt the heating unit from side to side.
   c Set the temperature as the nurse directs (usually 105° F [40.5° C]). Remove the key. (Give the key to the nurse after the procedure.)
   d Place the pad in the cover.
   e Plug in the unit. Let water warm to the desired temperature.
   f Set the heating unit on the bedside stand. Keep the pad and connecting hoses level with the unit. Hoses must not have kinks.
   g Apply the pad to the part. Note the time.
   h Secure the pad in place with ties, tape, or rolled gauze. Do not use pins.

13 For an *ice bag, collar,* or *glove:*
   a Fill the device with water. Put in the stopper. Turn the device upside down to check for leaks.
   b Empty the device.
   c Fill the device ½ to ⅔ full with crushed ice or ice chips.
   d Remove excess air. Bend, twist, or squeeze the device. Or press it against a firm surface.
   e Place the cap or stopper on securely.
   f Dry the device with paper towels.
   g Place the device in the cover.
   h Apply the device. Note the time.
   i Secure the device in place with ties, tape, or rolled gauze.

14 For a *cold compress:*
   a Place the small basin with cold water into the large basin with ice.
   b Place the compresses into the cold water.
   c Wring out a compress.
   d Apply the compress to the part. Note the time.

15 Place the signal light within reach. Unscreen the person.

16 Raise or lower bed rails. Follow the care plan.

17 Check the person every 5 minutes. Check for signs and symptoms of complications (see *Delegation Guidelines: Applying Heat and Cold,* p. 424). Remove the application if any occur. Tell the nurse at once.

18 Check the application every 5 minutes. Change the application if cooling (hot applications) or warming (cold applications) occurs.

19 Remove the application at the specified time. Heat and cold applications are usually left on for 15 to 20 minutes. (If bed rails are up, lower the near one for this step.)

POST-PROCEDURE

20 Provide for comfort. (See the inside of the front book cover.)

21 Place the signal light within reach.

22 Raise or lower bed rails. Follow the care plan.

23 Unscreen the person.

24 Clean and return re-usable items to their proper place. Follow agency policy for soiled linen. Wear gloves for this step.

25 Complete a safety check of the room. (See the inside of the front book cover.)

26 Remove and discard the gloves. Decontaminate your hands.

27 Report and record your observations.

Focus on P R I D E
The Person, Family, and Yourself

Personal and Professional Responsibility—You are responsible for the tasks you perform. Before applying an elastic bandage, changing a dressing, or applying heat and cold, make sure that:

- Your state allows you to perform the procedure.
- The procedure is in your job description.
- You have the necessary training.
- You are familiar with the equipment.
- You review the procedure with the nurse.
- A nurse is available to answer questions and to supervise you.

If you are unsure of any of the above, tell the nurse. Never perform a task you are not comfortable doing. The person may be harmed. Do not be afraid, embarrassed, or ashamed to talk to the nurse about your concerns. Take pride in acting responsibly.

Rights and Respect—Some wounds are large and disfiguring. Wound drainage may have odors. The person may feel embarrassed. Body image is often impacted. Love, belonging, and self-esteem needs are also affected.

Do not judge the person by the size, site, odor, or cause of the wound. Be sensitive to the person's feelings. The person may be sad and tearful or angry and hostile. Treat the person with dignity and respect. Be gentle and kind, give thoughtful care, and practice good communication.

Independence and Social Interaction—Patients, residents, and visitors may be disturbed by the sight of wounds and dressings. Some wounds are connected to drainage devices. Drainage in the container or odors from wounds may disgust some persons. Family and friends may feel uncomfortable when visiting. To promote comfort and interaction with family and friends:

- Keep the wound or dressing covered if able.
- Ask visitors to leave the room during dressing changes or when exposing the wound or dressing.
- Remove soiled dressings from the room promptly.
- Keep drainage containers out of sight if able. Some large containers can be covered with a towel as directed by the nurse.
- Use a room deodorizer for odors as directed.

Delegation and Teamwork—The entire nursing team must prevent pressure ulcers. As you walk down hallways, look into rooms to see if a person has slid down in bed. Do the same when people are in dining and lounge areas. Help reposition the person. Ask a co-worker to help you as needed. Help co-workers when they need help repositioning persons. Take pride in working as a team to promote safety and comfort to prevent pressure ulcers.

Ethics and Laws—The Joint Commission (TJC) certifies and accredits health care programs and organizations nationally. Its mission is to improve safety and quality of care. To earn TJC approval, ethical and safety standards must be met.

Every year TJC develops National Patient Safety Goals for hospitals, nursing centers, and other agencies. The goals focus on ways to solve health care safety problems. Preventing pressure ulcers is an example. Agencies must have a plan to predict, prevent, and treat pressure ulcers early. Many agencies use a form or screening tool to identify persons at risk. Assessments are done on admission and regularly. The agency must take action to address risks.

Know your agency's policies and procedures for identifying those at risk for pressure ulcers. Follow the measures in Box 23-1 to do your part to prevent pressure ulcers.

REVIEW QUESTIONS

Circle the BEST answer.

1 Which can cause skin tears?
   a Keeping your nails trim and smooth
   b Dressing the person in soft clothing
   c Wearing rings
   d Padding wheelchair footplates

2 The first sign of a pressure ulcer is
   a A blister   c Drainage
   b A reddened area   d Gangrene

3 Which can cause pressure ulcers?
   a Repositioning the person every 2 hours
   b Scrubbing and rubbing the skin
   c Applying lotion to dry areas
   d Keeping linens clean, dry, and wrinkle-free

4 Pressure ulcers usually occur
   a On the feet
   b Over a bony area
   c On the buttocks
   d Where skin has contact with skin

5 What is the preferred position for preventing pressure ulcers?
   a 30-degree lateral position   c Prone position
   b Semi-Fowler's position   d Supine position

6 A person is at risk for pressure ulcers. Which measure should you question?
   a Apply lotion to the hands, elbows, legs, ankles, and heels.
   b Massage bony areas.
   c Give a back massage when repositioning the person.
   d Apply powder under the breasts.

7 A person has a circulatory ulcer. Which measure should you question?
   a Hold socks in place with elastic garters.
   b Do not cut or trim toenails.
   c Apply elastic stockings.
   d Reposition the person every hour.

8 Persons with diabetes are at risk for diabetic foot ulcers because of
   a Gangrene   d Nerve and blood
   b Amputation   vessel damage
   c Infection

9 A person has diabetes. You should check the person's feet every
   a 2 hours   c Week
   b Day   d Month

10 Elastic stockings are applied
   a Before the person gets out of bed
   b When the person is standing
   c After the person's shower or bath
   d For 30 minutes and then removed

11 When applying an elastic bandage
   a Position the part in good alignment
   b Cover the fingers or toes if possible
   c Apply it from the largest to smallest part of the extremity
   d Apply it from the upper to lower part of the extremity

12 To secure a dressing, apply tape
   a Around the entire part
   b Along the sides of the dressing
   c To the top, middle, and bottom of the dressing
   d As the person prefers

13 To remove tape
   a Pull it toward the wound
   b Pull it away from the wound
   c Use an adhesive remover
   d Use a saline solution

14 An abdominal binder is used to
   a Prevent blood clots
   b Prevent wound infection
   c Provide support and hold dressings in place
   d Decrease swelling and circulation

15 The *greatest* threat from heat applications is
   a Infection   c Chilling
   b Burns   d Pressure ulcers

16 A person uses an aquathermia pad. Which is *false*?
   a It is a dry heat application.
   b A flannel cover is used.
   c Electrical safety precautions are practiced.
   d Pins secure the pad in place.

17 Before applying an ice bag
   a Place the bag in the freezer
   b Measure the temperature of the bag
   c Place the bag in a cover
   d Provide perineal care

18 Moist cold compresses are left in place no longer than
   a 20 minutes   c 45 minutes
   b 30 minutes   d 60 minutes

Answers to these questions are on p. 528.

24

ASSISTING WITH OXYGEN NEEDS

PROCEDURE

Assisting With Deep-Breathing and Coughing Exercises

OBJECTIVES

- Define the key terms and key abbreviations listed in this chapter.
- Describe hypoxia and abnormal respirations.
- Explain the measures that promote oxygenation.
- Describe the devices used in oxygen therapy.
- Explain how to safely assist with oxygen therapy.
- Explain how to promote PRIDE in the person, the family, and yourself.
- Perform the procedure described in this chapter.

KEY TERMS

apnea Lack or absence (*a*) of breathing (*pnea*)

bradypnea Slow (*brady*) breathing (*pnea*); respirations are fewer than 12 per minute

Cheyne-Stokes respirations Respirations gradually increase in rate and depth and then become shallow and slow; breathing may stop (*apnea*) for 10 to 20 seconds

dyspnea Difficult, labored, or painful (*dys*) breathing (*pnea*)

hyperventilation Respirations (*ventilation*) are rapid (*hyper*) and deeper than normal

hypoventilation Respirations (*ventilation*) are slow (*hypo*), shallow, and sometimes irregular

hypoxia Cells do not have enough (*hypo*) oxygen (*oxia*)

Kussmaul respirations Very deep and rapid respirations

orthopnea Breathing (*pnea*) deeply and comfortably only when sitting (*ortho*)

orthopneic position Sitting up (*ortho*) and leaning over a table to breathe

tachypnea Rapid (*tachy*) breathing (*pnea*); respirations are more than 20 per minute

KEY ABBREVIATIONS

L/min Liters per minute

O$_2$ Oxygen

Oxygen (O$_2$) is a gas. It has no taste, odor, or color. It is a basic need required for life. Death occurs within minutes if breathing stops. Brain damage and serious illnesses can occur without enough oxygen. Illness, surgery, and injuries affect the amount of oxygen in the blood and cells.

ALTERED RESPIRATORY FUNCTION

Hypoxia means that cells do not have enough (*hypo*) oxygen (*oxia*). When cells do not have enough oxygen, they cannot function properly. Hypoxia is life-threatening. Anything that affects respiratory function can cause hypoxia. The brain is very sensitive to low levels of O$_2$. Restlessness is an early sign. So are dizziness and disorientation. Report the signs and symptoms in Box 24-1 to the nurse at once.

BOX 24-1	Signs and Symptoms of Hypoxia

- Restlessness
- Dizziness
- Disorientation
- Confusion
- Behavior and personality changes
- Concentrating and following directions: problems with
- Apprehension
- Anxiety
- Fatigue
- Agitation
- Pulse rate: increased
- Respirations: increased rate and depth
- Sitting position: often leaning forward
- Cyanosis (bluish color to the skin, lips, mucous membranes, and nail beds)
- Dyspnea

Abnormal Respirations

Adults normally have 12 to 20 respirations per minute. Normal respirations are quiet, effortless, and regular. Both sides of the chest rise and fall equally. These breathing patterns are abnormal (Fig. 24-1):

- **Tachypnea**—rapid (*tachy*) breathing (*pnea*). Respirations are more than 20 per minute.
- **Bradypnea**—slow (*brady*) breathing (*pnea*). Respirations are fewer than 12 per minute.
- **Apnea**—lack or absence (*a*) of breathing (*pnea*).
- **Hypoventilation**—respirations (*ventilation*) are slow (*hypo*), shallow, and sometimes irregular.
- **Hyperventilation**—respirations (*ventilation*) are rapid (*hyper*) and deeper than normal.
- **Dyspnea**—difficult, labored, or painful (*dys*) breathing (*pnea*).
- **Cheyne-Stokes respirations**—respirations gradually increase in rate and depth. Then they become shallow and slow. Breathing may stop (*apnea*) for 10 to 20 seconds.
- **Orthopnea**—breathing (*pnea*) deeply and comfortably only when sitting (*ortho*).
- **Kussmaul respirations**—very deep and rapid respirations.

PROMOTING OXYGENATION

Disease and injury can prevent air from reaching the alveoli. Pain, immobility, and some drugs interfere with deep breathing and coughing and coughing up secretions. Oxygen needs must be met. The following measures are common in care plans.

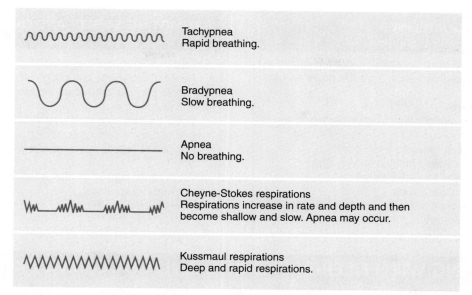

FIGURE 24-1 Some abnormal breathing patterns. (*Modified from Talbot L, Meyers-Marquardt M: Pocket guide to critical care assessment, ed 3, St Louis, 1997, Mosby.*)

Positioning

Breathing is usually easier in semi-Fowler's and Fowler's positions. Persons with difficulty breathing often prefer sitting up and leaning over a table to breathe. This is called the **orthopneic position**. (*Ortho* means *sitting* or *standing*. *Pneic* means *breathing*.) Place a pillow on the table to increase the person's comfort (Fig. 24-2).

Position changes are needed at least every 2 hours. Follow the care plan.

Deep Breathing and Coughing

Deep breathing moves air into most parts of the lungs. Coughing removes mucus. Deep-breathing and coughing exercises help persons with respiratory problems. They are done after surgery or injury and during bedrest. The exercises are painful after surgery or injury. Breaking an incision open while coughing is a fear.

Deep breathing and coughing are usually done every 2 hours while the person is awake. Sometimes they are done every hour while the person is awake.

See *Focus on Communication: Deep Breathing and Coughing.*

See *Delegation Guidelines: Deep Breathing and Coughing*, p. 432.

See *Promoting Safety and Comfort: Deep Breathing and Coughing*, p. 432.

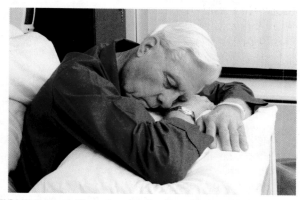

FIGURE 24-2 The person is in the orthopneic position. A pillow is on the overbed table for the person's comfort.

> **FOCUS ON COMMUNICATION**
> Deep Breathing and Coughing
>
> To encourage cough etiquette, you can say: "Please remember to cover your nose and mouth when coughing. I'll put these tissues where you can reach them. Here is a waste container to dispose of your tissues. Where would you like me to place it? Also, please remember to disinfect or wash your hands often. Let me know if you need help."

DELEGATION GUIDELINES
Deep Breathing and Coughing

When delegated deep-breathing and coughing exercises, you need this information from the nurse and the care plan:
- When to do them
- How many deep breaths and coughs the person needs to do
- What observations to report and record:
  - The number of deep breaths and coughs
  - How the person tolerated the procedure
- When to report observations
- What specific patient or resident concerns to report at once

PROMOTING SAFETY AND COMFORT
Deep Breathing and Coughing

Safety

Respiratory hygiene and cough etiquette are needed if the person has a productive cough (Chapter 11). The person needs to:
- Cover the nose and mouth when coughing or sneezing.
- Use tissues to contain respiratory secretions.
- Dispose of tissues in the nearest waste container after use.
- Wash his or her hands after coughing or contact with respiratory secretions.

ASSISTING WITH DEEP-BREATHING AND COUGHING EXERCISES

QUALITY OF LIFE

Remember to:
- Knock before entering the person's room.
- Address the person by name.
- Introduce yourself by name and title.
- Explain the procedure to the person before beginning and during the procedure.
- Protect the person's rights during the procedure.
- Handle the person gently during the procedure.

PRE-PROCEDURE

1 Follow *Delegation Guidelines: Deep Breathing and Coughing.* See *Promoting Safety and Comfort: Deep Breathing and Coughing.*
2 Practice hand hygiene.
3 Identify the person. Check the ID (identification) bracelet against the assignment sheet. Also call the person by name.
4 Provide for privacy.

PROCEDURE

5 Lower the bed rail if up.
6 Help the person to a comfortable sitting position: sitting on the side of the bed, semi-Fowler's, or Fowler's.
7 Have the person deep breathe:
  a Have the person place the hands over the rib cage (Fig. 24-3).
  b Have the person take a deep breath. It should be as deep as possible. Remind the person to inhale through the nose.
  c Ask the person to hold the breath for 2 to 3 seconds.

  d Ask the person to exhale slowly through pursed lips (Fig. 24-4). Ask the person to exhale until the ribs move as far down as possible.
  e Repeat this step 4 more times.
8 Ask the person to cough:
  a Have the person place both hands over the incision. One hand is on top of the other (Fig. 24-5, *A*). The person can hold a pillow or folded towel over the incision (Fig. 24-5, *B*).
  b Have the person take in a deep breath as in step 7.
  c Ask the person to cough strongly twice with the mouth open.

POST-PROCEDURE

9 Provide for comfort. (See the inside of the front book cover.)
10 Place the signal light within reach.
11 Raise or lower bed rails. Follow the care plan.
12 Unscreen the person.
13 Complete a safety check of the room. (See the inside of the front book cover.)
14 Decontaminate your hands.
15 Report and record your observations.

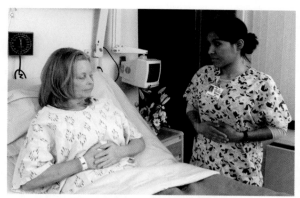

FIGURE 24-3 The hands are over the rib cage for deep breathing.

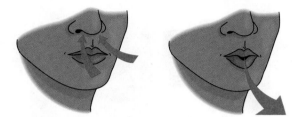

FIGURE 24-4 The person inhales through the nose and exhales through pursed lips during the deep-breathing exercise.

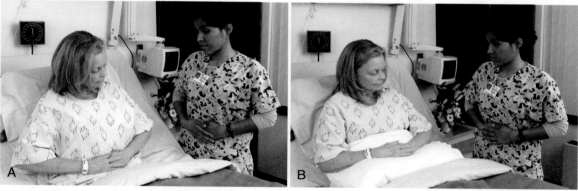

FIGURE 24-5 The person supports an incision for the coughing exercises. **A,** The hands are over the incision. **B,** A pillow is held over the incision.

ASSISTING WITH OXYGEN THERAPY

Disease, injury, and surgery often interfere with breathing. The amount of O_2 in the blood may be less than normal *(hypoxemia)*. If so, the doctor orders oxygen therapy.

Oxygen is treated as a drug. The doctor orders the amount of oxygen to give, the device to use, and when to give it. Some people need oxygen constantly. Others need it for symptom relief—chest pain or shortness of breath. Oxygen helps relieve chest pain. Persons with respiratory diseases may have enough oxygen at rest. With mild exercise or activity, they become short of breath. Oxygen helps to relieve shortness of breath.

Pulse Oximetry

Pulse oximetry measures *(metry)* the oxygen *(oxi)* concentration in arterial blood. *Oxygen concentration is the amount (percent) of hemoglobin containing* oxygen. Measurements are used for oxygen therapy. The normal range is 95% to 100%. For example, if 97% of all the hemoglobin (100%) carries O_2, tissues get enough oxygen. If only 90% contains O_2, tissues do not get enough oxygen.

A sensor attaches to a finger, toe, earlobe, nose, or forehead (Fig. 24-6, p. 434). Light beams on one side of the sensor pass through the tissues. A detector on the other side measures the amount of light passing through the tissues. With this information, the oximeter measures the O_2 concentration. The value and pulse rate are shown. Oximeter alarms are set for continuous monitoring.

A good sensor site is needed. Swollen sites are avoided. So are sites with skin breaks. Aging and vascular disease often cause poor circulation. Sometimes blood flow to the fingers or toes is poor. Then the earlobe, nose, and forehead sites are used.

See *Promoting Safety and Comfort: Pulse Oximetry,* p. 434.

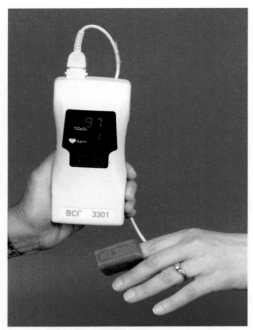

FIGURE 24-6 A pulse oximetry sensor is attached to a finger.

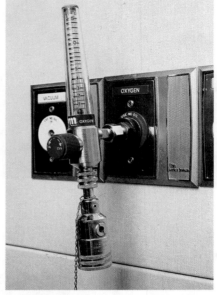

FIGURE 24-7 Wall oxygen outlet.

PROMOTING SAFETY AND COMFORT
Pulse Oximetry

Safety
  The person's condition can change rapidly. Pulse oximetry does not lessen the need for good observations. Observe for signs and symptoms of hypoxia (see Box 24-1).

Oxygen Sources

Oxygen is supplied as follows:
- *Wall outlet.* O$_2$ is piped into each person's unit (Fig. 24-7).
- *Oxygen tank.* The oxygen tank is placed at the bedside. Small tanks are used during emergencies and transfers. They also are used by persons who walk or use wheelchairs (Fig. 24-8). A gauge tells how much oxygen is left (Fig. 24-9). Tell the nurse if the tank is low.
- *Oxygen concentrator.* The machine removes oxygen from the air (Fig. 24-10). A power source is needed. A portable oxygen tank is needed for power failures and mobility.
- *Liquid oxygen system.* A portable unit is filled from a stationary unit. The portable unit has enough oxygen for about 8 hours of use. A dial shows the amount of oxygen in the unit. Tell the nurse if the unit is low. The portable unit can be worn over the shoulder (Fig. 24-11).

See *Promoting Safety and Comfort: Oxygen Sources.*

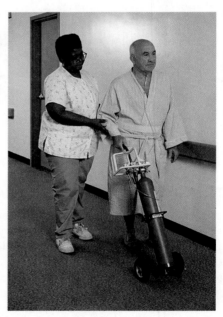

FIGURE 24-8 A portable oxygen tank is used when walking.

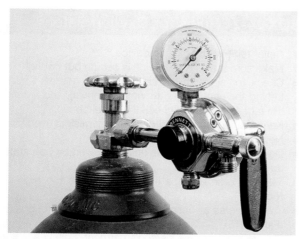

FIGURE 24-9 The gauge shows the amount of oxygen in the tank.

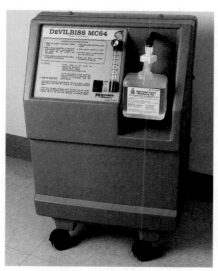

FIGURE 24-10 Oxygen concentrator.

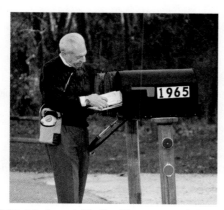

FIGURE 24-11 A portable liquid oxygen unit is worn over the shoulder. *(Image used by permission from Nellcor Puritan Bennett LLC, Boulder, Colorado, part of Covidien.)*

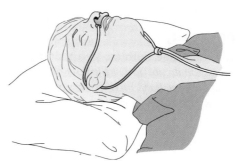

FIGURE 24-12 Nasal cannula.

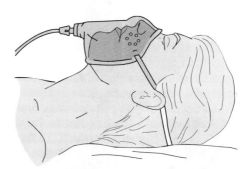

FIGURE 24-13 Simple face mask.

Oxygen Devices

The doctor orders the device to give oxygen. These devices are common:

- *Nasal cannula* (Fig. 24-12). The prongs are inserted into the nostrils. A band goes behind the ears and under the chin to keep the device in place. A cannula allows eating and drinking. Tight prongs can irritate the nose. Pressure on the ears and cheekbones is possible.
- *Simple face mask* (Fig. 24-13). It covers the nose and mouth. The mask has small holes in the sides. Carbon dioxide escapes when exhaling. Talking and eating are hard to do with a mask. Listen carefully. Moisture can build up under the mask. Keep the face clean and dry. This helps prevent irritation from the mask. Masks are removed for eating. Usually oxygen is given by cannula during meals.

Oxygen Flow Rates

The *flow rate* is the amount of oxygen given. It is measured in liters per minute (L/min). The doctor orders 2 to 15 L/min. The nurse or respiratory therapist sets the flow rate (Fig. 24-14).

The nurse and care plan tell you the person's flow rate. When giving care and checking the person, always check the flow rate. Tell the nurse at once if it is too high or too low. A nurse or respiratory therapist will adjust the flow rate.

Oxygen Safety

You assist the nurse with oxygen therapy. *You do not give oxygen. You do not adjust the flow rate unless allowed by your state and agency.* However, you must give safe care. Follow the rules in Box 24-2.

BOX 24-2	Rules for Oxygen Safety

- Never remove the oxygen device.
- Make sure the oxygen device is secure but not tight.
- Check for signs of irritation from the device. Check behind the ears, under the nose (cannula), and around the face (mask). Also check the cheekbones.
- Keep the face clean and dry when a mask is used.
- Never shut off the oxygen flow.
- Do not adjust the flow rate unless allowed by your state and agency.
- Tell the nurse at once if the flow rate is too high or too low.
- Tell the nurse at once if the humidifier is not bubbling (Fig. 24-15).
- Secure tubing to the person's garment. Follow agency policy.
- Make sure there are no kinks in the tubing.
- Make sure the person does not lie on any part of the tubing.
- Make sure the oxygen tank is secure in its holder.
- Report signs and symptoms of hypoxia, respiratory distress, or abnormal breathing patterns at once.
- Give oral hygiene as directed. Follow the care plan.
- Make sure the oxygen device is clean and free of mucus.
- Follow the safety measures for fire and the use of oxygen (Chapter 8).

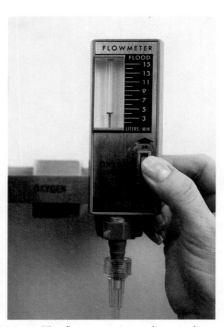

FIGURE 24-14 The flowmeter is used to set the oxygen flow rate.

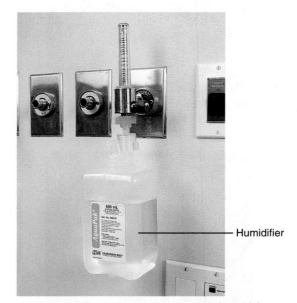

Humidifier

FIGURE 24-15 Oxygen set-up with humidifier.

Focus on P R I D E
The Person, Family, and Yourself

Personal and Professional Responsibility—You are responsible for reporting patient and resident complaints to the nurse. A person may say: "I can't breathe" or "I'm not getting enough air." Yet you see the person breathing. Do not dismiss the person's complaint. Tell the nurse at once. You cannot feel what the person does. Trust what the person tells you.

Rights and Respect—Persons have the right to a safe setting. To protect the person, smoking is not allowed where oxygen is used and stored. "No Smoking" signs in the room and hallways are often used. You may need to remind the person or visitors not to smoke. Be polite and respectful. Show the person where smoking is allowed.

Independence and Social Interaction—Portable oxygen sources increase the person's independence. Small oxygen tanks are examples. The person can wheel the tank (see Fig. 24-8) or attach it to a wheelchair. A portable liquid oxygen unit can be worn over the shoulder (see Fig. 24-11). Using such devices allows freedom and promotes quality of life.

Delegation and Teamwork—Oxygen tanks and liquid oxygen systems only contain a certain amount of oxygen. When the oxygen level is low, another tank is needed or the liquid oxygen system refilled. Always check the oxygen level when you are with or near all persons using these oxygen sources. Even if the person is not assigned to you, report a low oxygen level to the person's nurse at once.

Ethics and Laws—Oxygen is treated as a drug. State nurse practice acts allow nurses to give drugs. You assist the nurse with oxygen therapy. You do not give oxygen. You do not adjust the flow rate unless allowed by your state and agency and instructed to by the nurse. Know the limits of your role and provide safe care.

REVIEW QUESTIONS

Circle the BEST answer.

1 Hypoxia is
   a Not enough oxygen in the blood
   b The amount of hemoglobin that affects oxygen
   c Not enough oxygen in the cells
   d The lack of carbon dioxide
2 An early sign of hypoxia is
   a Cyanosis
   b Increased pulse and respiratory rates
   c Restlessness
   d Dyspnea
3 A person can breathe deeply and comfortably only while sitting. This is called
   a Apnea   c Bradypnea
   b Orthopnea   d Kussmaul respirations
4 The nurse tells you that a person has tachypnea. You know that the person's respirations are
   a Slow   c Absent
   b Rapid   d Difficult or painful
5 To promote oxygenation, position changes are needed at least every
   a 30 minutes   c 90 minutes
   b Hour   d 2 hours

6 You are assisting with deep breathing and coughing. Which is *false*?
   a The person inhales through pursed lips.
   b The person sits in a comfortable sitting position.
   c The person inhales deeply through the nose.
   d The person holds a pillow over an incision.
7 When assisting with oxygen therapy, you can
   a Turn the oxygen on and off
   b Start the oxygen
   c Decide what device to use
   d Keep connecting tubing secure and free of kinks
8 These statements are about oxygen flow rates. Which is *true*?
   a You can check the flow rate.
   b The flow rate is measured in milliliters (mL).
   c The flow rate is the amount of oxygen given in 1 hour.
   d The flow rate is the same for all persons.

Answers to these questions are on p. 528.

25

ASSISTING WITH REHABILITATION AND RESTORATIVE NURSING CARE

OBJECTIVES

- Define the key terms and key abbreviation listed in this chapter.
- Describe how rehabilitation and restorative care involve the whole person.
- Identify the complications to prevent.
- List the common rehabilitation programs and services.
- Explain your role in rehabilitation and restorative nursing care.
- Explain how to promote PRIDE in the person, the family, and yourself.

KEY TERMS

activities of daily living (ADL) The activities usually done during a normal day in a person's life

disability Any lost, absent, or impaired physical or mental function

prosthesis An artificial replacement for a missing body part

rehabilitation The process of restoring the person to his or her highest possible level of physical, psychological, social, and economic function

restorative aide A nursing assistant with special training in restorative nursing and rehabilitation skills

restorative nursing care Care that helps persons regain health, strength, and independence

KEY ABBREVIATION

ADL Activities of daily living

Disease, injury, birth defects and injuries, and surgery can affect body function. Often more than one function is lost. A **disability** is any lost, absent, or impaired physical or mental function. Disabilities are short-term or long-term. Some are permanent. Daily activities are hard or seem impossible. The person may depend totally or in part on others for basic needs. The degree of disability affects how much function is possible.

Rehabilitation is the process of restoring the person to his or her highest possible level of physical, psychological, social, and economic function. The focus is on improving abilities. This promotes function at the highest level of independence. For some persons the goal is to return to a job. For others, self-care is the goal. Sometimes improved function is not possible. Then the goal is to prevent further loss of function. This helps the person maintain the best possible quality of life.

Some people have suffered strokes, fractures, amputations, or other diseases and injuries. They need to regain function or adjust to a long-term disability. Some need home care or nursing center care.

RESTORATIVE NURSING

Some persons are weak. Many cannot perform daily functions. **Restorative nursing care** is care that helps persons regain health, strength, and independence.

Some illnesses are progressive. The person becomes more and more disabled. Restorative nursing:
- Helps maintain the highest level of function
- Prevents unnecessary decline in function

Restorative nursing may involve measures that promote:
- Self-care
- Elimination
- Positioning
- Mobility
- Communication
- Cognitive function

Many persons need restorative nursing and rehabilitation. Often it is hard to separate them. In many agencies, they mean the same thing. Both focus on the whole person.

Restorative Aides

Some agencies have restorative aides. A **restorative aide** is a nursing assistant with special training in restorative nursing and rehabilitation skills. These aides assist the nursing and health teams as needed.

Usually nursing assistants are promoted to restorative aide positions. Those chosen have excellent work ethics, job performance, and skills. Required training varies among states. If there are no state requirements, the agency provides needed training.

REHABILITATION AND THE WHOLE PERSON

An illness or injury has physical, psychological, and social effects. So does a disability. The person needs to adjust physically, psychologically, socially, and economically. Abilities—what the person can do—are stressed. Complications are prevented. They can cause further disability.

Rehabilitation often takes longer in older persons than in other age-groups. Changes from aging affect healing, mobility, vision, hearing, and other functions. Chronic health problems can slow recovery. Older persons also are at risk for injuries. Fast-paced rehabilitation programs are hard for them. Their programs usually are slower-paced.

Physical Aspects

Rehabilitation starts when the person seeks health care. Complications are prevented. They can occur from bedrest, a long illness, or recovery from surgery or injury. Bowel and bladder problems are prevented. So are contractures and pressure ulcers. Good alignment (Chapter 12), turning and repositioning (Chapter 13), and range-of-motion exercises and supportive devices (Chapter 22) are needed. Good skin care also prevents pressure ulcers (Chapter 15).

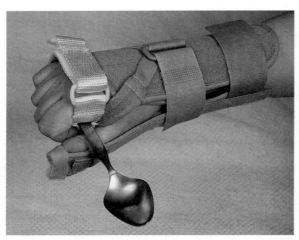

FIGURE 25-1 Eating device attached to a splint.

Self-Care. Self-care is a major goal. **Activities of daily living (ADL)** are the activities usually done during a normal day in a person's life. ADL include bathing, oral hygiene, dressing, eating, elimination, and moving about. The health team evaluates the person's ability to perform ADL. They consider the need for self-help devices.

Sometimes the hands, wrists, and arms are affected. Self-help devices are often needed. Equipment is changed, made, or bought to meet the person's needs.

- Eating devices include glass holders, plate guards, and silverware with curved handles or cuffs (Chapter 19). Some devices attach to splints (Fig. 25-1).
- Electric toothbrushes are helpful. They have back-and-forth brushing motions for oral hygiene.
- Longer handles attach to combs, brushes, and sponges. Or the devices have long handles (Fig. 25-2).
- Self-help devices are useful for cooking, dressing, writing, phone calls, and other tasks. Some are shown in Figure 25-3.

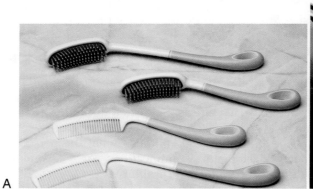

A

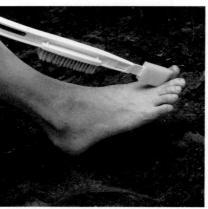

B

C

FIGURE 25-2 **A,** Long-handled combs and brushes for hair care. **B,** Long-handled brush for bathing. **C,** Brush with a curved handle. (**A** and **B** *courtesy North Coast Medical, Inc., Morgan Hill, Calif;* **C** *courtesy Sammons Preston Roylan, An AbilityOne Company, Bolingbrook, Ill.*)

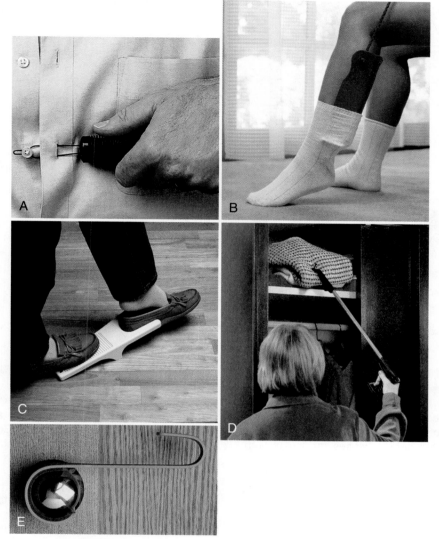

FIGURE 25-3 A, A button hook is used to button and zip clothing. **B,** A sock assist is used to pull on socks and stockings. **C,** A shoe remover is used to take off shoes. **D,** A reacher is helpful to remove items from high shelves. **E,** A doorknob turner increases leverage to help turn the knob. (*A, B, C, and E courtesy North Coast Medical, Inc., Morgan Hill, Calif; D courtesy Sammons Preston Roylan, An AbilityOne Company, Bolingbrook, Ill.*)

Elimination. Some persons need bladder training (Chapter 17). The method depends on the person's problems, abilities, and needs. Some need bowel training (Chapter 18). Control of bowel movements and regular elimination are goals. Fecal impaction, constipation, and fecal incontinence are prevented. Follow the care plan and the nurse's instructions.

Mobility. The person may need crutches or a walker, cane, or brace (Chapter 22). Physical and occupational therapies are common for musculoskeletal and nervous system problems. Some people need wheelchairs. If possible, they learn wheelchair transfers. Such transfers include to and from the bed, toilet, bathtub, sofa, and chair and in and out of vehicles (Fig. 25-4, p. 442).

A **prosthesis** is an artificial replacement for a missing body part. The person learns how to use the artificial arm or leg (Chapter 26). The goal is for the device to be like the missing body part in function and appearance.

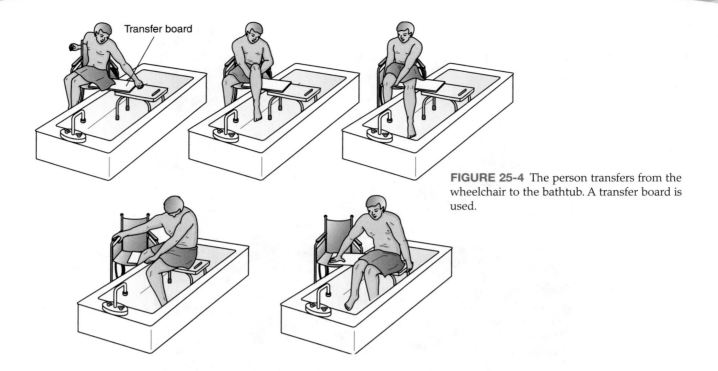

FIGURE 25-4 The person transfers from the wheelchair to the bathtub. A transfer board is used.

FOCUS ON COMMUNICATION
Communication

Speaking is difficult or impossible for some persons. Alternate methods of communication may be needed for persons with speech disorders. Pictures, reading, writing, facial expressions, and gestures are examples. The person and nursing team decide on a method. All members of the nursing team use the same method with the person. Changing methods can cause confusion and delay progress.

Nutrition. Difficulty swallowing *(dysphagia)* may occur after a stroke. The person may need a dysphagia diet (Chapter 19). When possible, exercises are taught to improve swallowing. Some persons cannot swallow. They need enteral nutrition (Chapter 19).

Communication. *Aphasia* may occur from a stroke (Chapter 26). Aphasia means the inability to have normal speech. Speech therapy and communication devices are helpful (Chapter 5).

See *Focus on Communication: Communication.*

Psychological and Social Aspects

A disability can affect function and appearance. Self-esteem and relationships may suffer. The person may feel unwhole, useless, unattractive, unclean, or undesirable. The person may deny the disability. The person may expect therapy to correct the problem. He or she may be depressed, angry, and hostile.

FOCUS ON COMMUNICATION
Psychological and Social Aspects

Denial, anger, depression, fear, and frustration are commonly felt during rehabilitation. Good communication and support provide encouragement. To deal with such emotions:
- Listen to the person.
- Show concern, not pity.
- Focus on what the person is able to do. Point out even slight progress.
- Be polite but firm. Do not allow the person to control you.
- Do not shout at or insult the person. Such behaviors are abuse and mistreatment.
- Do not argue with the person.
- Tell the nurse. Other support measures may be needed.

Successful rehabilitation depends on the person's attitude. The person must accept his or her limits and be motivated. The focus is on abilities and strengths. Despair and frustration are common. Progress may be slow. Learning a new task is a reminder of the disability. Old fears and emotions may recur.

Remind persons of their *progress.* They need help accepting disabilities and limits. Give support, reassurance, and encouragement. Psychological and social needs are part of the care plan. Spiritual support helps some persons.

See *Focus on Communication: Psychological and Social Aspects.*

THE REHABILITATION TEAM

Rehabilitation is a team effort. The person is the key team member. The family, doctor, nursing team, and other health team members help the person set goals and plan care. All help the person regain function and independence.

The team meets often to discuss the person's progress. Changes in the rehabilitation plan are made as needed. The person and family attend the meetings when possible. Families are important. They provide support and encouragement. Often they help with care when the person returns home.

Your Role

Every part of your job focuses on promoting the person's independence. Preventing decline in function also is a goal. The many procedures, care measures, and rules in this book apply. Safety, communication, and legal and ethical aspects apply. So do the measures in Box 25-1.

See *Focus on Communication: Your Role.*

REHABILITATION PROGRAMS AND SERVICES

Rehabilitation begins when the person first needs health care. Often this is in the hospital. Common rehabilitation programs include:

- Cardiac rehabilitation for heart disorders
- Brain injury rehabilitation for nervous system disorders including traumatic brain injury
- Spinal cord rehabilitation for spinal cord injuries
- Stroke rehabilitation after a stroke
- Respiratory rehabilitation for respiratory system disorders such as chronic obstructive pulmonary disease, after lung surgery, for respiratory complications from other health problems
- Musculoskeletal rehabilitation for fractures, joint replacement surgery, and so on
- Rehabilitation for complex medical and surgical conditions—for wound care, diabetes, burns, and so on

Depending on the person's needs and problems, the process may continue after the person leaves the hospital. The person may need home care or nursing center care. Some persons transfer to rehabilitation agencies. There are agencies for persons who are blind or deaf, have intellectual disabilities (formerly known as mental retardation), are physically disabled, or have speech problems. Some agencies are for persons who are mentally ill. Many substance abuse programs are available.

BOX 25-1 Assisting With Rehabilitation and Restorative Care

- Follow the nurse's instructions carefully.
- Follow the person's care plan.
- Follow the person's daily routine.
- Provide for safety.
- Protect the person's rights. Privacy and personal choice are very important.
- Report early signs and symptoms of complications. They include pressure ulcers, contractures, and bowel and bladder problems.
- Keep the person in good alignment at all times.
- Turn and reposition the person as directed.
- Use safe transfer methods.
- Practice measures to prevent pressure ulcers.
- Perform range-of-motion exercises as instructed.
- Apply assistive devices as ordered.
- Do not pity the person or give sympathy.
- Encourage the person to perform ADL to the extent possible.
- Allow the person time to complete tasks. Do not rush the person.
- Give praise when even a little progress is made.
- Provide emotional support and reassurance.
- Try to understand and appreciate the person's situation, feelings, and concerns.
- Provide for spiritual needs.
- Practice the methods developed by the rehabilitation team. This helps you better assist the person.
- Practice the task that the person must do. This helps you guide and direct the person.
- Know how to apply the person's self-help devices.
- Know how to use and operate equipment used by the person.
- Stress what the person can do. Focus on abilities and strengths. Do not focus on disabilities and weaknesses.
- Remember that muscles will atrophy if not used. And contractures can develop.
- Have a hopeful outlook.

FOCUS ON COMMUNICATION
Your Role

You may need to guide and direct the person during care measures. First, listen to how the nurse or therapist guides and directs the person. Use those words. Hearing the same thing helps the person learn and remember what to do.

QUALITY OF LIFE

Successful rehabilitation and restorative care improves the person's quality of life. A hopeful and winning outlook is needed. Promoting quality of life helps the person's attitude. The more the person can do alone, the better his or her quality of life. To promote quality of life:

- *Protect the right to privacy.* The person relearns old skills or practices new skills in private. No one needs to watch. They do not need to see mistakes, falls, spills, or clumsiness. Nor do they need to see anger or tears. Privacy protects dignity and promotes self-respect.
- *Encourage personal choice.* This gives the person control. Not being able to control body movements or functions is very frustrating. Allow and encourage persons to control their lives to the extent possible. Persons who are sad and depressed may not want to make choices. Encourage them to do so. It can help them feel in control of those things that affect them. Personal choice is important in planning care.
- *Protect the right to be free from abuse and mistreatment.* Sometimes improvement is not seen for weeks. Learning to use a self-help device takes time. Learning to speak again can take a long time. So can learning how to dress when there is paralysis. What seems simple is often very hard to do. Repeated explanations and demonstrations may have no or little results. You may become upset and short-tempered. Other staff or the family may have such behaviors. Protect the person from abuse and mistreatment. No one can shout, scream, or yell at the person. Nor can they call the person names. They cannot hit or strike the person. Unkind remarks are not allowed. Report signs of abuse or mistreatment to the nurse.
- *Learn to deal with your anger and frustration.* The person does not choose loss of function. If the process upsets you, think how the person must feel. Discuss your feelings with the nurse. The nurse can suggest ways to help you control or express your feelings. Perhaps you can assist other persons for a while.
- *Encourage activities.* Often a person worries about how others view the disability. Provide support and reassurance. Remind the person that others have disabilities. They can give support and understanding. Allow personal choice. Let the person do what interests him or her. The person usually chooses activities that he or she can do.

- *Provide a safe setting.* It must meet the person's needs. Needed changes are made. The overbed table, bedside stand, and signal light are moved to the person's strong side. If unable to use the signal light, another way is needed to communicate with the staff. The person may need a special chair. The rehabilitation team suggests these and other changes. They explain the need and purpose to the person and family.
- *Show patience, understanding, and sensitivity.* Progress may be slow and hard to see. The person may be upset and discouraged. Give support, encouragement, and praise when needed. Stress the person's abilities and strengths. Do not give pity or sympathy.

Focus on P R I D E
The Person, Family, and Yourself

Personal and Professional Responsibility—Some agencies have opportunities for nursing assistants to advance to restorative aides. Special training is needed for certification. Restorative aide training teaches the knowledge and skills needed to assist with rehabilitation.

Often nursing assistants are promoted to restorative aide positions. Professional behaviors are highly valued when considering persons to promote. Restorative aides require patience, kindness, and good communication skills. Persons with a positive attitude, good work ethic, and excellent job performance are considered first.

Opportunities are available to advance as a nursing assistant. Becoming a restorative aide is one rewarding option. Seek out learning opportunities and practice positive work habits. Take pride in continuing to learn, improve, and grow as a nursing assistant.

Rights and Respect—Disability affects the person as a whole. Many emotions are felt. Often feelings are expressed as anger and frustration. Some persons have trouble controlling such feelings. Persons may have outbursts. You may feel short-tempered. You still must show respect. Remain calm. Act in a professional manner. Control your words and actions. And tell the nurse.

Independence and Social Interaction—The more the person can do for himself or herself, the better his or her quality of life. Independence to the greatest extent possible is the goal of rehabilitation and restorative care. To promote independence:

- Focus on what the person can do.
- Offer encouragement and support.
- Remain patient. Avoid rushing the person.
- Resist the urge to do things for the person that he or she is able to do. This hinders the person's ability to regain function. Remind the family to resist as well.
- Use self-help devices as needed.

Delegation and Teamwork—The rehabilitation process can frustrate the person, you, and other nursing team members. Nursing teamwork is not just about helping with care. It is also about providing emotional support to each other. Sometimes it helps to talk about your feelings. The nursing team can help you control or express your feelings. In the same manner, allow team members to voice their feelings and concerns. Listen and offer to help the person if you are able. Sometimes it is helpful to change care assignments for a while. Take pride in being a part of a strong, supportive team.

Ethics and Laws—The person may not want to practice rehabilitation procedures or methods. He or she may want you to provide care instead. Personal choice is important. However, the person needs to follow the rehabilitation plan. Otherwise, he or she will not make progress. Do not let the person control you. Letting the person control you is the wrong thing to do. Report any problems to the nurse.

REVIEW QUESTIONS

Circle the BEST answer.

1 Rehabilitation and restorative nursing care focus on
   a What the person cannot do
   b Self-care
   c The whole person
   d The person's rights
2 A person's rehabilitation begins with preventing
   a Angry feelings   c Illness and injury
   b Contractures and   d Loss of self-esteem
      pressure ulcers
3 A person has weakness on the right side. ADL are
   a Done by the person to the extent possible
   b Done by you
   c Postponed until the right side can be used
   d Supervised by a therapist
4 Persons with disabilities are likely to feel the following *except*
   a Undesirable   c Depressed
   b Angry and hostile   d Relief
5 Which statement is *false*?
   a Sympathy and pity help the person adjust.
   b You should know how to apply self-help devices.
   c You should know how to use equipment used in the person's care.
   d You need to convey hopefulness to the person.
6 During a therapy, a person asks to have music played. You should
   a Explain that music is not allowed
   b Choose some music
   c Ask the person to choose some music
   d Ask a therapist to choose some music

7 A person's right side is weak. You move the signal light to the left side. You have promoted quality of life by
   a Protecting the person from abuse and mistreatment
   b Allowing personal choice
   c Providing for safety
   d Taking part in activities

Circle T if the statement is *true*. Circle F if the statement is *false*.

8 T F You should give praise even when slight progress is made.
9 T F A person's speech therapy should be done in private.
10 T F You tell a person that dessert is not allowed until exercises are done. This is abuse and mistreatment.
11 T F A person refuses to attend a concert at the nursing center. The person must attend. It is part of the rehabilitation plan.
12 T F Rehabilitation programs for older persons are usually slower paced than those for younger persons.
13 T F Nursing assistants and restorative aides are involved in the person's rehabilitation program.
14 T F You need to stress the person's abilities and strengths.

Answers to these questions are on p. 528.

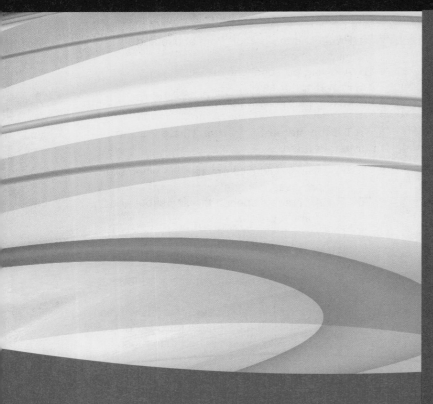

26

CARING FOR PERSONS WITH COMMON HEALTH PROBLEMS

OBJECTIVES

- Define the key terms and key abbreviations listed in this chapter.
- Describe how cancer is treated.
- Describe musculoskeletal disorders and the care required.
- Describe nervous system disorders and the care required.
- Describe hearing loss and the care required.
- Describe eye disorders and the care required.
- Describe cardiovascular disorders and the care required.
- Describe respiratory disorders and the care required.
- Describe digestive disorders and the care required.
- Describe urinary disorders and the care required.
- Describe reproductive disorders and the care required.
- Describe endocrine disorders and the care required.
- Describe immune system disorders and the care required.
- Explain how to promote PRIDE in the person, the family, and yourself.

KEY TERMS

aphasia The total or partial loss (*a*) of the ability to use or understand language (*phasia*)

arthroplasty The surgical replacement (*plasty*) of a joint (*arthr*)

benign tumor A tumor that does not spread to other body parts

cancer See "malignant tumor"

emesis See "vomitus"

fracture A broken bone

hemiplegia Paralysis (*plegia*) on one side (*hemi*) of the body

malignant tumor A tumor that invades and destroys nearby tissue and can spread to other body parts; cancer

metastasis The spread of cancer to other body parts

paraplegia Paralysis in the legs and trunk

quadriplegia Paralysis in the arms, legs, and trunk; tetraplegia

tetraplegia See "quadriplegia"

tumor A new growth of abnormal cells

vomitus The food and fluids expelled from the stomach through the mouth; emesis

KEY ABBREVIATIONS

ADL Activities of daily living

AIDS Acquired immunodeficiency syndrome

ALS Amyotrophic lateral sclerosis

BPH Benign prostatic hyperplasia

CAD Coronary artery disease

CHF Congestive heart failure

CO₂ Carbon dioxide

COPD Chronic obstructive pulmonary disease

CVA Cerebrovascular accident

HBV Hepatitis B virus

HIV Human immunodeficiency virus

I&O Intake and output

IV Intravenous

MI Myocardial infarction

mm Hg Millimeters of mercury

MS Multiple sclerosis

O₂ Oxygen

RA Rheumatoid arthritis

STD Sexually transmitted disease

TB Tuberculosis

TBI Traumatic brain injury

TIA Transient ischemic attack

UTI Urinary tract infection

Understanding common health problems gives meaning to the required care. The nurse gives you more information as needed. Refer to Chapter 6 while you study this chapter.

CANCER

Sometimes cell division and growth are out of control. A mass or clump of cells develops. This new growth of abnormal cells is called a **tumor.** Tumors are benign or malignant (Fig. 26-1).

Benign tumors do not spread to other body parts. They usually do not grow back when removed. **Malignant tumors (cancer)** invade and destroy nearby tissue. They can spread to other body parts. Sometimes they grow back after removal. **Metastasis** is the spread of cancer to other body parts (Fig. 26-2, p. 448). Cancer cells break off the tumor and travel to other body parts. New tumors grow in other body parts. This occurs if cancer is not treated and controlled.

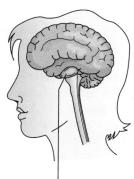

A   Benign tumor

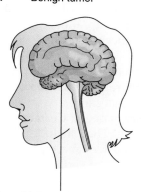

B   Malignant tumor

FIGURE 26-1 Tumors. **A,** A benign tumor grows within a local area. **B,** A malignant tumor invades other tissues.

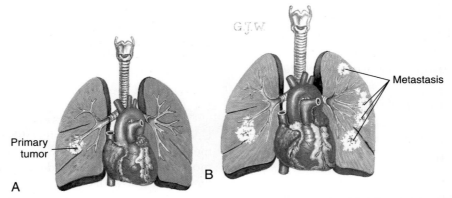

FIGURE 26-2 A, Tumor in the lung. **B,** Tumor has metastasized to the other lung. *(Modified from Belcher AE: Cancer nursing, St Louis, 1992, Mosby.)*

Common sites are the skin, lung and bronchus, colon and rectum, breast, prostate, uterus, ovary, urinary bladder, kidney, mouth and pharynx, pancreas, and thyroid gland. Cancer is the second leading cause of death in the United States.

Certain factors increase the risk of cancer. The National Cancer Institute describes these risk factors:

- *Growing older.* Cancer occurs in all age-groups. However, most cancers occur in persons over 65 years of age.
- *Tobacco.* This includes using tobacco (smoking, snuff, and chewing tobacco) and being around tobacco (second-hand smoke).
- *Sunlight.* Sun, sunlamps, and tanning booths cause early aging of the skin and skin damage. These can lead to skin cancer.
- *Ionizing radiation.* This can cause cell damage that leads to cancer. Sources are x-rays and radon gas that forms in the soil and some rocks. Radioactive fallout is another source. It can come from nuclear power plant accidents and from the production, testing, or use of atomic weapons.
- *Certain chemicals and other substances.* Examples include paint, pesticides, and used engine oil.
- *Some viruses and bacteria.* Being infected with certain viruses increases the risk of these cancers: cervical, liver, lymphoma, leukemia, and Kaposi's sarcoma (a cancer associated with acquired immunodeficiency syndrome [AIDS]).
- *Certain hormones.* One example is hormone replacement therapy for menopause. It may increase the risk of breast cancer.
- *Family history of cancer.* Certain cancers tend to occur in families. They include melanoma and cancers of the breast, ovary, prostate, and colon.
- *Alcohol.* The risk of certain cancers increases with more than two drinks a day. Such cancers are of the mouth, throat, esophagus, larynx, liver, and breast.
- *Poor diet, lack of physical activity, and being overweight.* A high fat diet increases the risk of cancers of the colon, uterus, and prostate. Lack of physical activity and being over-weight increase the risk for cancers of the breast, colon, esophagus, kidney, and uterus.

If detected early, cancer can be treated and controlled (Box 26-1). Sometimes the treatment goal is to reduce symptoms for as long as possible. Surgery, radiation therapy, and chemotherapy are the most common treatments.

- *Surgery.* Tumors are removed.
- *Radiation therapy.* X-ray beams are aimed at the tumor. Cancer cells and normal cells receive radiation. Both are destroyed. Burns, skin breakdown, and hair loss can occur at the treatment site. The doctor may order special skin care measures. Fatigue is common. Extra rest is needed. Discomfort, nausea and vomiting, diarrhea, and loss of appetite *(anorexia)* are other side effects.
- *Chemotherapy.* Drugs are given that kill cancer cells and normal cells. Side effects include hair loss *(alopecia)*, poor appetite, nausea, vomiting, diarrhea, and *stomatitis*—an inflammation *(itis)* of the mouth *(stomat)*. Bleeding and infection are risks from decreased blood cell production.

Persons with cancer have many needs. They include:

- Pain relief or control
- Rest and exercise
- Fluids and nutrition
- Preventing skin breakdown
- Preventing bowel problems (Constipation occurs from pain-relief drugs. Diarrhea occurs from some cancer treatments.)
- Dealing with treatment side effects
- Psychological and social needs
- Spiritual needs
- Sexual needs

BOX 26-1   Some Signs and Symptoms of Cancer

- Thickening or lump in the breast or any other part of the body
- New mole or change in an existing mole
- A sore that does not heal
- Hoarseness or cough that does not go away
- Changes in bowel or bladder habits
- Discomfort after eating
- A hard time swallowing
- Weight gain or loss with no known reason
- Unusual bleeding or discharge
- Feeling weak or very tired

From National Cancer Institute: *What you need to know about cancer: an overview*, NIH Publication Number 06-1566, Bethesda, Md, posted October 4, 2006.

Anger, fear, and depression are common. Some surgeries are disfiguring. The person may feel unwhole, unattractive, or unclean. The person and family need support.

Talk to the person. Do not avoid the person because you are uncomfortable. Use touch and listening to show that you care. Often the person needs to talk and have someone listen. You may not have to say anything. Just listen. A spiritual leader may provide comfort.

MUSCULOSKELETAL DISORDERS

Musculoskeletal disorders affect movement. Injury and age-related changes are common causes.

Arthritis

Arthritis means joint *(arthr)* inflammation *(itis)*. Pain, swelling, and stiffness occur in the affected joints.

Osteoarthritis (Degenerative Joint Disease). This occurs with aging, being over-weight, and joint injury. The fingers, spine (neck and lower back), and weight-bearing joints (hips, knees, and feet) are often affected.

Joint stiffness occurs with rest and lack of motion. Pain occurs with weight-bearing and joint motion. Or pain can be constant or occur from lack of motion. Pain can affect rest, sleep, and mobility. Cold weather and dampness seem to increase symptoms.

Treatment involves:

- *Pain relief.* Drugs decrease swelling and inflammation and relieve pain.
- *Heat or cold applications.* Heat relieves pain, increases blood flow to the part, and reduces swelling. Sometimes cold applications are used after joint use.
- *Exercise.* Exercise decreases pain, increases flexibility, and improves blood flow. It helps with weight control and promotes fitness. Mental well-being improves. The person is taught what exercises to do.
- *Rest and joint care.* Good body mechanics, posture, and regular rest protect the joints. Canes and walkers provide support. Splints support weak joints and keep them in alignment.
- *Weight control.* If over-weight, weight loss reduces stress and injury on weight-bearing joints.
- *Healthy life-style.* The focus is on fitness, exercise, rest, managing stress, and good nutrition.

Falls are prevented. Needed help is given with activities of daily living (ADL). Toilet seat risers are helpful when hips and knees are affected. So are chairs with higher seats and armrests. Some people need joint replacement surgery (p. 450).

Rheumatoid Arthritis. Rheumatoid arthritis (RA) is a chronic inflammatory disease. It causes joint pain, swelling, stiffness, and loss of function. More common in women than in men, it generally develops between the ages of 20 and 50.

RA occurs on both sides of the body. For example, if the right wrist is involved, so is the left wrist. The wrist and finger joints closest to the hand are often affected (Fig. 26-3). Other joints affected are the neck, shoulders, elbows, hips, knees, ankles, and feet. Joints are tender, warm, and swollen. Other body parts may be affected. Fatigue and fever are common. The person does not feel well. Symptoms may last for many years.

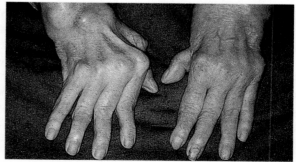

FIGURE 26-3 Deformities caused by rheumatoid arthritis. *(From Stevens A, Lowe J: Pathology: illustrated review in color, ed 2, London, 2000, Mosby.)*

Treatment goals are to relieve pain, reduce inflammation, and slow down or stop joint damage. The person's care plan may include:

- *Rest balanced with exercise.* Short rest periods during the day are better than long times in bed. Range-of-motion exercises are ordered. Exercise promotes sleep, reduces pain, and helps weight control.
- *Proper positioning.* Contractures and deformities are prevented. Bedboards, a bed cradle, trochanter rolls, and pillows are used.
- *Joint care.* Good body mechanics and body alignment, wrist and hand splints, and self-help devices for ADL reduce stress on the joints. Walking aids may be needed.
- *Weight control.* Excess weight places stress on the weight-bearing joints. Exercise and a healthy diet help control weight.
- *Measures to reduce stress.* Relaxation, distraction, exercise, and regular rest help reduce stress.
- *Measures to prevent falls.* See Chapter 9.

Drugs are ordered for pain relief and to reduce inflammation. Heat and cold applications may be ordered. Some persons need joint replacement surgery.

Emotional support is needed. A good outlook is important. Persons with RA need to stay as active as possible. The more they can do for themselves, the better off they are. Give encouragement and praise. Listen when the person needs to talk.

Total Joint Replacement Surgery. **Arthroplasty**
is the surgical replacement *(plasty)* of a joint *(arthro)*. The damaged joint is removed and replaced with an artificial joint *(prosthesis)*.

Hip and knee replacements are the most common. Ankle, foot, shoulder, elbow, and finger joints also can be replaced. See Box 26-2 for care of the person after hip and knee replacement surgeries.

Osteoporosis

With osteoporosis, the bone *(osteo)* becomes porous and brittle *(porosis)*. Bones are fragile and break easily. Spine, hip, wrist, and rib fractures are common.

Older persons of all ethnic groups are at risk. The risk for women increases after menopause. The ovaries do not produce estrogen after menopause. The lack of estrogen causes bone changes. So do low levels of dietary calcium. Other risk factors include a family history of the disease, being thin or having a

---

BOX 26-2	**Care of the Person After Total Joint Replacement Surgery—Hip and Knee**

- Deep-breathing and coughing exercises to prevent respiratory complications.
- Elastic stockings to prevent thrombi (blood clots) in the legs.
- Exercises to strengthen the hip or knee. These are taught by a physical therapist.
- Measures to protect the hip as shown in Figure 26-4.
- Food and fluids for tissue healing and to restore strength.
- Safety measures to prevent falls.
- Measures to prevent infection. Wound, urinary tract, and skin infections must be prevented.
- Measures to prevent pressure ulcers.
- Assist devices for moving, turning, repositioning, and transfers.
- Assistance with walking and a walking aid. The person may need a cane, walker, or crutches.

---

small frame, eating disorders, tobacco use, alcoholism, lack of exercise, bedrest, and immobility. Exercise and activity are needed for bone strength. For bone to form properly, it must bear weight. If not, calcium is lost from the bone. The bone becomes porous and brittle.

Back pain, gradual loss of height, and stooped posture occur. Fractures are a major threat. Even slight activity can cause a fracture. Fractures can occur from turning in bed, getting up from a chair, coughing, and from falls and accidents.

Prevention is important. Doctors often order calcium and vitamin supplements. Estrogen is ordered for some women. Other preventive measures include:

- Exercising weight-bearing joints—walking, jogging, stair climbing
- Strength-training (lifting weights)
- No smoking
- Limiting alcohol and caffeine
- Back supports or corsets if needed for good posture
- Walking aids if needed
- Safety measures to prevent falls and accidents
- Good body mechanics
- Safe handling, moving, transfer, and turning and positioning procedures

Do

Do Not

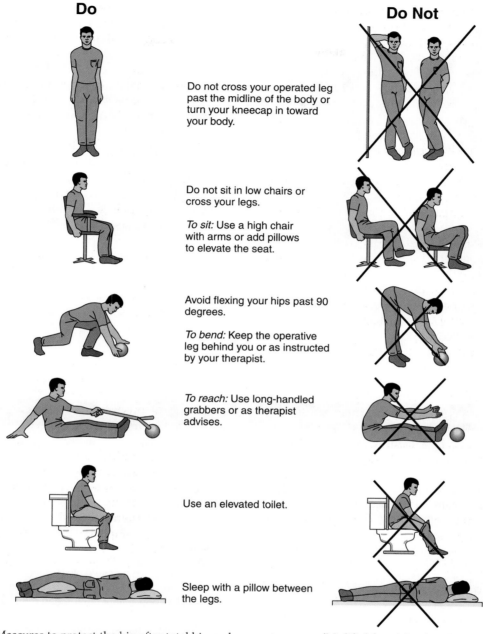

Do not cross your operated leg past the midline of the body or turn your kneecap in toward your body.

Do not sit in low chairs or cross your legs.

To sit: Use a high chair with arms or add pillows to elevate the seat.

Avoid flexing your hips past 90 degrees.

To bend: Keep the operative leg behind you or as instructed by your therapist.

To reach: Use long-handled grabbers or as therapist advises.

Use an elevated toilet.

Sleep with a pillow between the legs.

FIGURE 26-4 Measures to protect the hip after total hip replacement surgery. (*Modified from Monahan FD and others:* Phipps' medical-surgical nursing: health and illness perspectives, *ed 8, St Louis, 2007, Mosby.*)

Fractures

A **fracture** is a broken bone (Fig. 26-5, p. 452). A *closed fracture (simple fracture)* means the bone is broken but the skin is intact. In an *open fracture (compound fracture)*, the broken bone has come through the skin.

Falls, accidents, bone tumors, and osteoporosis are other causes. Signs and symptoms include pain, swelling, limited or no movement of the part, skin color changes, and bleeding. Sometimes the part is deformed—in an abnormal position.

For healing, bone ends are brought into and held in normal position. This is called *reduction* or *fixation:*
- *Closed reduction or external fixation.* The bone is moved back into place. The bone is not exposed.
- *Open reduction or internal fixation.* This requires surgery. The bone is exposed and moved into alignment. Nails, rods, pins, screws, plates, or wires keep the bone in place.

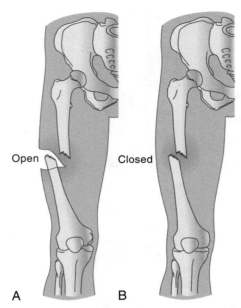

FIGURE 26-5 A, Open fracture. **B,** Closed fracture. *(From Thibodeau GA, Patton KT: The human body in health & disease, ed 4, St Louis, 2005, Mosby.)*

After reduction, movement of the bone ends is prevented. This is done with a cast or traction. Other devices—splints, walking boots, external fixators—also are used.

- *Casts.* Casts are made of plaster of paris, plastic, or fiberglass. Plastic and fiberglass casts dry quickly. A plaster of paris cast dries in 24 to 48 hours. It is odorless, white, and shiny when dry. When wet, it is gray and cool and has a musty smell. The nurse may ask you to assist with care (Box 26-3).
- *Traction.* A steady pull from two directions keeps the bone in place. Weights, ropes, and pulleys are used (Fig. 26-8). Traction is applied to the neck, arms, legs, or pelvis. The nurse may ask you to assist with the person's care (Box 26-4).

BOX 26-3   Rules for Cast Care

- Do not cover the cast with blankets, plastic, or other material. A cast gives off heat as it dries. Covers prevent the escape of heat. Burns can occur if heat cannot escape.
- Turn the person every 2 hours or as often as directed by the nurse and the care plan. All cast surfaces are exposed to the air at one time or another. Turning promotes even drying.
- Do not place a wet cast on a hard surface. It flattens the cast. The cast must keep its shape. Use pillows to support the entire length of the cast (Fig. 26-6).
- Support the wet cast with your palms when turning and positioning the person (Fig. 26-7). Fingertips can dent the cast. The dents can cause pressure areas that lead to skin breakdown.
- Report rough cast edges. The nurse will need to cover the cast edges with tape.
- Keep the cast dry. A wet cast loses its shape. Some casts are near the perineal area. The nurse may apply a waterproof material around the perineal area after the cast dries.
- Do not let the person insert anything into the cast. Itching under the cast causes an intense desire to scratch. Items used for scratching (pencils, coat hangers, knitting needles, back scratchers, and so on) can open the skin. An infection can develop. Scratching items can wrinkle the stockinette or cotton padding. Or scratching items can be lost into the cast. Both can cause pressure and lead to skin breakdown.

- Elevate a casted arm or leg on pillows. This reduces swelling.
- Have enough help when turning and repositioning the person. Plaster casts are heavy and awkward. Balance is lost easily.
- Position the person as directed.
- Follow the care plan for elimination needs. Some persons use a fracture pan.
- Report these signs and symptoms at once:
  - Pain: means a pressure ulcer, poor circulation, or nerve damage
  - Swelling and a tight cast: mean reduced blood flow to the part
  - Pale skin: means reduced blood flow to the part
  - Cyanosis (bluish skin color): means reduced blood flow to the part
  - Odor: means infection
  - Inability to move the fingers or toes: means pressure on a nerve
  - Numbness: means pressure on a nerve or reduced blood flow to the part
  - Temperature changes: cool skin means poor circulation; hot skin means inflammation
  - Drainage on or under the cast: means infection or bleeding
  - Chills, fever, nausea, and vomiting: mean infection
- Complete a safety check before leaving the room. (See the inside of the front book cover.)

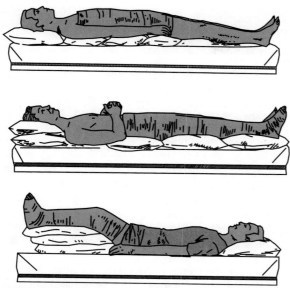

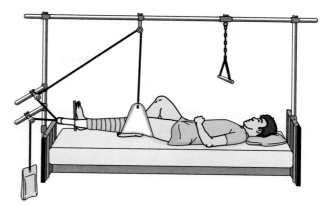

FIGURE 26-8 Traction set-up. Note the weights, pulleys, and ropes. *(From Monahan FD and others: Phipps' medical-surgical nursing: health and illness perspectives, ed 8, St Louis, 2007, Mosby.)*

FIGURE 26-6 Pillows support the entire length of the wet cast. *(From Harkness GA, Dincher JR: Medical-surgical nursing: total patient care, ed 10, St Louis, 1999, Mosby.)*

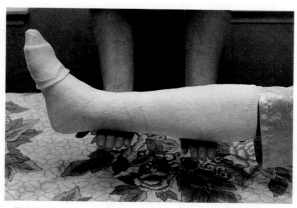

FIGURE 26-7 The cast is supported with the palms.

BOX 26-4   Caring for Persons in Traction

- Keep the person in good alignment.
- Do not remove the traction.
- Keep the weights off the floor. Weights must hang freely from the traction set-up (see Fig. 26-8).
- Do not add or remove weights from the traction set-up.
- Check for frayed ropes. Report fraying to the nurse at once.
- Perform range-of-motion exercises for the uninvolved joints as directed.
- Position the person as directed. Usually only the back-lying position is allowed. Sometimes slight turning is allowed.
- Provide the fracture pan for elimination.
- Give skin care as directed.
- Put bottom linens on the bed from the top down. The person uses a trapeze to raise the body off the bed.
- Check pin, nail, wire, or tong sites for redness, drainage, and odors. Report any observations to the nurse at once.
- Observe for the signs and symptoms listed under cast care (see Box 26-3). Report them to the nurse at once.
- Complete a safety check before leaving the room. (See the inside of the front book cover.)

Hip Fractures. Fractured hips are common in older persons (Fig. 26-9). The fracture requires internal fixation (p. 451) or partial or total hip replacement. Adduction, internal rotation, external rotation, and severe hip flexion are avoided after surgery. Rehabilitation is usually needed.

Post-operative problems present life-threatening risks. They include pneumonia, atelectasis (collapse of a part of a lung), urinary tract infections, and thrombi (blood clots) in the leg veins. Pressure ulcers, constipation, and confusion are other risks. Box 26-5 describes the required care.

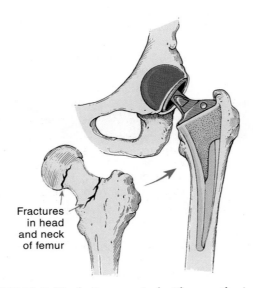

Fractures in head and neck of femur

FIGURE 26-9 Hip fracture repaired with a prosthesis. (*Modified from Christensen BL, Kockrow EO:* Adult health nursing, *ed 5, St Louis, 2006, Mosby.*)

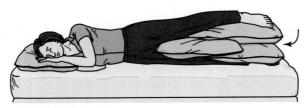

FIGURE 26-10 Pillows are used to keep the hip in abduction. (*From Monahan FD and others:* Phipps' medical-surgical nursing: health and illness perspectives, *ed 8, St Louis, 2007, Mosby.*)

BOX 26-5	**Care of the Person With a Hip Fracture**

- Give good skin care. Skin breakdown can occur rapidly.
- Follow the care plan to prevent pressure ulcers.
- Follow the care plan to prevent wound, skin, and urinary tract infections.
- Encourage deep-breathing and coughing exercises as directed.
- Turn and position the person as directed. Turning and positioning depend on the type of fracture and the surgery performed. Usually the person is not positioned on the operative side.
- Use trochanter rolls, pillows, and sandbags as directed. These prevent external rotation when the person is in bed.
- Keep the operated leg abducted at all times. The leg is abducted when the person is supine, being turned, or in a side-lying position. Use pillows (Fig. 26-10) or a hip abduction wedge (abductor splint) as directed. Do not exercise the affected leg.
- Provide a straight-back chair with armrests. The person needs a high, firm seat. A low, soft chair is not used.
- Place the chair on the unaffected side.
- Assist the nurse in transferring the person.
- Use assist devices for moving, turning, repositioning, and transfers.
- Do not let the person stand on the operated leg unless allowed by the doctor.
- Follow the care plan for when to elevate the leg. If the person has an internal fixation device, the leg is not elevated when the person sits in a chair. Elevating the leg puts strain on the device.
- Apply elastic stockings to prevent thrombi (blood clots) in the legs.
- Remind the person not to cross his or her legs.
- Assist with ambulation according to the care plan. The person uses a walker or crutches.
- Follow measures to protect the hip. See Box 26-2 and Figure 26-4.
- Practice safety measures to prevent falls.

Loss of Limb

An *amputation* is the removal of all or part of an extremity. Severe injuries, tumors, severe infection, gangrene, and vascular disorders are common causes. Diabetes is a common cause of vascular changes that can lead to amputation.

Gangrene is a condition in which there is death of tissue. Causes include infection, injuries, and vascular disorders. Blood flow is affected. Tissues do not get enough oxygen and nutrients. They become black, cold, and shriveled (Fig. 26-11). Surgery is needed to remove dead tissue. Gangrene can cause death.

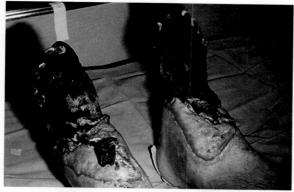

FIGURE 26-11 Gangrene. *(Courtesy Cameron Bangs, MD. From Auerbach PS:* Wilderness medicine, management of wilderness and environmental emergencies, *ed 3, St Louis, 1995, Mosby.)*

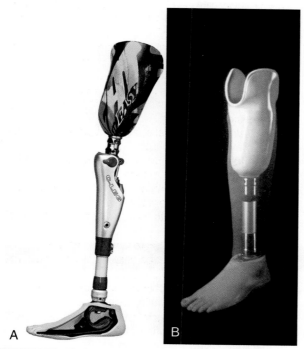

A   B

FIGURE 26-12 Leg prostheses. **A,** Above-the-knee prosthesis. **B,** Below-the-knee prostheses. *(Courtesy Otto Bock Health Care, Minneapolis, Minn.)*

The person is fitted with a prosthesis—an artificial replacement for a missing body part (Fig. 26-12). Occupational and physical therapists help the person use the prosthesis.

The person may feel that the limb is still there. Aching, tingling, and itching are common sensations. Or the person may complain of pain in the amputated part. This is called *phantom limb pain.* This is a normal reaction.

NERVOUS SYSTEM DISORDERS

Nervous system disorders can affect mental and physical function. They can affect the ability to speak, understand, feel, see, hear, touch, think, control bowels and bladder, and move.

Stroke

Stroke is the third leading cause of death in the United States. It is a leading cause of disability in adults. Stroke is a disease that affects the arteries that supply blood to the brain. It also is called a *brain attack* or *cerebrovascular accident (CVA).* The two major types of strokes are:

- A blood vessel in the brain bursts. Bleeding occurs in the brain (cerebral hemorrhage).
- A blood clot blocks blood flow to the brain.

Brain cells in the affected area do not get enough oxygen and nutrients. Brain cells die. Brain damage occurs. Functions lost depend on the area of damage (Fig. 26-13, p. 456).

Stroke can occur suddenly. The person may have warning signs (Box 26-6, p. 456). Sometimes warning signs last a few minutes. This is called a *transient ischemic attack (TIA).* (*Transient* means temporary or short term. *Ischemic* means to hold back [*ischein*] blood [*hemic*].) Blood supply to the brain is interrupted for a short time. Sometimes a TIA occurs before a stroke.

The person also may have nausea, vomiting, and memory loss. Unconsciousness, noisy breathing, high blood pressure, slow pulse, redness of the face, and seizures may occur. So can **hemiplegia**—paralysis *(plegia)* on one side *(hemi)* of the body. The person may lose bowel and bladder control and the ability to speak. (See "Aphasia" on p. 457.) All stroke-like symptoms signal the need for emergency care.

The effects of stroke include:
- Loss of face, hand, arm, leg, or body control
- Hemiplegia
- Changing emotions (crying easily or mood swings, sometimes for no reason)
- Difficulty swallowing (dysphagia)
- Aphasia or slowed or slurred speech
- Changes in sight, touch, movement, and thought
- Impaired memory
- Urinary frequency, urgency, or incontinence
- Loss of bowel control or constipation
- Depression and frustration

Rehabilitation starts at once. The person may depend in part or totally on others for care. The health team helps the person regain the highest possible level of function (Box 26-7, p. 456).

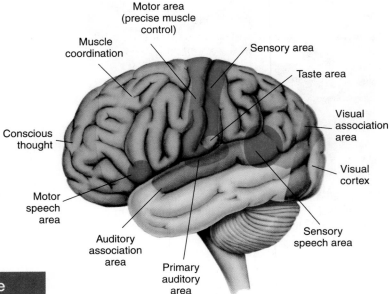

FIGURE 26-13 Functions lost from a stroke depend on the area of brain damage. *(From Thibodeau GA, Patton KT: The human body in health & disease, ed 5, St Louis, 2010, Mosby.)*

BOX 26-6	Warning Signs of Stroke

- Sudden numbness or weakness of the face, arm, or leg, especially on one side of the body
- Sudden confusion, trouble speaking or understanding speech
- Sudden trouble seeing in one or both eyes
- Sudden trouble walking, dizziness, loss of balance or coordination
- Sudden, severe headache with no known cause

From National Institute for Neurological Disorders and Stroke: *Know stroke. Know the signs. Act in time,* National Institutes of Health, NIH Publication Number 08-4872, Bethesda, Md, January 2008.

BOX 26-7	Care of the Person With a Stroke

- The lateral (side-lying) position prevents aspiration.
- The bed is kept in semi-Fowler's position.
- The person is approached from the strong (unaffected) side. Objects are placed on the strong (unaffected) side. The person may have loss of vision on the affected side.
- Turning and repositioning are done at least every 2 hours.
- Assist devices are used for moving, turning, repositioning, and transfers.
- Deep breathing and coughing are encouraged.
- Contractures are prevented.
- Food and fluid needs are met. The person may need a dysphagia diet.
- Elastic stockings prevent thrombi (blood clots) in the legs.
- Range-of-motion exercises prevent contractures. They also strengthen affected extremities.
- Elimination needs are met:
  - A catheter is inserted, or a bladder training program is started if needed.
  - A bowel training program is started if needed.

- Safety precautions are practiced:
  - The signal light is kept within reach. It is on the person's strong (unaffected) side.
  - The person is checked often if he or she cannot use the signal light. Follow the care plan.
  - Bed rails are used according to the care plan.
  - Falls are prevented.
- The person does as much self-care as possible. This includes turning, positioning, and transfers.
- Communication methods are established.
- Speech, physical, and occupational therapies are ordered.
- Assistive and self-help devices are used as needed.
- Ambulation aids are used as needed.
- Support, encourage, and praise are given.
- A safety check is completed before leaving the room. (See the inside of the front book cover.)

Aphasia

Aphasia is the total or partial loss (*a*) of the ability to use or understand language (*phasia*). Parts of the brain responsible for language are damaged. Two types of aphasia are:

- *Expressive aphasia (motor aphasia, Broca's aphasia)* relates to difficulty expressing or sending out thoughts. Thinking is clear. The person knows what to say but has difficulty or cannot speak the words. There are problems speaking, spelling, counting, gesturing, or writing. The person may:
  - Speak in single words or short sentences. For example, a person says "Walk dog." It can mean "I will take the dog for a walk" or "You take the dog for a walk."
  - Put words in the wrong order. For example, the persons says "room bath," not "bathroom."
  - Think one thing but say another. For example, the person wants food but asks for a book.
  - Call people by the wrong names.
  - Produce sounds and no words.
  - Cry or swear for no reason.
- *Receptive aphasia (Wernicke's aphasia)* relates to difficulty understanding language. The person has trouble understanding what is said or read. People and common objects are not recognized. The person may not know how to use a fork, toilet, cup, TV, phone, or other items.

Some people have both types. This is called *expressive-receptive aphasia (global aphasia, mixed aphasia).* The person has problems speaking and understanding language.

Parkinson's Disease

Parkinson's disease is a slow, progressive disorder with no cure. The area of the brain that controls muscle movement is affected. Persons over the age of 50 are at risk. Signs and symptoms become worse over time (Fig. 26-14). They include:

- *Tremors*—often start in one finger and spread to the whole arm. Pill-rolling movements—rubbing the thumb and index finger—may occur. The person may have trembling in the hands, arms, legs, jaw, and face.
- *Rigid, stiff muscles*—in the arms, legs, neck, and trunk.
- *Slow movements*—the person has a slow, shuffling gait.
- *Stooped posture and impaired balance*—it is hard to walk. Falls are a risk.
- *Mask-like expression*—the person cannot blink and smile. A fixed stare is common.

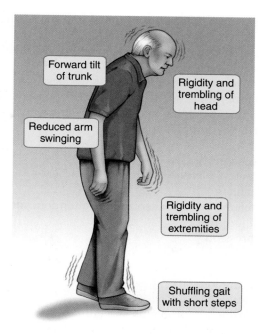

Forward tilt of trunk

Rigidity and trembling of head

Reduced arm swinging

Rigidity and trembling of extremities

Shuffling gait with short steps

FIGURE 26-14 Signs of Parkinson's disease. (*From Thibodeau GA, Patton KT: The human body in health & disease, ed 5, St Louis, 2010, Mosby.*)

Other signs and symptoms develop over time. They include swallowing and chewing problems, constipation, and bladder problems. Sleep problems, depression, and emotional changes (fear, insecurity) can occur. So can memory loss and slow thinking. The person may have slurred, monotone, and soft speech. Some people talk too fast or repeat what they say.

The doctor orders drugs to treat and control the disease. Exercise and physical therapy are ordered to improve strength, posture, balance, and mobility. Therapy is needed for speech and swallowing problems. The person may need help with eating and self-care. Normal elimination is a goal. Safety measures are needed to prevent falls and injury.

Multiple Sclerosis

Multiple sclerosis (MS) is a chronic disease. *Multiple* means many. *Sclerosis* means hardening or scarring. The myelin (which covers nerve fibers) in the brain and spinal cord is destroyed. Nerve impulses are not sent to and from the brain in a normal manner. Functions are impaired or lost. There is no cure.

Symptoms usually start between the ages of 20 and 40. A person's risk increases if a family member has MS.

Signs and symptoms depend on the damaged area. They may include:

- Vision problems—blurred or double vision, blindness in one eye
- Muscle weakness in the arms and legs
- Balance problems that affect standing and walking
- Tingling, prickling, or numb sensations
- Partial or complete paralysis
- Pain
- Speech problems
- Tremors
- Dizziness
- Problems with concentration, attention, memory, and judgment
- Depression
- Bowel and bladder problems
- Problems with sexual function
- Hearing loss
- Fatigue
- Coordination problems and clumsiness

In some people, symptoms do not progress after the first attack. For others, symptoms lessen or disappear (remission). At some point, there are flare-ups (relapses). With each flare-up, more symptoms occur. Some people have no remissions. Their conditions gradually decline. New attacks present new symptoms and more damage.

Persons with MS are kept active as long as possible and as independent as possible. The care plan reflects the person's changing needs. Skin care, hygiene, and range-of-motion exercises are important. So are turning, positioning, and deep breathing and coughing. Bowel and bladder elimination is promoted. Injuries and complications from bedrest are prevented.

Amyotrophic Lateral Sclerosis

Amyotrophic lateral sclerosis (ALS) attacks the nerve cells that control voluntary muscles. Commonly called *Lou Gehrig's disease,* it is rapidly progressive and fatal. (Lou Gehrig was a New York Yankees baseball player. He died of the disease in 1941.)

ALS usually strikes between 40 and 60 years of age. The person usually dies within 3 to 5 years after onset.

Motor nerve cells in the brain, brainstem, and spinal cord are affected. They stop sending messages to the muscles. The muscles weaken, waste away (atrophy), and twitch. Over time, the brain cannot start voluntary movements or control them. The person cannot move the arms, legs, and body. Muscles for speaking, chewing, swallowing, and breathing also are affected. Eventually muscles in the chest wall fail.

The disease usually does not affect the mind, intelligence, or memory. Sight, smell, taste, hearing, and touch are not affected. Usually bowel and bladder functions remain intact.

ALS has no cure. Some drugs can slow disease progression. However, damage cannot be reversed. Persons with ALS are kept active as long as possible and as independent as possible. The care plan reflects the person's changing needs.

Traumatic Brain Injury

Traumatic brain injury (TBI) occurs when a sudden trauma damages the brain. Brain tissue is bruised or torn. Bleeding can be in the brain or in nearby tissues. Spinal cord injuries are likely. Motor vehicle crashes, falls, and firearms are common causes. So are assaults and sports and recreation injuries.

If the person survives TBI, some permanent damage is likely. Disabilities depend on the severity and location of the injury. They include:

- Cognitive problems—thinking, memory, and reasoning
- Sensory problems—sight, hearing, touch, taste, and smell
- Communication problems—expressing or understanding language
- Behavior or mental health problems—depression, anxiety, personality changes, aggressive behavior, socially inappropriate behavior
- Stupor—an unresponsive state; the person can be briefly aroused
- Coma—the person is unconscious, does not respond, is unaware, and cannot be aroused
- Vegetative state—the person is unconscious and unaware of surroundings; he or she has sleep-wake cycles and periods of being alert
- Persistent vegetative state (PVS)—the person is in a vegetative state for more than one month

Rehabilitation is required. Nursing care depends on the person's needs and remaining abilities.

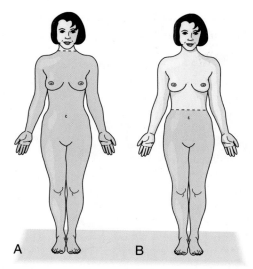

FIGURE 26-15 The *shaded areas* show the area of paralysis. **A,** Quadriplegia. **B,** Paraplegia.

Spinal Cord Injury

Spinal cord injuries can permanently damage the nervous system. Common causes are stab or gunshot wounds, motor vehicle crashes, falls, and sports injuries. Problems depend on the amount of damage to the spinal cord and the level of injury. The higher the level of injury, the more functions lost (Fig. 26-15).

- Lumbar injuries—sensory and muscle function in the legs is lost. The person has paraplegia. **Paraplegia** is paralysis in the legs and trunk. (*Para* means beside or beyond; *plegia* means paralysis.)
- Thoracic injuries—sensory and muscle function below the chest is lost. The person has paraplegia.
- Cervical injuries—sensory and muscle function of the arms, legs, and trunk is lost. Paralysis in the arms, legs, and trunk is called **quadriplegia (tetraplegia).** (*Quad* and *tetra* mean four.)

Cervical traction may be needed (p. 452). Care measures are listed in Box 26-8. Emotional needs require attention. Reactions to paralysis and loss of function are often severe. If the person survives, rehabilitation is necessary.

BOX 26-8 Care of Persons With Paralysis

- Prevent falls. Follow the care plan for safety measures and bed rail use.
- Keep the bed in the low position.
- Keep the signal light within reach. If unable to use the signal light, check the person often.
- Prevent burns. Check bath water, heat applications, and food for proper temperature.
- Turn and reposition the person at least every 2 hours. Follow the care plan.
- Prevent pressure ulcers. Follow the care plan.
- Maintain good alignment at all times. Use supportive devices according to the care plan.
- Follow bowel and bladder training programs.
- Keep intake and output (I&O) records.
- Maintain muscle function and prevent contractures. Assist with range-of-motion exercises as directed.
- Assist with food and fluids as needed. Provide self-help devices as ordered.
- Give emotional and psychological support.
- Follow the person's rehabilitation plan.
- Complete a safety check of the room. (See the inside of the front book cover.)

HEARING LOSS

Hearing loss is not being able to hear the normal range of sounds associated with normal hearing. Deafness is the most severe form. *Deafness* is hearing loss in which it is impossible for the person to understand speech through hearing alone. Clear speech, responding to others, safety, and awareness of surroundings require hearing.

A person may not notice gradual hearing loss. Others may see changes in the person's behavior or attitude. Obvious signs and symptoms of hearing loss include:

- Speaking too loudly
- Leaning forward to hear
- Turning and cupping the better ear toward the speaker
- Answering questions or responding inappropriately
- Asking for words to be repeated
- Asking others to speak louder or to speak more slowly and clearly
- Having trouble hearing over the phone
- Finding it hard to follow conversations when two or more people are talking
- Turning up the TV, radio, or music volume so loud that others complain

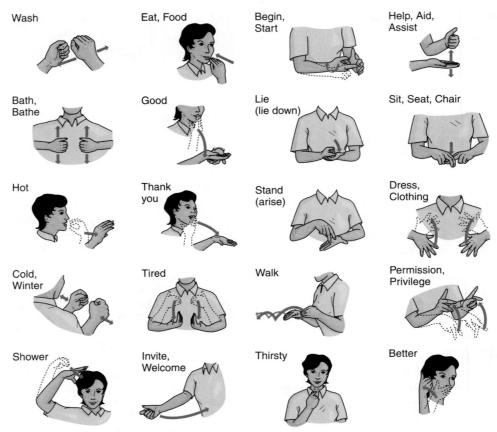

Wash Eat, Food Begin, Start Help, Aid, Assist

Bath, Bathe Good Lie (lie down) Sit, Seat, Chair

Hot Thank you Stand (arise) Dress, Clothing

Cold, Winter Tired Walk Permission, Privilege

Shower Invite, Welcome Thirsty Better

FIGURE 26-16 American Sign Language examples.

Persons with hearing loss may wear hearing aids or lip-read (speech-read). They watch facial expressions, gestures, and body language. Some people learn American Sign Language (ASL) (Fig. 26-16).

Some people have *hearing assistance dogs* (hearing dogs). The dog alerts the person to sounds. Examples include phones, doorbells, smoke detectors, alarm clocks, sirens and on-coming cars.

See *Focus on Communication: Hearing Loss.*

FOCUS ON COMMUNICATION
Hearing Loss

The National Association of the Deaf (NAD) uses the terms *deaf* and *hard-of-hearing* to describe persons with hearing loss. Do not use the terms "deaf and dumb," "deaf-mute," or "hearing-impaired." Such terms offend persons who are deaf or hard-of-hearing.

There are many ways to communicate with persons who are deaf or hard-of-hearing. Some use American Sign Language (ASL). The nurse can contact a sign language interpreter. Some persons write notes or use a computer. Pictures may also be used. Others are able to lip-read (speech-read). Another method may be used with lip-reading to be sure that messages are understood.

Check the care plan or ask the nurse which communication method to use. See Box 26-9 for measures to promote communication.

BOX 26-9 Measures to Promote Hearing

The Environment

- Reduce or eliminate background noises. For example, turn off radios, stereos, music players, TVs, air conditioners, fans, and so on.
- Provide a quiet place to talk.
- Have the person sit in small groups or where he or she can hear best.

The Person

- Have the person wear his or her hearing aid. It must be turned on and working.
- Have the person wear needed eyeglasses or contact lenses. The person needs to see your face for lip-reading (speech-reading).

You

- Gain attention. Alert the person to your presence. Raise an arm or hand, or lightly touch the person's arm. Do not startle or approach the person from behind.
- Position yourself at the person's level. If the person is sitting, you sit. If the person is standing, you stand.
- Face the person when speaking. Do not turn or walk away while you are talking. Do not talk to the person from the doorway or another room.
- Stand or sit in good light. Shadows and glares affect the person's ability to see your face clearly.
- Speak clearly, distinctly, and slowly.
- Speak in a normal tone of voice. Do not shout.

You—cont'd

- Adjust the pitch of your voice as needed. Ask the person if he or she can hear you better:
  - If the person does not wear a hearing aid, lower the pitch if you are a female. Women's voices are higher-pitched and harder to hear than lower-pitched male voices.
  - If the person wears a hearing aid, raise the pitch slightly.
- Do not cover your mouth, smoke, eat, or chew gum while talking. Mouth movements are affected.
- Keep your hands away from your face. The person must be able to clearly see your face.
- Stand or sit on the side of the better ear.
- State the topic of conversation first.
- Tell the person when you are changing the subject. State the new subject of conversation.
- Use short sentences and simple words.
- Use gestures and facial expressions to give useful clues.
- Write out important names and words.
- Say things in another way if the person does not seem to understand.
- Keep conversations and discussions short. This avoids tiring the person.
- Repeat and rephrase statements as needed.
- Be alert to messages sent by your facial expressions, gestures, and body language.

Hearing Aids. *Hearing aids* are electronic devices that fit inside or behind the ear (Fig. 26-17). They make sounds louder. They do not correct, restore, or cure hearing problems. Background noise and speech are louder. The measures in Box 26-9 apply.

Hearing aids are battery-operated. Sometimes they do not seem to work properly. Try these simple measures:

- Check if the hearing aid is *on*. It has an *on* and *off* switch.
- Check the battery position.
- Insert a new battery if needed.
- Clean the hearing aid. *Follow the nurse's directions and the manufacturer's instructions.*

Hearing aids are turned off when not in use. And the battery is removed.

Hearing aids are costly. Handle and care for them properly. When not in the person's ear, store a hearing aid in its case. Place the case in the top drawer of the bedside stand. Report lost or damaged hearing aids to the nurse at once.

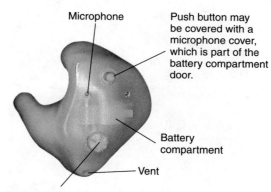

Microphone

Push button may be covered with a microphone cover, which is part of the battery compartment door.

Battery compartment

Vent

On/Off switch/Volume control

FIGURE 26-17 A hearing aid. (*Courtesy Siemens Hearing Instruments, Inc., Piscataway, NJ.*)

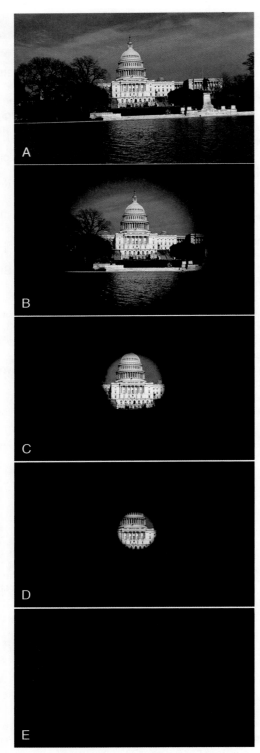

FIGURE 26-18 Vision loss from glaucoma. **A,** Normal vision. **B,** Loss of peripheral vision begins. **C, D,** and **E,** Vision loss continues, with eventual blindness.

EYE DISORDERS

Vision loss occurs at all ages—from mild vision loss to complete blindness. *Blind* is the absence of sight. Vision loss is sudden or gradual. One or both eyes are affected. The following are common.

- *Glaucoma*—results when fluid builds up in the eye and causes pressure on the optic nerve. The optic nerve is damaged. Vision loss with eventual blindness occurs. Glaucoma can develop in one or both eyes. Peripheral vision (side vision) is lost. The person sees through a tunnel (Fig. 26-18), has blurred vision, and sees halos around lights. Drugs and surgery can control glaucoma and prevent further damage to the optic nerve. Prior damage cannot be reversed.
- *Cataract*—is a clouding of the lens (Fig. 26-19). Normally the lens is clear. Cataract comes from the Greek word that means *waterfall*. Trying to see is like looking through a waterfall. Surgery is the only treatment (Box 26-10). Signs and symptoms of cataract are:
  - Cloudy, blurry, or dimmed vision (Fig. 26-20). Colors seem faded. Blues and purples are hard to see.
  - Sensitivity to light and glares.
  - Poor vision at night.
  - Halos around lights.
  - Double vision in one eye.
- *Age-related macular degeneration (AMD)*—is a disease that blurs central vision. *Central vision* is what you see "straight-ahead." It causes a blind spot in the center of vision (Fig. 26-21). Some people benefit from laser surgery.
- *Diabetic retinopathy*—tiny blood vessels in the retina are damaged. A complication of diabetes, it is a leading cause of blindness. Usually both eyes are affected. Vision blurs (Fig. 26-22). The person may see spots "floating." Often there are no early warning signs. The person needs to control diabetes, blood pressure, and blood cholesterol. Laser surgery may help.

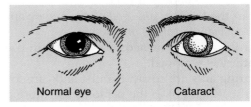

Normal eye   Cataract

FIGURE 26-19 One eye is normal. The other has a cataract. *(From Phipps WJ and others:* Medical-surgical nursing: concepts and clinical practice, *ed 5, St Louis, 1995, Mosby.)*

BOX 26-10   Nursing Measures After Cataract Surgery

- Keep the eye shield in place as directed. The shield is worn for sleep, including naps.
- Follow measures for persons who are visually impaired or blind when an eye shield is worn (p. 464). The person may have vision loss in the other eye.
- Remind the person not to rub or press the affected eye.

- Do not bump the eye.
- Place the overbed table and the bedside stand on the unoperative side.
- Place the signal light within reach.
- Report eye drainage or complaints of pain at once.

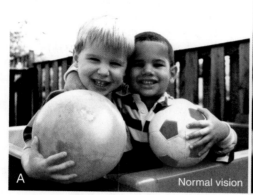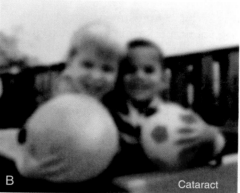

FIGURE 26-20 Vision loss from a cataract. **A,** Normal vision. **B,** Scene viewed with a cataract. *(From National Eye Institute: Cataract: what you should know, National Institutes of Health, Bethesda, Md.)*

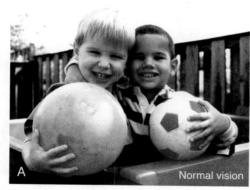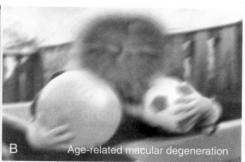

FIGURE 26-21 Vision loss from macular degeneration. **A,** Normal vision. **B,** Central vision is blurred. *(From National Eye Institute: Age-related macular degeneration: what you should know, National Institutes of Health, Bethesda, Md.)*

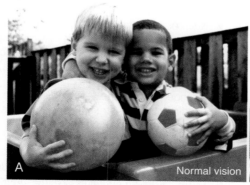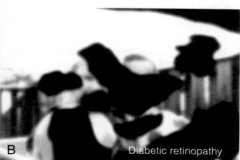

FIGURE 26-22 Vision loss from diabetic retinopathy. **A,** Normal vision. **B,** Vision with diabetic retinopathy. *(From National Eye Institute: Diabetic retinopathy: what you should know, National Institutes of Health, Bethesda, Md.)*

Impaired Vision and Blindness

Birth defects, accidents, and eye diseases are among the many causes of impaired vision and blindness. They also are complications of some diseases. Some people are totally blind. Others sense some light but have no usable vision. Still others have some usable vision but cannot read newsprint. The legally blind person sees at 20 feet what a person with normal vision sees at 200 feet.

Loss of sight is serious. Adjustments can be hard and long. Moving about, performing daily activities, reading and writing, communication, and using a dog guide require training.

Rehabilitation programs help the person adjust to the vision loss and to learn to be independent. The goal is for the person to be as active as possible and to have quality of life. The person learns how to use visual and adaptive devices, braille, long canes, and dog guides.

Braille is a touch reading and writing system that uses raised dots for each letter of the alphabet (Fig. 26-23). The first 10 letters also represent the numbers 0 through 9. Braille is read by moving the hands along each braille line.

Special devices allow computer access. There are braille keyboards. A "braille display" lets the person read information. Braille printers allow printing computer information in braille.

Blind and visually impaired persons learn to move about using a long cane with a red tip or using a dog guide. Both are used worldwide by persons who are blind.

Follow the practices in Box 26-11.

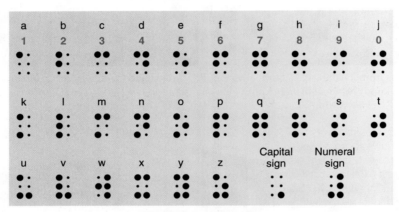

FIGURE 26-23 Braille.

BOX 26-11 | **Caring for Blind and Visually Impaired Persons**

The Environment

- Report worn carpeting and other flooring.
- Keep furniture, equipment, and electrical cords out of areas where the person will walk.
- Keep table and desk chairs pushed in under the table or desk.
- Keep doors fully open or fully closed. This includes room, closet, and cabinet doors.
- Keep drawers fully closed.
- Report burnt out bulbs.
- Provide lighting as the person prefers. Tell the person when the lights are on or off.
- Adjust window coverings to prevent glares.

The Environment—cont'd

- Provide a consistent mealtime setting:
  - Use plates, napkins, placemats, and tablecloths in solid colors that provide contrast. For example, place a white plate on a dark placemat or tablecloth.
  - Provide good light above the table where the person will sit to eat.
  - Keep place settings the same. The knife and spoon are to the right of the plate. The fork and napkin are to the left of the plate. For a right-handed person, the glass or cup is to the right of the plate. For a left-handed person, it is to the left of the plate.
  - Arrange main dishes, side dishes, seasonings, and condiments in a straight line or in a semi-circle just beyond the person's place setting.
  - Explain the location of food and beverages. Use the face of a clock (Chapter 19). Or guide the person's hand to each item on the tray or place setting.
  - Cut meat, open containers, butter bread, and perform other tasks as needed.

BOX 26-11   Caring for Blind and Visually Impaired Persons—cont'd

The Environment—cont'd

- Keep the signal light and TV, light, and other controls within the person's reach.
- Turn on night-lights in the person's room, bathroom, and hallways.
- Practice safety measures to prevent falls (Chapter 9).
- Orient the person to the room. Describe the layout. Also describe the location and purpose of furniture and equipment.
- Let the person move about. Let him or her touch and find furniture and equipment.
- Do not leave the person in the middle of a room. Make sure he or she can reach a wall or furniture.
- Do not re-arrange furniture and equipment.
- Tell the person when you are coming to a curb or steps. State if the steps are up or down.
- Tell the person about doors, turns, furniture, and other obstructions when assisting with ambulation.
- Complete a safety check before leaving the room. (See the inside of the front book cover.)

The Person

- Have the person use railings when climbing stairs.
- Make sure the person wears comfortable shoes that fit correctly.
- Assist with walking as needed. Have the person lightly hold onto your arm just above the elbow (Fig. 26-24, p. 466). Tell the person which arm is offered. Have the person walk about a half step behind you. Never push, pull, or guide the person in front of you. Walk at a normal pace.
- Let the person do as much for himself or herself as possible.
- Provide visual and adaptive devices—radio, compact discs, audio books, TV, braille books, and so on. Follow the care plan.

You

- Face the person when speaking. Speak slowly and clearly.
- Use a normal tone of voice. Do not shout or speak loudly. Vision loss does not mean the person has hearing loss.
- Identify yourself when you enter the room. Give your name, title, and reason for being there. Do not touch the person until he or she knows you are there.
- Ask the person how much he or she can see. Do not assume the person is totally blind or that the person has some vision.
- Identify others. Explain where each person is located and what the person is doing.
- Address the person by name. This tells the person that you are directing a comment or question to him or her.

You—cont'd

- Speak directly to the person. Do not just talk to family and friends who are present.
- Encourage the person to do as much for himself or herself as possible.
- Feel free to use words such as "see," "look," "read," or "watch TV."
- Feel free to refer to colors, sizes, shapes, patterns, designs, and so on.
- Describe people, places, and things completely. Do not leave out a detail because you do not think it is important.
- Offer to help. Simply say "May I help you?" Respect the person's answer.
- Warn the person of dangers. Provide a calm and clear warning.
- Leave the person's belongings where you found them. Do not move or re-arrange things.
- Greet the person by name when he or she enters a room. Tell the person who you are. Also identify others in the room.
- Listen to the person. Give the person verbal cues that you are listening. Say "yes," "ok," "I see," "tell me more," "I don't understand," and so on.
- Answer the person's questions. Give specific and descriptive responses.
- Assist in food selection. Read menus to the person.
- Give step-by-step explanations of procedures as you perform them. Say when the procedure is over.
- Give specific directions. Say "right behind you," "on your left," or "in front of you." Avoid phrases like "over here" or "over there."
- Tell the person when you are ending a conversation. For example, "I enjoyed hearing about your children. Thank you for sharing stories with me."
- Guide the person to a seat by placing your guiding arm on the seat. The person will move his or her hand down your arm to the seat.
- Do the following if the person uses a long cane:
  - Announce your presence.
  - Ask if you can assist before trying to help.
  - Do not interfere with the arm used to hold the cane.
  - Let the person store his or her cane. If you store the cane, tell the person where to find it.
- Do not pet, feed, or distract a dog guide. Such actions can place the person in danger.
- Tell the person when you are leaving the room or the area. If appropriate, tell the person where you are going. For example, "I'm going to go into your bathroom now."

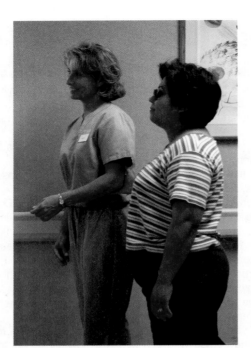

FIGURE 26-24 The blind person walks slightly behind the nursing assistant. She touches the assistant's arm lightly.

Corrective Lenses

Eyeglasses and contact lenses can correct many vision problems. Some people wear eyeglasses for reading or seeing at a distance. Others wear them for all activities. Contact lenses are usually worn while awake. Some contacts can be worn day and night for up to 30 days.

Eyeglass lenses are hardened glass or plastic. Clean them daily and as needed. Wash glass lenses with warm water. Dry them with a lens cloth or cotton cloth. Plastic lenses scratch easily. Use special cleaning solutions and cloths.

Contact lenses fit on the eye. They are cleaned, removed, and stored according to the manufacturer's instructions.

See *Delegation Guidelines: Corrective Lenses.*
See *Promoting Safety and Comfort: Corrective Lenses.*

DELEGATION GUIDELINES
Corrective Lenses

Cleaning eyeglasses is a routine care measure. Do not wait until the nurse tells you to clean them. Clean them daily and as needed.

When you need to clean eyeglasses, find out if a special cleaning solution is needed. Then follow the manufacturer's instructions.

PROMOTING SAFETY AND COMFORT
Corrective Lenses

Safety

Eyeglasses are costly. Protect them from loss or damage (Fig. 26-25). When not worn, put them in their case. Place the case in the top drawer of the bedside stand or in the drawer of the overbed table.

Some agencies let nursing assistants remove and insert contact lenses. Others do not. Know your agency's policies. If allowed to insert and remove contacts, follow the agency's procedures.

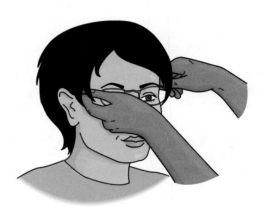

A

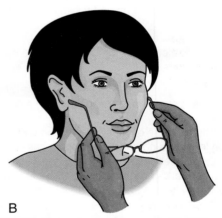

B

FIGURE 26-25 Removing eyeglasses. **A,** Hold the frames in the front of the ear on both sides. **B,** Lift the frames from the ears. Bring the glasses down away from the face.

CARDIOVASCULAR DISORDERS

Cardiovascular disorders are leading causes of death in the United States. Problems occur in the heart or blood vessels.

Hypertension

With hypertension *(high blood pressure),* the resting blood pressure is too high. The systolic pressure is 140 mm Hg (millimeters of mercury) or higher *(hyper).* Or the diastolic pressure is 90 mm Hg or higher. Such measurements must occur several times. *Pre-hypertension* is when the systolic pressure is between 120 and 139 mm Hg or the diastolic pressure is between 80 and 89 mm Hg. The person with pre-hypertension will likely develop hypertension in the future. See Box 26-12 for risk factors.

Narrowed blood vessels are a common cause. The heart pumps with more force to move blood through narrowed vessels. Kidney disorders, head injuries, some pregnancy problems, and adrenal gland tumors are causes.

Signs and symptoms develop over time. Headache, blurred vision, dizziness, and nose bleeds occur. Hypertension can lead to stroke, hardening of the arteries, heart attack, heart failure, kidney failure, and blindness.

Life-style changes can lower blood pressure. A diet low in fat and salt, a healthy weight, and regular exercise are needed. No smoking is allowed. Alcohol and caffeine are limited. Managing stress and sleeping well also lower blood pressure. Certain drugs can lower blood pressure.

Coronary Artery Disease

The coronary arteries supply the heart with blood. In coronary artery disease (CAD), the coronary arteries become hardened and narrow. One or all are affected. Therefore the heart muscle gets less blood and oxygen.

The most common cause is atherosclerosis (Fig. 26-26, p. 468). Plaque—made up of fat, cholesterol, and other substances—collects on the arterial walls. The narrowed arteries block blood flow. Blockage may be total or partial. Blood clots also can form along the plaque and block blood flow.

The major complications of CAD are angina, myocardial infarction (heart attack), irregular heartbeats, and sudden death. See Box 26-12 for risk factors.

CAD can be treated. The goals of treatment are to:
- Relieve symptoms (see "Angina," p. 468)
- Slow or stop atherosclerosis
- Lower the risk of blood clots forming
- Widen or bypass clogged arteries
- Reduce cardiac events (see "Angina" and "Myocardial Infarction," p. 469)

Persons with CAD need to make life-style changes to reduce risk factors. Drug therapy may be used to decrease the heart's workload, relieve symptoms, prevent a heart attack or sudden death, or to delay the need for procedures that open or bypass diseased arteries (Fig. 26-27, p. 468).

BOX 26-12   Risk Factors for Cardiovascular Disorders

Hypertension

Factors You *Cannot* Change
- Age—45 years or older for men; 55 years or older for women
- Gender—younger men are at greater risk than younger women; the risk increases for women after menopause
- Race—African-Americans are at greater risk than whites
- Family history—tends to run in families

Factors You *Can* Change
- Being over-weight
- Stress
- Tobacco use
- High-salt diet
- Excessive alcohol
- Lack of exercise
- Atherosclerosis
- Pre-hypertension

Coronary Artery Disease

Factors You *Cannot* Change
- Gender—men are at greater risk than women
- Age—in men, the risk increases after age 45; in women, the risk increases after age 55
- Family history
- Race—African-Americans are at greater risk than other groups

Factors You *Can* Change
- Being over-weight
- Lack of exercise
- High blood cholesterol
- Hypertension
- Smoking
- Diabetes

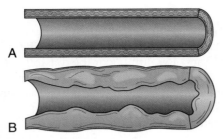

FIGURE 26-26 A, Normal artery. **B,** Plaque (fatty deposits) on the artery wall in atherosclerosis.

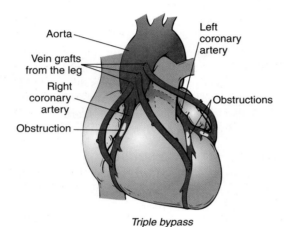

Triple bypass

FIGURE 26-27 Coronary artery bypass surgery. *(Modified from Thibodeau GA, Patton KT: The human body in health & disease, ed 5, St Louis, 2010, Mosby.)*

Angina

Angina *(pain)* is chest pain. It is from reduced blood flow to part of the heart muscle (myocardium). It occurs when the heart needs more oxygen. Normally blood flow to the heart increases when the need for oxygen increases. Exertion, a heavy meal, stress, and excitement increase the heart's need for oxygen. So does smoking and exposure to very hot or cold temperatures. In CAD, narrowed vessels prevent increased blood flow.

Chest pain is described as a tightness, pressure, squeezing, or burning in the chest (Fig. 26-28). Pain can occur in the shoulders, arms, neck, jaw, or back. Pain in the jaw, neck, and down one or both arms is common. The person may be pale, feel faint, and perspire. Dyspnea is common. Nausea, fatigue, and weakness may occur. Some persons complain of "gas" or indigestion. Rest often relieves symptoms in 3 to 15 minutes.

Besides rest, a *nitroglycerin* tablet is taken when angina occurs. It is placed under the tongue. There it dissolves and is rapidly absorbed into the bloodstream. Tablets are kept within the person's reach at all times. The person takes a tablet and then tells the nurse. Some persons have nitroglycerin patches. These are applied and removed by the nurse.

Things that cause angina are avoided. These include over-exertion, heavy meals and over-eating, and emotional stress. The person needs to stay indoors during cold weather or during hot, humid weather. Doctor-supervised exercise programs are helpful.

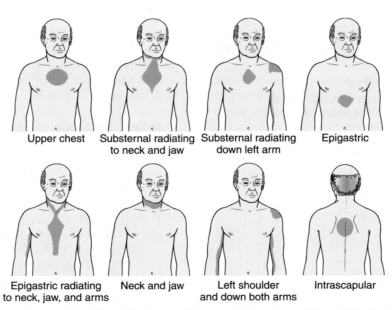

Upper chest   Substernal radiating to neck and jaw   Substernal radiating down left arm   Epigastric

Epigastric radiating to neck, jaw, and arms   Neck and jaw   Left shoulder and down both arms   Intrascapular

FIGURE 26-28 Shaded areas show where the pain of angina is located. *(From Lewis SM et al: Medical-surgical nursing: assessment and management of clinical problems, ed 7, St Louis, 2007, Mosby.)*

See "Coronary Artery Disease" (p. 467) for the treatment of angina. Increased blood flow to the heart is the goal. Doing so may prevent or lower the risk of heart attack and death. Chest pain lasting longer than a few minutes and not relieved by rest and nitroglycerin may signal a heart attack. The person needs emergency care.

Myocardial Infarction

Myocardial refers to the heart muscle. *Infarction* means tissue death. With myocardial infarction (MI), blood flow to the heart muscle is suddenly blocked. Part of the heart muscle dies. Sudden cardiac death *(sudden cardiac arrest)* can occur (Chapter 29). MI also is called *heart attack, acute myocardial infarction (AMI),* and *acute coronary syndrome (ACS).*

Signs and symptoms are listed in Box 26-13. MI is an emergency. Efforts are made to:
- Relieve pain
- Restore blood flow to the heart
- Stabilize vital signs
- Give oxygen
- Calm the person
- Prevent life-threatening problems

If the person survives, he or she may need medical or surgical procedures to open or bypass the diseased artery. Cardiac rehabilitation is needed. The goals are to:
- Recover and resume normal activities
- Prevent another MI
- Prevent complications such as heart failure or sudden cardiac arrest

---

BOX 26-13 Signs and Symptoms of Myocardial Infarction

- Chest pain
  - Sudden, severe; usually on the left side
  - Described as crushing, stabbing, or squeezing; some describe it as someone sitting on the chest
  - More severe and lasts longer than angina
  - Not relieved by rest and nitroglycerin
- Pain or numbness in one or both arms, the back, neck, jaw, or stomach
- Indigestion or "heartburn"
- Dyspnea
- Nausea
- Dizziness
- Perspiration and cold, clammy skin
- Pallor or cyanosis
- Blood pressure: low
- Pulse: weak and irregular
- Fear, apprehension, and a feeling of doom

Heart Failure

Heart failure or congestive heart failure (CHF) occurs when the heart is weakened and cannot pump normally. Blood backs up. Tissue congestion occurs.

When the left side of the heart cannot pump blood normally, blood backs up into the lungs. Respiratory congestion occurs. The person has dyspnea, increased sputum, cough, and gurgling sounds in the lungs. Also, the rest of the body does not get enough blood. Signs and symptoms occur from the effects on other organs. Poor blood flow to the brain causes confusion, dizziness, and fainting. The kidneys produce less urine. The skin is pale. Blood pressure falls.

When the right side of the heart cannot pump blood normally, blood backs up into the venous system. Feet and ankles swell. Neck veins bulge. Liver congestion affects liver function. The abdomen becomes congested with fluid. The right side of the heart pumps less blood to the lungs. Normal blood flow does not occur from the lungs to the left side of the heart. The left side has less blood to pump to the body. As with left-sided heart failure, organs receive less blood. The signs and symptoms described for left-sided failure occur.

A very severe form of heart failure is *pulmonary edema* (fluid in the lungs). It is an emergency. The person can die.

Drugs strengthen the heart. They also reduce the amount of fluid in the body. A sodium-controlled diet is ordered. Oxygen is given. Semi-Fowler's position is preferred for breathing. I&O, daily weight, elastic stockings, and range-of-motion exercises are part of the care plan.

RESPIRATORY DISORDERS

The respiratory system brings oxygen (O_2) into the lungs and removes carbon dioxide (CO_2) from the body. Respiratory disorders interfere with this function and threaten life.

Chronic Obstructive Pulmonary Disease

Two disorders are grouped under chronic obstructive pulmonary disease (COPD). They are chronic bronchitis and emphysema. These disorders affect O_2 and CO_2 exchange in the lungs. They obstruct airflow. Less air gets into the lungs; less air goes out of the lungs. Lung function is gradually lost.

Cigarette smoking is the most important risk factor. Pipe, cigar, and other smoking tobaccos are also risk factors. So is exposure to second-hand smoke. Not smoking is the best way to prevent COPD. COPD has no cure.

Chronic Bronchitis. Chronic bronchitis occurs after repeated episodes of bronchitis. Bronchitis means inflammation (*itis*) of the bronchi (*bronch*). Smoking is the major cause.

Smoker's cough in the morning is often the first symptom. At first the cough is dry. Over time, the person coughs up mucus. Mucus may contain pus. The cough becomes more frequent. The person has difficulty breathing and tires easily. Mucus and inflamed breathing passages *obstruct* airflow into the lungs. The body cannot get normal amounts of oxygen.

The person must stop smoking. Oxygen therapy and breathing exercises are often ordered. Respiratory tract infections are prevented. If one occurs, the person needs prompt treatment.

Emphysema. In emphysema, the alveoli enlarge. They become less elastic. They do not expand and shrink normally with breathing in and out. As a result, some air is trapped in the alveoli when exhaling. Trapped air is not exhaled. Over time, more alveoli are involved. O_2 and CO_2 exchange cannot occur in affected alveoli. As more air is trapped in the lungs, the person develops a *barrel chest* (Fig. 26-29).

Smoking is the most common cause. The person has shortness of breath and a cough. At first, shortness of breath occurs with exertion. Over time, it occurs at rest. Sputum may contain pus. Fatigue is common. The person works hard to breathe in and

out. And the body does not get enough oxygen. Breathing is easier in the orthopneic position (Chapter 24).

The person must stop smoking. Respiratory therapy, breathing exercises, oxygen, and drug therapy are ordered.

Asthma

In asthma, the airway becomes inflamed and narrow. Extra mucus is produced. Dyspnea results. Wheezing and coughing are common. So are pain and tightening in the chest. Symptoms are mild to severe.

Asthma usually is triggered by allergies. Other triggers include air pollutants and irritants, smoking and second-hand smoke, respiratory infections, exertion, and cold air.

Sudden attacks (*asthma attacks*) can occur. There is shortness of breath, wheezing, coughing, rapid pulse, sweating, and cyanosis. The person gasps for air and is very frightened.

Asthma is treated with drugs. Severe attacks may require emergency care.

Pneumonia

Pneumonia is an inflammation and infection of lung tissue. (*Pneumo* means lungs.) Affected tissues fill with fluid. O_2 and CO_2 exchange is affected.

Bacteria, viruses, and other microbes are causes. The person is very ill. High fever, chills, painful cough, chest pain on breathing, and rapid pulse occur. Shortness of breath and rapid breathing also occur. Cyanosis may be present. Sputum is thick and white, green, yellow, or rust-colored. Other signs and symptoms are nausea, vomiting, headache, tiredness, and muscle aches.

Drugs are ordered for infection and pain. Fluid intake is increased because of fever and to thin secretions. Thin secretions are easier to cough up. Intravenous therapy and oxygen may be needed. Semi-Fowler's position eases breathing. Rest is important. Standard Precautions are followed. Isolation precautions are used depending on the cause.

Tuberculosis

Tuberculosis (TB) is a bacterial infection in the lungs. TB is spread by airborne droplets with coughing, sneezing, speaking, singing, or laughing (Chapter 11). Nearby persons can inhale the bacteria. Those who have close, frequent contact with an infected person are at risk. TB is more likely to occur in close, crowded areas. Age, poor nutrition, and HIV (human immunodeficiency virus) infection are other risk factors.

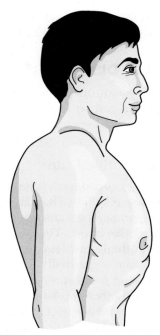

FIGURE 26-29 Barrel chest from emphysema.

TB can be present in the body but not cause signs and symptoms. An active infection may not occur for many years. Chest x-rays and TB testing can detect the disease. Signs and symptoms are tiredness, loss of appetite, weight loss, fever, and night sweats. Cough and sputum production increase over time. Sputum may contain blood. Chest pain occurs.

Drugs for TB are given. Standard Precautions and isolation precautions are needed (Chapter 11). The person must cover the mouth and nose with tissues when sneezing, coughing, or producing sputum. Tissues are flushed down the toilet, placed in a BIO-HAZARD bag, or placed in a paper bag and burned. Hand washing after contact with sputum is essential.

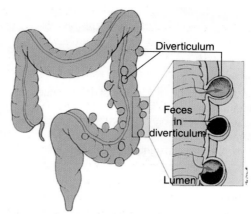

FIGURE 26-30 Diverticulosis. (*From Christensen BL, Kockrow EO: Adult health nursing, ed 5, St Louis, 2007, Mosby.*)

DIGESTIVE DISORDERS

The digestive system breaks down food so the body can absorb it. Solid wastes are eliminated. Diarrhea, constipation, flatulence, and fecal incontinence are discussed in Chapter 18. So is the care of persons with colostomies and ileostomies.

Vomiting

Vomiting means expelling stomach contents through the mouth. It signals illness or injury. **Vomitus (emesis)** is the food and fluids expelled from the stomach through the mouth. Aspirated vomitus can obstruct the airway. Vomiting large amounts of blood can lead to shock. These measures are needed:

- Follow Standard Precautions and the Bloodborne Pathogen Standard.
- Turn the person's head well to one side. This prevents aspiration.
- Place a kidney basin under the person's chin.
- Move vomitus away from the person.
- Provide oral hygiene. This helps remove the bitter taste of vomitus.
- Observe vomitus for color, odor, and undigested food. If it looks like coffee grounds, it contains undigested blood. This signals bleeding. Report your observations.
- Measure, report, and record the amount of vomitus. Also record the amount on the I&O record.
- Save a specimen for laboratory study.
- Dispose of vomitus after the nurse observes it.
- Eliminate odors.
- Provide for comfort. (See the inside of the front book cover.)

Diverticular Disease

Many people have small pouches in their colons (Fig. 26-30). Each pouch is called a *diverticulum*. (*Diverticulare* means *to turn inside out*.) The condition of having these pouches is called *diverticulosis*. (*Osis* means *condition of*.) The pouches can become infected or inflamed. This is called *diverticulitis*. (*Itis* means *inflammation*.)

About half of all people over 60 years of age have diverticulosis. A low-fiber diet and constipation are risk factors.

When feces enter the pouches, they can become inflamed and infected. The person has abdominal pain and tenderness in the lower left abdomen. Fever, nausea and vomiting, chills, cramping, and constipation are likely. Bloating, rectal bleeding, frequent urination, and pain while voiding can occur.

The doctor orders needed dietary changes. Sometimes antibiotics are ordered. Surgery is needed for severe disease, obstruction, and ruptured pouches. The diseased part of the bowel is removed. Sometimes a colostomy is necessary (Chapter 18).

Hepatitis

Hepatitis is an inflammation *(itis)* of the liver *(hepat)*. It can be mild or cause death. Signs and symptoms are listed in Box 26-14, p. 472. Some people do not have symptoms. Treatment involves rest, a healthy diet, fluids, and no alcohol. Recovery takes about 8 weeks.

Protect yourself and others. Follow Standard Precautions and the Bloodborne Pathogen Standard. Isolation precautions are ordered as necessary (Chapter 11). Assist the person with hygiene and hand washing as needed.

BOX 26-14   Signs and Symptoms of Hepatitis

- Jaundice (yellowish color of the skin or whites of the eyes)
- Fatigue, weakness
- Pain and discomfort: abdominal, joint, muscle
- Appetite: loss of
- Nausea and vomiting
- Diarrhea
- Bowel movements: light, clay-colored

- Urine: dark
- Fever
- Chills
- Headache
- Itching
- Weight loss
- Skin rash

There are five major types of hepatitis.

- *Hepatitis A* is spread by the fecal-oral route. The hepatitis A virus is ingested when eating or drinking food or water contaminated with feces. It is also ingested when eating or drinking from vessels contaminated with feces. Causes include poor sanitation, crowded living conditions, poor nutrition, and poor hygiene. Anal sex and intravenous (IV) drug abuse also are causes. Handle bedpans, feces, and rectal thermometers carefully. Good hand washing is needed by everyone, including the person.
- *Hepatitis B* is caused by the hepatitis B virus (HBV). It is present in the blood and body fluids (saliva, semen, vaginal secretions) of infected persons. It is spread by:
  - IV drug use and sharing needles
  - Accidental needle sticks
  - Sex without a condom, especially anal sex
  - Contaminated tools used for tattoos or body piercings
  - Sharing a toothbrush, razor, or nail clippers with an infected person
- *Hepatitis C* is spread by blood contaminated with the hepatitis C virus. A person may have the virus but no symptoms. Serious liver disease and damage may show up years later. Even without symptoms, the person can transmit the disease. The virus is spread by:
  - Blood contaminated with the virus
  - IV drug use and sharing needles
  - Inhaling cocaine through contaminated straws
  - Contaminated tools used for tattoos or body piercings
  - High-risk sexual activity—sex with an infected person, multiple sex partners
  - Sharing a toothbrush, razor, or nail clippers with an infected person
- *Hepatitis D* occurs only in people infected with hepatitis B. It is spread the same way as HBV.
- *Hepatitis E* is spread through food or water contaminated by feces from an infected person. It is spread by the fecal-oral route. This disease is not common in the United States.

URINARY SYSTEM DISORDERS

The kidneys, ureters, bladder, and urethra are the major urinary system structures. Disorders can occur in these structures.

- *Urinary tract infection (UTI).* UTIs are common. Microbes can enter the system through the urethra. Catheters, poor perineal hygiene, immobility, and poor fluid intake are common causes. UTI is a common healthcare-associated infection (Chapter 11).
  - *Cystitis* is a bladder *(cyst)* infection *(itis)*. Urinary frequency, urgency, pain or burning on urination, foul-smelling urine, blood or pus in the urine, and fever may occur. Antibiotics are ordered. Fluids are encouraged. If untreated, cystitis can lead to pyelonephritis.
  - *Pyelonephritis* is inflammation *(itis)* of the kidney *(nephr)* pelvis *(pyelo)*. Cloudy urine may contain pus, mucus, and blood. Chills, fever, back pain, and nausea and vomiting occur. So do the signs and symptoms of cystitis. Treatment involves antibiotics and fluids.
- *Renal calculi.* These are kidney *(renal)* stones *(calculi)*. Bedrest, immobility, and poor fluid intake are risk factors. Stones vary in size (Fig. 26-31). Some are as small as grains of sand; some are as big as golf balls. Signs and symptoms are listed in Box 26-15. Drugs are given for pain relief. The person needs to drink 2000 to 3000 mL (milliliters) of fluid a day. Increased fluids help stones pass from the body through the urine. All urine is strained. Surgical removal of the stone may be necessary. Some dietary changes can prevent stones.
- *Renal failure.* The kidneys do not function or are severely impaired. Waste products are not removed from the blood. The body retains fluid. Heart failure and hypertension easily result. Renal failure may be acute or chronic. The person is very ill.

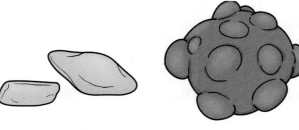

Smooth   Golf-ball-sized and brown

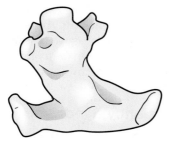 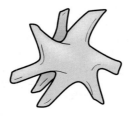

Staghorn   Jagged and yellow

FIGURE 26-31 Kidney stones.

BOX 26-15	**Signs and Symptoms of Renal Calculi**

- Severe, cramping pain in the back and side just below the ribs
- Pain in the abdomen, thigh, and urethra
- Nausea and vomiting
- Fever and chills
- Dysuria—difficult or painful *(dys)* urination *(uria)*
- Urinary frequency
- Urinary urgency
- Burning on urination
- Oliguria—scant *(olig)* urine *(uria)*
- Hematuria—blood *(hemat)* in the urine *(uria)*
- Cloudy urine
- Foul-smelling urine

Prostate Enlargement

The prostate is a gland in men. It lies in front of the rectum and just below the bladder (Chapter 6). The prostate also surrounds the urethra. In young men, the prostate is about the size of a walnut. The prostate grows larger (enlarges) as the man grows older. This is called benign prostatic hyperplasia (BPH). (*Benign* means non-malignant. *Hyper* means excessive. *Plasia* means formation or development.) Most men older than 60 have some symptoms of BPH.

The enlarged prostate presses against the urethra. This obstructs urine flow through the urethra. Bladder function is gradually lost. These problems are common:
- A weak urine stream
- Frequent voidings of small amounts of urine
- Urgency and leaking or dribbling of urine
- Frequent urination at night
- Urinary retention (The man cannot void. Urine remains in the bladder.)

The doctor may order drugs to shrink the prostate or stop its growth. Some microwave and laser treatments destroy the excess prostate tissue. Or surgery is done to remove tissue.

REPRODUCTIVE DISORDERS

Aging affects the structures and functions of the reproductive system. Many injuries, diseases, and surgeries can affect reproductive structures and functions.

Sexually Transmitted Diseases

A sexually transmitted disease (STD) is spread by oral, vaginal, or anal sex. Some people do not have signs and symptoms or are not aware of an infection. Others know but do not seek treatment because of embarrassment.

STDs often occur in the genital and rectal areas. They also occur in the ears, mouth, nipples, throat, tongue, eyes, and nose. Using condoms helps prevent the spread of STDs, especially HIV and AIDS (p. 474). Some STDs are also spread through skin breaks, by contact with infected body fluids (blood, semen, saliva), or by contaminated blood or needles.

Standard Precautions and the Bloodborne Pathogen Standard are followed.

ENDOCRINE DISORDERS

The endocrine system is made up of glands. The endocrine glands secrete hormones that affect other organs and glands. Diabetes is the most common endocrine disorder.

Diabetes

In this disorder the body cannot produce or use insulin properly. Insulin is needed for glucose to move from the blood into the cells. The pancreas secretes insulin. Without enough insulin, sugar builds up in the blood. Blood glucose (sugar) is high. Cells do not have enough sugar for energy and cannot function.

Signs and symptoms of diabetes are:
- Being very thirsty
- Urinating often
- Feeling very hungry or tired
- Losing weight without trying
- Having sores that heal slowly
- Having dry, itchy skin
- Tingling or loss of feeling in the feet
- Blurred vision

The three types of diabetes are:
- *Type 1*—occurs most often in children, teenagers, and young adults. The pancreas produces little or no insulin. Onset is rapid.
- *Type 2*—can occur at any age, even during childhood. Persons over 45 years of age are at risk. Being over-weight, lack of exercise, and hypertension are risk factors. The pancreas secretes insulin. However, the body cannot use it well. Onset is slow. Infections are frequent. Wounds heal slowly. Gum disease (Chapter 15) is common.
- *Gestational diabetes*—develops during pregnancy. (Gestation comes from *gestare*. It means to *bear*.) It usually goes away after the baby is born. However, the mother is at risk for type 2 diabetes later in life.

Diabetes must be controlled to prevent complications. They include blindness, renal failure, nerve damage, and damage to the gums and teeth. Heart and blood vessel diseases are very serious problems. They can lead to stroke, heart attack, and slow healing. Foot and leg wounds and ulcers are very serious (Chapter 23). Infection and gangrene can occur. Sometimes amputation is necessary.

Risk factors include a family history of the disease. For type 1, whites are at greater risk than non-whites. Type 2 is more common in older and over-weight persons. African-Americans, Native Americans, and Hispanics are at risk for type 2.

Type 1 is treated with daily insulin therapy, healthy eating (Chapter 19), and exercise. Type 2 is treated with healthy eating and exercise. Many persons with type 2 take oral drugs. Some need insulin. Over-weight persons need to lose weight. Types 1 and 2 involve controlling blood pressure, cholesterol, and the risk factors for CAD.

Good foot care is needed. Corns, blisters, calluses, and other foot problems can lead to an infection and amputation.

The person's blood sugar level can fall too low or go too high. Blood glucose is monitored daily or 3 or 4 times a day for:
- *Hypoglycemia* means low (*hypo*) sugar (*glyc*) in the blood (*emia*).
- *Hyperglycemia* means high (*hyper*) sugar (*glyc*) in the blood (*emia*).

See Table 26-1 for the causes, signs, and symptoms of hypoglycemia and hyperglycemia. Both can lead to death if not corrected. You must call for the nurse at once.

IMMUNE SYSTEM DISORDERS

The immune system protects the body from microbes, cancer cells, and other harmful substances. The immune system defends against threats inside and outside the body.

Immune system disorders occur when there is a problem with the immune response. The response may be inappropriate, too strong, or lacking. *Autoimmune disorders* can occur. The immune system can cause disease by attacking the body's own (*auto*) normal cells, tissues, or organs. Most autoimmune disorders are chronic.

Acquired Immunodeficiency Syndrome

Acquired immunodeficiency syndrome (AIDS) is caused by a virus. The virus is called the *human immunodeficiency virus (HIV)*. It attacks the immune system. Therefore it destroys the body's ability to fight infections and certain cancers. Some infections are life-threatening.

The virus is spread through body fluids—blood, semen, vaginal secretions, and breast milk. HIV is not spread by saliva, tears, sweat, sneezing, coughing, insects, or casual contact. The virus is transmitted mainly by:
- Unprotected anal, vaginal, or oral sex with an infected person ("Unprotected" is without a new latex or polyurethane condom.)
- Needle and syringe sharing among IV drug users
- HIV-infected mothers before or during childbirth
- HIV-infected mothers through breast-feeding

Box 26-16 lists the signs and symptoms of AIDS. Some persons infected with HIV have symptoms within a few months. Others are symptom-free for more than 10 years. However, they carry the virus. They can spread it to others.

Persons with AIDS are at risk for pneumonia, TB, and Kaposi's sarcoma (a cancer). Memory loss, loss of coordination, paralysis, mental health disorders, and dementia signal nervous system damage.

Many new drugs help slow the spread of HIV in the body. They also reduce complications and prolong life. AIDS has no vaccine and no cure at present. It is a life-threatening disease.

You may care for persons with AIDS or those who are HIV carriers (Box 26-17, p. 476). Protect yourself and others from the virus. Follow Standard Precautions and the Bloodborne Pathogen Standard. A

TABLE 26-1   Hypoglycemia and Hyperglycemia

	Causes	Signs and Symptoms
Hypoglycemia (low blood sugar)	Too much insulin or diabetic drugs Omitting or missing a meal Delayed meal Eating too little food Increased exercise Vomiting Drinking alcohol	Hunger Fatigue; weakness Trembling; shakiness Sweating Headache Dizziness Faintness Pulse: rapid Blood pressure: low Respirations: rapid and shallow Motions: clumsy and jerky Tingling around the mouth Confusion Vision: changes in Skin: cold and clammy Convulsions Unconsciousness
Hyperglycemia (high blood sugar)	Undiagnosed diabetes Not enough insulin or diabetic drugs Eating too much food Too little exercise Emotional stress Infection or sickness	Weakness Drowsiness Thirst Dry mouth (very) Hunger Urination: frequent Leg cramps Face: flushed Breath odor: sweet Respirations: rapid, deep, and labored Pulse: rapid, weak Blood pressure: low Skin: dry Vision: blurred Headache Nausea and vomiting Convulsions Coma

BOX 26-16   Signs and Symptoms of AIDS

- Appetite: loss of
- Cough
- Depression
- Diarrhea lasting more than a week
- Energy: lack of
- Fever
- Headache
- Memory loss, confusion, and forgetfulness
- Mouth or tongue:
  - Brown, red, pink, or purple spots or blotches
  - Sores or white patches
- Night sweats
- Pneumonia

- Shortness of breath
- Skin:
  - Rashes or flaky skin
  - Brown, red, pink, or purple spots or blotches on the skin, eyelids, or nose
- Swallowing: painful or difficult
- Swollen glands: neck, underarms, and groin
- Tiredness: may be extreme
- Vision loss
- Weight loss

person may have the HIV virus but no symptoms. In some persons, HIV or AIDS is not yet diagnosed.

Persons 45 years old and older also get AIDS. They get and spread HIV through sexual contact and IV drug use. Aging and some diseases can mask the signs and symptoms of AIDS. Older persons are less likely to be tested for HIV/AIDS. Often the person dies without the disease being diagnosed.

BOX 26-17   Caring for the Person With AIDS

- Practice Standard Precautions.
- Follow the Bloodborne Pathogen Standard.
- Provide daily hygiene. Avoid irritating soaps.
- Provide oral hygiene according to the care plan. A toothbrush with soft bristles is best.
- Provide oral fluids as ordered.
- Measure and record intake and output.
- Measure weight daily.
- Encourage deep-breathing and coughing exercises as ordered.
- Prevent pressure ulcers.
- Assist with range-of-motion exercises and ambulation as ordered.
- Encourage self-care as able. The person may need assistive devices (walker, commode, eating devices).
- Encourage the person to be as active as possible.
- Change linens and garments as often as needed when fever or night sweats are present.
- Be a good listener. Provide emotional support.

Focus on P R I D E
The Person, Family, and Yourself

Personal and Professional Responsibility—A basic understanding of common health problems is a professional responsibility. This knowledge allows you to safely assist with care. Only the common health problems were presented in this chapter. And only basic information was given.

You may want to know more about a health problem. Or a person may have a disorder not discussed in this chapter. Ask the nurse to explain the problem and the care required. Also look up the problem in a medical dictionary. Take pride in seeking to know more. Learning produces personal and professional rewards.

Rights and Respect—Some disorders, accidents, and injuries result from life-style choices. Poor diet, lack of exercise, and alcohol and drug abuse are examples. Whatever the cause or contributing factors, do not judge the person or the person's actions. Always treat the person with dignity and respect.

Independence and Social Interaction—Many persons require rehabilitation after illness, injury, or surgery. For example, persons often need physical, occupational, and speech therapy after a stroke. The goal is for the person to function at his or her highest possible level. Independence improves the person's quality of life. Follow the rehabilitation plan (Chapter 25).

Delegation and Teamwork—A person's condition can change very quickly. A person with angina may have an MI. A person with hypertension may have a stroke. A person may develop complications after surgery. Sudden changes in a person's condition require the nurse's attention. You may need to assist the nurse. Help as the nurse directs. Or you may need to help with other patients or residents. Always help willingly. The entire nursing team may need to make that "extra effort" to meet patient and resident needs.

Ethics and Laws—You must protect the person's privacy and confidentiality. This is required by the Omnibus Budget Reconciliation Act of 1987 (OBRA) and the Health Insurance Portability and Accountability Act of 1996 (HIPAA). See Chapter 2.

A patient or resident may be your family member or friend. If you are not involved in that person's care, you have no right to information about that person. Or friends or family members may ask you about patients and residents whom they know. You cannot share information with them. Simply say: "I'm sorry. I cannot tell you. That would be unprofessional, illegal, and unethical conduct." Take pride in protecting the privacy of others.

REVIEW QUESTIONS

Circle the BEST answer.

1 Which is *not* a warning sign of cancer?
   a Painful, swollen joints
   b A sore that does not heal
   c Unusual bleeding or discharge
   d Discomfort after eating
2 A person receiving chemotherapy will likely experience
   a Diarrhea   c Skin breakdown
   b Burns   d Weight gain
3 A person has arthritis. Care includes the following *except*
   a Preventing contractures
   b Range-of-motion exercises
   c A cast or traction
   d Assisting with ADL
4 A person had hip replacement surgery. Which measure should you question?
   a Provide a chair with a low seat.
   b Do not cross the legs.
   c Keep a hip abduction wedge between the legs.
   d Provide a long-handled brush for bathing.
5 A person with osteoporosis is at risk for
   a Fractures   c Phantom limb pain
   b An amputation   d Paralysis
6 A cast needs to dry. Which is *false?*
   a The cast is covered with blankets and plastic.
   b The person is turned so the cast dries evenly.
   c The entire cast is supported with pillows.
   d The cast is supported by the palms when lifted.
7 A person is in traction. You should do the following *except*
   a Perform range-of-motion exercises as directed
   b Keep the weights off the floor
   c Remove the weights if the person is uncomfortable
   d Give skin care at frequent intervals
8 After a hip pinning, the operated leg is
   a Abducted at all times
   b Adducted at all times
   c Externally rotated at all times
   d Flexed at all times
9 A person has aphasia. You know that
   a The person cannot use the muscles of speech
   b Mouth and face muscles are affected
   c The person has a language disorder
   d The person cannot speak
10 A person had a stroke. Which measure should you question?
   a Semi-Fowler's position
   b Range-of-motion exercises every 2 hours
   c Turn, reposition, and skin care every 2 hours
   d Bed in the highest horizontal position

11 A person has Parkinson's disease. Which is *false?*
   a The part of the brain controlling muscle movements is affected.
   b Mental function is affected first.
   c Tremors, slow movements, and a shuffling gait occur.
   d The person needs protection from injury.
12 A person has multiple sclerosis. Which is *false?*
   a There is no cure.
   b Only voluntary muscles are affected.
   c Symptoms begin in young adulthood.
   d Over time, the person depends on others for care.
13 A person has quadriplegia following a spinal cord injury. Which care measure should you question?
   a Keep the bed in the low position.
   b Assist with active range-of-motion exercises.
   c Follow the bowel training program.
   d Turn and reposition every hour.
14 You are talking to a person with hearing loss. You can do the following *except*
   a State the topic
   b Change the subject if the person does not seem to understand
   c Use short sentences and simple words
   d Write out key words and names
15 A person's hearing aid does not seem to be working. Your *first* action is to
   a See if it is turned on
   b Wash it with soap and water
   c Have it repaired
   d Remove the batteries
16 A person has a cataract. Which is *false?*
   a Vision is cloudy, blurry, or dimmed.
   b Colors seem faded.
   c Central vision is lost.
   d The person is sensitive to light and glares.
17 A person is not wearing eyeglasses. They should be
   a Soaked in a cleansing solution
   b Kept within the person's reach
   c Put in the eyeglass case
   d Placed on the overbed table
18 Which presents dangers to persons who are blind or visually impaired?
   a Drawers that are fully closed
   b Doors that are fully open
   c Burnt out bulbs
   d Night-lights

Continued

19 A person is blind. You should do the following *except*

  a Identify yourself

  b Assume that the person has no sight

  c Explain procedures step by step

  d Have the person walk behind you

20 A person has hypertension. You know that the person's systolic blood pressure is

  a Over 140 mm Hg   c Over 90 mm Hg

  b Over 120 mm Hg   d Over 80 mm Hg

21 A person has hypertension. Treatment will likely include the following *except*

  a No smoking and regular exercise

  b A high-sodium diet

  c A low-calorie diet if the person is obese

  d Drugs to lower blood pressure

22 A person has angina. Which is *true?*

  a There is heart muscle damage.

  b Pain is described as crushing, stabbing, or squeezing.

  c Pain is relieved with rest and nitroglycerin.

  d Pain is always on the left side of the chest.

23 A person is having a myocardial infarction. Which is *false?*

  a The person is having a heart attack.

  b This is an emergency.

  c The person may have a cardiac arrest.

  d The person does not have enough blood to provide needed oxygen.

24 A person has heart failure. Which measure should you question?

  a Encourage fluids.

  b Measure I&O.

  c Measure weight daily.

  d Perform range-of-motion exercises.

25 The most common cause of COPD is

  a Smoking   c Being over-weight

  b Allergies   d A high-sodium diet

26 A person has emphysema. Which is *false?*

  a The person has dyspnea.

  b The person has an infection.

  c Breathing is usually easier sitting upright and slightly forward.

  d Sputum may contain pus.

27 Which position is usually best for the person with pneumonia?

  a Supine

  b Prone

  c Semi-Fowler's

  d Trendelenburg's

28 Tuberculosis is spread by

  a Coughing and sneezing

  b Contaminated drinking water

  c Contact with wound drainage

  d The fecal-oral route

29 A person has TB. You had contact with the person's sputum. What should you do?

  a Wash your hands.

  b Put on gloves.

  c Use an alcohol-based hand rub.

  d Tell the nurse.

30 A person is vomiting. How should you position the person?

  a Supine   c Semi-Fowler's

  b Prone   d With the head turned to the side

31 Hepatitis is an inflammation of the

  a Liver   c Pancreas

  b Gallbladder   d Stomach

32 Hepatitis A is spread by

  a Needle sharing   c Contaminated blood

  b IV drug use   d The fecal-oral route

33 Hepatitis requires

  a Sterile gloves   c Standard Precautions

  b Double-bagging   d Masks, gowns, and goggles

34 A person has cystitis. This is a

  a Kidney infection   c Failing kidney

  b Kidney stone   d Bladder infection

35 Benign prostatic hyperplasia causes urinary problems because

  a The person has a weak urine stream

  b The person voids frequently at night

  c The enlarged prostate presses against the urethra

  d Voidings are in small amounts

36 These statements are about STDs. Which is *false?*

  a They are usually spread by sexual contact.

  b They can affect the genital area and other body parts.

  c Signs and symptoms are obvious.

  d Standard Precautions are needed.

37 A person with diabetes needs the following *except*

  a Exercise   c A sodium-controlled diet

  b Good foot care   d Healthy eating

38 A person with diabetes is vomiting after a meal. The person is at risk for

  a Hypoglycemia   c Jaundice

  b Hyperglycemia   d Bleeding

39 HIV is spread through

  a Body fluids

  b Coughing and sneezing

  c Using public telephones and restrooms

  d Hugging or dancing with an infected person

40 Which of the following is used to prevent the spread of HIV and AIDS?

  a Isolation precautions   c Chemotherapy

  b Radiation therapy   d Standard Precautions

Answers to these questions are on p. 528.

27

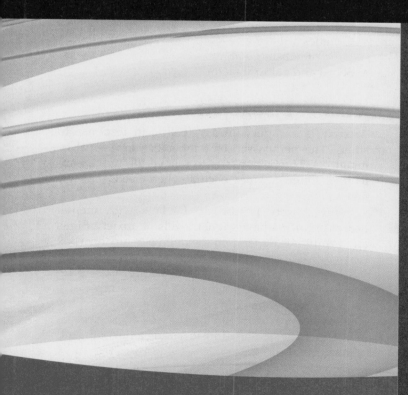

CARING FOR PERSONS WITH MENTAL HEALTH PROBLEMS

OBJECTIVES

- Define the key terms and key abbreviation listed in this chapter.
- Explain the difference between mental health and mental illness.
- List the causes of mental illness.
- Describe four anxiety disorders.
- Explain the defense mechanisms used to relieve anxiety.
- Explain schizophrenia.
- Describe bipolar disorder and depression.
- Describe personality disorders.
- Describe substance abuse.
- Describe suicide and the persons at risk.
- Describe the care required by persons with mental health disorders.
- Explain how to promote PRIDE in the person, the family, and yourself.

KEY TERMS

anxiety A vague, uneasy feeling in response to stress

compulsion Repeating an act over and over again

defense mechanism An unconscious reaction that blocks unpleasant or threatening feelings

delusion A false belief

delusion of grandeur An exaggerated belief about one's importance, wealth, power, or talents

delusion of persecution A false belief that one is being mistreated, abused, or harassed

flashback Reliving the trauma in thoughts during the day and in nightmares during sleep

hallucination Seeing, hearing, smelling, or feeling something that is not real

mental Relating to the mind; something that exists in the mind or is done by the mind

mental health The person copes with and adjusts to everyday stresses in ways accepted by society

mental illness A disturbance in the ability to cope with or adjust to stress; behavior and function are impaired; mental disorder, emotional illness, psychiatric disorder

obsession A recurrent, unwanted thought, idea, or image

panic An intense and sudden feeling of fear, anxiety, terror, or dread

paranoia A disorder (*para*) of the mind (*noia*); false beliefs (delusions) and suspicion about a person or situation

phobia An intense fear

psychosis A state of severe mental impairment

stress The response or change in the body caused by any emotional, physical, social, or economic factor

suicide To kill oneself

suicide contagion Exposure to suicide or suicidal behaviors within one's family, one's peer group, or media reports of suicide

withdrawal syndrome The person's physical and mental response after stopping or severely reducing the use of a substance that was used regularly

KEY ABBREVIATION

PTSD Post-traumatic stress disorder

The whole person has physical, social, psychological, and spiritual parts. Each part affects the other.

- A physical problem has social, mental, and spiritual effects.
- A mental health problem can affect the person physically, socially, and spiritually.
- A social problem can have physical, mental health, and spiritual effects.

Mental relates to the mind. It is something that exists in the mind or is done by the mind. Therefore mental health involves the mind. Mental health and mental illness involve stress:

- **Stress**—is the response or change in the body caused by any emotional, physical, social, or economic factor.
- **Mental health**—means that the person copes with and adjusts to everyday stresses in ways accepted by society.
- **Mental illness**—is a disturbance in the ability to cope with or adjust to stress. Behavior and function are impaired. *Mental disorder, emotional illness,* and *psychiatric disorder* also mean mental illness.

Causes of mental health disorders include:

- Not being able to cope or adjust to stress
- Chemical imbalances
- Genetics
- Drug or substance abuse
- Social and cultural factors

ANXIETY DISORDERS

Anxiety is a vague, uneasy feeling in response to stress. The person senses danger or harm—real or imagined. The person acts to relieve the unpleasant feeling. Often anxiety occurs when needs are not met.

Some anxiety is normal. Persons with mental health problems have higher levels of anxiety. Signs and symptoms depend on the degree of anxiety (Box 27-1).

Coping and defense mechanisms are used to relieve anxiety. Some are healthy. Others are not—eating, drinking, smoking, and fighting are examples. Healthy ways to cope include discussing the problem, exercising, playing music, taking a hot bath, and wanting to be alone.

Defense mechanisms are unconscious reactions that block unpleasant or threatening feelings (Box 27-2). Some use of defense mechanisms is normal. With mental health problems, they are used poorly.

BOX 27-1   Signs and Symptoms of Anxiety

- A "lump" in the throat
- "Butterflies" in the stomach
- Pulse: rapid
- Respirations: rapid
- Blood pressure: increased
- Speech: rapid, voice changes
- Mouth: dry
- Sweating

- Nausea
- Diarrhea
- Urinary frequency and urgency
- Attention span: poor
- Directions: difficulty following
- Sleep: difficulty
- Appetite: loss of

BOX 27-2   Defense Mechanisms

Compensation. *Compensate* means to make up for, replace, or substitute. The person makes up for or substitutes a strength for a weakness.
EXAMPLE: Not good in sports, a child develops another talent.

Conversion. *Convert* means to change. An emotion is shown as a physical symptom or changed into a physical symptom.
EXAMPLE: Not wanting to read out loud in school, a child complains of a headache.

Denial. *Deny* means refusing to accept or believe something that is true. The person refuses to face or accept unpleasant or threatening things.
EXAMPLE: After a heart attack, a person continues to smoke.

Displacement. *Displace* means to move or take the place of. An individual moves behaviors or emotions from one person, place, or thing to a safe person, place, or thing.
EXAMPLE: Angry at your boss, you yell at a friend.

Identification. *Identify* means to relate or recognize. A person assumes the ideas, behaviors, and traits of another person.
EXAMPLE: A neighbor is a high school cheerleader. A little girl practices cheerleading in her backyard.

Projection. *Project* means to blame another. An individual blames another person or object for unacceptable behaviors, emotions, ideas, or wishes.
EXAMPLE: Sleeping too long, a worker blames the traffic when late for work.

Rationalization. *Rational* means sensible, reasonable, or logical. An acceptable reason or excuse is given for behaviors or actions. The real reason is not given.
EXAMPLE: Often late for work, an employee does not get a raise. The employee thinks "My boss doesn't like me."

Reaction formation. A person acts in a way opposite to what he or she truly feels.
EXAMPLE: A worker does not like his boss. He buys the boss an expensive gift.

Regression. *Regress* means to move back or to retreat. The person retreats or moves back to an earlier time or condition.
EXAMPLE: A 3-year-old wants a baby bottle when a new baby comes into the family.

Repression. *Repress* means to hold down or keep back. The person keeps unpleasant or painful thoughts or experiences from the conscious mind. They cannot be recalled or remembered.
EXAMPLE: A child was sexually abused. Now 33 years old, there is no memory of the event.

Some common anxiety disorders are:

- *Panic disorder.* **Panic** is an intense and sudden feeling of fear, anxiety, terror, or dread. Onset is sudden with no obvious reason. The person cannot function. Signs and symptoms of anxiety are severe. The person may feel that he or she is having a heart attack, losing his or her mind, or on the verge of death. Attacks can occur at any time, even during sleep. *Panic attacks* can last for 10 minutes or longer.
- *Phobias.* **Phobia** means an intense fear. The person has an intense fear of an object, situation, or activity that has little or no actual danger. The person avoids what is feared. When faced with the fear, the person has high anxiety and cannot function. Common phobias are fear of:
  - Being in an open, crowded, or public place (agoraphobia—*agora* means marketplace)
  - Water (aquaphobia—*aqua* means water)
  - Being in or being trapped in an enclosed or narrow space (claustrophobia—*claustro* means closing)
  - The slightest uncleanliness (mysophobia—*myso* means anything that is disgusting)
- *Obsessive-compulsive disorder (OCD).* An **obsession** is a recurrent, unwanted thought, idea, or image. **Compulsion** is repeating an act over and over again (a ritual). The act may not make sense. However, the person has much anxiety if the act is not done. Common rituals are hand washing, cleaning, and counting things to a certain number. Such activities can take over an hour every day. They are very distressing and affect daily life.
- *Post-traumatic stress disorder (PTSD).* PTSD occurs after a terrifying ordeal. It involved physical harm or the threat of physical harm. See Box 27-3 for signs and symptoms. PTSD can result from many traumatic events. They include war, a terrorist attack, rape, torture, child abuse, a crash (vehicle, train, plane), a natural disaster (flood, tornado, hurricane), and so on. Flashbacks are common. A **flashback** is reliving the trauma in thoughts during the day and in nightmares during sleep. During a flashback, the person may lose touch with reality. He or she may believe that the trauma is happening all over again. Signs and symptoms usually develop about 3 months after the harmful event. Or they may emerge years later. Some people recover within 6 months. PTSD lasts longer in other people and may become chronic. PTSD can develop at any age.

SCHIZOPHRENIA

Schizophrenia means split *(schizo)* mind *(phrenia).* It is a severe, chronic, disabling brain disorder. It involves:

- **Psychosis**—a state of severe mental impairment. The person does not view the real or unreal correctly.
- **Delusion**—a false belief. For example, the person believes that a radio station is broadcasting the person's thoughts.
- **Hallucination**—seeing, hearing, smelling, or feeling something that is not real. A person may see animals, insects, or people that are not real. "Voices" are the most common type of hallucination in schizophrenia. "Voices" may comment on behavior, order the person to do things, warn of danger, or talk to other voices.
- **Paranoia**—a disorder *(para)* of the mind *(noia).* The person has false beliefs (delusions). He or she is suspicious about a person or situation. For example, a person may believe that others are cheating, harassing, poisoning, spying upon, or plotting against him or her.
- **Delusion of grandeur**—an exaggerated belief about one's importance, wealth, power, or talents. For example, a man believes he is Superman. Or a woman believes she is the Queen of England.
- **Delusion of persecution**—the false belief that one is being mistreated, abused, or harassed. For example, a person believes that someone is "out to get" him or her.

Thinking and behavior are disturbed. The person has problems relating to others. He or she may be paranoid. Responses are inappropriate. Communication is disturbed. The person may ramble or repeat what another says. Sometimes speech is not understood. He or she may make up words. The person may withdraw and lacks interest in others. He or she is not involved with people or society.

Disorders of movement occur. These include:

- Being clumsy and uncoordinated
- Involuntary movements
- Grimacing
- Unusual mannerisms
- Sitting for hours without moving, speaking, or responding

Some persons regress. To *regress* means to retreat or move back to an earlier time or condition. For example, an adult may act like an infant or child.

In men, the symptoms usually begin in the late teens or early 20s. In women, symptoms usually begin in the mid-20s and early 30s. People with schizophrenia do not tend to be violent. However, if a

BOX 27-3 Signs and Symptoms of Post-Traumatic Stress Disorder

- Startles easily
- Emotionally numb—especially to those with whom the person used to be close
- Difficulty trusting people
- Difficulty feeling close to people
- Loss of interest in things he or she used to enjoy
- Problems being affectionate
- Feelings of intense guilt
- Irritability
- Avoiding situations that are reminders of the harmful event
- Difficulty around the anniversary of the harmful event

- Gets mad easily
- Outbursts of anger
- Problems sleeping
- Increasingly aggressive
- Becoming more violent
- Physical symptoms:
  - Headache
  - Gastro-intestinal distress
  - Immune system problems
  - Dizziness
  - Chest pain
  - Discomfort in other body parts

BOX 27-4 Signs and Symptoms of Bipolar Disorder

Mania (Manic Episode)

- Increased energy, activity, and restlessness
- Excessively "high," overly good mood
- Extreme irritability
- Racing thoughts and talking very fast
- Jumping from one idea to another
- Easily distracted; problems concentrating
- Little sleep needed
- Unrealistic beliefs in one's abilities and powers
- Poor judgment
- Spending sprees
- A lasting period of behavior that is different from usual
- Increased sexual drive
- Drug abuse (particularly cocaine, alcohol, and sleeping pills)
- Aggressive behavior
- Denial that anything is wrong

Depression (Depressive Episode)

- Lasting sad, anxious, or empty mood
- Feelings of hopelessness
- Feelings of guilt, worthlessness, or helplessness
- Loss of interest or pleasure in activities once enjoyed
- Loss of interest in sex
- Decreased energy; a feeling of fatigue or being "slowed down"
- Problems concentrating, remembering, or making decisions
- Restlessness or irritability
- Sleeping too much, or unable to sleep
- Change in appetite
- Unintended weight loss or gain
- Chronic pain or other symptoms not caused by physical illness or injury
- Thoughts of death or suicide
- Suicide attempts

person with paranoid schizophrenia becomes violent, it is often directed at family members. Some persons with schizophrenia attempt suicide (p. 485).

See *Focus on Communication: Schizophrenia.*

MOOD DISORDERS

Mood relates to feelings and emotions. Mood disorders involve feelings, emotions, and moods. Two common mood disorders are bipolar disorder and major depression.

Bipolar Disorder

Bipolar means two (*bi*) poles or ends (*polar*). The person with bipolar disorder has severe extremes in mood, energy, and ability to function (Box 27-4).

FOCUS ON COMMUNICATION
Schizophrenia

Delusions, hallucinations, and paranoia can frighten a person. Good communication is important. Remember to:

- Speak slowly and calmly.
- Do not pretend you experience what the person does. Help the person focus on reality.
- Do not try to convince the person that the experience is not real. To the person, it is real. For example, a person is hearing voices. You can say: "I don't hear the voices, but I believe that you do. Try to listen to my voice and not the other voices."

There are emotional lows (*depression*) and emotional highs (*mania*). The disorder also is called manic-depressive illness. The disorder tends to run in families. It usually develops in the late teens or in early adulthood. The disorder requires life-long management. Signs and symptoms can range from mild to severe. Some people are suicidal.

Major Depression

Depression involves the body, mood, and thoughts (see Box 27-4). The person is very sad. He or she loses interest in daily activities. Body functions are depressed. Depression may occur because of a stressful event such as the death of a partner, parent, or child. Divorce and job loss are other stressful events. Some physical disorders can cause depression. Stroke, myocardial infarction (heart attack), and cancer are examples. Hormonal factors may cause depression in women—menstrual cycle changes, pregnancy, miscarriage, after birth (post-partum depression), and before and during menopause.

Depression in Older Persons. Depression is common in older persons. They have many losses—death of family and friends, loss of health, loss of body functions, loss of independence. Loneliness and the side effects of some drugs also are causes. See Box 27-5 for the signs and symptoms of depression in older persons. Depression in older persons is often overlooked or a wrong diagnosis is made. Often the person is thought to have a cognitive disorder (Chapter 28). Therefore depression is often not treated.

PERSONALITY DISORDERS

Personality disorders involve rigid and maladaptive behaviors. To *adapt* means to change or adjust. *Mal* means bad, wrong, or ill. *Maladaptive* means to change or adjust in the wrong way. Because of their behaviors, those with personality disorders cannot function well in society. Personality disorders include:

- *Antisocial personality disorder.* The person has poor judgment. He or she lacks responsibility and is hostile. The person is not loyal to any person or group. Morals and ethics are lacking. The person lies or cons others for personal gain or pleasure. Others are blamed for actions and behaviors. The rights of others do not matter. The person has no guilt. He or she does not learn from experiences or punishment. The person is often in trouble with the police.

BOX 27-5	Signs and Symptoms of Depression in Older Persons

- Fatigue and lack of interest
- Inability to experience pleasure
- Feelings of uselessness, hopelessness, and helplessness
- Decreased sexual interest
- Increased dependency
- Anxiety
- Slow or unreliable memory
- Paranoia
- Agitation
- Focus on the past
- Thoughts of death and suicide
- Difficulty completing activities of daily living
- Changes in sleep patterns
- Poor grooming
- Withdrawal from people and interests
- Muscle aches, abdominal pain, and headaches
- Nausea and vomiting
- Dry mouth
- Loss of appetite and weight loss

- *Borderline personality disorder (BPD).* The person has problems with moods, interpersonal relationships, self-image, and behavior. The person has intense bouts of anger, depression, and anxiety. Aggression, self-injury, and drug or alcohol abuse may occur. The person may greatly admire and love family and friends and then suddenly shift to intense anger and dislike.

SUBSTANCE ABUSE AND ADDICTION

Substance abuse or addiction occurs when a person overuses or depends on alcohol or drugs. The person's physical and mental health are affected. The welfare of others is affected too.

Substances involved in abuse and addiction affect the nervous system. Some depress the nervous system. Others stimulate it. All affect the mind and thinking.

Alcoholism

Alcohol slows down brain activity. It affects alertness, judgment, coordination, and reaction time. Over time, heavy drinking damages the brain, central nervous system, liver, heart, blood vessels, kidneys, and stomach. It also can cause forgetfulness and confusion.

Alcoholism includes these symptoms:

- *Craving.* The person has a strong need or urge to drink.
- *Loss of control.* The person cannot stop drinking once drinking has begun.
- *Physical dependence.* The person has withdrawal symptoms when he or she stops drinking. They include nausea, sweating, shakiness, and anxiety.
- *Tolerance.* The person needs to drink greater amounts of alcohol to get "high."

Alcoholism is a chronic disease lasting throughout life. It can be treated but not cured. Counseling and drugs are used to help the person stop drinking. The person must avoid all alcohol to avoid a relapse.

Alcohol and Older Persons. Alcohol effects vary with age. Even small amounts can make older persons feel "high." Older persons are at risk for falls, vehicle crashes, and other injuries from drinking. They have:

- Slower reaction times
- Hearing and vision problems
- A lower tolerance for alcohol

Older people tend to take more drugs than younger persons. Mixing alcohol with some drugs can be harmful, even fatal. Alcohol also makes some health problems worse. High blood pressure is an example.

Drug Abuse and Addiction

Drugs interfere with normal brain function. They create powerful feelings of pleasure.

- *Drug abuse*—is the overuse of a drug for non-medical or non-therapy effects.
- *Drug addiction*—is a chronic, relapsing brain disease. The person has an overwhelming desire to take a drug. The person repeatedly takes the drug because of its effect. Usually the effect is altered mental awareness. The person has to have the drug. Often higher doses are needed. The person cannot stop taking the drug without treatment.

A diagnosis of drug abuse or addiction is based on three or more of the following. They must have occurred any time during a 12-month period.

- The substance is often taken in larger amounts. Or it is taken over a longer period than intended.
- The person has a constant desire for the substance. Or the person cannot cut down or control substance use.
- A great deal of time is spent using the substance or recovering from its effects. Or a great deal of time is spent trying to obtain the substance.
- The person gave up or reduced important social, occupational, or recreational activities because of substance abuse.

- The person continues to use the substance. The person does so despite knowing that a constant or recurring problem is caused by or made worse by using the substance.
- The person has tolerance to the substance:
  - Increased amounts are needed to achieve intoxication or the desired effect.
  - Continued use of the same amount has a greatly reduced effect on the person.
- Withdrawal from the substance (*withdraw* means to stop, remove, or take away):
  - **Withdrawal syndrome** is the physical and mental response after stopping or severely reducing the use of a substance that was used regularly. The body responds with anxiety, restlessness, insomnia, irritability, impaired attention, and physical illness.
  - The same (or similar) substance is taken to relieve or avoid withdrawal symptoms.

Drug abuse and addiction affect social and mental function. Drug abuse and addiction are linked to crimes, violence, and motor vehicle crashes.

There also are physical effects. The following can occur from one use, high doses, or prolonged use:

- Human immunodeficiency virus (HIV) and acquired immunodeficiency syndrome (AIDS)
- Cardiovascular and lung diseases
- Stroke
- Sudden death
- Hepatitis

Legal and illegal drugs are abused. Legal drugs are approved for use in the United States. Doctors prescribe them. Illegal drugs are not approved for use. They are obtained through illegal means. Often legal drugs also are obtained through illegal means.

A drug treatment program combines various therapies and services to meet the person's needs. Drug abuse and addiction are chronic problems. Relapses can occur. A short-term, one-time treatment is often not enough. Treatment is a long-term process.

SUICIDE

Suicide means to kill oneself. People think about suicide when they feel hopeless or when they cannot see solutions to their problems. Suicide is most often linked to:

- Depression
- Alcohol or substance abuse
- Stressful events (Major losses and jail are examples.)

Risk factors for suicide are listed in Box 27-6. If a person mentions or talks about suicide, take the person seriously. Call for the nurse at once. Do not leave the person alone.

Agencies that treat persons with mental health problems must identify persons at risk for suicide. They must:

- Identify specific factors or features that increase or decrease the risk for suicide.
- Meet the person's immediate safety needs.
- Provide the most appropriate setting for treating the person.
- Provide crisis information to the person and family. A crisis "hotline" phone number is an example.

See *Focus on Communication: Suicide.*

BOX 27-6   Risk Factors for Suicide

- Depression and other mental health disorders
- Substance abuse disorder
- Stressful life events (in combination with other risk factors)
- Prior suicide attempt
- Family history of a mental health disorder or substance abuse
- Family history of suicide
- Family violence (including physical or sexual abuse)
- Firearms in the home
- Incarceration
- Exposure to suicidal behavior of others (family, peers, media figures)

From National Institute of Mental Health: *Suicide in the U.S.: statistics and prevention,* National Institutes of Health, NIH publication number 06-4594, reviewed July 27, 2009.

FOCUS ON COMMUNICATION
Suicide

Persons thinking of suicide may talk about their thoughts. For example, the person may say:

- "I just don't want to live anymore."
- "I wish I was dead."
- "I wish I had never been born."
- "Everyone would be better off without me."

Call for the nurse at once if a person mentions thoughts of suicide.

Suicide Contagion

Suicide contagion is exposure to suicide or suicidal behaviors within one's family, one's peer group, or media reports of suicide. The exposure has led to an increase in suicide and suicidal behaviors in persons at risk for suicide. Adolescents and young adults are at risk for suicide contagion.

Following suicide exposure, those close to the victim should be evaluated by a mental health professional. They include family, friends, peers, and co-workers. Persons at risk for suicide need mental health services.

CARE AND TREATMENT

Treatment of mental health problems involves having the person explore his or her thoughts and feelings. This is done through psychotherapy and behavior, group, occupational, art, and family therapies. Often drugs are ordered.

The care plan reflects the person's needs. The needs of the total person must be met. This includes physical, safety and security, and emotional needs.

Communication is important. Be alert to nonverbal communication. This includes the person's nonverbal communication and your own.

See *Focus on Communication: Care and Treatment.*

FOCUS ON COMMUNICATION
Care and Treatment

Nonverbal communication involves eye contact, tone of voice, facial expressions, body movements, and posture. Persons with major depression often have little eye contact, poor posture, and speak softly. Some do not speak much at all. Facial expressions may not change. Some persons cry.

Persons with anxiety feel uneasy. They may be restless and unable to sit still. Anxious persons often speak quickly. Eye contact may be prolonged and intense. Others have poor eye contact. The eyes may move quickly from one place to another. Be alert to nonverbal cues. Tell the nurse what you observe.

Your nonverbal communication is important as well. When interacting with persons with mental health problems:

- Face the person.
- Maintain eye contact.
- Position yourself near the person but not too close. Do not invade the person's space.
- Crouch, sit, or stand at the person's level if it is safe to do so.
- Show interest and concern through your posture and facial expressions.
- Speak calmly.

Focus on P R I D E
The Person, Family, and Yourself

Personal and Professional Responsibility—Persons with mental health problems may respond to stress with anxiety, panic, or anger. Some may become violent. To protect yourself:

- Call for help. Do not try to handle the situation on your own.
- Keep a safe distance between you and the person.
- Be aware of your surroundings. Do not let the person between you and the exit.

You must take responsibility for your safety. Your first priority is to protect yourself. Once you are safe, the health team can work together to protect the person and others.

Rights and Respect—The common health problems presented in Chapter 26 are physical illnesses. This chapter discussed mental health problems. People do not choose to have physical or mental health problems. Just as a person does not choose to have diabetes, a person does not choose to have anxiety or depression. How you view the person's illness affects the way you treat the person. Persons with mental illnesses deserve the same dignity and respect given to persons with physical illnesses.

Persons with mental health problems respond to stress in different ways. The person may say or do things that seem strange or odd to you. Do not laugh at or insult the person. Do not joke with others about the person. Treat the person with kindness and respect.

Independence and Social Interaction—Social support is important in the treatment of mental illness. Interacting with others offers a healthy way to deal with stress. Family and friends provide a sense of worth and belonging. The care plan includes how family and friends are involved in the person's care.

Providing support for a person with a mental health problem can be demanding. Family and friends often feel stress. They need support as well. Many communities offer support groups. You can also offer encouragement. Tell family and friends that you value the support they give.

Delegation and Teamwork—Caring for persons with mental health problems requires great teamwork. A person may become hostile or violent. Or the person may threaten or attempt suicide. The team must react quickly to protect the person and others. If someone calls for help, respond at once. Assist as the nurse directs. Follow agency policy. Take pride in working as a team to ensure safety.

Ethics and Laws—Persons thinking of suicide may confide in you. A person may ask you not to tell anyone about his or her suicidal thoughts. Protecting personal information is important. But the person's safety must be the priority. Never promise the person that you will not tell anyone. Report the statements to the nurse at once. It is the right thing to do.

REVIEW QUESTIONS

Circle the BEST answer.

1 Stress is
 a The way a person copes with and adjusts to everyday living
 b A response or change in the body caused by some factor
 c A mental illness
 d A thought or idea

2 Defense mechanisms are used to
 a Blame others
 b Make excuses for behavior
 c Return to an earlier time
 d Block unpleasant feelings

3 These statements are about defense mechanisms. Which is *false*?
 a Mentally healthy persons use them.
 b They relieve anxiety.
 c They prevent mental illness.
 d Persons with mental illness use them.

4 A phobia is
 a The event that causes stress
 b A false belief
 c An intense fear of something
 d Feelings and emotions

Continued

5 A person cleans and cleans. This behavior is
   a A delusion
   b A hallucination
   c A compulsion
   d An obsession

6 A person has nightmares about a trauma. The person is having
   a Phobias
   b Panic attacks
   c Flashbacks
   d Anxiety

7 Seeing, hearing, smelling, or feeling something that is not real is called a
   a Fantasy
   b Delusion
   c Psychosis
   d Hallucination

8 These statements are about schizophrenia. Which is *false?*
   a It is a brain disorder.
   b It can be cured with drugs and therapy.
   c Thinking and behavior are disturbed.
   d Suicide is a risk.

9 Bipolar disorder means that the person
   a Is very suspicious
   b Has anxiety
   c Is very unhappy and feels unwanted
   d Has severe mood swings

10 In bipolar disorder, an "emotional high" is called
   a Depression
   b Psychosis
   c An obsession
   d Mania

11 These statements are about antisocial personality disorder. Which is *false?*
   a The person has poor judgment.
   b The person blames others.
   c The person lies or cons others for pleasure.
   d The person is loyal to others.

12 These statements are about alcoholism. Which is *false?*
   a The person has a strong craving for alcohol.
   b The disease lasts throughout life.
   c After treatment, the person can have a social drink.
   d The person physically depends on alcohol.

13 These statements are about drug addiction. Which is *false?*
   a Physical and mental function are affected.
   b Higher doses of the drug may be needed.
   c The person has to have the drug.
   d The person can stop taking the drug without treatment.

14 A hospital patient talks about suicide. What should you do?
   a Call for the nurse.
   b Identify factors that increase the risk of suicide.
   c Ask what method the person intends to use.
   d Restrain the person.

Answers to these questions are on p. 528.

28

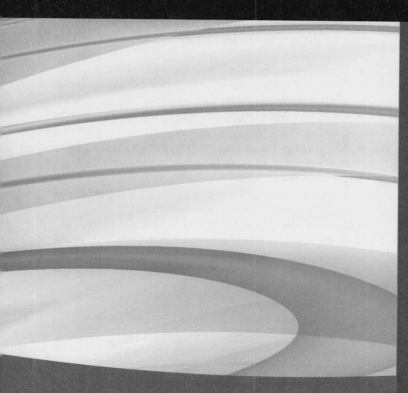

CARING FOR PERSONS WITH CONFUSION AND DEMENTIA

OBJECTIVES

- Define the key terms and key abbreviations listed in this chapter.
- Describe confusion and its causes.
- List the measures that help confused persons.
- Explain the differences between delirium, depression, and dementia.
- Describe Alzheimer's disease (AD).
- Describe the signs, symptoms, and behaviors of AD.
- Explain the care required by persons with AD and other dementias.
- Describe the effects of AD on the family.
- Explain validation therapy.
- Explain how to promote quality of life for persons with AD.
- Explain how to promote PRIDE in the person, the family, and yourself.

KEY TERMS

cognitive function Involves memory, thinking, reasoning, ability to understand, judgment, and behavior

delirium A state of temporary but acute mental confusion

delusion A false belief

dementia The loss of cognitive function that interferes with routine personal, social, and occupational activities

hallucination Seeing, hearing, smelling, or feeling something that is not real

pseudodementia False (*pseudo*) dementia

sundowning Signs, symptoms, and behaviors of AD increase during hours of darkness

KEY ABBREVIATIONS

AD Alzheimer's disease

ADL Activities of daily living

OBRA Omnibus Budget Reconciliation Act of 1987

Changes in the brain and nervous system occur with aging (Box 28-1). Certain diseases affect the brain. Changes in the brain can affect cognitive function. (*Cognitive* relates to knowledge.) Quality of life is affected. **Cognitive function** involves, memory, thinking, reasoning, ability to understand, judgment, and behavior.

CONFUSION

Confusion has many causes. Diseases, infections, hearing and vision loss, and drug side effects are some causes. So is brain injury. With aging, there is reduced blood supply to the brain. Personality and mental changes can result. Memory and the ability to make good judgments are lost. A person may not know people, the time, or the place. Some people gradually lose the ability to perform daily activities. Behavior changes are common. The person may be angry, restless, depressed, and irritable.

Acute confusion (*delirium*) occurs suddenly. It is usually temporary. Causes include infection, illness, injury, drugs, and surgery. Treatment is aimed at the cause.

Confusion caused by physical changes cannot be cured. Some measures help to improve function (Box 28-2). You must meet the person's basic needs.

BOX 28-1	Changes in the Nervous System From Aging

- Nerve cells are lost.
- Nerve conduction slows.
- Responses and reaction times are slower.
- Reflexes are slower.
- Vision and hearing decrease.
- Taste and smell decrease.
- Touch and sensitivity to pain decrease.
- Blood flow to the brain is reduced.
- Sleep patterns change.
- Memory is shorter.
- Forgetfulness occurs.
- Dizziness can occur.

DEMENTIA

Dementia is the loss of cognitive function that interferes with routine personal, social, and occupational activities. (*De* means from. *Mentia* means mind.) The person may have changes in personality, mood, or behavior. Dementia is a group of symptoms that may occur with certain diseases or conditions.

Dementia is not a normal part of aging. Most older people do not have dementia. Some early warning signs include:

- Recent memory loss that affects job skills
- Problems with common tasks (for example, dressing, cooking, driving)
- Problems with language; forgetting simple words
- Getting lost in familiar places
- Misplacing things and putting things in odd places (for example, putting a watch in the oven)
- Personality changes
- Poor or decreased judgment (for example, going outdoors in the snow without shoes)
- Loss of interest in life

If changes in the brain have not occurred, some dementias can be reversed. When the cause is removed, so are the signs and symptoms. Treatable causes include:

- Drugs and alcohol
- Delirium and depression
- Tumors
- Heart, lung, and blood vessel problems
- Head injuries
- Infection
- Vision and hearing problems

Permanent dementias result from changes in the brain. They have no cure. Function declines over time. Causes of permanent dementia are listed in Box 28-3. Alzheimer's disease is the most common type of permanent dementia.

BOX 28-2   Caring for the Confused Person

- Follow the person's care plan.
- Provide for safety.
- Face the person. Speak clearly.
- Call the person by name every time you are in contact with him or her.
- State your name. Show your name tag.
- Give the date and time each morning. Repeat as needed during the day or evening.
- Explain what you are going to do and why.
- Give clear, simple directions and answers to questions.
- Ask clear and simple questions. Give the person time to respond.
- Keep calendars and clocks with large numbers in the person's room and in nursing areas (Fig. 28-1). Remind the person of holidays, birthdays, and special events.
- Have the person wear eyeglasses and hearing aids as needed.
- Use touch to communicate (Chapter 5).
- Place familiar objects and pictures within the person's view.
- Provide newspapers, magazines, TV, and radio. Read to the person if appropriate.
- Discuss current events with the person.
- Maintain the day-night cycle.
  - Open window coverings during the day. Close them at night.
  - Use night-lights at night. Use them in rooms, bathrooms, hallways, and other areas.
  - Have the person wear regular clothes during the day—not sleepwear.
- Provide a calm, relaxed, and peaceful setting. Prevent loud noises, rushing, and congested hallways and dining rooms.
- Follow the person's routine. Meals, bathing, exercise, TV, bedtime, and other activities have a schedule. This promotes a sense of order and what to expect.
- Break tasks into small steps when helping the person.
- Do not re-arrange furniture or the person's belongings.
- Encourage the person to take part in self-care.
- Be consistent.

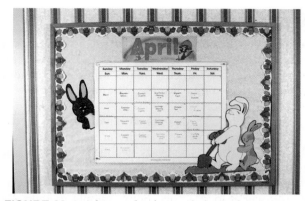

FIGURE 28-1 A large calendar can help confused persons.

BOX 28-3   Causes of Permanent Dementia

- Alcohol-related dementia and Korsakoff's syndrome
- Alzheimer's disease
- AIDS-related dementia
- Brain tumors
- Cerebrovascular disease
- Huntington's disease (a nervous system disease)
- Multi-infarct dementia (MID) (many [*multi*] strokes leave areas of damage [*infarct*])
- Multiple sclerosis
- Parkinson's disease
- Stroke
- Syphilis
- Trauma and head injury

Pseudodementia means false (*pseudo*) dementia. The person has signs and symptoms of dementia. However, there are no changes in the brain. This can occur with delirium and depression.

Delirium and Depression

Delirium and depression can be mistaken for dementia. **Delirium** is a state of temporary but acute mental confusion. Onset is sudden. It is common in older persons with acute or chronic illnesses. Infections, heart and lung diseases, and poor nutrition are common causes. So are hormone disorders. Hypoglycemia is also a cause (Chapter 26). Alcohol and many drugs can cause delirium. Delirium has a short course. It can last for a few hours to as long as 1 month.

Delirium signals physical illness in older persons and in persons with dementia. It is an emergency. The cause must be found and treated. Signs and symptoms include:

- Anxiety
- Disorientation
- Tremors
- Hallucinations (p. 494)
- Delusions (p. 494)
- Attention problems
- Decline in level of consciousness
- Memory problems

Depression is the most common mental health problem in older persons. It is often overlooked. Depression, aging, and some drug side effects have similar signs and symptoms. See Chapter 27 for signs and symptoms of depression in older persons.

ALZHEIMER'S DISEASE

Alzheimer's disease (AD) is a brain disease. Nerve cells that control intellectual and social function are damaged. These functions are affected: memory, thinking, reasoning, judgment, language, behavior, mood, and personality.

The person has problems with work and everyday functions. Problems with family and social relationships occur. There is a steady decline in memory and mental function.

The disease is gradual in onset. It gets worse and worse over 3 to 20 years. Some people in their 40s and 50s have AD. However, it usually occurs after the age of 60. The risk increases with age. It is often diagnosed around the age of 80. Nearly half of the persons age 85 and older have AD.

The cause is unknown. A family history of AD increases a person's risk of developing the disease. More women than men have AD. Women live longer than men.

Signs of AD

The classic sign of AD is *gradual loss of short-term memory*. At first, the only symptom may be forgetfulness. Box 28-4 lists the warning signs and other signs of AD.

BOX 28-4   Signs of Alzheimer's Disease

Warning Signs

- Gradual loss of short-term memory.
- Asking the same question over and over again.
- Repeating the same story—word for word, again and again.
- Forgetting how to cook, how to make repairs, or how to play cards. The person forgets activities that were once done regularly and with ease.
- Losing the ability to pay bills or balance a checkbook.
- Getting lost in familiar places. Or misplacing household objects.
- Neglecting to bathe. Or wearing the same clothes over and over again. Meanwhile, the person insists that a bath was taken or that clothes are clean.
- Relying on someone else to make decisions or answer questions that he or she would have handled.

Other Signs

- Forgets recent events, conversations, and appointments.
- Forgets simple directions.
- Forgets names (including family members).
- Forgets the names of everyday things (clock, radio, TV, and so on).
- Forgets words, loses train of thought.
- Substitutes unusual words and names for what is forgotten.
- Speaks in a native language.

Other Signs—cont'd

- Curses or swears.
- Misplaces things; puts things in odd places.
- Has problems writing checks.
- Gives away large amounts of money.
- Does not recognize or understand numbers.
- Has problems following conversations.
- Has problems reading and writing.
- Becomes lost in familiar settings.
- Forgets where he or she is.
- Does not know how to get back home.
- Wanders from home.
- Cannot tell or understand time or dates.
- Cannot solve everyday problems (iron is left on, stove burners left on, food burning on the stove, and so on).
- Cannot perform everyday tasks (dressing, bathing, brushing teeth, and so on).
- Distrusts others.
- Is stubborn.
- Withdraws socially.
- Is restless.
- Becomes suspicious.
- Becomes fearful.
- Does not want to do things.
- Sleeps more than usual.

Warning signs written by Eric Pfeiffer, MD, the director of the University of South Florida Suncoast Alzheimer's and Gerontology Center. Reprinted with permission.

Stages of AD

Signs and symptoms become more severe as the disease progresses. The disease ends in death. AD is often described in terms of 3 stages (Box 28-5, p. 494). The Alzheimer's Association describes seven stages:

- *No impairment.* The person does not show signs of memory problems.
- *Very mild cognitive decline.* The person thinks that he or she has memory lapses. Familiar words or names are forgotten. The person does not know where to find keys, eyeglasses, or other objects. These problems are not apparent to family, friends, or the health team.
- *Mild cognitive decline.* Family, friends, and others notice problems. The person has problems with memory or concentration and with words or names. The person loses or misplaces something valuable. Functioning in social or work settings declines.
- *Moderate cognitive decline.* Memory of recent or current events declines. There are problems with shopping, paying bills, and managing money. The person may withdraw or be quiet in social situations.
- *Moderately severe decline.* The person has major memory problems. There may be confusion about the date or day of the week. He or she may need help choosing the correct clothing to wear. The person knows his or her own name, a partner's name, and children's names. Usually help is not needed with eating or elimination.
- *Severe cognitive decline.* Memory problems are worse. Personality and behavior changes develop—delusions, hallucinations, repetitive behavior. The person needs much help with daily activities, including dressing and elimination. Names may be forgotten, but faces may be recognized. Sleep problems, incontinence (urinary and fecal), and wandering are common.
- *Very severe decline.* The person cannot respond to his or her environment, speak, or control movement. The person cannot walk without help. Over time, he or she cannot sit up without support or hold the head up. Muscles become rigid. Swallowing is impaired.

Behaviors

The following behaviors are common with AD.

Wandering. Persons with AD are not oriented to person, time, and place. They may wander away and not find their way back. Wandering may be by foot, car, bike, or other means. They may be with you one moment and gone the next.

Judgment is poor. They cannot tell what is safe or dangerous. Life-threatening accidents are great risks. They can walk into traffic or into a nearby river, lake, ocean, or forest. If not properly dressed, heat or cold exposure is a risk.

Wandering may have no cause. Or the person may be looking for something or someone—the bathroom, the bedroom, a child, or a partner. Pain, drug side effects, stress, restlessness, and anxiety are possible causes. Sometimes finding the cause prevents wandering.

MedicAlert + Safe Return. *MedicAlert + Safe Return* is a 24-hour emergency service for persons who wander or have a medical emergency. It was formed by the MedicAlert Foundation International and the Alzheimer's Association. The program is nationwide.

It serves to identify and safely return persons who wander and become lost. A small fee is charged. A family member completes a form and provides a photo. These are entered into a national database. The person receives an ID (wallet card, bracelet, or necklace).

When reported missing, the person's information is sent to the police. The toll-free number on the ID is called when the person is found. *MedicAlert + Safe Return* then calls the family member or caregiver and safely returns the person home.

Sundowning. With **sundowning,** signs, symptoms, and behaviors of AD increase during hours of darkness. It occurs in the late afternoon and evening hours. As daylight ends and darkness starts, confusion and restlessness increase. So do anxiety, agitation, and other symptoms. Behavior is worse after the sun goes down. It may continue throughout the night.

Sundowning may relate to being tired or hungry. Poor light and shadows may cause the person to see things that are not there. Persons with AD may be afraid of the dark.

BOX 28-5 Stages of Alzheimer's Disease

Stage 1: Mild AD

- Memory loss—forgetfulness; forgets recent events
- Problems finding words, finishing thoughts, following directions, and remembering names
- Repeats questions
- Poor judgment; bad decisions (including when driving)
- Disoriented to time and place
- Lack of spontaneity—less outgoing or interested in things
- Blames others for mistakes, forgetfulness, and other problems
- Moodiness
- Personality changes
- Problems performing everyday tasks; takes longer than usual to complete tasks
- Loses things; puts things in odd places
- Gets lost
- Has trouble handling money and paying bills

Stage 2: Moderate AD

- Restlessness—increases during the evening hours
- Sleep problems
- Memory loss increases—may not know family and friends
- Cannot learn new things
- Confusion
- Dulled senses—cannot tell the difference between hot and cold; cannot recognize dangers
- Fecal and urinary incontinence
- Needs help with activities of daily living (ADL)—bathing, feeding, and dressing self; afraid of bathing; will not change clothes

Stage 2: Moderate AD—cont'd

- Loses impulse control—foul language, poor table manners, sexual aggression, rudeness
- Movement and gait problems—walks slowly, has a shuffling gait
- Communication problems—cannot follow directions; problems with reading, writing, and math; speaks in short sentences or single words; statements may not make sense
- Repeats motions and statements—moves things back and forth constantly; says the same thing over and over again
- Agitation—behavior may be violent
- Delusions; paranoia

Stage 3: Severe AD

- Seizures (Chapter 29)
- Cannot speak—may groan, grunt, or scream
- Does not recognize self or family members
- Depends totally on others for all ADL
- Disoriented to person, time, and place
- Totally incontinent of urine and feces
- Cannot swallow—choking and aspiration are risks
- Sleeps more
- Becomes bed bound—cannot sit or walk
- Weight loss
- Skin infections
- Coma
- Death

Hallucinations. A **hallucination** is seeing, hearing, smelling, or feeling something that is not real. Senses are dulled. Affected persons see animals, insects, or people that are not present. Some hear voices. They may feel bugs crawling or feel that they are being touched.

Sometimes the problem is caused by impaired vision or hearing. The person needs to wear eyeglasses and hearing aids as prescribed.

Delusions. **Delusions** are false beliefs. People with AD may think they are some other person. Some believe they are in jail, are being killed, or are being attacked. A person may believe that the caregiver is someone else. Many other false beliefs can occur.

Catastrophic Reactions. These are extreme responses. The person reacts as if there is a disaster or tragedy. The person may scream, cry, or be agitated or combative. These reactions are common from too many stimuli. Eating, music or TV playing, and being asked questions all at once can overwhelm the person.

Agitation and Restlessness. The person may pace, hit, or yell. Common causes are pain or discomfort, anxiety, lack of sleep, and too many or too few stimuli. Hunger and the need to eliminate also are causes. A calm, quiet setting helps calm the person. So does meeting basic needs.

Caregivers can cause these behaviors. A caregiver may rush the person or be impatient. Or mixed verbal and nonverbal messages are sent. For example, a caregiver may talk too fast or too loud. Caregivers always need to look at how their behaviors affect other persons.

Aggression and Combativeness. These behaviors include hitting, pinching, grabbing, biting, or swearing. They may result from agitation and restlessness. They frighten others.

Sometimes these behaviors are personality traits. Or pain, fatigue, too much stimulation, caregiver stress, and feeling lost or abandoned are causes. The behaviors can occur during care measures (bathing, dressing) that upset or frighten the person. See Chapter 5 for dealing with the angry person. See Chapter 8 for workplace violence. Also follow the person's care plan.

Screaming. Persons with AD have communication problems. At first, it is hard to find the right words. As AD progresses, the person speaks in short sentences or in words. Often speech is not understandable.

The person screams to communicate. This is common in persons who are very confused and have poor communication skills. The person may scream a word or a name. Or the person just makes screaming sounds.

Possible causes include hearing and vision problems, pain or discomfort, fear, and fatigue. Too much or not enough stimulation is another cause. The person may react to a caregiver or family member by screaming.

Sometimes these measures are helpful:

- Providing a calm, quiet setting
- Playing soft music
- Having the person wear hearing aids and eyeglasses
- Having a family member or favorite caregiver comfort and calm the person
- Using touch to calm the person

Abnormal Sexual Behaviors. Sexual behaviors are labeled abnormal because of how and when they occur. Persons with AD are not oriented to person, time, and place. Sexual behaviors may involve the wrong person, the wrong place, and the wrong time. Also, persons with AD cannot control behavior.

Healthy persons do not undress or expose themselves in front of others. They do not masturbate or engage in sexual pleasures in public. They know their sexual partners. Persons with AD often mistake someone else for a sexual partner. The person kisses and hugs the other person.

Some behaviors are not sexual. Touching, scratching, and rubbing the genitals can signal infection, pain, or discomfort in the urinary or reproductive systems. Poor hygiene is another cause. So is being wet or soiled from urine or feces.

The nurse encourages the person's sexual partner to show affection. Their normal practices are encouraged. Examples include hand holding, hugging, kissing, and touching. When a person masturbates in public, lead the person to his or her room. Provide for privacy and safety. Good hygiene prevents itching. Clean the person quickly and thoroughly after elimination. Do not let the person stay wet or soiled.

The nurse assesses the person for urinary or reproductive system problems. The doctor is contacted as necessary.

Repetitive Behaviors. *Repetitive* means to repeat over and over again. Persons with AD repeat the same motions over and over again. For example, the person folds the same napkin over and over. Or the person says the same words over and over. Or the same question is asked. Such behaviors do not harm the person. However, they can annoy caregivers and the family.

Harmless acts are allowed. Music, picture books, exercise, and movies are distracting. Taking the person for a walk can help. Such measures help when words or questions are repeated.

CARE OF PERSONS WITH AD AND OTHER DEMENTIAS

Usually the person is cared for at home until symptoms are severe. Adult day care may help. Often assisted living or nursing center care is required. Sometimes hospital care is needed for other illnesses. You may care for persons with AD or other dementias in such settings. The person and family need your support and understanding.

People with AD do not choose to be forgetful, incontinent, agitated, or rude. Nor do they choose to have other behaviors, signs, and symptoms of the disease. They cannot control what is happening to them. The disease causes the behaviors. *The disease is responsible, not the person.*

Currently AD has no cure. Symptoms worsen over many years. The rate varies from person to person. Over time, persons with AD depend on others for care. Safety, hygiene, nutrition and fluids, elimination, and activity needs must be met. So must comfort and sleep needs. The person's care plan will include many of the measures listed in Box 28-6, p. 496.

Comfort and safety are important. Good skin care and alignment prevent skin breakdown and contractures. You must treat these persons with dignity and respect. They have the same rights as persons who are alert and active. Talk to them in a calm voice. Always explain what you are going to do. Massage, soothing touch, music, and aroma therapy are comforting and relaxing. Range-of-motion exercises and touch are also important therapies. The person may need hospice care as death nears (Chapter 30).

The person can have other health problems and injuries. However, the person may not be aware of pain, fever, constipation, incontinence, or other signs and symptoms. Carefully observe the person. Report any change in the person's usual behavior to the nurse.

Infection is a risk. The person cannot fully tend to self-care. Infection can occur from poor hygiene. This includes poor skin care, oral hygiene, and perineal care after bowel and bladder elimination. Inactivity and immobility can cause pneumonia and pressure ulcers.

The person needs to feel useful, worthwhile, and active. This promotes self-esteem. Therapists work with one person, a small group, or a large group. Therapies and activities focus on the person's strengths and past successes. For example:

- A woman used to cook. She helps clean fruit.
- A man was a good dancer. Activities are planned so he can dance.
- A man likes to clean. He helps with dusting.

Supervised activities meet the person's needs and cognitive abilities. The person's interests are considered. Activities are based on what the person enjoys and can do. Some people like crafts, exercise, gardening, and listening and moving to music. Others like sing-alongs, reminiscing, and board games. Some like to string beads, fold towels, or roll dough.

See *Focus on Communication: Care of Persons With AD and Other Dementias*, p. 499.

BOX 28-6	Care of Persons With AD and Other Dementias

Environment

- Follow established routines.
- Avoid changing rooms or roommates.
- Place picture signs by room doors, bathrooms, dining rooms, and other areas (Fig. 28-2, p. 498).
- Keep personal items where the person can see them.
- Stay within the person's sight to the extent possible.
- Place memory aids (large clocks and calendars) where the person can see them.
- Keep noise levels low.
- Play music and show movies from the person's past.
- Select tasks and activities that fit the person's cognitive abilities and interests.

Communication

- Approach the person in a calm, quiet manner.
- Approach the person from the front. Do not approach the person from the side or the back. This can startle the person.
- Call the person by name. Have the person's attention before you start speaking.
- Identify other people by their names. Avoid pronouns (he, she, them, and so on).
- Follow the rules of communication (Chapters 4 and 5).
- Practice measures to promote communication (Chapter 5).
- Use gestures or cues. Point to objects.
- Speak in a calm, gentle voice.
- Speak slowly. Use simple words and short sentences.
- Let the person speak. Do not interrupt or rush the person.
- Give the person time to respond.
- Do not criticize, correct, interrupt, or argue with the person.
- Present one idea, question, or instruction at a time.
- Ask simple questions having simple answers. Do not ask complex questions.
- Do not present the person with many questions.
- Provide simple explanations of all procedures and activities.
- Give consistent responses.
- Practice measures to promote hearing (Chapter 26).
- Practice measures for blind and visually impaired persons (Chapter 26).

Safety

- Remove harmful, sharp, and breakable objects from the area. This includes knives, scissors, glass, dishes, razors, and tools.
- Provide plastic eating and drinking utensils. This helps prevent breakage and cuts.
- Place safety plugs in electric outlets.
- Keep cords and electric equipment out of reach.
- Remove electric appliances from the bathroom. Examples include hair dryers, curling irons, make-up mirrors, and electric shavers.
- Store personal care items (shampoo, deodorant, lotion, and so on) in a safe place.
- Keep child-proof caps on medicine containers and household cleaners.
- Store household cleaners and drugs in locked storage areas.
- Store dangerous equipment and tools in a safe place.
- Remove knobs from stoves or place child-proof covers on the knobs.
- Remove dangerous appliances and power tools from the home.
- Remove firearms from the home.
- Store car keys in a safe place.
- Supervise the person who smokes.
- Store cigarettes, cigars, pipes, matches, and other smoking materials in a safe place.
- Practice safety measures to prevent falls (Chapter 9).
- Practice safety measures to prevent fires (Chapter 8).
- Practice safety measures to prevent burns (Chapters 8 and 15).
- Practice safety measures to prevent poisoning (Chapter 8).
- Lock all doors to kitchens, utility rooms, and housekeeping closets. Keep them locked.

Wandering

- Follow agency policy for locking doors and windows. Locks are often placed at the top and bottom of doors (Fig. 28-3, p. 498). The person is not likely to look for a lock in such places.

BOX 28-6 Care of Persons With AD and Other Dementias—cont'd

Wandering—cont'd

- Keep door alarms and electronic doors turned on. The alarm goes off when the door is opened. Respond to door alarms at once.
- Follow agency policy for fire exits. Everyone must be able to leave the building if there is a fire.
- Make sure the person wears an ID bracelet or *MedicAlert + Safe Return* ID at all times.
- Exercise the person as ordered. Adequate exercise often reduces wandering.
- Involve the person in activities—folding napkins, dusting a table, sorting socks, rolling yarn, sweeping, sanding blocks of wood, or watering plants.
- Do not use restraints. Restraints require a doctor's order. They also tend to increase confusion and disorientation.
- Do not argue with the person who wants to leave. The person does not understand what you are saying.
- Go with the person who insists on going outside. Make sure he or she is properly dressed. Guide the person inside after a few minutes (Fig. 28-4, p. 498).
- Let the person wander in enclosed areas. The agency may have enclosed areas where the person can walk about (Fig. 28-5, p. 498). They provide a safe place for the person to wander.

Sundowning

- Complete treatments and activities early in the day.
- Provide a calm, quiet setting late in the day.
- Do not restrain the person.
- Encourage exercise and activity early in the day.
- Meet nutrition needs. Hunger can increase restlessness.
- Promote elimination. The need to eliminate can increase restlessness.
- Do not try to reason with the person. He or she cannot understand what you are saying.
- Do not ask the person to tell you what is bothering him or her. Communication is impaired. The person does not understand what you are asking. He or she cannot think or speak clearly.

Hallucinations and Delusions

- Make sure the person wears eyeglasses and hearing aids as needed. Follow the care plan.
- Do not argue with the person. He or she does not understand what you are saying.
- Reassure the person. Tell him or her that you will provide protection from harm.
- Distract the person with some item or activity. Taking the person for a walk may be helpful.
- Turn off TV or movies when violent and disturbing programs are on. The person may believe that the story is real.
- Use touch to calm and reassure the person (Fig. 28-6, p. 498).
- Eliminate noises that the person could misinterpret. TV, radio, music, furnaces, air conditioners, and other things could affect the person.
- Check lighting. Make sure there are no glares, shadows, or reflections.

Hallucinations and Delusions—cont'd

- Cover or remove mirrors. The person could misinterpret his or her reflection.

Sleep

- Develop a regular bedtime. Keep the bedtime at the same time each evening.
- Follow bedtime rituals.
- Use night-lights so the person can see. Use them in rooms, hallways, bathrooms, and other areas. They help prevent accidents and disorientation.
- Limit caffeine during the day.
- Discourage naps during the day.
- Reduce noises.
- Provide oral hygiene (Chapter 15).
- Choose clothing that is comfortable and simple to put on. Front opening garments are easy to put on. Pullover tops are harder to put on. And the person may become frightened when his or her head is inside the pullover top.
- Select clothing that closes with Velcro. Such items are easy to put on and take off. Buttons, zippers, snaps, and other closures can frustrate the person.
- Offer simple clothing choices (Fig. 28-7, p. 498). Let the person choose between two shirts or two blouses, two pants or two slacks, and so on.
- Lay clothing out in the order it will be put on. Hand the person one clothing item at a time. Tell or show the person what to do. Do not rush him or her.
- Have equipment ready for any procedure. This reduces the amount of time the person is involved in care measures.
- Observe for signs and symptoms of health problems (Chapter 4).
- Prevent infection (Chapter 11).

Basic Needs

- Meet food and fluid needs (Chapter 19). Provide finger foods. Cut food and pour liquids as needed.
- Provide good skin care (Chapters 15 and 23). Keep the person's skin free of urine and feces.
- Promote urinary and bowel elimination (Chapters 17 and 18).
- Provide incontinence care as needed (Chapters 17 and 18).
- Promote exercise and activity during the day (Chapter 22). This helps reduce wandering and sundowning behaviors. The person may also sleep better.
- Reduce intake of coffee, tea, and cola drinks. These contain caffeine. Caffeine is a stimulant. It can increase restlessness, confusion, and agitation.
- Provide a quiet, restful setting. Soft music is better than loud TV programs.
- Play music during care activities such as bathing and during meals.
- Promote personal hygiene (Chapter 15). Do not force the person into a shower or tub. People with AD are often afraid of bathing. Try bathing the person when he or she is calm. Use the person's preferred bathing method (tub bath, shower). Provide privacy and keep the person warm. Do not rush the person.

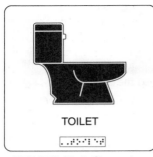
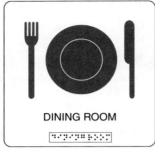

FIGURE 28-2 Signs give cues to persons with dementia.

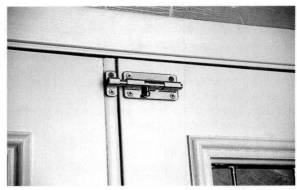

FIGURE 28-3 A slide lock is at the top of the door.

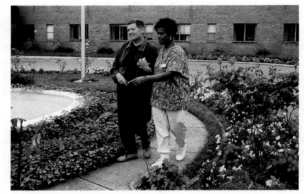

FIGURE 28-4 Walk outside with the person who wanders. Then guide the person back inside after a few minutes.

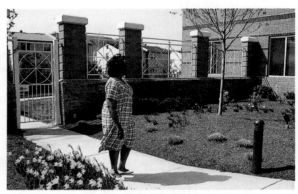

FIGURE 28-5 An enclosed garden allows persons with AD to wander in a safe setting.

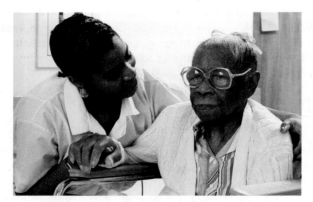

FIGURE 28-6 Use touch to calm the person.

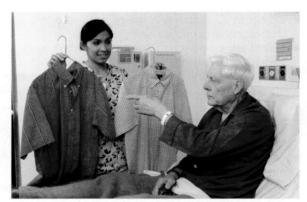

FIGURE 28-7 The person with AD is offered simple clothing choices.

FOCUS ON COMMUNICATION
Care of Persons With AD and Other Dementias

Impaired communication is a common problem among persons with AD and other dementias. Communication abilities decline over time. Some persons can have brief conversations. To promote communication, practice the measures in Box 28-6, p. 495. Avoid the following:

- Giving orders. For example: "Sit down and eat." The statement is bossy. It does not show respect for the person.
- Wanting the truth. For example, do not say: "Don't you remember?" "What's my name?" "What day is it?"
- Correcting the person's errors. For example, do not say: "No, that is your daughter Rose. That's not Mary." Or, "I just told you that it's time to get dressed. You already had breakfast."

Special Care Units

Many nursing centers have special units for persons with AD and other dementias. Some units are secured. This means that entrances and exits are locked. Persons in these units have a safe setting to move about in. They cannot wander away. Some persons have aggressive behaviors that disrupt or threaten others. They may need a secured unit.

At some point, the secured unit is no longer needed for safe care. For example, the person's condition progresses from stage 2 to stage 3. The person cannot sit or walk. Wandering is not a concern. The person is transferred to another unit.

The Family

The person may live at home or with a partner, children, or other family members. The family gives care. Or someone stays with the person. Health care is sought when the family cannot deal with the situation or meet the person's needs. Home health care may help for a while. Adult day care is an option. Long-term care is needed when:

- Family members cannot meet the person's needs.
- The person no longer knows the caregiver.
- Family members have health problems.
- Money problems occur.
- The person's behavior presents dangers to self and others.

Diagnostic tests, doctor's visits, drugs, and home care are costly. So is long-term care. The person's medical care can drain family finances.

The family has special needs. Caring for the person at home or in a nursing center is stressful. There are physical, emotional, social, and financial stresses. Adult children are in the *sandwich generation.* They are caught between their own children who need attention and an ill parent who needs care. Caring for two families is stressful. Often adult children have jobs too.

Caregivers can suffer from anger, anxiety, depression, and sleeplessness. Some cannot concentrate or are irritable. They can develop health problems. They need to take care of their own health. A healthy diet, exercise, and plenty of rest are needed. Asking for help is important. The caregiver needs to feel free to ask family and friends for help.

Caregivers need much support and encouragement. Many join AD support groups. The groups are sponsored by hospitals, nursing centers, and the Alzheimer's Association. The Alzheimer's Association has chapters in cities and towns across the country. Support groups offer encouragement and advice. People in similar situations share their feelings, anger, frustration, guilt, and other emotions. They also share coping and caregiving ideas.

The family often feels hopeless. No matter what is done, the person only gets worse. Much time, money, energy, and emotion are needed to care for the person. Anger and resentment may result. Guilt feelings are common. The family also knows that the person did not choose the disease. They know that the person does not choose to have its signs, symptoms, and behaviors. Sometimes behaviors are embarrassing. The family may be upset and angry that the loved one cannot show love or affection.

The family is an important part of the health team. They help plan the person's care whenever possible. They need to learn how to bathe, feed, dress, and give oral hygiene to the person. They also need to learn how to provide a safe setting. The nurse and support group help the family learn how to give necessary care.

Some family members take part in unit activities. For many persons, family members provide comfort. They also need support and understanding from the health team.

Validation Therapy

Validation therapy may be part of the person's care plan. The therapy is based on these principles:

- All behavior has meaning.
- Development occurs in a sequence, order, and pattern (Chapter 7). Certain tasks must be completed during a stage of development. A stage cannot be skipped. Each stage is the basis of the next stage.
- If a person does not successfully complete a stage of development, unresolved issues and emotions may surface later in life.
- A person may return to the past to resolve such issues and emotions.
- Caregivers need to listen and provide empathy.
- Attempts are not made to correct the person's thoughts or bring the person back to reality. For example:
  - While going from room to room, Mrs. Bell calls for her daughter. In reality, her daughter died 20 years ago. The caregiver does not tell Mrs. Bell that her daughter died. Instead, the caregiver says: "Tell me about your daughter."
  - Mrs. Brown sits all day on a bench by the window. She says that she is at the train station waiting to meet her husband. In reality, her husband was killed during World War II. Buried in England, he never returned home. The caregiver does not remind Mrs. Brown of what happened. Instead, the caregiver encourages Mrs. Brown to talk about her husband.
  - Mr. Garcia was 3 years old when his father died. He holds a ball constantly. He is very upset when anyone tries to remove it from his hand. He calls for his father and repeats "play ball, play ball." The caregiver does not remind Mr. Garcia that he is 80 years old and that his father died many years ago. Instead, the caregiver says, "Tell me about playing ball."

The health team decides if validation therapy might help a person. If so, it will be part of the person's care plan. Proper use of validation therapy requires special training. If used in your agency, you will receive the training needed to use it correctly.

QUALITY OF LIFE

Quality of life is important for all persons with confusion and dementia. Nursing center residents have rights under the Omnibus Budget Reconciliation Act of 1987 (OBRA). They may not know or be able to exercise their rights. However, the family knows the person's rights. They want those rights protected. They want respect and dignity for the loved one.

The person has the right to privacy and confidentiality. Protect the person from exposure. Only those involved in the person's care are present for care and procedures. The person is allowed to visit in private. Protect confidentiality. Do not share information about the person's care and condition with others.

Personal choice is important. If able, simple choices are encouraged. For example, a person chooses to wear a shirt or sweater. Watching or not watching TV may be a simple choice. The family makes choices if the person cannot. They choose bath times, menus, clothing, activities, and other care.

The person has the right to keep and use personal items. Some items provide comfort. A pillow, blanket, afghan, or sweater may have meaning to the person. The person may not know why or even recognize the item. Still, it is important. Keep personal items safe. Protect the person's property from loss or damage.

These persons must be kept free from abuse, mistreatment, and neglect. Caring for persons with confusion and dementia is often very frustrating. Some behaviors are hard to deal with. Family and staff can become short-tempered and angry. Protect the person from abuse. Report any signs and symptoms of abuse to the nurse at once. Be patient and calm when caring for these persons. Talk with the nurse if you are becoming upset. Sometimes an assignment change is needed for a while.

All persons have the right to be free from restraints. Restraints require a doctor's order. They are used only if it is the best way to protect the person. They are not used for staff convenience. Restraints can make confusion and demented behaviors worse. The nurse tells you when to use restraints.

Activity and a safe setting promote quality of life (see Box 28-6, p. 496). Safe, calm, and quiet activities are needed. The recreational therapist and other health team members will find activities that are best for each person. These are part of the person's care plan.

Focus on P R I D E
The Person, Family, and Yourself

Personal and Professional Responsibility—Confusion has many causes. The person may have an infection. Or the cause may be hypoglycemia or a drug side effect. You are responsible for reporting changes in the person's condition. If you observe signs of confusion, do not assume the person has AD. Report changes to the nurse at once.

Rights and Respect—Persons with AD often have changes in mood, behavior, and personality. The person may become easily agitated or angry. The person does not have control over his or her words and actions. The person deserves quality care. Treat the person with dignity and respect.

Behavior changes also impact family members. They know the person well. The person's conduct is unlike his or her normal character. The changes may frustrate or sadden the family. Show kindness to the family.

Independence and Social Interaction—Persons with dementia have problems with ADL. Eating, bathing, dressing, and elimination are examples. The care plan includes measures to help the person remain independent as long as possible. Maintaining the person's routines is an example. For example, Mrs. Lund follows this order after getting out of bed: uses the bathroom, washes hands, brushes teeth, showers, puts on make-up, brushes hair, dresses, and has breakfast. You may need to break down each task into simple steps. Allow extra time for the person to complete a task. Let the person do as much for himself or herself as possible.

Delegation and Teamwork—Every staff member must be alert to persons who wander. Such persons are allowed to wander in safe areas. However, the person may wander into another person's room or unsafe area. Kitchens, shower rooms, and utility rooms are examples.

Patients or residents may try to wander to another nursing unit or out of the agency. Leaving the agency without staff knowledge is known as *elopement*. Serious injury and death have resulted from elopement. Agencies must follow state and federal guidelines to prevent elopement.

Tell your team members when you are caring for a person who wanders. You cannot be around the person all of the time. The team can assist and monitor the person. Help your team members in the same way. If you see a person wandering to an unsafe area, gently guide the person back to a safe area. Report the problem to the nurse.

Ethics and Laws—According to OBRA, secured nursing units are physical restraints. Certain conditions must be met for a person to be placed on a secured unit. A dementia diagnosis and a doctor's order are examples. The health team reviews the person's need for a secured unit on a regular basis. Centers must follow OBRA rules. The center must use the least-restrictive approach to care. The person's rights are always protected.

REVIEW QUESTIONS

Circle the BEST answer.

1   Cognitive function relates to the following *except*
    a   Memory loss and personality
    b   Thinking and reasoning
    c   Ability to understand
    d   Judgment and behavior

2   A person is confused after surgery. The confusion is likely to be
    a   Permanent
    b   Temporary
    c   Caused by an infection
    d   Caused by a brain injury

3   A person is confused. The care plan includes the following. Which should you question?
    a   Restrain in bed at night.
    b   Give clear, simple directions.
    c   Use touch to communicate.
    d   Open drapes during the day.

4   A person has delusions. A delusion is
    a   A false belief
    b   An illness caused by changes in the brain
    c   Seeing, hearing, or feeling something that is not real
    d   Alzheimer's disease

5   A person has AD. Which is *true?*
    a   AD occurs only in older persons.
    b   Diet and drugs can cure the disease.
    c   AD and delirium are the same.
    d   AD ends in death.

6   The following are common in persons with AD *except*
    a   Memory loss, poor judgment, and sleep disturbances
    b   Loss of impulse control and communication abilities
    c   Wandering, delusions, and hallucinations
    d   Paralysis, dyspnea, and pain

7   Sundowning means that
    a   The person becomes sleepy when the sun sets
    b   Behaviors become worse in the late afternoon and evening hours
    c   Behavior improves at night
    d   The person goes to bed when the sun sets

8   A person with AD is screaming. You know that this is
    a   An agitated reaction
    b   A way to communicate
    c   Caused by a delusion
    d   A repetitive behavior

9   AD support groups do the following *except*
    a   Provide care
    b   Offer encouragement and care ideas
    c   Provide support for the family
    d   Promote the sharing of feelings and frustrations

10 A person with AD tends to wander. You should do the following *except*
    a   Make sure door alarms are turned on
    b   Make sure an ID bracelet is worn
    c   Assist with exercise as ordered
    d   Tell the person where to wander safely

11 Safety is important for the person with AD. Which is *false?*
    a   Safety plugs are placed in electric outlets.
    b   Cleaners and drugs are kept locked up.
    c   The person can keep smoking materials.
    d   Sharp and breakable objects are removed from the person's setting.

12 You are caring for a person with AD. Which is *false?*
    a   You can reason with the person.
    b   Touch can calm and reassure the person.
    c   A calm, quiet setting is important.
    d   Help is needed with ADL.

Answers to these questions are on p. 528.

29

ASSISTING WITH EMERGENCY CARE

PROCEDURES

- Adult CPR—One Rescuer
- Adult CPR—Two Rescuers
- Adult CPR With AED—Two Rescuers

OBJECTIVES

- Define the key terms and key abbreviations listed in this chapter.
- Describe the rules of emergency care.
- Identify the signs of sudden cardiac arrest and the emergency care required.
- Describe the signs, symptoms, and emergency care for hemorrhage.
- Identify the signs, symptoms, and emergency care for shock.
- Describe the causes and types of seizures and how to care for a person during a seizure.
- Identify the common causes and emergency care for fainting.
- Describe the signs, symptoms, and emergency care for stroke.
- Explain how to promote PRIDE in the person, the family, and yourself.
- Perform the procedures described in this chapter.

KEY TERMS

anaphylaxis A life-threatening sensitivity to an antigen

cardiac arrest See "sudden cardiac arrest"

convulsion See "seizure"

fainting The sudden loss of consciousness from an inadequate blood supply to the brain

first aid Emergency care given to an ill or injured person before medical help arrives

hemorrhage The excessive loss of blood in a short time

respiratory arrest Breathing stops but heart action continues for several minutes

seizure Violent and sudden contractions or tremors of muscle groups; convulsion

shock Results when organs and tissues do not get enough blood

sudden cardiac arrest (SCA) The heart stops suddenly and without warning; cardiac arrest

KEY ABBREVIATIONS

AED Automated external defibrillator

AHA American Heart Association

BLS Basic Life Support

CPR Cardiopulmonary resuscitation

EMS Emergency Medical Services

RRT Rapid Response Team

SCA Sudden cardiac arrest

VF Ventricular fibrillation

V-fib Ventricular fibrillation

Emergencies can occur anywhere. Sometimes you can save a life if you know what to do. You are encouraged to take a first aid course and a Basic Life Support (BLS) course. These courses prepare you to give emergency care.

The Basic Life Support procedures in this chapter are given as basic information. They do not replace certification training. You need a Basic Life Support course for health care providers.

EMERGENCY CARE

First aid is the emergency care given to an ill or injured person before medical help arrives. The goals of first aid are to:

- Prevent death
- Prevent injuries from becoming worse

For emergencies in out-of-hospital settings, the Emergency Medical Services (EMS) system is activated. Emergency personnel (paramedics, emergency medical technicians) rush to the scene. They treat, stabilize, and transport persons with life-threatening problems. Their ambulances have emergency drugs, equipment, and supplies. They have guidelines for care and communicate with doctors in hospital emergency departments. The doctors can tell them what to do. To activate the EMS system, do one of the following:

- Dial 911
- Call the local fire or police department
- Call the phone operator

Each emergency is different. The rules in Box 29-1 apply to any emergency. Hospitals and other agencies have procedures for emergencies. A Rapid Response Team (RRT) is called to the bedside when a person shows warning signs of a life-threatening condition. The team may include a doctor, one or more nurses, and a respiratory therapist. The RRT's goal is to prevent death.

See *Promoting Safety and Comfort: Emergency Care.*

PROMOTING SAFETY AND COMFORT
Emergency Care

Safety

During emergencies, contact with blood, body fluids, secretions, and excretions is likely. Follow Standard Precautions and the Bloodborne Pathogen Standard to the extent possible.

When an emergency occurs in a hospital or health care agency, call for the nurse at once. You may need to activate the RRT or take the person's vital signs (Chapter 20).

Comfort

Mental comfort is important during emergencies. Help the person feel safe and secure. Provide reassurance and explanations about care. Use a calm approach.

BOX 29-1	Rules of Emergency Care

- Know your limits. Do not do more than you are able. Do not perform an unfamiliar procedure. Do what you can under the circumstances.
- Stay calm. This helps the person feel more secure.
- Know where to find emergency supplies.
- Follow Standard Precautions and the Bloodborne Pathogen Standard to the extent possible.
- Check for life-threatening problems. Check for breathing, a pulse, and bleeding.
- Keep the person lying down or as you found him or her. Moving the person could make an injury worse.
- Move the person only if the setting is unsafe. Examples include:
  - A burning building or car
  - A building that might collapse
  - Stormy conditions with lightning
  - In water
  - Near electrical wires
- Wait for help to arrive if the scene is not safe enough for you to approach.
- Perform necessary emergency measures.

- Call for help. Or have someone activate the EMS system. *Do not hang up until the operator has hung up.* Give the operator the following information:
  - Your location: street address and city, cross streets or roads, and landmarks
  - Phone number you are calling from
  - What seems to have happened (for example: heart attack, crash, fire)—police, fire equipment, and ambulances may be needed
  - How many people need help
  - Conditions of victims, obvious injuries, and life-threatening situations
  - What aid is being given
- Do not remove clothes unless you have to. If you must remove clothing, tear or cut garments along the seams.
- Keep the person warm. Cover the person with a blanket, coats, or sweaters.
- Reassure the person. Explain what is happening and that help was called.
- Do not give the person food or fluids.
- Keep onlookers away. They invade privacy, and tend to stare, give advice, and comment about the person's condition. The person may think the situation is worse than it really is.

BASIC LIFE SUPPORT FOR ADULTS

When the heart and breathing stop, the person is clinically dead. Blood is not circulated through the body. Heart, brain, and other organ damage occurs within minutes. The American Heart Association's (AHA) Basic Life Support (BLS) procedures support breathing and circulation.

Chain of Survival for Adults

The AHA's BLS courses teach the adult *Chain of Survival.* These actions are taken for heart attack (Chapter 26), sudden cardiac arrest (p. 506), respiratory arrest (p. 506), stroke (Chapter 26 and p. 516), and choking (Chapter 8). They also apply to other life-threatening problems. They are done as soon as possible. Any delay reduces the person's chance of surviving.

Chain of Survival actions for the adult are:
- *Recognizing cardiac arrest and activating the EMS system at once.*
- *Early cardiopulmonary resuscitation (CPR).*
- *Early defibrillation.* See p. 509.

FOCUS ON COMMUNICATION
Chain of Survival for Adults

Calling for help is a critical step in the Chain of Survival. If others are around, tell a certain person to activate the EMS system. You may not know the person's name. Point at the person. Make eye contact. You can say: "Call 911 and get an AED." Begin care. Follow up soon. Make sure the person was able to contact help.

Different systems are used to contact the RRT in the hospital setting. Many agencies use a telephone or paging system. Know your agency's procedure for activating the RRT.

- *Early advanced care.* This is given by EMS staff, doctors, and nurses. They give drugs and perform life-saving measures.
- *Organized post-cardiac arrest care.* This is care given to improve survival following cardiac arrest.

You will learn the Chain of Survival for children in the AHA's *BLS for Healthcare Providers* course.

See *Focus on Communication: Chain of Survival for Adults.*

Sudden Cardiac Arrest

Sudden cardiac arrest (SCA) or **cardiac arrest** is when the heart stops suddenly and without warning. Within moments, breathing stops as well. Permanent brain and other organ damage occurs unless circulation and breathing are restored. There are three major signs of SCA:

- No response.
- No breathing or no normal breathing. The person may have *agonal gasps* or *agonal respirations* early during SCA. (*Agonal* comes from the Greek word that means to *struggle*. Agonal is used in relation to death and dying.) Agonal gasps do not bring enough oxygen into the lungs. Gasps are not normal breathing.
- No pulse.

The person's skin is cool, pale, and gray. The person is not coughing or moving.

SCA is a sudden, unexpected, and dramatic event. It can occur anywhere and at any time—while driving, shoveling snow, playing golf or tennis, watching TV, eating, or sleeping. Common causes include heart disease, drowning, electric shock, severe injury, choking (Chapter 8), and drug overdose. These causes lead to an abnormal heart rhythm called ventricular fibrillation (p. 509). The heart cannot pump blood. A normal rhythm must be restored. Otherwise the person will die.

Respiratory Arrest

Respiratory arrest is when breathing stops but heart action continues for several minutes. If breathing is not restored, cardiac arrest occurs. Causes of respiratory arrest include:

- Drowning
- Stroke
- Choking
- Drug overdose
- Electric shock (including lightning strikes)
- Smoke inhalation
- Suffocation
- Heart attack
- Coma
- Other injuries

Rescue Breathing. Rescue breaths are given when there is a pulse but no breathing or only gasping. To give rescue breaths:

- Open the airway.
- Give 1 breath every 5 to 6 seconds for adults.

- Give each breath over 1 second. The chest should rise when breaths are given.
- Check the pulse every 2 minutes. If there is no pulse, begin CPR.

Cardiopulmonary Resuscitation for Adults

When the heart and breathing stop, blood and oxygen are not supplied to the body. Brain and other organ damage occurs within minutes.

Cardiopulmonary resuscitation (CPR) must be started at once when a person has SCA. CPR supports circulation and breathing. It provides blood and oxygen to the heart, brain, and other organs until advanced emergency care is given. CPR involves:

- Chest compressions
- Airway
- Breathing
- Defibrillation

CPR procedures require speed, skill, and efficiency. Chest compressions and airway and breathing procedures are done until a defibrillator arrives. The defibrillator is used as soon as possible.

See *Promoting Safety and Comfort: Cardiopulmonary Resuscitation for Adults.*

PROMOTING SAFETY AND COMFORT
Cardiopulmonary Resuscitation for Adults

Safety

The discussion and procedures that follow assume that the person does not have injuries from trauma. If injuries are present, special measures are needed to position the person and open the airway. Such measures are learned during a BLS certification course.

Chest Compressions. The heart, brain, and other organs must receive blood. Otherwise, permanent damage results. In cardiac arrest, the heart has stopped beating. Blood must be pumped through the body in some other way. Chest compressions force blood through the circulatory system.

Before starting chest compressions, check for a pulse. Use the carotid artery on the side near you. To find the carotid pulse, place 2 or 3 fingertips on the trachea (windpipe). Then slide your fingertips down off the trachea to the groove of the neck (Fig. 29-1, p. 507). Check for a pulse for at least 5 seconds but no more than 10 seconds. While checking for a pulse, look for signs of circulation. See if the person has started breathing or is coughing or moving.

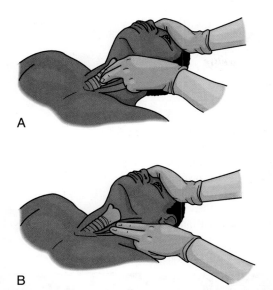

A

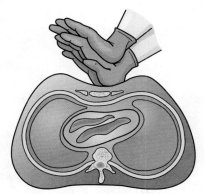

B

FIGURE 29-1 Locating the carotid pulse. **A,** Two fingers are placed on the trachea. **B,** The fingertips are moved down into the groove of the neck to the carotid artery.

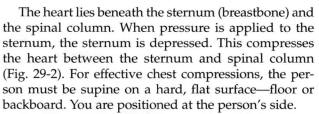

FIGURE 29-2 The heart lies between the sternum and the spinal column. The heart is compressed when pressure is applied to the sternum.

The heart lies beneath the sternum (breastbone) and the spinal column. When pressure is applied to the sternum, the sternum is depressed. This compresses the heart between the sternum and spinal column (Fig. 29-2). For effective chest compressions, the person must be supine on a hard, flat surface—floor or backboard. You are positioned at the person's side.

Hand position is important for effective chest compressions (Fig. 29-3). You use the heels of your hands—one on top of the other—for chest compressions. For proper placement:

* Expose the person's chest. Remove clothing or move it out of the way. You need to be able to see the person's bare skin for proper hand position.
* Place the heel of one hand (usually your dominant hand) in the center of the bare chest. The heel of this hand is placed on the sternum between the nipples.
* Place the heel of your other hand on top of the heel of the first hand.

To give chest compressions, your arms are straight. Your shoulders are directly over your hands. And your fingers are interlocked (Fig. 29-4, p. 508). Exert firm downward pressure to depress the adult sternum at least 2 inches. Then release pressure without removing your hands from the chest. Releasing pressure allows the chest to recoil—to return to its normal position. Recoil lets the heart fill with blood.

The AHA recommends that you:

* Give compressions at a rate of at least 100 per minute.
* Push hard, and push fast.
* Push deeply into the chest.
* Interrupt chest compressions only when necessary. Interruptions should be less than 10 seconds. When there are no chest compressions, blood does not flow to the heart, brain, and other organs.

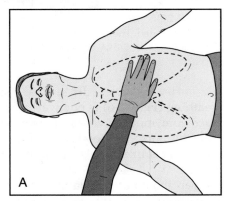

A

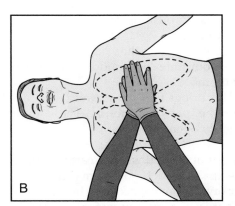

B

FIGURE 29-3 Proper hand position for CPR. **A,** The heel of the dominant hand is placed in the center of the chest between the nipples. **B,** The heel of the non-dominant hand is placed on top of the dominant hand.

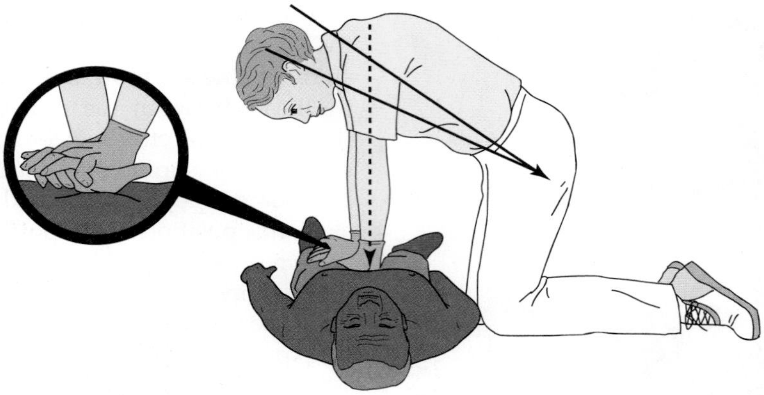

FIGURE 29-4 Giving chest compressions. The arms are straight. The shoulders are over the hands. The fingers are interlocked.

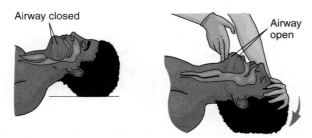

FIGURE 29-5 The head tilt-chin lift method opens the airway. One hand is on the person's forehead. Pressure is applied to tilt the head back. The chin is lifted with the fingers of the other hand.

Airway. The respiratory passages (airway) must be open to restore breathing. The airway is often obstructed (blocked) during SCA. The person's tongue falls toward the back of the throat and blocks the airway. The head tilt-chin lift method opens the airway (Fig. 29-5):

- Place the palm of one hand on the forehead.
- Tilt the head back by pushing down on the forehead with your palm.
- Place the fingers of your other hand under the lower jaw. Use your index and middle fingers. Do not use your thumb.
- Lift the jaw. This brings the chin forward.
- Do not close the person's mouth. The mouth should be slightly open.

Breathing. Air is not inhaled when breathing stops. The person must get oxygen. If not, permanent heart, brain, and other organ damage occurs. The person is given *breaths.* That is, a rescuer inflates the person's lungs.

Each breath should take 1 second. *You should see the chest rise with each breath.* Then two breaths are given after every 30 chest compressions.

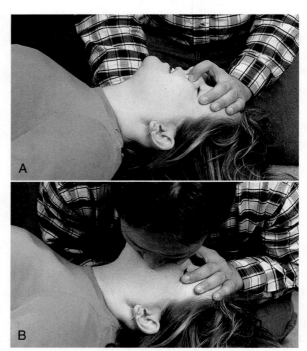

FIGURE 29-6 Mouth-to-mouth breathing. **A,** The person's airway is opened. The nostrils are pinched shut. **B,** The person's mouth is sealed by the rescuer's mouth.

Mouth-to-Mouth Breathing. Mouth-to-mouth breathing (Fig. 29-6) is one way to give breaths. You place your mouth over the person's mouth. Contact with the person's blood, body fluids, secretions, or excretions is likely. To give mouth-to-mouth breathing:

- Keep the airway open with the head tilt-chin lift method.
- Pinch the person's nostrils shut. Use your thumb and index finger. Use the hand on the forehead. Shutting the nostrils prevents air from escaping through the nose.

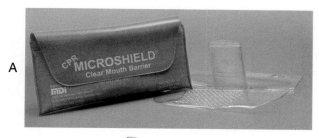

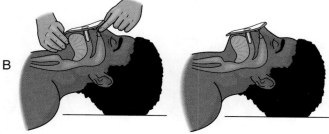

FIGURE 29-7 A, Face shield. **B,** The face shield is in place.

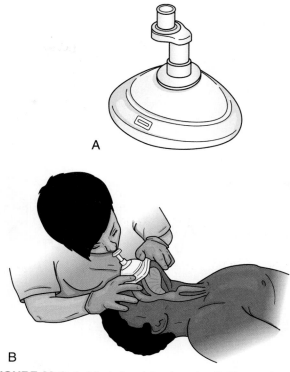

FIGURE 29-8 A, Mask for giving breaths. **B,** The mask is in place.

- Take a breath. A regular breath is needed, not a deep breath.
- Place your mouth tightly over the person's mouth. Seal the person's mouth with your lips.
- Blow air into the person's mouth. You should see the chest rise as the lungs fill with air. You should also hear air escape when the person exhales.
- Repeat the head tilt-chin lift method if the person's chest did not rise.
- Remove your mouth from the person's mouth. Then take in a quick breath.
- Give another breath. You should see the chest rise.

Barrier Device Breathing. A barrier device is used for giving breaths whenever possible. The device prevents contact with the person's mouth and blood, body fluids, secretions, or excretions. A face shield may be used (Fig. 29-7). A face shield is replaced with a face mask as soon as possible (Fig. 29-8, A). The mask is placed over the person's mouth and nose (Fig. 29-8, *B*). When using a barrier device, seal the device against the person's face. The seal must be tight. Then open the airway with the head tilt-chin lift method.

Defibrillation. Ventricular fibrillation (VF, V-fib) is an abnormal heart rhythm (Fig. 29-9, p. 510). It causes sudden cardiac arrest. Rather than beating in a regular rhythm, the heart shakes and quivers like a bowl of Jell-O. The heart does not pump blood. The heart, brain, and other organs do not receive blood and oxygen.

A *defibrillator* is used to deliver a shock to the heart. The shock stops the VF (V-fib). This allows the return of a regular heart rhythm. Defibrillation as soon as possible after the onset of VF (V-fib) increases the person's chance of survival.

For adults, the AHA recommends that rescuers:
- Attach and use the AED as soon as it is available.
- Minimize interruptions in chest compressions before and after a shock is delivered.
- Give one shock. Then resume CPR at once. Begin with compressions. Do 5 cycles of 30 compressions and 2 breaths.
- Check for a heart rhythm.

Automated external defibrillators (AEDs) are found in hospitals, nursing centers, dental offices, and other health care agencies (Fig. 29-10, p. 510). They are on airplanes and in airports, health clubs, malls, and many other public places. Many people have them in their homes.

You will learn more about using an AED in the AHA's *BLS for health care providers* course.

❧ Performing Adult CPR CPR is done only for cardiac arrest. You must determine if cardiac arrest or fainting has occurred. *CPR is done if the person does not respond, is not breathing (or has no normal breathing), and has no pulse.*

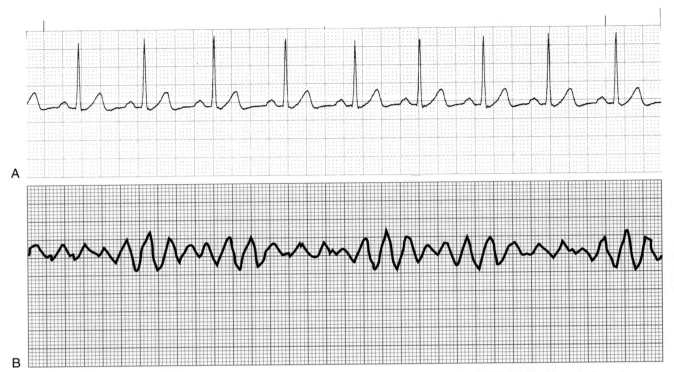

FIGURE 29-9 A, Normal rhythm. **B,** Ventricular fibrillation. *(From Ignatavicius DD, Workman ML: Medical-surgical nursing: critical thinking for collaborative care, ed 5, Philadelphia, 2006, Saunders.)*

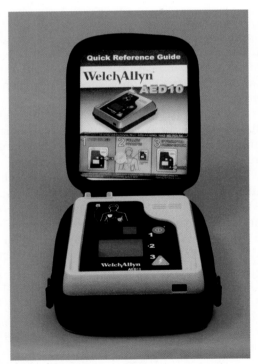

FIGURE 29-10 An automated external defibrillator (AED).

CPR is done alone or with another person. When done alone, chest compressions and rescue breathing are done by the one rescuer. With two rescuers, one person gives chest compressions and the other does rescue breathing. Rescuers switch tasks about every 2 minutes to avoid fatigue and inadequate compressions. The second rescuer uses the AED if one is available.

See *Promoting Safety and Comfort: Performing Adult CPR.*

PROMOTING SAFETY AND COMFORT
Performing Adult CPR

Safety

Never practice CPR on another person. Serious damage can be done. Mannequins are used to learn and practice CPR.

Make sure you have a safe setting for CPR. Move the person only if the setting is unsafe (see Box 29-1, p. 505). Do not approach the person if the scene is unsafe for you.

The person must be on a hard, flat surface for CPR. If the person is in bed, place a board under the person. Or move the person to the floor.

Hands-Only CPR. When an adult has sudden cardiac arrest, the person's survival depends on others nearby. Outside of the health care setting, persons trained in BLS are often not available. Bystanders commonly worry that they will not do CPR correctly or they may injure the person.

The AHA developed "Hands-Only CPR" to improve the response of bystanders who witness an adult collapse suddenly in the out-of-hospital setting. In "Hands-Only CPR", CPR is simplified to 2 steps:
1. Call 911.
2. Push hard and fast in the center of the chest.

"Hands-Only CPR" is used to educate persons not trained in BLS. As a health care provider, use the CPR method presented in this chapter and in a BLS course.

ADULT CPR—ONE RESCUER

PROCEDURE

1 Make sure the scene is safe.
2 Take 5 to 10 seconds to check for a response and breathing:
   a Check if the person is responding. Tap or gently shake the person. Call the person by name, if known. Shout, "Are you OK?"
   b Check for no breathing or no normal breathing (gasping).
3 Call for help. Activate the EMS system or the agency's RRT if the person is not responding and not breathing or not breathing normally (gasping).
4 Get or ask someone to bring an AED if available.
5 Position the person supine on a hard, flat surface. Logroll the person so there is no twisting of the spine. Place the arms alongside the body.
6 Check for a carotid pulse. This should take 5 to 10 seconds. Start chest compressions if you do not feel a pulse.
7 Expose the person's chest.

8 Give chest compressions at a rate of at least 100 per minute. Push hard and fast. Establish a regular rhythm. Count out loud. Press down at least 2 inches. Allow the chest to recoil between compressions. Give 30 chest compressions.
9 Open the airway. Use the head tilt-chin lift method.
10 Give 2 breaths. Each breath should take only 1 second. Each breath must make the chest rise. (If the first breath does not make the chest rise, try opening the airway again. Use the head tilt-chin lift method.)
11 Continue the cycle of 30 chest compressions followed by 2 breaths. Limit interruptions in compressions to less than 10 seconds. Continue cycles until the AED arrives. See procedure *Adult CPR With AED—Two Rescuers* (p. 512). Or continue until help arrives or the person begins to move. If movement occurs, place the person in the recovery position (p. 513).

ADULT CPR—TWO RESCUERS

PROCEDURE

1 Make sure the scene is safe.
2 *Rescuer 1*—take 5 to 10 seconds to check for a response and breathing:
   a Check if the person is responding. Tap or gently shake the person. Call the person by name, if known. Shout, "Are you OK?"
   b Check for no breathing or no normal breathing (gasping).
3 *Rescuer 2:*
   a Activate the EMS system or the agency's RRT if the person is not responding and not breathing or not breathing normally (gasping).
   b Get a defibrillator (AED) if one is available. See procedure *Adult CPR With AED—Two Rescuers*, p. 512.

4 *Rescuer 1:* Position the person supine on a hard, flat surface. Logroll the person so there is no twisting of the spine. Place the arms alongside the body. Begin 1-rescuer CPR until the second rescuer returns. (See procedure *Adult CPR—One Rescuer*, steps 6 to 11.)
5 When the second rescuer returns, perform 2-rescuer CPR (Fig. 29-11).
   a *Rescuer 1:* Give chest compressions at a rate of at least 100 per minute. Push hard and fast. Establish a regular rhythm. Count out loud. Press down at least 2 inches. Allow the chest to recoil between compressions. Give 30 chest compressions. Pause to allow the other rescuer to give 2 breaths.

Continued

ADULT CPR—TWO RESCUERS—cont'd

PROCEDURE—cont'd

b *Rescuer 2:*
    (1) Open the airway. Use the head tilt-chin lift method.
    (2) Give 2 breaths after every 30 compressions. Each breath should take only 1 second and make the chest rise. (If the first breath does not make the chest rise, try opening the airway again. Use the head tilt-chin lift method.)

c Continue cycles of 30 compressions and 2 breaths.

d Change positions every 2 minutes (after about 5 cycles of 30 compressions and 2 breaths). The switch should take no more than 5 seconds.

e Continue until the AED arrives. See procedure *Adult CPR With AED—Two Rescuers.* Or continue until help takes over or the person begins to move. If movement occurs, place the person in the recovery position (p. 513).

ADULT CPR WITH AED—TWO RESCUERS

PROCEDURE

1 Make sure the scene is safe.

2 *Rescuer 1*—Take 5 to 10 seconds to check for a response and breathing:
    a Check if the person is responding. Tap or gently shake the person. Call the person by name, if known. Shout, "Are you OK?"
    b Check for no breathing or no normal breathing (gasping).

3 *Rescuer 2:*
    a Activate the EMS system or the agency's RRT if the person is not responding and not breathing or not breathing normally (gasping).
    b Get a defibrillator (AED) if one is available.

4 *Rescuer 1:*
    a Position the person supine on a hard, flat surface. Logroll the person so there is no twisting of the spine. Place the arms alongside the body.
    b Check for a carotid pulse. This should take 5 to 10 seconds. Start chest compressions if you do not feel a pulse.
    c Expose the person's chest.
    d Give chest compressions at a rate of at least 100 per minute. Push hard and fast. Establish a regular rhythm. Count out loud. Press down at least 2 inches. Allow the chest to recoil between compressions. Give 30 chest compressions.
    e Open the airway. Use the head tilt-chin lift method.
    f Give 2 breaths. Each breath should take only 1 second. Each breath must make the chest rise. (If the first breath does not make the chest rise, try opening the airway again. Use the head tilt-chin lift method.)
    g Continue the cycle of 30 chest compressions followed by 2 breaths. Limit interruptions in compressions to less than 10 seconds.

5 *Rescuer 2:*
    a Open the case with the AED.
    b Turn on the AED.
    c Apply adult electrode pads to the person's chest. Follow the instructions and diagram provided with the AED.
    d Attach the connecting cables to the AED.
    e Clear away from the person. Make sure no one is touching the person.
    f Let the AED check the person's heart rhythm.
    g Make sure everyone is clear of the person if the AED advises a "shock." Loudly instruct others not to touch the person. Say: "I am clear, you are clear, everyone is clear!" Look to make sure no one is touching the person.
    h Press the "SHOCK" button if the AED advises a "shock."

6 *Rescuers 1 and 2:*
    a Perform 2-person CPR:
        (1) Begin with compressions. One rescuer gives chest compressions at a rate of at least 100 per minute. Push hard and fast. Establish a regular rhythm. Count out loud. Allow the chest to recoil between compressions. Give 30 chest compressions. Pause to allow the other rescuer to give 2 breaths.
        (2) The other rescuer gives 2 breaths after every 30 chest compressions.

7 Repeat step 5 e, f, g, and h after 2 minutes of CPR (5 cycles of 30 compressions and 2 breaths). Change positions and continue CPR beginning with compressions.

8 Continue until help takes over or the person begins to move. If movement occurs, place the person in the recovery position (p. 513).

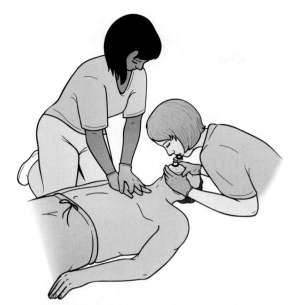

FIGURE 29-11 Two people perform CPR.

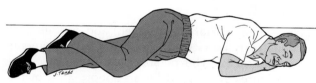

FIGURE 29-12 Recovery position.

Recovery Position

The recovery position is used when the person is breathing and has a pulse but is not responding (Fig. 29-12). The position helps keep the airway open and prevents aspiration.

Logroll the person into the recovery position. Keep the head, neck, and spine straight. A hand supports the head. *Do not use this position if the person might have neck injuries or other trauma.*

HEMORRHAGE

Life and body functions require an adequate blood supply. If a blood vessel is cut or torn, bleeding occurs. The larger the blood vessel, the greater the bleeding and blood loss. **Hemorrhage** is the excessive loss of blood in a short time. If bleeding is not stopped, the person will die.

Hemorrhage is internal or external. You cannot see internal hemorrhage. The bleeding is inside body tissues and body cavities. Pain, shock (p. 514), vomiting blood, coughing up blood, and loss of consciousness signal internal hemorrhage. There is little you can do for internal bleeding.

* Follow the rules in Box 29-1, p. 505. This includes activating the EMS system.
* Keep the person warm, flat, and quiet until help arrives.
* Do not give fluids.

If not hidden by clothing, external bleeding is usually seen. Bleeding from an artery occurs in spurts. There is a steady flow of blood from a vein. To control external bleeding:

* Follow the rules in Box 29-1. This includes activating the EMS system.
* Do not remove any objects that have pierced or stabbed the person.
* Elevate the affected part—hand, arm, foot, or leg.
* Place a sterile dressing directly over the wound. Or use any clean material (handkerchief, towel, cloth, or sanitary napkin).
* Apply pressure with your hand directly over the bleeding site (Fig. 29-13). Do not release pressure until bleeding stops.
* If direct pressure does not control bleeding, apply pressure over the artery above the bleeding site (Fig. 29-14, p. 514). For example, if bleeding is from the lower arm, apply pressure over the brachial artery.
* Bind the wound when bleeding stops. Tape or tie the dressing in place. You can tie the dressing with such things as clothing, a scarf, a necktie, or a belt.

See *Promoting Safety and Comfort: Hemorrhage,* p. 514.

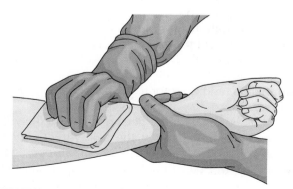

FIGURE 29-13 Direct pressure is applied to the wound to stop bleeding.

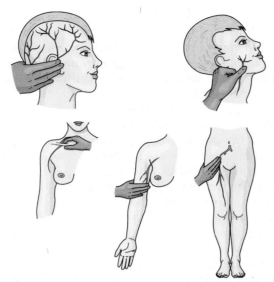

FIGURE 29-14 Pressure points to control bleeding.

PROMOTING SAFETY AND COMFORT
Hemorrhage

Safety

Contact with blood is likely with hemorrhage. Follow Standard Precautions and the Bloodborne Pathogen Standard to the extent possible. Wear gloves if possible. Practice hand hygiene as soon as you can.

SHOCK

Shock results when organs and tissues do not get enough blood. Blood loss, heart attack (myocardial infarction), burns, and severe infection are causes. Signs and symptoms include:

- Low or falling blood pressure
- Rapid and weak pulse
- Rapid respirations
- Cold, moist, and pale skin
- Thirst
- Restlessness
- Confusion and loss of consciousness as shock worsens

Shock is possible in any person who is acutely ill or severely injured. Follow the rules in Box 29-1. Keep the person lying down, maintain an open airway, and control bleeding. Begin CPR if cardiac arrest occurs.

Anaphylactic Shock

Some people are allergic or sensitive to foods, insects, chemicals, and drugs. For example, many people are allergic to the drug penicillin. An *antigen* is a substance that the body reacts to. The body releases chemicals to fight or attack the antigen. The person may react with an area of redness, swelling, or itching. Or the reaction can involve the entire body.

Anaphylaxis is a life-threatening sensitivity to an antigen. (*Ana* means without. *Phylaxis* means protection.) It can occur within seconds. Signs and symptoms include:

- Sweating
- Shortness of breath
- Low blood pressure
- Irregular pulse
- Respiratory congestion
- Swelling of the larynx (laryngeal edema)
- Hoarseness
- Dyspnea

Anaphylactic shock is an emergency. The EMS system must be activated. The person needs special drugs to reverse the allergic reaction. Keep the person lying down and the airway open. Start CPR if cardiac arrest occurs.

SEIZURES

Seizures (convulsions) are violent and sudden contractions or tremors of muscle groups. Movements are uncontrolled. The person may lose consciousness. Seizures are caused by an abnormality in the brain. Causes include head injury, high fever, brain tumors, poisoning, and nervous system disorders or infections. Lack of blood flow to the brain can also cause seizures.

The major types of seizures are:

- *Partial seizure.* Only one part of the brain is involved. A body part may jerk. Or the person has a hearing or vision problem or stomach discomfort. The person does not lose consciousness.
- *Generalized tonic-clonic seizure (grand mal seizure).* This type has two phases. In the *tonic phase*, the person loses consciousness. If standing or sitting, the person falls to the floor. The body is rigid because all muscles contract at once. The *clonic phase* follows. Muscle groups contract and relax. This causes jerking and twitching movements. Urinary and fecal incontinence may occur. A deep sleep is common after the seizure. Confusion and headache may occur on awakening.
- *Generalized absence (petit mal) seizure.* This type usually lasts a few seconds. There is loss of consciousness, twitching of the eyelids, and staring. No first aid is necessary. However, you should guide the person away from dangers—stairs, streets, a hot stove, fireplaces, and so on.

Emergency Care for Seizures

You cannot stop a seizure. However, you can protect the person from injury:

- Follow the rules in Box 29-1. This includes activating the EMS system.
- Do not leave the person alone.
- Lower the person to the floor. This protects the person from falling.
- Note the time the seizure started.
- Place something soft under the person's head (Fig. 29-15). It prevents the person's head from striking the floor. You can use a pillow, a cushion, or a folded blanket, towel, or jacket. Or cradle the person's head in your lap.
- Loosen tight jewelry and clothing around the person's neck. Ties, scarves, collars, and necklaces are examples.
- Turn the person onto his or her side. Make sure the head is turned to the side.
- Do not put any object or your fingers between the person's teeth. The person can bite down on your fingers during the seizure.
- Do not try to stop the seizure or control the person's movements.
- Move furniture, equipment, and sharp objects away from the person. He or she may strike these objects during the seizure.
- Note the time when the seizure ends.
- Make sure the mouth is clear of food, fluids, and saliva after the seizure.
- Provide BLS if the person is not breathing after the seizure.

FAINTING

Fainting is the sudden loss of consciousness from an inadequate blood supply to the brain. Hunger, fatigue, fear, and pain are common causes. Some people faint at the sight of blood or injury. Standing in one position for a long time and being in a warm, crowded room are other causes. Dizziness, perspiration, and blackness before the eyes are warning signals. The person looks pale. The pulse is weak. Respirations are shallow if consciousness is lost. Emergency care for fainting includes the following:

- Have the person sit or lie down before fainting occurs.
- If sitting, the person bends forward and places the head between the knees (Fig. 29-16).
- If the person is lying down, raise the legs.
- Loosen tight clothing (belts, ties, scarves, collars, and so on).
- Keep the person lying down if fainting has occurred. Raise the legs.
- Do not let the person get up until symptoms have subsided for about 5 minutes.
- Help the person to a sitting position after recovery from fainting. Observe for fainting.

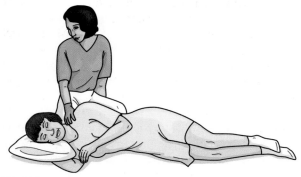

FIGURE 29-15 A pillow protects the person's head during a seizure.

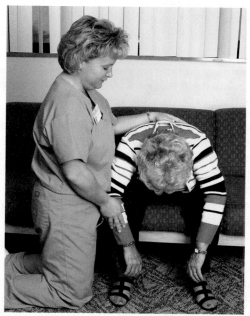

FIGURE 29-16 The person bends forward and lowers her head between her knees to prevent fainting.

STROKE

Stroke (cerebrovascular accident) occurs when the brain is suddenly deprived of its blood supply (Chapter 26). Usually only part of the brain is affected. A stroke may be caused by a thrombus, an embolus, or hemorrhage if a blood vessel in the brain ruptures.

Signs of stroke vary (Chapter 26). They depend on the size and location of brain injury. Loss of consciousness or semi-consciousness, rapid pulse, labored respirations, high blood pressure, facial drooping on one side, and hemiplegia (paralysis on one side of the body) are signs of a stroke. The person may have slurred speech or aphasia (the inability to have normal speech). Loss of vision in one eye, unsteadiness, and falling also are signs. Seizures may occur.

Emergency care includes the following:

* Follow the rules in Box 29-1. This includes activating the EMS system.
* Position the person in the recovery position on the affected side (see Fig. 29-12, p. 513). The affected side is limp, and the cheek appears puffy.
* Raise the head without flexing the neck.
* Loosen tight clothing (belts, ties, scarves, collars, and so on).
* Keep the person quiet and warm.
* Reassure the person.
* Provide CPR if necessary.
* Provide emergency care for seizures if necessary.

Focus on P R I D E
The Person, Family, and Yourself

Personal and Professional Responsibility—Having an understanding of emergency care is a professional responsibility. This knowledge allows you to safely assist in an emergency situation. This chapter includes basic information on emergency care. BLS courses for health care providers offer further training. The courses allow you to practice emergency procedures. CPR and the use of an AED are examples.

Most agencies require nursing assistants to be certified in BLS. Certification courses often involve a written and skills test. During the skills test, you demonstrate your ability to provide BLS. Take the course seriously. And take pride in receiving this training. What you learn can save a life.

Rights and Respect—During emergencies, protect the right to privacy. Do not expose the person unnecessarily. You may be in a place where you cannot close doors or window coverings. The person may be in a lounge, dining area, or public place. Do what you can to provide privacy. As always, treat the person with dignity and respect.

Independence and Social Interaction—Promoting quality of life and independence in an emergency is important. Choices may be few. However, they are given when possible. Hospital care may be required. The person has the right to choose a hospital.

Sometimes the person may refuse care. EMS have guidelines to follow for persons refusing care. For example, the person must be competent and able to legally make his or her own medical decisions. The person must also be informed of the risks, benefits, and alternatives to the care recommended.

Delegation and Teamwork—Onlookers can threaten privacy and confidentiality. During an emergency, your main concern is the person's illness or injuries. You cannot give care and manage onlookers at the same time. Ask someone to deal with onlookers. If someone else is giving care, keep onlookers away from the person. Take pride in working as a team to protect the person's privacy in an emergency situation.

Ethics and Laws—People are curious. They want to know what happened, the extent of injuries or illness, and if the person will be okay. Do not discuss the situation. Do not offer ideas of what is wrong with the person. Information about the person's care, treatment, and condition is confidential. Keep the person's information private. It is the right thing to do.

REVIEW QUESTIONS

Circle the BEST answer.

1 When giving first aid, you should
   a Be aware of your own limits
   b Move the person
   c Give the person fluids
   d Remove clothing
2 The signs of sudden cardiac arrest are
   a Confusion, hemiplegia, and slurred speech
   b Restlessness, rapid breathing, and a weak pulse
   c No response, no normal breathing, and no pulse
   d Dizziness, pale skin, and rapid breathing
3 Rescue breathing for an adult involves
   a Giving each breath over 2 seconds
   b Watching the abdomen rise with each breath
   c Giving a breath every 3 to 5 seconds
   d Giving a breath every 5 to 6 seconds
4 In adult CPR, the chest is compressed
   a 1½ inches with the index and middle fingers
   b 2 inches with the heel of one hand
   c At least 2 inches with two hands
   d At least 1 inch with two hands
5 When checking for breathing,
   a Use the head tilt-chin lift method to open the airway
   b Look for no breathing or gasping
   c Look, listen, and feel for air moving in and out of the lungs
   d Take 10 to 15 seconds to listen for breathing
6 Which pulse is used during adult CPR?
   a The apical pulse
   b The brachial pulse
   c The carotid pulse
   d The femoral pulse
7 Which compression rate is used for CPR?
   a At least 150 compressions per minute
   b At least 100 compressions per minute
   c At least 30 compressions per minute
   d At least 15 compressions per minute
8 When doing adult CPR alone,
   a Give 2 breaths after every 15 compressions
   b Give 2 breaths after every 30 compressions
   c Give 1 breath after every 5 compressions
   d Give 2 breaths when you are tired from giving compressions

9 After delivering a shock with an AED, you should
   a Deliver another shock
   b Place the person in the recovery position
   c Look, listen, and feel for breathing
   d Perform CPR beginning with compressions
10 Arterial bleeding
   a Cannot be seen
   b Occurs in spurts
   c Is dark red
   d Oozes from the wound
11 A person is hemorrhaging from the left forearm. Your first action is to
   a Lower the arm
   b Apply pressure to the brachial artery
   c Apply direct pressure to the wound
   d Tape a dressing in place
12 Which is *not* a sign of shock?
   a High blood pressure
   b Rapid pulse
   c Rapid respirations
   d Cold, moist, and pale skin
13 A person in shock needs
   a Rescue breathing
   b To be kept lying down
   c Clothes removed
   d The head raised
14 These statements relate to tonic-clonic seizures. Which is *false?*
   a There is contraction of all muscles at once.
   b Incontinence may occur.
   c The seizure lasts 5 seconds.
   d There is loss of consciousness.
15 A person is about to faint. Which is *false?*
   a Take the person outside for fresh air.
   b Have the person sit or lie down.
   c Loosen tight clothing.
   d Raise the legs if the person is lying down.
16 A person is having a stroke. Emergency care involves the following *except*
   a Positioning the person on the affected side
   b Giving the person sips of water
   c Loosening tight clothing
   d Keeping the person quiet and warm

Answers to these questions are on p. 528.

30

CARING FOR THE DYING PERSON

PROCEDURE

- Assisting with Post-Mortem Care

OBJECTIVES

- Define the key terms and key abbreviations listed in this chapter.
- Describe the factors that affect attitudes about death.
- Describe the five stages of dying.
- Explain how to meet the needs of the dying person and family.
- Describe hospice care.
- Describe three advance directives and their purposes.
- Identify the signs of approaching death and the signs of death.
- Explain how to promote PRIDE in the person, the family, and yourself.
- Perform the procedure described in this chapter.

KEY TERMS

advance directive A document stating a person's wishes about health care when that person cannot make his or her own decisions

autopsy The examination of the body after death

post-mortem care Care of the body after (*post*) death (*mortem*)

reincarnation The belief that the spirit or soul is reborn in another human body or in another form of life

rigor mortis The stiffness or rigidity (*rigor*) of skeletal muscles that occurs after death (*mortis*)

terminal illness An illness or injury from which the person will not likely recover

KEY ABBREVIATIONS

CPR Cardiopulmonary resuscitation

DNR Do not resuscitate

OBRA Omnibus Budget Reconciliation Act of 1987

Sometimes death is sudden. Often it is expected. Many illnesses and diseases have no cure. Some injuries are so serious that the body cannot function. The disease or injury ends in death. An illness or injury from which the person will not likely recover is a **terminal illness.**

Your feelings about death affect the care you give. You will help meet the dying person's physical, psychological, social, and spiritual needs. Therefore you must understand the dying process. Then you can approach the dying person with caring, kindness, and respect.

ATTITUDES ABOUT DEATH

Many people fear death. Some look forward to and accept death. Attitudes about death often change as a person grows older and with changing circumstances.

Culture and Religion

Practices and attitudes about death differ among cultures. See *Caring About Culture: Death Rites*. In some cultures, dying people are cared for at home by the family. Some families prepare the body for burial.

Attitudes about death are closely related to religion. Some believe that life after death is free of suffering and hardship. They also believe in reunion with loved ones. Many believe sins and misdeeds are punished in the afterlife. Others do not believe in the afterlife. To them, death is the end of life.

There also are religious beliefs about the body's form after death. Some believe the body keeps its physical form. Others believe that only the spirit or soul is present in the afterlife. **Reincarnation** is the belief that the spirit or soul is reborn in another human body or in another form of life.

See *Focus on Communication: Culture and Religion.*

⊘ CARING ABOUT CULTURE
Death Rites

In *Vietnam,* dying persons are helped to recall past good deeds and to achieve a fitting mental state. Death at home is preferred over death in the hospital. In some areas, a coin or jewels (a wealthy family) and rice (a poor family) are put in the dead person's mouth. This is from the belief that they will help the soul go through encounters with gods and devils and the soul will be born rich in the next life.

The *Chinese* have an aversion to death and anything concerning death. Autopsy and disposal of the body are not prescribed by religion. Donating body parts is encouraged. The eldest son makes all arrangements. The body is buried in a coffin. After 7 years, the body is exhumed and cremated. The urn, containing the ashes, is buried in the family tomb. White, yellow, or black clothing is worn for mourning.

In *India,* Hindu persons are often accepting of God's will. The person's desire to be clear-headed as death nears must be assessed in planning medical treatment. A time and place for prayer are essential for the family and the person. Prayer helps them deal with anxiety and conflict. The Hindu priest reads from Holy Sanskrit books. Some priests tie strings (meaning a blessing) around the neck or wrist. After death, the son pours water into the mouth of the deceased. Blood transfusions, organ transplants, and autopsies are allowed. Cremation is preferred.

From D'Avanzo CE: *Pocket guide to cultural health assessment,* ed 4, St Louis, 2008, Mosby.

FOCUS ON COMMUNICATION
Culture and Religion

You may have different cultural or religious practices and beliefs about death. You must not judge the person by your standards. Do not make negative comments or insult the person's beliefs. Respect the person as a whole. This includes his or her beliefs and customs.

Age

Infants and toddlers do not understand the nature or meaning of death. They are aware of or sense that something is different. They sense that a caregiver is absent or that there is a different caregiver. They also sense changes in when and how their needs are met. They may feel a sense of loss.

Between 2 and 6 years old, children think death is temporary. The dead person can come back to life. These ideas come from fairy tales, cartoons, movies, video games, and TV. Children this age often blame themselves when someone or something dies. To them, death is punishment for being bad. They know when family members or pets die. They notice dead birds or bugs. Answers to questions about death often cause fear and confusion. Children who are told "He is sleeping" may be afraid to go to sleep.

Between 6 and 11 years, children learn that death is final. They do not think that they will die. Death happens to other people, especially adults. It can be avoided. Children relate death to punishment and body mutilation. It also involves witches, ghosts, goblins, and monsters. Understanding increases as children grow older and have more experiences with death.

Adults fear pain and suffering, dying alone, and the invasion of privacy. They also fear loneliness and separation from loved ones. They worry about the care and support of those left behind. Adults often resent death because it affects plans, hopes, dreams, and ambitions.

Older persons usually have fewer fears than younger adults. They know death will occur. Some welcome death as freedom from pain, suffering, and disability. Death also means reunion with those who have died. Like younger adults, they often fear dying alone.

THE STAGES OF DYING

Dr. Elisabeth Kubler-Ross described five stages of dying.

- *Stage 1: Denial*. The person refuses to believe that he or she is dying. "No, not me" is a common response. The person believes a mistake was made.
- *Stage 2: Anger*. The person thinks "Why me?" There is anger and rage. Dying persons envy and resent those with life and health. Family, friends, and the health team are often targets of anger.
- *Stage 3: Bargaining*. Anger has passed. The person now says "Yes, me, but...." Often the person bargains with God for more time. Promises are made in exchange for more time. Bargaining is usually private and spiritual.
- *Stage 4: Depression*. The person thinks "Yes, me" and is very sad. The person mourns things that were lost and the future loss of life.
- *Stage 5: Acceptance*. The person is calm and at peace. The person has said what needs to be said. Unfinished business is completed.

Dying persons do not always pass through all five stages. A person may never get beyond a certain stage. Some move back and forth between stages. For example, Mr. Jones reached acceptance but moves back to bargaining. Then he moves forward to acceptance. Some people stay in one stage.

THE PERSON'S NEEDS

Dying people have psychological, social, and spiritual needs. They may want family and friends present. They may want to talk about their fears, worries, and anxieties. Some want to be alone. Often they need to talk during the night. Things are quiet. There are few distractions, and there is more time to think. You need to listen and use touch.

- *Listening*. The person needs to talk and share worries and concerns. Let the person express feelings and emotions in his or her own way. Do not worry about saying the wrong thing or finding comforting words. You do not need to say anything. Being there for the person is what counts.
- *Touch*. Touch shows caring and concern when words cannot. Sometimes the person does not want to talk but needs you nearby. Do not feel that you need to talk. Silence, along with touch, is a powerful and meaningful way to communicate.

Some people may want to see a spiritual leader. Or they want to take part in religious practices. Provide privacy during prayer and spiritual moments. Be courteous to the spiritual leader. The person has the right to have religious objects nearby—medals, pictures, statues, writings, and so on. Handle these valuables with care and respect.

Every effort is made to promote physical and psychological comfort. The person is allowed to die in peace and with dignity.

See *Focus on Communication: Psychological and Spiritual Needs*.

Vision, Hearing, and Speech

Vision blurs and gradually fails. The person naturally turns toward light. A darkened room may frighten the person. The eyes may be half-open. Secretions may collect in the eye corners.

Because of failing vision, explain what you are doing to the person or in the room. The room should be

> ### FOCUS ON COMMUNICATION
> #### Psychological and Spiritual Needs
>
> You may not know what to say to the dying person. That is hard for many experienced health team members. Unless you have been near death yourself, do not say "I understand what you are going through." The statement is a communication barrier. Instead you can say:
> - "Would you like to talk? I have time to listen."
> - "You seem sad. Can I help?"
> - "Is it okay if I quietly sit with you for a while?"

well lit. However, avoid bright lights and glares. Good eye care is essential.

Hearing is one of the last functions lost. Many people hear until the moment of death. Even unconscious persons may hear. Always assume that the person can hear. Speak in a normal voice. Provide reassurance and explanations about care. Offer words of comfort. Avoid topics that could upset the person.

Speech becomes harder. It may be hard to understand the person. Sometimes the person cannot speak. Anticipate the person's needs. Do not ask questions that need long answers. Ask "yes" or "no" questions. These should be few in number. Despite speech problems, you must talk to the person.

Mouth, Nose, and Skin

Oral hygiene promotes comfort. Give routine mouth care if the person can eat and drink. Frequent oral hygiene is given as death nears and when taking oral fluids is difficult. Oral hygiene is needed if mucus collects in the mouth and the person cannot swallow.

Crusting and irritation of the nostrils can occur. Nasal secretions, an oxygen cannula, and an NG (naso-gastric) tube are common causes. Carefully clean the nose. Apply lubricant as directed by the nurse and the care plan.

Circulation fails and body temperature rises as death nears. The skin feels cool, pale, and mottled (blotchy). Perspiration increases. Skin care, bathing, and preventing pressure ulcers are necessary. Linens and gowns are changed whenever needed. Although the skin feels cool, only light bed coverings are needed. Blankets may make the person feel warm and cause restlessness.

Elimination

Urinary and fecal incontinence may occur. Use incontinence products or bed protectors as directed. Give perineal care as needed. Constipation and urinary retention are common. Enemas and catheters may be needed. Provide catheter care according to the care plan.

Comfort and Positioning

Skin care, personal and oral hygiene, back massages, and good alignment promote comfort. Some persons have severe pain. The nurse gives pain-relief drugs ordered by the doctor. Frequent position changes and supportive devices promote comfort. Turn the person slowly and gently. Semi-Fowler's position is usually best for breathing problems.

The Person's Room

Provide a comfortable and pleasant room. It should be well lit and well ventilated. Remove unnecessary equipment. Some equipment is upsetting to look at (suction machines, drainage containers). If possible, keep these items out of the person's sight.

Mementos, pictures, cards, flowers, and religious items provide comfort. The person and family arrange the room as they wish. This helps meet love, belonging, and self-esteem needs. The room should reflect the person's choices.

THE FAMILY

This is a hard time for the family. It may be very hard to find comforting words. Show you care by being available, courteous, and considerate. Use touch to show your concern.

The health team makes the family as comfortable as possible. Respect the right to privacy. The person and family need time together. However, do not neglect care because the family is present. Most agencies let family members help give care. Or you can suggest that they take a break for a beverage or meal.

The family may be very tired, sad, and tearful. Watching a loved one die is very painful. So is dealing with the eventual loss of that person. The family goes through stages like the dying person. They need support, understanding, courtesy, and respect. A spiritual leader may provide comfort. Communicate this request to the nurse at once.

HOSPICE CARE

Hospice care focuses on the physical, emotional, social, and spiritual needs of dying persons and their families (Chapter 1). It is not concerned with cure or life-saving measures. Pain relief and comfort are stressed. The goal is to improve the dying person's quality of life.

Follow-up care and support groups for survivors are hospice services. Hospice also provides support for the health team to help deal with a person's death.

LEGAL ISSUES

Much attention is given to the right to die. Some people make end-of-life wishes known.

The Patient Self-Determination Act and the Omnibus Budget Reconciliation Act of 1987 (OBRA) give persons the right to accept or refuse medical treatment. They also give the right to make advance directives. An **advance directive** is a document stating a person's wishes about health care when that person cannot make his or her own decisions. Advance directives usually forbid certain care if there is no hope of recovery. These laws protect quality of care. Quality of care cannot be less because of the person's advance directives.

- *Living wills.* A living will is a document about measures that support or maintain life when death is likely. Tube feedings, ventilators, and CPR (cardiopulmonary resuscitation) are examples. A living will may instruct doctors:
  - Not to start measures that prolong dying
  - To remove measures that prolong dying
- *Durable power of attorney for health care.* This gives the power to make health care decisions to another person. Usually this is a family member, friend, or lawyer. When a person cannot make health care decisions, the person with durable power of attorney can do so.
- *"Do Not Resuscitate" (DNR) order.* This means that the person will not be resuscitated. The person is allowed to die with peace and dignity. The DNR order is written after consulting with the person and family. The family and doctor make the decision if the person is not mentally able to do so.

SIGNS OF DEATH

There are signs that death is near. These signs may occur rapidly or slowly:

- Movement, muscle tone, and sensation are lost. This usually starts in the feet and legs. When mouth muscles relax, the jaw drops. The mouth may stay open. The facial expression is often peaceful.
- Peristalsis and other gastro-intestinal functions slow down. Abdominal distention, fecal incontinence, nausea, and vomiting are common.
- Body temperature rises. The person feels cool or cold, looks pale, and perspires heavily.
- Circulation fails. The pulse is fast, weak, and irregular. Blood pressure starts to fall.

- The respiratory system fails. Slow or rapid and shallow respirations are observed. Mucus collects in the airway. This causes the *death rattle* that is heard.
- Pain decreases as the person loses consciousness. However, some people are conscious until the moment of death.

The signs of death include no pulse, no respirations, and no blood pressure. The pupils are fixed and dilated. A doctor determines that death has occurred. He or she pronounces the person dead.

❖ CARE OF THE BODY AFTER DEATH

Care of the body after *(post)* death *(mortem)* is called **post-mortem care.** A nurse gives post-mortem care. You may be asked to assist. Post-mortem care begins when the doctor pronounces the person dead.

Post-mortem care is done to maintain a good appearance of the body. Discoloration and skin damage are prevented. Valuables and personal items are gathered for the family. The right to privacy and the right to be treated with dignity and respect apply after death.

Within 2 to 4 hours after death, rigor mortis develops. **Rigor mortis** is the stiffness or rigidity *(rigor)* of skeletal muscles that occurs after death *(mortis).* The body is positioned in normal alignment before rigor mortis sets in. The family may want to see the body. The body should appear in a comfortable and natural position for this viewing.

In some agencies, the body is prepared only for viewing by the family. The funeral director completes post-mortem care.

Sometimes an autopsy is done. An **autopsy** is the examination of the body after death. (*Autos* means *self. Opsis* means *view.*) Its purpose is to determine the cause of death. The coroner or medical examiner can order an autopsy. Or the family can request one. Follow agency procedures when an autopsy is to be done. Post-mortem care is not done. Doing so could remove or destroy evidence.

Post-mortem care involves moving the body. For example, soiled areas are bathed and the body is placed in good alignment. Moving the body can cause remaining air in the lungs, stomach, and intestines to be expelled. When air is expelled, sounds are produced. Do not let these sounds alarm or frighten you. They are normal and expected.

See *Delegation Guidelines: Post-Mortem Care.*
See *Promoting Safety and Comfort: Post-Mortem Care.*

When assisting with post-mortem care, you need this information from the nurse:
- If dentures will be inserted or placed in a denture cup
- If tubes and dressings will be removed or left in place
- If rings will be removed or left in place
- If the family wants to view the body
- Special agency policies and procedures

Safety

Standard Precautions and the Bloodborne Pathogen Standard are followed. You may have contact with blood, body fluids, secretions, or excretions.

ASSISTING WITH POST-MORTEM CARE

PRE-PROCEDURE

1 Follow *Delegation Guidelines: Post-Mortem Care.* See *Promoting Safety and Comfort: Post-Mortem Care.*
2 Practice hand hygiene.
3 Collect the following:
   - Post-mortem kit (shroud or body bag, gown, ID tags, gauze squares, safety pins)
   - Bed protectors
   - Wash basin
   - Bath towel and washcloths
   - Denture cup
   - Tape
   - Dressings
   - Gloves
   - Cotton balls
   - Valuables envelope
4 Provide for privacy.
5 Raise the bed for body mechanics.
6 Make sure the bed is flat.

PROCEDURE

7 Put on the gloves.
8 Position the body supine. Arms and legs are straight. A pillow is under the head and shoulders. Or raise the head of the bed 15 to 20 degrees if this is agency policy.
9 Close the eyes. Gently pull the eyelids over the eyes. Apply moist cotton balls gently over the eyelids if the eyes will not stay closed.
10 Insert dentures if it is agency policy to do so. If not, put them in a labeled denture cup.
11 Close the mouth. If necessary, place a rolled towel under the chin to keep the mouth closed.
12 Follow agency policy for jewelry. Remove all jewelry, except for wedding rings if this is agency policy. List the jewelry that you removed. Place the jewelry and the list in a valuables envelope.
13 Place a cotton ball over the rings. Tape them in place.
14 Remove drainage containers.
15 Remove tubes and catheters. Use the gauze squares as needed.
16 Bathe soiled areas with plain water. Dry thoroughly.
17 Place a bed protector under the buttocks.
18 Remove soiled dressings. Replace them with clean ones.
19 Put a clean gown on the body. Position the body as in step 8.
20 Brush and comb the hair if necessary.
21 Cover the body to the shoulders with a sheet if the family will view the body.
22 Gather the person's belongings. Put them in a bag labeled with the person's name. Make sure you include eyeglasses, hearing aids, and other valuables.
23 Remove supplies, equipment, and linens. Straighten the room. Provide soft lighting.
24 Remove the gloves. Decontaminate your hands.
25 Let the family view the body. Provide for privacy. Return to the room after they leave.
26 Decontaminate your hands. Put on gloves.
27 Fill out the ID tags. Tie one to the ankle or to the right big toe.
28 Place the body in the body bag or cover it with a sheet. Or apply the shroud (Fig. 30-1, p. 524).
   a Position the shroud under the body.
   b Bring the top down over the head.
   c Fold the bottom up over the feet.
   d Fold the sides over the body.
   e Pin or tape the shroud in place.
29 Attach the second ID tag to the shroud, sheet, or body bag.
30 Leave the denture cup with the body.
31 Pull the privacy curtain around the bed. Or close the door.

Continued

ASSISTING WITH POST-MORTEM CARE—cont'd

POST-PROCEDURE

32 Remove the gloves. Decontaminate your hands.
33 Strip the unit after the body has been removed. Wear gloves for this step.
34 Remove the gloves. Decontaminate your hands.

35 Report the following:
   • The time the body was taken by the funeral director
   • What was done with jewelry, other valuables, and personal items
   • What was done with dentures

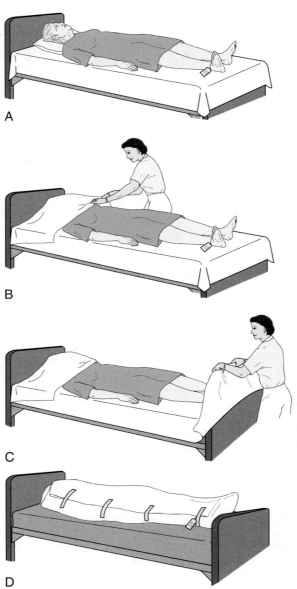

A

B

C

D

FIGURE 30-1 Applying a shroud. **A,** Position the shroud under the body. **B,** Bring the top of the shroud down over the head. **C,** Fold the bottom up over the feet. **D,** Fold the sides over the body. Tape or pin the sides together. Attach the ID tag.

Focus on P R I D E
The Person, Family, and Yourself

Personal and Professional Responsibility—You are responsible for assisting the nurse with the dying person's care. The person has the right to die with peace and dignity. To give quality care:
• Promote comfort. Report the person's complaints of pain or signs of pain to the nurse at once. Follow the comfort measures in the care plan.
• Protect the person's privacy.
• Provide support to the person and family. Be kind. Show compassion and respect.
• Offer time alone with family.
   Take pride in being a support to the person and family during a difficult time.

Rights and Respect—You may not agree with advance directive or resuscitation decisions. However, you must respect the person's or family's wishes. The doctor's orders must be followed. The decision may be against your personal, religious, and cultural values. If so, discuss the matter with the nurse. An assignment change may be needed.

Independence and Social Interaction—The person is encouraged to take part in his or her care to the extent possible. Some days the person can do more than on other days. Follow the nurse's directions and the care plan. Do not force the person to do more than he or she can physically or mentally do.

Delegation and Teamwork—The nurse may need to spend a lot of time with the dying person. Often it is a busy time before and after someone dies. Offer to take equipment and supplies to and from the room. Also offer to help with other patients and residents.

Ethics and Laws—The dying person has rights under OBRA:

- *The right to privacy before and after death.* The person has the right not to have his or her body seen by others. Proper draping and screening are important.
- *The right to confidentiality before and after death.* The final moments and cause of death are kept confidential. So are statements, conversations, and family reactions.
- *The right to be free from abuse, mistreatment, and neglect.* The person has the right to receive kind and respectful care before and after death. Always report signs of abuse, mistreatment, or neglect to the nurse at once.

- *Freedom from restraint.* Restraints are used only if ordered by the doctor. Dying persons are often too weak to be dangerous to themselves or others.
- *The right to have personal possessions.* The person may want photos and religious items nearby. Protect the person's property from loss or damage before and after death. They may be family treasures or mementos.
- *The right to personal choice.* The person has the right to be involved in treatment and care. The dying person may refuse treatment. Advance directives are common. The health team must respect choices to refuse treatment or not prolong life.

REVIEW QUESTIONS

Circle the BEST answer.

1 Which is *true?*
 a Death from terminal illness is sudden and unexpected.
 b Doctors know when death will occur.
 c An illness is terminal when recovery is not likely.
 d All severe injuries end in death.
2 Reincarnation is the belief that
 a There is no afterlife
 b The spirit or soul is reborn into another human body or another form of life
 c The body keeps its physical form in the afterlife
 d Only the spirit or soul is present in the afterlife
3 Adults and older persons usually fear
 a Dying alone   c The five stages of dying
 b Reincarnation   d Advance directives
4 Persons in the stage of denial
 a Are angry
 b Make "deals" with God
 c Are sad and quiet
 d Refuse to believe they are dying
5 A dying person tries to gain more time during the stage of
 a Anger   c Depression
 b Bargaining   d Acceptance
6 When caring for the dying person, you should
 a Use touch and listen
 b Do most of the talking
 c Keep the room darkened
 d Speak in a loud voice

7 As death nears, the last sense lost is
 a Sight   c Smell
 b Taste   d Hearing
8 The dying person's care includes the following *except*
 a Eye care
 b Mouth care
 c Active range-of-motion exercises
 d Position changes
9 The dying person is positioned in
 a The supine position
 b The Fowler's position
 c Good body alignment
 d The dorsal recumbent position
10 A "DNR" order was written. This means that
 a CPR will not be done
 b The person has a living will
 c Life-prolonging measures will be carried out
 d The person is kept alive as long as possible
11 The signs of death are
 a Convulsions and incontinence
 b No pulse, respirations, or blood pressure
 c Loss of consciousness and convulsions
 d The eyes stay open, no muscle movements, and the body is rigid
12 Post-mortem care is done
 a After rigor mortis sets in
 b After the doctor pronounces the person dead
 c When the funeral director arrives for the body
 d After the family has viewed the body

Answers to these questions are on p. 528.

REVIEW QUESTION ANSWERS

Chapter 1
1 b
2 b
3 a
4 b
5 a
6 b
7 a
8 a
9 a
10 d
11 T
12 T
13 T
14 F
15 F
16 T
17 F
18 T
19 T
20 T
21 F
22 T
23 F
24 T
25 T

Chapter 2
1 d
2 c
3 c
4 b
5 c
6 c
7 a
8 a
9 b
10 c
11 b
12 b
13 c
14 a
15 c
16 c
17 d
18 a
19 d
20 c
21 b
22 a
23 d
24 b
25 a
26 c

Chapter 3
1 T
2 T
3 F

4 T
5 T
6 F
7 F
8 F
9 F
10 c
11 d
12 d
13 d
14 c
15 c
16 d
17 c
18 a
19 a
20 c
21 d
22 b
23 a
24 d

Chapter 4
1 a
2 d
3 b
4 c
5 b
6 c
7 d
8 b
9 b
10 c
11 c
12 d
13 d
14 b
15 a
16 d
17 b
18 b

Chapter 5
1 c
2 d
3 b
4 b
5 c
6 b
7 d
8 c
9 a
10 d
11 d
12 d
13 c
14 b

Chapter 6
1 a
2 b
3 c
4 c
5 a
6 b
7 c
8 d
9 d
10 b
11 a
12 b
13 b
14 b
15 c
16 d
17 a
18 b

Chapter 7
1 b
2 a
3 d
4 b
5 c
6 b
7 a
8 d
9 c
10 a
11 a
12 a
13 b
14 b

Chapter 8
1 d
2 c
3 c
4 d
5 d
6 b
7 a
8 b
9 b
10 c
11 b
12 d
13 b
14 b
15 b
16 c
17 b
18 c
19 b
20 d

Chapter 9
1 a
2 d
3 c
4 a
5 a
6 c
7 d
8 c
9 a
10 b
11 a
12 c
13 c
14 a

Chapter 10
1 F
2 T
3 T
4 F
5 F
6 T
7 T
8 T
9 F
10 F
11 F
12 T
13 F
14 T
15 F
16 a
17 c
18 b
19 c
20 a
21 d
22 c
23 c
24 d

Chapter 11
1 T
2 F
3 F
4 F
5 F
6 T
7 b
8 d
9 d
10 a
11 d
12 a
13 d
14 a
15 c
16 a

17 d
18 d

Chapter 12
1 d
2 b
3 a
4 a
5 c
6 c
7 b
8 b
9 c
10 a

Chapter 13
1 b
2 a
3 a
4 b
5 a
6 b
7 a
8 a
9 a
10 a
11 a
12 a
13 d
14 b
15 c

Chapter 14
1 d
2 b
3 d
4 b
5 d
6 d
7 a
8 c
9 b
10 b
11 a
12 a
13 d
14 c
15 a
16 b
17 T
18 T
19 F
20 T
21 T
22 T

Chapter 15
1 T
2 T

3 F
4 F
5 F
6 F
7 F
8 F
9 F
10 T
11 T
12 T
13 d
14 d
15 b
16 c
17 c
18 d

Chapter 16
1 d
2 b
3 c
4 a
5 d
6 d
7 b
8 d
9 a
10 f
11 T
12 T
13 T
14 F

Chapter 17
1 b
2 d
3 a
4 b
5 d
6 d
7 a
8 a
9 a
10 a
11 d
12 c

Chapter 18
1 a
2 b
3 d
4 a
5 c
6 a
7 a
8 c
9 d
10 d

Chapter 19
1 a
2 a
3 d
4 d
5 c
6 a
7 c
8 a
9 d
10 c
11 d
12 c
13 c
14 b
15 c
16 a
17 a
18 c
19 b
20 a

Chapter 20
1 b
2 a
3 a
4 a
5 b
6 b
7 d
8 a
9 b
10 c
11 d
12 b
13 c
14 c

Chapter 21
1 d
2 b
3 c
4 d
5 d
6 a
7 b

Chapter 22
1 b
2 b
3 c
4 b
5 b
6 c
7 a
8 a
9 c
10 b
11 F
12 F
13 F
14 T

Chapter 23
1 c
2 b
3 b
4 b
5 a
6 b
7 a
8 d
9 b
10 a
11 a
12 c

13 a
14 c
15 b
16 d
17 c
18 a

Chapter 24
1 c
2 c
3 b
4 b
5 d
6 a
7 d
8 a

Chapter 25
1 c
2 b
3 a
4 d
5 a
6 c
7 c
8 T
9 T
10 T
11 F
12 T
13 T
14 T

Chapter 26
1 a
2 a
3 c
4 a

5 a
6 a
7 c
8 a
9 c
10 d
11 b
12 b
13 b
14 b
15 a
16 c
17 c
18 c
19 b
20 a
21 b
22 c
23 d
24 a
25 a
26 b
27 c
28 a
29 a
30 d
31 a
32 d
33 c
34 d
35 c
36 c
37 c
38 a
39 a
40 d

Chapter 27
1 b
2 d
3 c
4 c
5 c
6 c
7 d
8 b
9 d
10 d
11 d
12 c
13 d
14 a

Chapter 28
1 a
2 b
3 a
4 a
5 d
6 d
7 b
8 b
9 a
10 d
11 c
12 a

Chapter 29
1 a
2 c
3 d
4 c
5 b
6 c
7 b

8 b
9 d
10 b
11 c
12 a
13 b
14 c
15 a
16 b

Chapter 30
1 c
2 b
3 a
4 d
5 b
6 a
7 d
8 c
9 c
10 a
11 b
12 b

NATIONAL NURSE AIDE ASSESSMENT PROGRAM (NNAAP™) WRITTEN EXAMINATION CONTENT OUTLINE

The **NNAAP Written Examination** is comprised of seventy (70) multiple choice questions. Ten (10) of these questions are pre-test (non-scored) questions on which statistical information will be collected.

I. Physical Care Skills
    A. Activities of Daily Living *14% of exam*
       1. Hygiene
       2. Dressing and Grooming
       3. Nutrition and Hydration
       4. Elimination
       5. Rest/Sleep/Comfort
    B. Basic Nursing Skills *35% of exam*
       1. Infection Control
       2. Safety/Emergency
       3. Therapeutic/Technical Procedures
       4. Data Collection and Reporting
    C. Restorative Skills *8% of exam*
       1. Prevention
       2. Self Care/Independence

II. Psychosocial Care Skills
    A. Emotional and Mental Health Needs *10% of exam*
    B. Spiritual and Cultural Needs *4% of exam*

III. Role of the Nurse Aide
    A. Communication *7% of exam*
    B. Client Rights *7% of exam*
    C. Legal and Ethical Behavior *5% of exam*
    D. Member of the Health Care Team *10% of exam*

NATIONAL NURSE AID ASSESSMENT PROGRAM (NNAAP™) SKILLS EVALUATION

List of Skills

1. Washes Hands
2. Applies one knee high stocking
3. Assists to ambulate using transfer belt
4. Cleans upper or lower denture
5. Counts and records radial pulse
6. Counts and records respirations
7. Donning and removing PPE (gown and gloves)
8. Dresses client with affected (weak) right arm
9. Feeds client who cannot feed self
10. Gives modified bed bath (face and one arm, hand and underarm)
11. Makes an occupied bed (client does not need assistance to turn)
12. Measures and records blood pressure (two-step procedure)
13. Measures and records urinary output
14. Measures and records weight of ambulatory client
15. Performs passive range of motion (PROM) for one knee and ankle
16. Performs passive range of motion (PROM) for one shoulder
17. Positions on side
18. Provides catheter care for female
19. Provides fingernail care on one hand
20. Provides foot care on one foot
21. Provides mouth care
22. Provides perineal care (peri-care) for female
23. Transfers from bed to wheelchair using transfer belt

USEFUL SPANISH VOCABULARY AND PHRASES*

ENGLISH	SPANISH
A bowel movement.	Hacer del baño. (Ah-sehr dehl bah-nyoh)
A glass of juice?	¿Un vaso de jugo? (oon bah-soh deh hoo-goh)
A glass of water?	¿Un vaso de agua? (oon bah-soh deh ah-goo-ah)
A nurse will see you.	Una enfermera la atenderá. (Ooh-nah ehn-fehr-meh-rah lah ah-tehn-deh-rah)
A virus known as HIV . . .	El virus causal del SIDA se conoce como VIH . . . (Ehl bee-roos kah-oo-sahl dehl see-dah seh koh-noh- seh koh-moh beh-ee-ah- cheh [VIH])
abdomen	abdomen (ahb-doh-mehn)
Activities are part of the plan.	Las actividades son parte del plan. (Lahs ahk-tee-bee-dah-dehs sohn pahr-teh dehl plahn)
After meals.	Después de las comidas. (Dehs-poo-ehs deh lahs koh-mee-dahs)
AIDS has a high fatality rate approaching 100%.	El SIDA tiene una tasa cercana al cien por ciento de mortalidad. (Ehl see-dah tee-eh-neh oo-nah tah-sah sehr-kah-nah ahl see-ehn pohr see-ehn-toh deh mohr-tah-lee-dahd)
Among the vegetables that we serve are:	Entre los vegetales que servimos hay: (Ehn-treh lohs beh-heh-tah-lehs keh sehr-bee-mohs ah-ee)
anesthesia	anestesia (ah-nehs-teh-see-ah)
apple	manzana (mahn-sah-nah)
Are you cold?	¿Tiene frío? (Tee-eh-neh free-oh)
Are you comfortable?	¿Está cómoda? (Ehs tah koh-moh-dah)
Are you constipated?	¿Está estreñido? (Ehs-tah ehs-treh-nyee-doh)
Are you dizzy?	¿Tiene mareos? (Tee-eh-neh mah-reh-ohs)
Are you having problems breathing?	¿Tiene problemas al respirar? (Tee-eh-neh proh-bleh-mahs ahl rehs-pee-rahr)
Are you hot?	¿Tiene calor? (tee-eh-neh kah-lohr)
Are you hungry?	¿Tiene hambre? (Tee-eh-neh ahm-breh)
Are you hurting?	¿Tiene dolor? (Tee-eh-neh doh-lohr)
Are you nauseated?	¿Está nauseado?/¿Tiene náuseas? (Ehs-tah nah-oo-seh-ah-doh/Tee-eh-neh nah-oo-seh-ahs)
Are you okay?	¿Está bien?/¿Se siente bien? (Ehs-tah bee-ehn/ Seh see-ehn-teh bee-ehn)
Are you sleepy?	¿Tiene sueño? (Tee-eh-neh soo-eh-nyoh)
Are you thirsty?	¿Tiene sed? (Tee-eh-neh sehd)

ENGLISH	SPANISH
asthma	asma (ahs-mah)
at eleven thirty.	a las once y media. (ah lahs ohn-seh ee meh-dee-ah)
at five PM.	a las cinco de la tarde. (ah lahs seen-koh deh lah tahr-deh)
at seven AM.	a las siete de la mañana. (ah lahs see-eh-teh deh lah mah-nyah-nah)
At what time do you get up?	¿A qué hora se levanta? (Ah keh oh-rah seh leh-bahn-tah)
At what time do you go to bed?	¿A qué hora se acuesta? (Ah keh oh-rah seh ah-koo-ehs-tah)
At what time do you go to sleep?	¿A qué hora se acuesta a dormir? (Ah keh oh-rah seh ah-koo-ehs-tah ah dohr-meer)
aunt	tía (tee-ah)
Backward.	Atrás. (Ah-trahs)
bacteria	bacteria (bahk-teh-ree-ah)
baked chicken	pollo asado (poh-yoh ah-sah-doh)
baked potatoes	papas asadas (pah-pahs ah-sah-dahs)
beans	frijoles/habas (free-hoh-lehs/ah-bahs)
beef	res (rehs)
Bend it.	Dóblala. (Doh-blah-lah)
Bend the wrist.	Dobla la muñeca. (Doh-blah lah moo-nyeh-kah)
Bend your elbow.	Dobla el codo. (doh-blah ehl koh-doh)
Bend your hip.	Dobla tu cadera. (Doh-blah too kah-deh-rah)
Bend your toes.	Dobla sus dedos (del pie). (Doh-blah toos deh-dohs [dehl pee-eh]
black	negro (neh-groh)
blue	azul (ah-sool)
bradycardia	bradicardia (brah-dee-kahr-dee-ah)
breaded	empanizado (ehm-pah-nee-sah-doh)
breast	pechuga (peh-choo-gah)
breast-feeding?	¿tomando pecho? (toh-mahn-doh peh-choh)
Breathe in.	Respire. (Rehs-pee-reh)
Breathe out.	Saque el aire. (Sah-keh ehl ah-ee-reh)
broiled fish	pescado al horno (pehs-kah-doh ahl ohr-noh)
brother	hermano (ehr-mah-noh)

ENGLISH	SPANISH
brother-in-law	cuñado (koo-nyah-doh)
Call if you need help.	Llame si necesita ayuda. (Yah-meh see neh-seh-see-tah ah-yoo-dah)
Can casual contact cause AIDS?	¿Los contactos eventuales puden causar SIDA? (Lohs kohn-tahk-tohs eh-behn-too-ah-lehs poo-eh-dehn kah-oo-sahr see-dah)
cancer	cáncer (kahn-sehr)
candy	dulces (dool-sehs)
cardiac	cardíaco (kahr-dee-ah-koh)
Change into the gown.	Póngase esta bata. (Phn-gah-seh ehs-tah bah-tah)
chemotherapy	quimioterapia (kee-mee-oh-teh-rah-pee-ah)
chicken	pollo (poh-yoh)
children	hijos (eeh-hohs)
chocolate	chocolate (choh-koh-lah-teh)
chops	chuletas (choo-leh-tahs)
claustrophobia	claustrofobia (klah-oos-troh-foh-bee-ah)
clear	claro (klah-roh)
Close it.	Ciérrala. (See-eh-rah-lah)
coffee	café (kah-feh)
coma	coma (koh-mah)
comatose	comatoso (koh-mah-toh-soh)
communication	comunicación (koh-moo-nee-kah-see-ohn)
cookies	galletas (gah-yeh-tahs)
corn	maíz/elote (mah-ees/eh-loh-teh)
corn flakes	hojitas de maíz/corn flakes (oh-hee-tahs de mah-ees/hohrn fleh-ee-ks)
Cough!	¡Tosa! (Toh-sah)
Cough deeply.	Tosa más fuerte. (Toh-sah mahs foo-ehr-teh)
Cough harder!	¡Tosa más fuerte! (Toh-sah mahs foo-ehr-teh)
coughing, sneezing, kissing, or swimming with infected persons	tos, estornudo, besar, o nadar con personas infectadas (tohs, ehs-tohr-noo-doh, beh-sahr oh nah-dahr kohn pehr-soh-nahs een-fehk-tah-dahs)
cousin (female)	prima (pree-mah)
cousin (male)	primo (pree-moh)

ENGLISH	SPANISH
cousins	primos (pree-mohs)
cream of wheat	crema de trigo (kreh-mah deh tree-goh)
dad	papá (pah-pah)
daughter	hija (ee-hah)
decaffeinated	descafeinado (dehs-kah-feh-ee-nah-doh)
dehydration	deshidratación (deh-see-drah-tah-see-ohn)
delirious	delirio (deh-lee-ree-oh)
Dial 9, wait for the tone, then dial the number you want to call.	Marque el nueve, espere el tono, luego marque el número que quiera llamar. (mahr-keh ehl noo-eh-beh, ehs-peh-reh ehl toh-noh, loo-eh-doh mahr-key ehl noo-meh roh keh kee-eh-rah yah-mahr)
Did you bring a hearing aid?	¿Trajo un aparato para oír? (Trah-hoh oon ah-pah-rah-toh pah-rah oo-eer)
Did you bring an artificial eye?	¿Trajo un ojo artificial? (Trah-hoh oon prohs-teh tee-koh)
Did you bring an artificial limb?	¿Trajo un prostético? (Trah-hoh oon oh-hoh ahr-tee-fee-see-ahl)
Did you bring contact lenses?	¿Trajo lentes de contacto? (Trah-hoh lehn-tehs deh kohn-tahk-toh)
Did you bring dentures?	¿Trajo una dentadura postiza? (Trah-hoh oon-ah dehn-tah-doo-rah pohs-tee-sah)
Did you bring glasses?	¿Trajo anteojos/lentes? (Trah-hoh ahn-teh-oh-hohs/lehn-tehs)
Did you bring jewelry?/cash?	¿Trajo joyas?/diner? (Trah-hoh hoh-yahs/dee-neh-roh
Did you fall?	¿Se cay—? (Seh kah-yoh)
Difficulty in swallowing . . .	Diffcultad al tragar . . . (Dee-fee-kool-tahd ahl-trah-gahr)
Do not drink alcohol with this medicine.	No tome alcohol con esta medicina. (Noh toh-meh ahl-kohl kohn ehs-tah meh-dee-see-nah)
Do not drive!	¡No maneje/conduzca! (Noh mah-neh-heh/ kohn-doos-kah)
Do not operate machinery!	¡No maneje/opere una máquina/maquinaria! (Noh mah-neh-heh/oh-peh- reh oo-nah mah-kee-nah/ah-kee-nah-ree-ah)
Do not put on plastic pants!	¡No le ponga calzones de plástico! (Noh leh pohn-gah kahl-sohn-ehs deh plahs-tee-koh)
Do you feel dizzy?	¿Se siente mareado? (Seh see-ehn-teh mah-reh-ah-doh)
Do you feel nauseated?	¿Se siente nauseado? (Seh see-ehn-teh nah-oo-seh-ah-doh)

ENGLISH	SPANISH
Do you feel weak?	¿Se siente débril? (Seh see-ehn-teh deh-beel)
Do you have any symptoms: nausea, dizziness, other unusual feelings?	¿Tiene algún síntoma como náuseas, vértigo, otra sensación rara? (Tee-eh-neh ahl-goon seen-toh-mah koh-moh nah-oo-seh-ahs, behr-tee-goh, oh-trah sehn-sah-see-ohn rah-rah)
Do you have chest pain?	¿Tiene dolor en el pecho? (Tee-eh-neh doh-lohr ehn ehl peh-choh)
Do you have diarrhea?	¿Tiene diarrea? (Tee-eh-neh dee-ah-reh-ah)
Do you have dizzy spells?	¿Tiene mareos? (Tee-eh-neh mah-reh-ohs)
Do you have pain?	¿Tiene dolor? (Tee-eh-neh doh-lohr)
Do you have problems with starting to urinate?	¿Tiene dificultad para empezar a orinar? (Tee-eh-neh dee-fee-kool-tahd pah-rah ehm-peh-sahr ah oh-ree-nahr)
Do you have problems with your teeth?	¿Tienes problemas con los dientes? (Tee-eh-nehs proh-bleh-mahs kohn lohs dee-ehn-tehs)
Do you have vision problems?	¿Tienes problemas con la visión? (Tee-eh-nehs proh-bleh-mahs kohn lah bee-see-ohn)
Do you know the day?	¿Qué día es hoy? (Keh dee-ah ehs oh-ee)
Do you know where we are?	¿Sabe dónde está? (Sah-beh dohn-deh ehs-tah)
Do you like them hot/cold?	¿Le gustan calientes/fríos? (Leh goos-tahn kah-lee-ehn-tehs/free-ohs)
Do you need ice?	¿Necesita hielo? (Neh-seh-see-tah ee-eh-loh)
Do you need more pillows?	¿Necesita más almohadas? (Neh-seh-see-tah mahs ahl-moh-ah-dahs)
Do you need the headboard up?	¿Necesita levantar más la cabecera? (Neh-seh-see-tah leh-bahn-tahr mahs lah kah-beh-seh-rah)
Do you sleep during the day?	¿Duerme durante el día? (Doo-ehr-meh doo-rahn-teh ehl dee-ah)
Do you speak English?	¿Habla inglés? (Ah-blah een-glehs)
Do you take a special diet?	¿Toma dieta especial? (Toh-mah dee-eh-tah ehs-peh-see-ah-lehs)
Do you understand?	¿Comprende?/¿Entiende? (Kohm-prehn-deh/ Ehn-tee-ehn-deh)
Do you wake up at night?	¿Se despierta en la noche? (Seh dehs-pee-ehr-tah ehn lah noh-chen)
Do you want a cup of coffee?	¿Quiere una taza de café? (Kee-eh-reh oo-nah tah-sah deh-kah-feh)
Do you want a glass of juice?	¿Quiere un vaso con jugo? (Kee-eh-reh oon bah-soh kohn hoo-goh)

ENGLISH	SPANISH
Do you want a glass of water?	¿Quiere un vaso con agua? (Kee-eh-reh oon bah-soh kohn ah-goo-ah)
Do you want something to drink?	¿Quiere algo de tomar/beber? (Kee-eh-reh ahl-goh deh toh-mahr/beh-behr)
Do you want the bedpan?	¿Quiere el pato/el bacín? (Kee-eh-reh ehl pah-toh/ehl bah-seen)
Do you want to have a bowel movement?	¿Quiere evacuar?¿Quiere obrar? (Kee-eh-reh eh-bah-koo-ahr/Kee-eh-reh oh-brahr)
Do you want to pass urine?	¿Quiere orinar? (Kee-eh-reh oh-ree-nahr)
Do you want water?	¿Quiere agua? (Kee-eh-reh ah-goo-ah)
Do you want:	¿Quiere: (Kee-eh-reh)
Do you wear glasses?	¿Usa anteojos/lentes? (Oo-sahs ahn-teh-ohhohs/ lehn-tehs)
Do you wish to have a bowel movement?	¿Quiere evacuar/hacer del baño? (Kee-eh-reh eh-bah-koo-ahr/ ah-sehr dehl bah-nyoh)
Does he cry a lot?	¿Llora mucho? (Yoh-rah moo-choh)
Does he/she have: fever/diarrhea/ colic?	¿Tiene: fiebre/diarrea/cólico? (Tee-eh-neh: fee-eh-breh/dee-ah-rreh-ah/ koh-lee-koh)
Does it have undigested food?	¿Tiene restos de comida? (Tee-eh-neh rehs-tohs deh koh-mee-dah)
Does it hurt to breathe?	¿Te duele al respirar? (Teh doo-eh-leh ahl toh-sehr)
Does it hurt to cough?	¿Te duele al toser? (Teh doo-eh-leh ahl toh-sehr)
Does it smell bad?	¿Huele mal? (Oo-eh-leh mahl)
Does it still hurt?	¿Todavía le duele? (Toh-dah-bee-ah leh doo-eh-leh)
Does the baby sleep all night?	¿Duerme el bebé toda la noche? (Doo-ehr-meh ehl beh-beh toh-dah lah noh-cheh)
Does the pain get better if you stop and rest?	¿Se mejora el dolor si se detiene y descansa? (Seh meh-hoh-rah ehl doh-lohr see seh deh-tee-eh-neh ee dehs-kahn-sah)
Does the pain move from one place to another?	¿El dolor se mueve de un lugar a otro? (Ehl doh-lohr seh moo-eh-beh deh oon loo-gahr ah oh-trah)
Does the vomit have blood?	¿Tiene sangre el vómito? (Tee-eh-neh sahn-greh ehl boh-mee-toh)
eating food handled by persons with AIDS	comer comida preparada por personas infectadas con SIDA (koh-mehr koh-mee-dah preh-pah-rah-dah pohr pehr-soh-nahs een-fehk-tah-dahs kohn see-dah)
eggs	huevos (oo-eh-bohs)
embolism	embolismo (ehm-boh-lees-moh)
employ	emplear (ehm-pleh-ahr)

ENGLISH	SPANISH	ENGLISH	SPANISH
epilepsy	epilepsia (eh-peel-ehp-see-ah)	fried chicken	pollo frito (poh-yoh free-toh)
Every time you urinate, put it in the container.	Cada vez que orine, póngala en el frasco. (Kah-dah behs keh oh-ree-neh, pohn-gah-lah ehn ehl frahs-koh)	fruit	fruta (froo-tah)
Every two hours.	Cada dos horas. (Kah-dah dohs oh-rahs)	glaucoma	glaucoma (glah-oo-koh-mah)
Every time you go to the bathroom to void, you must place the urine in the container.	Cada vez que vaya al baño a orinar, debe poner la orina en el recipiente. (Kah-dah behs keh bah-yah ahl bah-nyoh ah oh-ree-nahr, deh-beh poh-nehr lah oh-ree-nah ehn ehl reh-see-pee-ehn-teh)	godfather	padrino (pah-dree-noh)
		godmother	madrina (mah-dree-nah)
		godparents	padrinos (pah-dree-nohs)
Excuse me.	Con permiso. (kohn pehr-mee-soh)	Good afternoon.	Buenas tardes. (Boo-eh-nahs tahr-dehs)
exercise	ejercicio (eh-hehr-see-see-oh)	Good afternoon, Miss González.	Buenas tardes, señorita González. (Boo-eh-nahs tahr-dehs, seh-nyoh-ree-tah Gohn-sah-lehs)
Extend it.	Extiéndelo. (Ehx-tee-ehn-deh-loh)	Good evening.	Buenas noches. (Boo-eh-nahs noh-chehs)
Extend your arm.	Extiende tu brazo. (Ehx-tee-ehn-deh too brah-soh)	Good luck!	¡Buena suerte! (Boo-eh-nah soo-ehr-teh)
Extend your leg and foot.	Extiende tu pierna y pie. (Ehx-tee-ehn-deh too pee-ehr-nah ee pee-eh)	Good morning.	Buenos días. (Boo-eh-nohs dee-ahs)
Extend your wrist.	Extiende tu muñeca. (Ehx-tee-ehn-deh too moo-nyeh-kay)	Good morning, doctor!	!Buenos días, doctor! (Boo-eh-nohs dee-ahs, dohk-tohr)
father	padre (pah-dreh)	Good morning, Mrs. Ortiz!	!Buenos días, señora Ortiz! (Boo-eh-nohs dee-ahs, seh-nyo-rah ohr-tees)
father-in-law	suegro (soo-eh-grah)	Good morning, sir.	Buenos días, señor. (Boo-eh-nohs dee-ahs, seh-nyohr)
fetus of infected mothers	fetos de madres contaminadas (feh-tohs deh mah-drehs kohn-tah-mee-nah-dahs)	Good!	¡Bueno! (Boo-eh-noh)
fever	fiebre (fee-eh-bray)	Good-bye!	¡Hasta luego! (Ahs-tah loo-eh-goh)
fish	pescado (pehs-kah-doh)	grandchildren	nietos (nee-eh-tohs)
Flex it.	Dóblalo. (Doh-blah-loh)	grandfather	abuelo (ah-boo-eh-loh)
Flex the foot upward.	Dobla el pie hacia arriba. (Doh-blah ehl pee-eh ah-see-ah ah-ree-bah)	grandmother	abuela (ah-boo-eh-lah)
Flex your arm.	Dobla tu brazo. (Doh-blah too brah-soh)	grandparents	abuelos (ah-boo-eh-lohs)
Flex your foot upward.	Dobla el pie para arriba. (Doh-blah ehl pee-eh pah-rah ah-ree-bah)	grape	uva (oo-bah)
		grapefruit	toronja (toh-rohn-hah)
For breakfast:	Para el desayuno: (Pah-rah ehl deh-sah-yoo-noh)	great-grandparents	bisabuelos (bee-sah-boo-eh-lohs)
for what?	¿para qué? (pah-rah keh)	green	verde (behr-deh)
for whom?	¿para quién? (pah-rah kee-ehn)	green beans	ejotes/habichuelas (eh-hoh-tehs/ah-bee-choo-eh-lahs)
Forward.	Adelante. (Ah-deh-lahn-teh)	hamburger	hamburguesa (ahm-boor-geh-sah)
french fries	papas fritas (pah-pahs free-tahs)	hard-boiled	duros (doo-rohs)
Friday	viernes (bee-ehr-nehs)	Has the pain gotten worse or gotten better?	¿Se ha puesto el dolor peor o mejor? (Seh ah poo-ehs-toh ehl doh-lohr peh-ohr oh meh-hohr)
fried	fritos (free-tohs)	Have a good day!	¡Pase un buen día! (Pah-seh oon boo-ehn dee-ah)
		Have you eaten?	¿Ha comido? (Ah koh-mee-doh)

ENGLISH	SPANISH
Have you had headaches?	¿Ha tenido dolor de cabeza? (Ah teh-nee-doh doh-lohr deh kah-beh-sah)
Have you seen blood in the urine?	¿Ha visto sangre en la orina? (Ah bees-toh sahn-greh ehn lah oh-ree-nah)
Hello.	Hola (Oh-lah)
Hello!	¡Hola! (Oh-lah)
Hello, I'm John Goodguy.	Hola, soy John Goodguy. (Oh-lah, soh-ee John Goodguy)
Hello, Mrs. Mora.	Hola, señora Mora. (Oh-lah, seh-nyoh-rah Moh-rah)
Help him to burp.	Póngalo a repetir/eructar. (Pohn-gah-loh ah reh-peh-teer/ eh-rook-tahr)
hematoma	hematoma (eh-mah-toh-mah)
hemophiliacs and recipients of blood/blood components	hemofílicos, donadores de sangre o transfusión con sangre contaminada (eh-moh-fee-lee-kohs, doh-nah-doh-rehs deh sahn-greh oh trahns-foo-see-ohn kohn sahn-greh kohn-tah-mee-nah-dah)
Here is a glass of water to rinse with.	Aquí está un vaso de agua para que se enjuague. (Ah-kee-ehs-tah oon bah-soh deh ah-goo-ah pah-rah keh seh ehn-hoo-ah-geh)
Hi!	¡Hola! (Oh-lah)
HIV is not transmissible by casual contact, nor . . .	El VIH no es transmitido en forma casual, ni por . . . (Ehl VIH noh ehs trahns-mee-tee-doh ehn fohr-mah kah-soo-ahl, nee pohr)
How are you?	¿Cómo está? (Koh-moh ehs-tah)
How do you feel?	¿Cómo se siente? (Koh-moh seh see-ehn-teh)
How do you feel now?	¿Cómo se siente ahora? (Koh-moh seh see-ehn-teh ah-oh-rah)
How do you like the eggs fixed?	¿Cómo le gustan los huevos? (Koh-moh leh goos-tahn lohs oo-eh-bohs)
How do you like your coffee?	¿Comó le gusta el café? (Koh-moh leh goos-tah ehl kah-feh)
How long?	¿Cuánto tiempo? (Koo-ahn-toh tee-ehm-poh)
How many diapers have you changed since yesterday?	¿Cuántos pañales le ha cambiado desde ayer? (Koo-ahn-tohs pah-nyah-lehs leh ah kahm-bee-ah-doh dehs-deh ah-yehr)
How many glasses of water do you drink?	¿Cuántos vasos de agua toma? (Koo-ahn-tohs bah-sohs de ah-goo-ah toh-mah)
How many hours do you sleep?	¿Cuántas horas duerme? (Koo-ahn-tahs oh Drahs doo-ehr-meh)

ENGLISH	SPANISH
How many ounces does he take?	¿Cuántas onzas toma? (Koo-ahn-tahs ohn sahs-toh-mah)
How many times do you eat per day?	¿Cuántas veces come por día? (Koo-ahn-tahs beh-sehs koh- meh pohr dee-ah)
How many times does he wake up?	¿Cuántas veces se despierta? (Koo-ahn-tahs beh-sehs seh dehs-pee-ehr-tah)
How many times has he vomited?	¿Cuántas veces ha vomitado? (Koo-ahn-tahs beh-sehs ah boh-mee-tah-doh)
how many?	¿cuántos? (koo-ahn-tohs)
How may I help you?	¿En qué puedo servirle? (Ehn keh poo-eh-doh sehr-beer-leh)
how much?	¿cuánto? (koo-ahn-toh)
How often do you feed the baby?	¿Qué tan a menudo alimenta al bebé? (keh tahn ah meh-noo-doh ah-lee-mehn-tah ahl beh-beh)
How often do you have the pain?	¿Qué tan seguido tiene el dolor? (Keh tahn seh-gee-doh tee-eh-neh ehl doh-lohr)
How often do you urinate?	¿Cuántas veces orina? (Koo-ahn-tahs beh-sehs oh-ree-nah)
How serious is AIDS?	¿Qué tan serio es el SIDA? (Keh tahn seh-ree-oh ehs-ehl see-dah)
How severe is the pain?	¿Qué tan severo es el dolor? (Keh tahn seh-beh-roh ehs ehl doh-lohr)
husband	esposo (ehs-poh-soh)
I also need a urine sample.	También necesito una muestra de orina. (Tahm-bee-ehn neh-seh-see-toh oo-nah moo-ehs-trah deh oh-ree-nah)
I am going to ask many questions!	¡Voy a hacerle muchas preguntas! (Boy ah ah-sehr-leh moo-chahs preh-goon-tahs)
I am going to clean your teeth.	Voy a limpiarle los dientes. (Boy ah leem-pee-ahr-leh lohs dee-ehn-tehs)
I am going to cover you.	Lo voy acubrir. (Loh boy ah-koo-breer)
I am going to explain how to collect the urine.	Le voy a explicar cómo juntar la orina. (Leh boy ah ehx-plee-kahr koh-moh hoon-tahr lah oh-ree-nah)
I am going to explain the collection of the urine.	Le voy a explicar la colección de orina. (Leh boy ah ehx-plee-kahr lah koh-lehk-see-ohn de oh-ree-nah)
I am going to give you a list.	Voy a darle una lista. (Boy ah dahr-leh oo-nah lees-tah)
I am going to give you a tour of the floor.	Voy a darle un recorrido por el piso. (Boy ah dahr-leh oon reh-koh-ree-doh pohr ehl pee-soh)

ENGLISH	SPANISH
I am going to help you lie down.	Voy a ayudarlo a acostarse. (Boy ah ah-yoo-dahr-loh ah ah-kohs-tahr-seh)
I am going to help you lie on the stretcher.	Voy a ayudarlo a acostarse en la camilla. (Boy ah ah-yoo-dahr-loh ah ah-kohs-tahr-seh ehn lah kah-mee-yah)
I am going to let you rest.	Voy a dejarlo descansar. (Boy ah deh-hahr-loh dehs-kahn-sahr)
I am through.	Ya terminé. (Yah tehr-mee-neh)
I need to ask you some questions.	Necesito hacerle unas preguntas. (Neh-seh-see-toh ah-sehr-leh oo-nahs preh-goon-tahs)
I will ask you to void.	Le diré que orine. (Leh dee-reh keh oh-ree-neh)
I will collect a sample of feces.	Voy a recoger una muestra de excremento. (Boy ah reh-koh-hehr oo-nah moo-ehs-trah deh ehx-kreh-mehn-toh)
I will help you sit.	Le ayudaré a sentarse. (Leh ah-yoo-dah-reh ah sehn-tahr-seh)
I will put you on the stretcher.	Voy a ponerlo en la camilla. (Boy ah poh-nher-loh ehn lah kah-mee-yah)
I will return shortly.	Regresaré en seguida. (Reh-greh-sah-reh ehn seh-ghee-dah)
I will see you tomorrow.	Le veré mañana. (Lah beh-reh mah-nyah-nah)
I will show you your room.	Le mostraré su cuarto. (Leh mohs-trah-reh soo koo-ahr-tah)
I will start by taking vital signs.	Voy a empezar por tomar los signos vitales. (Boy ah ehm-peh-sahr pohr toh-mahr lohs seeg-nohs bee-tah-lehs)
I will take the radial pulse.	Voy a tomar su pulso radial. (Boy ah toh-mahr soo pool-soh rah-dee-ahl)
I will take your blood pressure.	Voy a tomar tu presión de sangre. (Boy ah toh-mahr too preh-see-ohn deh sahn-greh)
ice cream	nieve/helado (nee-eh-beh/eh-lah-doh)
If it hurts, tell me.	Si duele, avísame. (See doo-eh-leh, ah-bee-sah-meh)
If there is no ice in the bucket, call me.	Si no hay hielo en la tina, llámeme. (See noh ah-ee ee-eh-loh ehn lah tee-nah, yah-meh-meh)
If you don't understand, please let me know.	Si no entiende, dígame por favor. (See noh ehn-tee-ehn-deh, dee-gah-meh pohr fah-bohr)
In case of fire, take the stairs.	En caso de fuego, use la escalera. (Ehn kah-soh deh foo-eh-goh, oo-seh lah ehs-kah-leh-rah)
independence	independencia (een-deh-pehn-dehn-see-ah)
infancy	infancia (een-fahn-see-ah)

ENGLISH	SPANISH
Infected persons can transmit the virus.	Las personas infectadas pueden transmitir el virus. (Lahs pehr-soh-nahs een-fehk-tah-dahs poo-ehdehn-trahns-mee-teer ehl bee-roos)
inflammation	inflamación (een-flah-mah-see-ohn)
instant	instantáneo (eens-tahn-tah-neh-oh)
insulin	insulina (een-soo-lee-nah)
intravenous drug abusers	los que abusan de las drogas intravenosas (lohs keh ah-boo-sah deh lahs droh-gahs een-trah-beh-noh-sahs)
Is he coughing?	¿Está tosiendo? (Ehs-tah toh-see-ehn-doh)
Is he urinating well?	¿Orina bien? (Oh-ree-nah bee-ehn)
Is he/she . . .	¿Está . . . (Ehs-tah)
Is it/that a lot?	¿Es mucho? (Ehs moo-choh)
Is that enough?	¿Es suficiente? (Ehs soo-fee-see-ehn-teh)
Is that too much?	¿Es demasiado? (Ehs deh-mah-see-ah-doh)
Is the pain there all the time, or does it come and go?	¿Está el dolor allí todo el tiempo, o va y viene? (Ehs-tah ehl doh-lohr ah-yee toh-doh ehl tee-ehm-poh, oh bah ee bee-ehn-eh?)
Is there a danger from donated blood?	¿Qué peligro hay por sangre donada? (Keh peh-lee-groh ah-ee pohr sahn-greh doh-nah-dah)
Is there any pain?	¿Tiene algún dolor? (Tee-eh-neh ahl-goon doh-lohr)
Is there anything else bothering you?	¿Hay otra cosa que le moleste? (Ah-ee oh-trah koh-sah keh-leh moh-lehs-teh)
Is there anything that worries you?	¿Hay algo que le preocupa? (Ah-ee ahl-goh keh leh preh-oh-koo-pah)
Is there numbness/a tingling sensation/burning in your leg/arm/foot/hand?	¿Está entumecido/adormecido/tiene ardor en su pierna/brazo/pie/mano? (Ehs-tah ehn-too-meh-see-doh/ah-dohr-meh-see-do/ tee-eh-neh ahr-dohr ehn soo pee-ehr-nah/brah-soh/ pee-eh/mah-noh)
It can cause drowsiness.	Le puede causar sueño. (Leh poo-eh-deh kah-oo-sahr soo-eh-nyoh)
It keeps the food warm.	Guarda la comida tibia. (Goo-ahr-dah lah koh-mee-dah tee-bee-ah)
juice	jugo (joo-goh)
leg	pierna (pee-ehr-nah)
Let it out.	Exhala. (Ehx-ah-lah)

ENGLISH	SPANISH	ENGLISH	SPANISH
Let me know how you feel.	Dígame cómo se siente. (Dee-gah-meh koh-moh seh see-ehn-teh)	no one, nobody	nadie (nah-dee-eh)
lettuce	lechuga (leh-choo-gah)	No smoking.	No se permite fumar. (Noh seh pehr-mee-teh foo-mahr)
Lift your arm.	Levanta su brazo. (leh-bahn-tah soo brah-soh)	no, not	no (noh)
Lift your foot.	Levanta su pie. (Leh-bahn-tah soo pee-eh)	normal	normal (nohr-mahl)
Lift your leg.	Levanta la pierna. (Leh-bahn-tah lah pee-ehr-nah)	not one, not any	ninguno (neen-goo-noh)
ligament	ligamento (lee-gah-mehn-toh)	nothing	nada (nah-dah)
linen	lino (lee-noh)	Now raise the left arm.	Ahora levante el brazo izquierdo. (Ah-oh-rah leh-bahn-teh ehl brah-soh ees-kee-ehr-doh)
living in the same house as infected persons	vivir en la misma casa con personas infectadas (bee-beer ehn lah mees-mah kah-sah kohn pehr-soh-nahs een-fehk-tah-dahs)	Now, take a deep breath.	Ahora, respira hondo. (Ah-oh-rah, rehs-pee-rah ohn-doh)
Lower your foot.	Baja el pie. (Bah-hah ehl pee-eh)	nutrition	nutrición (noo-tree-see-ohn)
mashed potatoes	puré de papas (poo-reh deh pah-pahs)	oatmeal	avena (ah-beh-nah)
medication	medicamento (meh-dee-kah-mehn-toh)	obsession	obsesión (ohb-seh-see-ohn)
medicine	medicina (meh-dee-see-nah)	On a scale from 1 [insignificant] to 10 [unbearable]	En una escala del uno [insignificante] al diez [intolerable] (Ehn oo-nah ehs-kah-lah dehl oo-noh [een-seeg-nee-fee-kahn-teh] ahl deeehs [een-toh-leh-rah-bleh])
milk	leche (leh-cheh)		
Miss	señorita (seh-nyoh-ree-tah)	Open the fingers wide.	Separa bien los dedos. (Seh-pah-rah bee-ehn lohs deh-dohs)
Monday	lunes (loo-nehs)	Open your hand.	Abre su mano. (Ah-breh soo mah-noh)
mother	madre (mah-dreh)	Open your mouth, please.	Abra la boca, por favor. (Ah-brah lah boh-kah, pohr fah-bohr)
mother-in-law	suegra (soo-eh-grah)		
Move your leg.	Mueve su pierna. (Moo-eh-beh soo pee-ehr-nah)	orange	naranja (nah-rah-hah)
Mr.	señor (seh-nyohr)	organ	órgano (ohr-gah-noh)
Mrs.	señora (seh-nyoh-rah)	over-easy	volteados (bohl-teh-ah-dohs)
Mrs. . . . , I need to help you change clothes.	Señora . . . , necesito ayudarle a cambiar su ropa. (Señora . . . , neh-seh-see-toh ah-yoo-dahr-leh ah kahm-bee-ahr soo roh-pah)	oxygen	oxígeno (ohx-ee-heh-noh)
		Pain?	¿Dolor? (Doh-lohr)
My name is . . .	Mi nombre es . . . /Me llamo . . . (Mee nohm-breh ehs/Meh yah-moh)	pancreas	páncreas (pahn-kreh-ahs)
nausea	náusea (nah-oo-seh-ah)	panic	pánico (pah-nee-koh)
neither	tampoco (tahm-poh-koh)	Pat his back gently.	Dé palmaditas en la espalda. (Deh pahl-mah-dee-tahs ehn lah ehs-pahl-dah)
neither . . . nor	ni . . . ni (nee . . . nee)	pathogen	patogénico (pah-toh-heh-nee-koh)
nephew	sobrino (soh-bree-noh)	peas	chícharos (chee-chah-rohs)
never, not ever	nunca, jamás (noon-kah, hah-mahs)	pecan	nuez (noo-ehs)
niece	sobrina (soh-bree-nah)	Phone for local calls.	Teléfono para llamadas locales. (Teh-leh-foh-noh pah-rah yah-mah-dahs loh-kah-lehs)

ENGLISH	SPANISH
pies	pasteles (pahs-teh-lehs)
pinto beans	frijol pinto (free-hohl peen-toh)
Please stay/remain in bed.	Por favor, quédese en la cama. (Pohr fah-bohr, keh-deh-seh ehn lah kan-mah)
Please!	¡Por favor! (Pohr fah-bohr)
Please walk.	Camina, por favor. (Kah-mee-nah, pohr fah-bohr)
Point.	Apunte./Señale. (Ah-poon-teh/Seh-nyah-leh)
Point where it hurts.	Señale donde duela. (Seh-nyah-leh koo-ahn-doh doo-eh-lah)
pork	puerco (poo-ehr-koh)
potatoes	papas (pah-pahs)
prune	ciruela (see-roo-eh-lah)
Pull the cord in the bathroom.	Jale el cordón en el baño. (Hah-leh ehl kohr-dohn ehn ehl bah-nyoh)
pulse	pulso (pool-soh)
rectal	rectal (rehk-tahl)
red	rojo (roh-hoh)
refried	refritos (reh-free-tohs)
regular	regular (reh-goo-lahr)
Remember that you will do this for 24 hours.	Recuerde que hará esto por veinticuatro horas. (Reh-koo-ehr-deh keh ah-rah ehs-toh pohr beh-een-tee-koo-ah-troh oh-rahs)
respect	respeto (rehs-peh-toh)
Rest.	Descanse. (Des-kahn-seh)
Rest now.	Descanse ahora. (Dehs-kahn-seh ah-oh-rah)
ribs	costillas (kohs-tee-yahs)
Rinse your mouth.	Enjuague su boca. (Ehn-hoo ah-geh soo boh-kah)
roast	rostizado (rohs-tee-sah-doh)
Rotate it.	Gíralo./Dale vuelta. (Hee-rah-loh/Dah-leh boo-ehl-tah)
salad	ensalada (ehn-sah-lah-dah)
saliva	saliva (sah-lee-bah)
salt	sal (sahl)
sanitary	sanitario (sah-nee-tah-ree-oh)
Saturday	sábado (sah-bah-doh)

ENGLISH	SPANISH
scrambled	revueltos (reh-boo-ehl-tohs)
Select your foods from the menu after breakfast.	Seleccione las comidas del menú después del desayuno. (Seh-lehk-see-oh-neh lahs koh-mee-dahs dehl meh-noo dehs-poo-ehs dehl deh-sah-yoo-noh)
sex	sexo (sehx-oh)
sexual	sexual (sehx-oo-ahl)
sexually active homosexual and bisexual males or females	homosexuales activos y hombres o mujeres bisexuales (oh-moh-sehx-oo-ah-lehs ahk-tee-bohs ee ohm-brehs oh moo-heh-rehs bee-sehx-oo-ah-lehs)
sister	hermana (ehr-mah-nah)
sister-in-law	cuñada (koo-nyah-dah)
Sit in the chair.	Siéntese en la silla. (See-ehn-teh-seh ehn lah see-yah)
something to drink?	¿algo de tomar/beber? (ahl-goh deh toh-mahr/beh-behr)
something to eat?	¿algo de comer? (ahl-goh deh koh-mehr)
something to read?	¿algo de leer? (ahl-goh deh leh-ehr)
son	hijo (ee-hoh)
spinal	espinal (ehs-pee-nahl)
steak	bistec (bees-tehk)
stepdaughter	hijastra (ee-hahs-trah)
stepfather	padrastro (pah-drahs-troh)
stepmother	madrastra (mah-drahs-trah)
stepson	hijastro (ee-hahs-troh)
Sterilize the bottles.	Esterilice las botellas/ los biberones. (Ehs-teh-ree-lee-seh lahs boh-teh-yahs/lohs bee-beh-roh-nehs)
stethoscope	estetoscopio (ehs-teh-tohs-koh-pee-oh)
Straighten your knee.	Endereza la rodilla. (Ehn-deh-reh-sah lah roh-dee-yah)
Straighten your leg.	Endereza su pierna. (Ehn-deh-reh-sah soo pee-ehr-nah)
strawberry	fresa (freh-sah)
Sunday	domingo (doh-meen-goh)
Swelling of the ankles?	¿Hinchazón en los tobillos? (Een-chah-sohn ehn lohs toh-bee-yohs)
syncope	síncope (seen-koh-peh)
systole	sístole (sees-toh-leh)

ENGLISH	SPANISH
Take it with a full glass of water.	Tómela con un vaso lleno de agua. (Toh-meh-lah kohn oon bah-soh yeh-noh deh ah-goo-a)
Take on an empty stomach.	Tómela con el estómago vacío. (Toh-meh-lah kohn ehl ehs-toh-mah-goh bah-see-oh)
Take one hour before eating.	Tómela una hora antes de comer. (Toh-meh-lah oo-nah oh-rah ahn-tehs de koh-mehr)
Take the medicine with food.	Tome la medicina con comida. (Toh-meh lah mehdee-see-nah kohn koh-mee-dah)
Take the medicine with juice.	Tome la medicina con jugo. (Toh-meh lah meh-dee-see-nah kohn joo-goh)
Take the temperature rectally.	Tome la temperatura por el recto. (Toh-meh lah tehm-peh-rah-too-rah pohr ehl rehk-toh)
taking formula?	¿tomando fórmula? (toh-mahn-doh fohr-moo-lah)
Tell me if it hurts.	Dime si esto le duele. (Dee-meh see ehs-toh leh doo-eh-leh)
Tell me if there is pain.	Dime si duele. (Dee-meh see doo-eh-leh)
Thank you for talking to me!	¡Gracias por hablar conmigo! (Grah-see-ahs pohr ah-blahr kohn-mee-goh)
Thank you very much!	¡Muchas gracias! (Moo-chahs grah-see-ahs)
Thank you!	¡Gracias! (Grah-see-ahs)
The bell will sound.	La campana sonará. (Lah kahm-pah-nah soh-nah-rah)
The chair turns into a bed.	Esta silla se hace cama. (Ehs-tah see-yah seh ah-seh kah-mah)
The container will be kept in the bucket with ice.	El frasco se mantendrá en una tina con hielo. (Ehl frahs-koh seh mahn-tehn-drah ehn oo-nah tee-nah kohn ee-eh-loh)
The cover is hot.	La cubierta está caliente. (Lah koo-bee-ehr-tah ehs-tah kah-lee-ehn-teh)
The elevators work twenty-four hours.	Los elevadores funcionan las veinticuatro horas. (Lohs eh-leh-bah-dohrehs foon-see-oh-nahn lahs beh-een-tee-koo-ah-troh oh-rahs)
the family	la familia (lah fah-mee-lee-ah)
The fork, spoon, and knife are wrapped in the napkin.	El tenedor, cuchara, y cuchillo están envueltos en la servilleta. (Ehl teh-neh-dohr, koo-chah-rah ee koo-chee-yoh ehs-tahn ehn-boo-ehl-tohs ehn lah sehr-bee-yeh-tah)
The meals are served	Los alimentos se sirven (Lohs ah-lee-mehn-tohs seh seer-behn)
The meals are served at . . .	Los alimentos se sirven a . . . (Lohs ah-lee-mehn-tohs seh seer-behn ah)

ENGLISH	SPANISH
The pain is in one place?	¿El dolor es fijo? (Ehl doh-lohr ehs fee-hoh)
The pain is localized, sharp.	El dolor está fijo, agudo. (Ehl doh-lohr ehs-tah ehn ehl lah-dohl kohs-tah-doh)
The pain is on the side.	El dolor está en el lado/costado. (Ehl doh-lohr ehs-tah ehn ehl lah-dohl kohs-tah-doh)
The pain is sharp?	¿El dolor es agudo? (Ehl doh-lohr ehs ah-goo-doh)
The rails lower down.	El barandal se baja. (Ehl bah-rahn-dahl seh bah-hah)
The risk of contracting HIV is not high. Blood banks and other centers use sterile equipment and disposable needles.	El riesgo de contraer VIH no es alto. Los bancos de sangre y otros centros usan equipos estériles y agujas desechables. (Ehl ree-ehs-goh deh kohn-trah-ehr VIH noh ehs ahl-toh. Lohns bahn-kohs deh sahn-greh ee oh-trohs sehn-trohs oo-sahn eh-kee-pohs ehs-teh-ree-lehs ee ah-goo-hahs deh-seh-chah-blehs)
The salt and pepper are in these packets.	La sal y pimienta están en estos paquetes. (Lah sahl ee pee-mee-ehn-tah ehs-tahn ehn ehs-tohn pah-keh-tehs)
The television has four channels.	El televisor tiene cuatro canales. (Ehl teh-leh-bee-sohr tee-eh-neh koo-ah-troh kay-nah-lehs)
The U.S. Public Health Service recommends:	El Departamento de Salud Pública de los Estados Unidos recomienda: (Ehl Deh-pahr-tah-mehn-toh deh Sah-lood Poo-blee-kah deh lohs Ehs-tah-dohs Oo- nee-dohs reh-koh-mee-ehn-dah)
1. Know sexual background/habits of partners.	1. Conozca los hábitos sexuales de su pareja. (Koh-nohs-kah lohs ah-bee-tohs sex-oo-ah-lehs deh soo pah-reh-hah)
2. Use a condom or prophylactic.	2. Use un condón o profiláctico. (Oo-seh oon kohn-dohn oh proh-fee-lahk-tee-koh)
3. If your partner is in a high risk group, cease sexual relations.	3. Si su compañera está en el grupo de alto riesgo, suspenda las relaciones sexuales. (See soo kohm-pah-nyeh-rah ehs-tah ehn ehl groo-pah deh ahl-toh ree-ehs-goh, soos-pehn-dah lahs reh-lah-see-ohn-ehs sehx-oo-ahl-ehs)
4. Eliminate multiple sexual partners.	4. Elimine múltiples compañeros sexuales. (Eh-lee-mee-neh mool-tee-plehs kohm-pha-nyeh-rohs sehx-oo-ah-lehs)
5. Don't use intravenous drugs with contaminated needles; don't share needles or syringes.	5. No use drogas intravenosas con agujas contaminadas; no comparta agujas o jeringas. (Noh oos-eh droh-gahs een-trah-veh-noh-sahs kohn ah-goo-hahs kohn-tah-mee-nah-dahs; noh kohm-pahr-tah ah-goo-hahs oh hehr-een-gahs)

ENGLISH	SPANISH	ENGLISH	SPANISH
The water is in the glass/pitcher.	El agua está en el vaso/la jarra. (Ehl ah-goo-ah ehs-tah ehn ehl bah-soh/lah hah-rah)	Turn your forearm.	Voltea el antebrazo. (Bohl-teh-ah ehl ahn-teh brah-soh)
There are bathrooms for guests in the corner.	Hay baños para las visitas en la esquina. (Hay bah-nyohs pah-rah lahs bee-see-tahs ehn lah ehs-kee-nah)	ulcer	úlcera (ool-seh-rah)
There is a shower.	Hay una ducha/regadera. (Ah-ee oo-nah doo-chah/ reh-gah-deh-rah)	uncle	tío (tee-oh)
There is a straw.	Hay un popote. (Ah-ee oon poh-poh-teh)	Use dental floss.	Use hilo dental. (Oo-seh ee-loh dehn-tahl)
There is also a bathtub/tub.	También hay una bañera/tina. (Tahm-bee-ehn ah-ee oo-nah bah-nyeh-rah/tee-nah)	vanilla	vainilla (bah-ee-nee-yah)
There is an emergency light.	Hay una luz para emergencias. (Ah-ee oo-nah loos pah-rah eh-mehr-hehn-see-ahs)	venereal	venéreo (beh-neh-reh-oh)
thermometer	termómetro (tehr-moh-meh-troh)	vertigo	vértigo (behr-tee-goh)
These buttons move the bed up/down.	Estos botones mueven la cama arriba/abajo. (Ehs-tohs boh-tah-nehs moo-eh-behn lah kay-mah ah-ree-bah/ah-bah-hoh)	vision	visión (bee-see-ohn)
This button lowers (raises) the headboard.	Este botón baha (sube) la cabecera de la cama. (Ehs-teh boh-tohn bah-hah (soo-beh) lah kah-beh-seh-rah deh lah kah-mah)	Visiting hours are from nine in the morning to nine at night.	Las horas de visita son de las nueve de la mañana a las nueve de la noche. (Lahs oh-rahs deh bee-see-tah shon deh lahs noo-eh-beh deh lah mah-nyah-nah ah lahs noo-eh-beh deh lah noh-cheh)
This is the call bell.	Este es el timbre. (Ehs-teh ehs ehl teem-breh)	Visiting hours are from two to eight PM.	Las horas de visita son de las dos a las ocho de la noche. (Lahs oh-rahs deh bee-see- tah sohn deh lahs dohs ah loahs oh-choh deh lah noh-cheh)
This is the call bell/buzzer.	Este es la campana/el timbre. (Ehs-teh ehs lah kahm- pah-nah/ehl teem-breh)	vomit	vómito (boh-mee-toh)
This is the lobby.	Esta es la sala de espera. (Ehs-tah ehs lah sah-lah deh ehs-peh-rah)	Wash hands before eating.	Lave las manos antes de comer. (Lah-beh lahs mah-nohs ahn-tehs deh koh-mehr)
This is the radio.	Este es el radio. (Ehs-teh ehs ehl rah-dee-oh)	Wash well all fruits and vegetables.	Lave bien frutas y verduras. (Lah-beh bee-ehn froo-tahs ee behr-doo-rahs)
This is your room.	Este es su cuarto. (Ehs-teh ehs soo koo-ahr-toh)	We also have desserts.	También tenemos postres: (Tahm-bee-ehn teh-neh-mohs pohs-trehs)
Thursday	jueves (hoo-eh-behs)	We are going in the ambulance.	Vamos en la ambulancia. (Bah-mohs ehn lah ahm-boo-lahn-see-ah)
toast	pan tostado (pahn tohs-tah-doh)	We are going to the hospital.	Vamos al hospital. (Bah-mohs ahl ohs-pee-tahl)
tomato	tomate (toh-mah-teh)	We have cereals.	Tenemos cereales. (Teh-neh-mohs seh-reh-ah-lehs)
Tuesday	martes (mahr-tehs)	We have meats.	Tenemos carnes. (Teh-nehmohs kahr-nehs)
Turn it to the left.	Voltéalo hacia la izquierda. (Bohl-teh-ah-loh ah-see-ah lah ees-kee-ehr-dah)	Wear this bracelet all the time.	Use esta pulsera todo el tiempo. (Oo-seh ehs-tah pool-seh-rah toh-doh ehl tee-ehm-poh)
Turn it to the right.	Voltéalo hacia la derecha. (Bohl-teh-ah-loh ah-see-ah lah deh-reh-chah)	Wednesday	miércoles (mee-ehr-koh-lehs)
Turn on your side.	Voltéese de lado. (Bhol-teh-eh-seh deh lah-doh)	What brought you to the hospital?	¿Qué lo trajo al hospital? (Keh loh trah-hoh ahl ohs-pee-tahl)
Turn the forearm.	Voltea el antebrazo. (Bhol-teh-ah ehl ahn-teh-brah-soh)	What can I help you with?	¿En qué puedo ayudarlo? (Ehn keh poo-eh-doh ah-yoo-dahr-loh)
Turn to your side.	Voltéate de lado. (Bhol-teh-ah-teh deh lah-doh)	What caused the pain?	¿Qué causó el dolor? (Keh kah-oo-soh ehl doh-lohr)
		What causes AIDS?	¿Qué causa el SIDA? (Keh kah-oo-sah ehl see-dah)

ENGLISH	SPANISH
What color?	¿De qué color? (Deh keh koh-lohr)
What did you do that caused the pain?	¿Qué hacía cuando apareció el dolor? (Keh ah-see-ah koo-ahn-doh ah-pah-reh-see-oh ehl doh-lohr)
What did you eat for breakfast?	¿Qué comió en el desayuno? (Keh koh-mee-oh ehn ehl deh-sah-yoo-noh)
What did you eat?	¿Qué comido? (Keh koh-mee-doh)
What foods do you dislike?	¿Qué alimentos le disgustan? (Keh ah-lee-mehn-tohs leh dees-goos-tahn)
What foods do you like?	¿Qué alimentos le gustan? (Keh ah-lee-mehn-tohs leh goos-tahn)
What formula does he take?	¿Qué fórmula toma? (Keh fohr-moo-lah toh-mah)
What is hurting you?	¿Qué le duele? (Keh leh doo-eh-leh)
What is the matter?	¿Qué le pasa/sucede? (Keh leh pah-sah/soo-seh-deh)
What is the pain like?	¿Qué tipo de dolor tiene? (Keh tee-oh deh doh-lohr tee-eh-neh)
What is wrong?	¿Qué pasa? (Keh pah-sah)
What kind of coffee?	¿Qué clase de café? (Keh klah-seh deh kah-feh)
What kind of juices?	¿Qué clase de jugos? (Keh klah-seh deh joo-gohs)
What makes the pain better?	¿Qué hace mejorar el dolor? (Keh ah-seh meh-hoh-rahr ehl doh-lohr)
What other discomfort do you have?	¿Qué otra molestia tiene? (Keh oh-trah moh-lehs-tee-ah tee-eh-neh)
What symptoms do you have?	¿Qué síntomas tiene? (Keh seen-toh-mahs tee-eh-neh)
what?	¿qué?/¿qué tal? (keh/keh tahl)
When did you notice the skin rash?	¿Cuándo se dico cuenta de la piel rosada? (Koo-ahn-doh seh dee-oh koo-ehn-tah deh lah pee-ehl roh-sah-dah)
When was the last time he had a bowel movement?	¿Cuándo fue la última vez que evacuó/hizo del baño? (Koo-ahn-doh foo-eh lah ool-tee-mah behs keh eh-bah-koo-oh/ee-soh dehl bah-nyoh)
When was the last time you ate?	¿Cuándo fue la última vez que comió? (Koo-ahn-doh foo-eh lah ool-tee-mah behs keh koh-mee-oh)
When was the last time you used the toilet?	¿Cuándo fue la última vez que hizo del baño/que obró? (Koo-ahn doh foo-eh lah ool-tee-mah behs keh ee-soh dehl bah-nyoh/keh oh-broh)
When you have pain, do you get nauseated?	¿Cuando tiene dolor, ¿le dan náuseas? (Koo-ahn-doh tee-eh-neh doh-lohr, leh dahn nah-oo-seh-ahs)

ENGLISH	SPANISH
when?	¿cuándo? (koo-ahn-doh)
Where does it hurt?	¿Dónde le duele? (Don-deh leh doo-eh-leh)
where?	¿dónde? (dohn-deh)
which?	¿cuál? (koo-ahl)
white	blanco (blahn-koh)
Who is at risk of getting AIDS?	¿Quién está en riesgo de contraer el SIDA? (Kee-ehn ehs-tah ehn ree-ehs-goh deh kohn-trah-ehr ehl see-dah)
who?	¿quién? (kee-ehn)
why?	¿por qué? (pohr keh)
wife	esposa (ehs-poh-sah)
wings	alas (ah-lahs)
with cream	con crema (kohn kreh-mah)
with ham	con jamón (kohn hah-mahn)
with sugar	con azúcar (kohn ah-soo-kahr)
without	sin (seen)
yellow	amarillo (ah-mah-ree-yoh)
Yes, sir.	Sí, señor. (See, seh-nyohr)
You are welcome.	De nada. (Deh nah-dah)
You can call collect.	Puede llamar por cobrar. (poo-eh-deh yah-mahr pohr koh-brahr)
You can have flowers.	Puede tener flores. (Poo-eh-deh teh-nehr floh-rehs)
You can make local phone calls.	Puede hacer llamadas locales. (Poo-eh-deh ah sehr-yah-mah-dahs loh-kah-lehs)
You can put cards on the shelf.	Puede poner trajetas en el estante. (Poo-eh-deh poh-nehr tahr-heh-tahs ehn ehl ehs- tahn-teh)
You can raise the feet.	Puede levantar los pies. (Poo-eh-deh leh-bahn-tahr lohs pee-ehs)
You can raise the head.	Puede levantar la cabeza. (Poo-eh-deh leh-bahn-tahr lah kah-beh-sah)
You can tape pictures to the wall.	Puede pegar retratos en la pared. (Poo-eh-deh peh-gahr reh-trah-tohs ehn lah pah-rehd)
You cannot smoke here.	No puede fumar aquí. (Noh poo-eh-deh foo-mahr ah-kee)
You cannot smoke in your room.	No puede fumar en el cuatro. (Noh poo-eh-deh foo-mahr ehn ehl koo-ahr-toh)
You have a private bathroom.	Tiene un baño/inodoro privado. (Tee-eh-neh oon bah-nyoh/ ee-noh-doh-roh pree-bah-doh)

ENGLISH	SPANISH
You have to choose three meals a day.	Tiene que escoger tres comidas diarias. (Tee-eh-neh keh ehs-koh-hehr trehs koh-mee-dahs dee-ah-ree-ahs)
Your clothes go in the closet.	Su ropa va en el closet/ropero. (Soo roh-pah bah ehn ehl kloh-seht/roh-peh-roh)
Your towels are in the bathroom.	Su toallas están en el baño. (Soo too-ahyahs ehs-tahn ehn ehl bah-nyoh)

Numbers

ENGLISH	SPANISH
one (1)	uno (oo-noh)
two (2)	dos (dohs)
three (3)	tres (trehs)
four (4)	cuatro (koo-ah-troh)
five (5)	cinco (seen-koh)
six (6)	seis (seh-ees)
seven (7)	siete (see-eh-teh)
eight (8)	ocho (oh-choh)
nine (9)	nueve (noo-eh-beh)
ten (10)	diez (dee-ehs)
eleven (11)	once (ohn-seh)
twelve (12)	doce (doh-seh)
thirteen (13)	trece (treh-seh)
fourteen (14)	catorce (kah-tohr-seh)
fifteen (15)	quince (keen-seh)
sixteen (16)	dieciséis (dee-ehs-ee-seh-ees)
seventeen (17)	diecisiete (dee-ehs-ee-see-eh-teh)
eighteen (18)	dieciocho (dee-ehs-ee-oh-choh)
nineteen (19)	diecinueve (dee-ehs-ee-noo-eh-beh)
twenty (20)	veinte (beh-een-teh)
thirty (30)	treinta (treh-een-tah)
forty (40)	cuarenta (koo-ah-rehn-tah)

ENGLISH	SPANISH
fifty (50)	cincuenta (seen-koo-ehn-tah)
sixty (60)	sesenta (seh-sehn-tah)
seventy (70)	setenta (seh-tehn-tah)
eighty (80)	ochenta (oh-chehn-tah)
ninety (90)	noventa (noh-behn-tah)
one hundred (100)	cien (see-ehn)

Time	Standard	Military (hours PM)
one o'clock	la una (la oo-nah)	las trece horas (lahs treh-seh oh-rahs)
two o'clock	las dos (lahs dohs)	las catorce horas (lahs kah-tohr-seh oh-rahs)
three o'clock	las tres (lahs trehs)	las quince horas (lahs keen-seh oh-rahs)
four o'clock	las cuatro (lahs koo-ah-troh)	las dieciséis horas (lahs dee-ehs-ee-seh-ees oh-rahs)
five o'clock	las cinco (lahs seen-koh)	las diecisiete horas (lahs dee-ehs-ee-see-eh-teh oh-rahs)
six o'clock	las seis (lahs seh-ees)	las dieciocho horas (lahs dee-ehs-ee-oh-choh oh-rahs)
seven o'clock	las siete (lahs see-eh-teh)	las diecinueve horas (lahs dee-ehs-ee-noo-eh-beh oh-rahs)
eight o'clock	las ocho (lahs oh-choh)	las veinte horas (lahs beh-een-teh oh-rahs)
nine o'clock	las nueve (lahs noo-eh-beh)	las veintiuna horas (lahs beh-een-tee-oo-nah oh-rahs)
ten o'clock	las diez (lahs dee-ehs)	las veintidós horas (lahs beh-een-tee-dohs oh-rahs)
eleven o'clock	las once (lahs ohn-seh)	las veintitrés horas (lahs beh-een-tee-trehs oh-rahs)
twelve o'clock/ midnight	las doce/la media noche (lahs doh-seh/lah meh-dee-ah non-cheh)	las cero horas (lahs seh-roh-oh-rahs) las veinticuatro horas (lahs beh-een-tee-koo-ah-troh oh-rahs)

*This appendix is presented for your convenience. Please note: This listing does not include all terms or address all chapters.
Translations taken from Joyce EV, Villanueva ME: *Say it in Spanish: a guide for health care professionals*, ed 3, St Louis, 2004, Saunders.

GLOSSARY

A

abduction Moving a body part away from the midline of the body

abuse The intentional mistreatment or harm of another person

acetone A substance that appears in urine from the rapid breakdown of fat for energy; ketone body or ketone

activities of daily living (ADL) The activities usually done during a normal day in a person's life

acute illness A sudden illness from which the person is expected to recover

adduction Moving a body part toward the midline of the body

advance directive A document stating a person's wishes about health care when that person cannot make his or her own decisions

alopecia Hair loss

ambulation The act of walking

anaphylaxis A life-threatening sensitivity to an antigen

anorexia The loss of appetite

anxiety A vague, uneasy feeling in response to stress

aphasia The total or partial loss *(a)* of the ability to use or understand language *(phasia)*

apnea Lack or absence *(a)* of breathing *(pnea)*

artery A blood vessel that carries blood away from the heart

arthroplasty The surgical replacement *(plasty)* of a joint *(arthr)*

asepsis Being free of disease-producing microbes

aspiration Breathing fluid, food, vomitus, or an object into the lungs

assault Intentionally attempting or threatening to touch a person's body without the person's consent

assisted living residence (ALR) Provides housing, personal care, support services, health care, and social activities in a home-like setting to persons needing help with daily activities

atrophy The decrease in size or the wasting away of tissue

autopsy The examination of the body after death

B

base of support The area on which an object rests

battery Touching a person's body without his or her consent

bed rail A device that serves as a guard or barrier along the side of the bed; side rail

benign tumor A tumor that does not spread to other body parts

biohazardous waste Items contaminated with blood, body fluids, secretions, or excretions; *bio* means life, and *hazardous* means dangerous or harmful

blood pressure The amount of force exerted against the walls of an artery by the blood

board and care home Provides a room, meals, laundry, and supervision

body alignment The way the head, trunk, arms, and legs are aligned with one another; posture

body language Messages sent through facial expressions, gestures, posture, hand and body movements, gait, eye contact, and appearance

body mechanics Using the body in an efficient and careful way

body temperature The amount of heat in the body that is a balance between the amount of heat produced and the amount lost by the body

boundary crossing A brief act or behavior outside of the helpful zone

boundary sign An act, behavior, or thought that warns of a boundary crossing or boundary violation

boundary violation An act or behavior that meets your needs, not the person's needs

bradypnea Slow *(brady)* breathing *(pnea)*; respirations are fewer than 12 per minute

C

calorie The amount of energy produced when the body burns food

cancer See "malignant tumor"

capillary A tiny blood vessel; food, oxygen, and other substances pass from the capillaries into the cells

cardiac arrest See "sudden cardiac arrest"

carrier A human or animal that is a reservoir for microbes but does not have the signs and symptoms of infection

catheter A tube used to drain or inject fluid through a body opening

cell The basic unit of body structure

chart See "medical record"

chemical restraint Any drug that is used for discipline or convenience and not required to treat medical symptoms

Cheyne-Stokes respirations Respirations gradually increase in rate and depth and then become shallow and slow; breathing may stop *(apnea)* for 10 to 20 seconds

chronic illness An on-going illness that is slow or gradual in onset; it has no known cure; it can be controlled and complications prevented with proper treatment

civil law Laws dealing with relationships between people

clean technique See "medical asepsis"

cognitive function Involves memory, thinking, reasoning, ability to understand, judgment, and behavior

colostomy A surgically created opening *(stomy)* between the colon *(colo)* and abdominal wall

coma A state of being unaware of one's surroundings and being unable to react or respond to people, places, or things

comatose Being unable to respond to verbal stimuli

communicable disease A disease caused by pathogens that spread easily; a contagious disease

communication The exchange of information—a message sent is received and correctly interpreted by the intended person

comprehensive care plan A written guide giving direction for the resident's care; required by OBRA

compulsion Repeating an act over and over again

confidentiality Trusting others with personal and private information

constipation The passage of a hard, dry stool

constrict To narrow

contagious disease See "communicable disease"

contamination The process of becoming unclean

contracture The lack of joint mobility caused by abnormal shortening of a muscle

convulsion See "seizure"

crime An act that violates a criminal law

criminal law Laws concerned with offenses against the public and society in general

culture The characteristics of a group of people—language, values, beliefs, habits, likes, dislikes, customs—passed from one generation to the next

D

dandruff Excessive amounts of dry, white flakes from the scalp

defamation Injuring a person's name and reputation by making false statements to a third person

defecation The process of excreting feces from the rectum through the anus; a bowel movement

defense mechanism An unconscious reaction that blocks unpleasant or threatening feelings

dehydration A decrease in the amount of water in body tissues

delegate To authorize another person to perform a nursing task in a certain situation

delirium A state of temporary but acute mental confusion

delusion A false belief

delusion of grandeur An exaggerated belief about one's importance, wealth, power, or talents

delusion of persecution A false belief that one is being mistreated, abused, or harassed

dementia The loss of cognitive and social function caused by changes in the brain; the loss of cognitive function that interferes with routine personal, social, and occupational activities

denture An artificial tooth or a set of artificial teeth

development Changes in mental, emotional, and social function

developmental task A skill that must be completed during a stage of development

diarrhea The frequent passage of liquid stools

diastolic pressure The pressure in the arteries when the heart is at rest

digestion The process of physically and chemically breaking down food so that it can be absorbed for use by the cells

dilate To expand or open wider

disability Any lost, absent, or impaired physical or mental function

disaster A sudden catastrophic event in which people are injured and killed and property is destroyed

disinfection The process of destroying pathogens

dorsal recumbent position See "supine position"

dorsiflexion Bending the toes and foot up at the ankle

dysphagia Difficulty *(dys)* swallowing *(phagia)*

dyspnea Difficult, labored, or painful *(dys)* breathing *(pnea)*

dysuria Painful or difficult *(dys)* urination *(uria)*

E

edema The swelling of body tissues with water

elder abuse Any knowing, intentional, or negligent act by a caregiver or any other person to an older adult

emesis See "vomitus"

enema The introduction of fluid into the rectum and lower colon

enteral nutrition Giving nutrients into the gastro-intestinal (GI) tract *(enteral)* through a feeding tube

ergonomics The science of designing a job to fit the worker

ethics Knowledge of what is right conduct and wrong conduct

extension Straightening a body part

external rotation Turning the joint outward

F

fainting The sudden loss of consciousness from an inadequate blood supply to the brain

false imprisonment Unlawful restraint or restriction of a person's freedom of movement

fecal impaction The prolonged retention and buildup of feces in the rectum

fecal incontinence The inability to control the passage of feces and gas through the anus

feces The semi-solid mass of waste products in the colon that is expelled through the anus

fever Elevated body temperature

first aid Emergency care given to an ill or injured person before medical help arrives

flashback Reliving the trauma in thoughts during the day and in nightmares during sleep

flatulence The excessive formation of gas or air in the stomach and intestines

flatus Gas or air passed through the anus

flexion Bending a body part

flow rate The number of drops per minute

footdrop The foot falls down at the ankle; permanent plantar flexion

Fowler's position A semi-sitting position; the head of the bed is raised between 45 and 60 degrees

fracture A broken bone

fraud Saying or doing something to trick, fool, or deceive a person

freedom of movement Any change in place or position of the body or any part of the body that the person is physically able to control

friction The rubbing of one surface against another

full visual privacy Having the means to be completely free from public view while in bed

functional incontinence The person has bladder control but cannot use the toilet in time

G

gait belt See "transfer belt"

gavage The process of giving a tube feeding

geriatrics The care of aging people

gerontology The study of the aging process

glucosuria Sugar *(glucos)* in the urine *(uria)*; glycosuria

glycosuria Sugar *(glycos)* in the urine *(uria)*; glucosuria

gossip To spread rumors or talk about the private matters of others

growth The physical changes that are measured and that occur in a steady, orderly manner

H

hallucination Seeing, hearing, smelling, or feeling something that is not real

harassment To trouble, torment, offend, or worry a person by one's behavior or comments

hazardous substance Any chemical in the workplace that can cause harm

healthcare-associated infection (HAI) An infection that develops in a person cared for in any setting where health care is given; the infection is related to receiving health care

health team The many health care workers whose skills and knowledge focus on the person's total care; interdisciplinary health care team

hematuria Blood *(hemat)* in the urine *(uria)*

hemiplegia Paralysis *(plegia)* on one side *(hemi)* of the body

hemoglobin The substance in red blood cells that carries oxygen and gives blood its color

hemoptysis Bloody *(hemo)* sputum *(ptysis* means *to spit)*

hemorrhage The excessive loss of blood in a short time

high-Fowler's position A semi-sitting position; the head of the bed is raised 60 to 90 degrees

hirsutism Excessive body hair

holism A concept that considers the whole person; the whole person has physical, social, psychological, and spiritual parts that are woven together and cannot be separated

hormone A chemical substance secreted by the endocrine glands into the bloodstream

hospice An agency or program for persons who are dying

hyperextension Excessive straightening of a body part

hypertension Blood pressure measurements that remain above *(hyper)* a systolic pressure of 140 mm Hg or a diastolic pressure above 90 mm Hg

hyperventilation Respirations *(ventilation)* are rapid *(hyper)* and deeper than normal

hypotension When the systolic blood pressure is below *(hypo)* 90 mm Hg and the diastolic pressure is below 60 mm Hg

hypoventilation Respirations *(ventilation)* are slow *(hypo)*, shallow, and sometimes irregular

hypoxia Cells do not have enough *(hypo)* oxygen *(oxia)*

I

ileostomy A surgically created opening *(stomy)* between the ileum (small intestine *[ileo]*) and the abdominal wall

immunity Protection against a disease or condition; the person will not get or be affected by the disease

infection A disease state resulting from the invasion and growth of microbes in the body

insomnia A chronic condition in which the person cannot sleep or stay asleep all night

intake The amount of fluid taken in

internal rotation Turning the joint inward

intravenous (IV) therapy Giving fluids through a needle or catheter inserted into a vein; IV and IV infusion

invasion of privacy Violating a person's right not to have his or her name, photo, or private affairs exposed or made public without giving consent

J

job description A document that describes what the agency expects you to do

K

ketone See "acetone"

ketone body See "acetone"

Kussmaul respirations Very deep and rapid respirations

L

lateral position The person lies on one side or the other; side-lying position

law A rule of conduct made by a government body

libel Making false statements in print, writing, or through pictures or drawings

lice See "pediculosis"

licensed practical nurse (LPN) A nurse who has completed a 1-year nursing program and has passed a licensing test; called *licensed vocational nurse (LVN)* in some states

licensed vocational nurse (LVN) See "licensed practical nurse"

logrolling Turning the person as a unit, in alignment, with one motion

M

malignant tumor A tumor that invades and destroys nearby tissue and can spread to other body parts; cancer

malpractice Negligence by a professional person

medical asepsis Practices used to remove or destroy pathogens and to prevent their spread from one person or place to another person or place; clean technique

medical record A written or electronic account of a person's condition and response to treatment and care; chart

medical symptom An indication or characteristic of a physical or psychological condition

menopause The time when menstruation stops and menstrual cycles end

menstruation The process in which the lining of the uterus breaks up and is discharged from the body through the vagina

mental Relating to the mind; something that exists in the mind or is done by the mind

mental health The person copes with and adjusts to everyday stresses in ways accepted by society

mental illness A disturbance in the ability to cope with or adjust to stress; behavior and function are impaired; mental disorder, emotional illness, psychiatric disorder

metabolism The burning of food for heat and energy by the cells

metastasis The spread of cancer to other body parts

microbe See "microorganism"

microorganism A small (micro) living plant or animal (organism) seen only with a microscope; a microbe

mixed incontinence Having more than one type of incontinence

N

need Something necessary or desired for maintaining life and mental well-being

neglect Failure to provide the person with the goods or services needed to avoid physical harm, mental anguish, or mental illness

negligence An unintentional wrong in which a person did not act in a reasonable and careful manner and a person or the person's property was harmed

nocturia Frequent urination (uria) at night (noct)

non-pathogen A microbe that does not usually cause an infection

nonverbal communication Communication that does not use words

nursing assistant A person who has passed a nursing assistant training and competency evaluation program; performs delegated nursing tasks under the supervision of a licensed nurse

nursing care plan A written guide about the person's care; care plan

nursing center A long-term care center that provides health care services to persons who need regular or continuous care; nursing facility or nursing home

nursing facility See "nursing center"

nursing home See "nursing center"

nursing process The method nurses use to plan and deliver nursing care; its five steps are assessment, nursing diagnosis, planning, implementation, and evaluation

nursing task Nursing care or a nursing function, procedure, activity, or work that can be delegated to nursing assistants when it does not require an RN's professional knowledge or judgment

nursing team Those who provide nursing care—RNs, LPNs/LVNs, and nursing assistants

nutrition The processes involved in the ingestion, digestion, absorption, and use of foods and fluids by the body

O

objective data Information that is seen, heard, felt, or smelled by an observer; signs

observation Using the senses of sight, hearing, touch, and smell to collect information

obsession A recurrent, unwanted thought, idea, or image

old Persons between 75 and 84 years of age

old-old Persons 85 years of age and older

oliguria Scant amount (olig) of urine (uria); less than 500 mL in 24 hours

ombudsman Someone who supports or promotes the needs and interests of another person

Omnibus Budget Reconciliation Act of 1987 (OBRA) A federal law requiring that nursing centers provide care in a manner and in a setting that maintains or improves each person's quality of life, health, and safety

oral hygiene Mouth care

organ Groups of tissues with the same function

orthopnea Breathing (pnea) deeply and comfortably only when sitting (ortho)

orthopneic position Sitting up (ortho) and leaning over a table to breathe

orthostatic hypotension Abnormally low (hypo) blood pressure when the person suddenly stands up (ortho and static); postural hypotension

ostomy A surgically created opening; see "colostomy" and "ileostomy"

output The amount of fluid lost

overflow incontinence Small amounts of urine leak from a bladder that is always full

P

pain To ache, hurt, or be sore

panic An intense and sudden feeling of fear, anxiety, terror, or dread

paralysis Loss of muscle function, loss of sensation, or loss of both muscle function and sensation

paranoia A disorder (para) of the mind (noia); false beliefs (delusions) and suspicion about a person or situation

paraplegia Paralysis in the legs and trunk

pathogen A microbe that is harmful and can cause an infection

pediculosis Infestation with wingless insects; lice

perineal care Cleaning the genital and anal areas; peri-care

peristalsis Involuntary muscle contractions in the digestive system that move food down the esophagus through the alimentary canal

phobia An intense fear

physical restraint Any manual method or physical or mechanical device, material, or equipment attached to or near the person's body that he or she cannot remove easily and which restricts freedom of movement or normal access to one's body

plantar flexion The foot *(plantar)* is bent *(flexion)*; bending the foot down at the ankle

polyuria Abnormally large amounts *(poly)* of urine *(uria)*

post-mortem care Care of the body after *(post)* death *(mortem)*

postural hypotension See "orthostatic hypotension"

posture See "body alignment"

pressure ulcer A localized injury to the skin and/or underlying tissue usually over a bony prominence; the result of pressure or pressure in combination with shear and/or friction

priority The most important thing at the time

professional boundary That which separates helpful behaviors from those that are not helpful

professionalism Following laws, being ethical, having good work ethics, and having the skills to do your work

professional sexual misconduct An act, behavior, or comment that is sexual in nature

pronation Turning the joint downward

prone position Lying on the abdomen with the head turned to one side

prosthesis An artificial replacement for a missing body part

protected health information Identifying information and information about the person's health care that is maintained or sent in any form (paper, electronic, oral)

pseudodementia False *(pseudo)* dementia

psychosis A state of severe mental impairment

pulse The beat of the heart felt at an artery as a wave of blood passes through the artery

pulse rate The number of heartbeats or pulses felt in 1 minute

Q

quadriplegia Paralysis in the arms, legs, and trunk; tetraplegia

R

range of motion (ROM) The movement of a joint to the extent possible without causing pain

recording The written account of care and observations; charting

reflex incontinence The loss of urine at predictable intervals when the bladder is full

registered nurse (RN) A nurse who has completed a 2-, 3-, or 4-year nursing program and has passed a licensing test

regurgitation The backward flow of stomach contents into the mouth

rehabilitation The process of restoring the person to his or her highest possible level of physical, psychological, social, and economic function

reincarnation The belief that the spirit or soul is reborn in another human body or in another form of life

religion Spiritual beliefs, needs, and practices

remove easily The manual method device, material, or equipment used to restrain the person that can be removed intentionally by the person in the same manner it was applied by the staff

reporting The oral account of care and observations

respiration The process of supplying the cells with oxygen and removing carbon dioxide from them; breathing air into *(inhalation)* and out of *(exhalation)* the lungs

respiratory arrest Breathing stops but heart action continues for several minutes

restorative aide A nursing assistant with special training in restorative nursing and rehabilitation skills

restorative nursing care Care that helps persons regain health, strength, and independence

reverse Trendelenburg's position The head of the bed is raised and the foot of the bed is lowered

rigor mortis The stiffness or rigidity *(rigor)* of skeletal muscles that occurs after death *(mortis)*

rotation Turning the joint

S

scabies A skin disorder caused by a female mite—a very small spider-like organism

seizure Violent and sudden contractions or tremors of muscle groups; convulsion

self-neglect A person's behaviors that threaten his or her health and safety

semi-Fowler's position The head of the bed is raised 30 degrees; or the head of the bed is raised 30 degrees and the knee portion is raised 15 degrees

semi-prone side position See "Sims' position"

sexuality The physical, emotional, social, cultural, and spiritual factors that affect a person's feelings and attitudes about his or her sex

shearing When skin sticks to a surface while muscles slide in the direction the body is moving

shock Results when organs and tissues do not get enough blood

side-lying position See "lateral position"

signs See "objective data"

Sims' position A left side-lying position in which the upper leg is sharply flexed so it is not on the lower leg and the lower arm is behind the person; semi-prone side position

skilled nursing facility (SNF) A long-term care center that provides complex care for severe health problems

skin tear A break or rip in the skin; the epidermis (top skin layer) separates from the underlying tissues

slander Making false statements orally

sleep deprivation The amount and quality of sleep are decreased

sleep-walking The sleeping person leaves the bed and walks about

sputum Mucus from the respiratory system that is expectorated *(expelled)* through the mouth

sterile The absence of *all* microbes

sterilization The process of destroying *all* microbes

stoma An opening; see "colostomy" and "ileostomy"

stool Excreted feces

stress The response or change in the body caused by any emotional, physical, social, or economic factor

stress incontinence When urine leaks during exercise and certain movements that cause pressure on the bladder

subacute care Complex medical care or rehabilitation when hospital care is no longer needed

subjective data Things a person tells you about that you cannot observe through your senses; symptoms

sudden cardiac arrest (SCA) The heart stops suddenly and without warning; cardiac arrest

suffocation When breathing stops from the lack of oxygen

suicide To kill oneself

suicide contagion Exposure to suicide or suicidal behaviors within one's family, one's peer group, or media reports of suicide

sundowning Signs, symptoms, and behaviors of Alzheimer's disease (AD) increase during hours of darkness

supination Turning the joint upward

supine position The back-lying position or dorsal recumbent position

suppository A cone-shaped, solid drug that is inserted into a body opening; it melts at body temperature

symptoms See "subjective data"

system Organs that work together to perform special functions

systolic pressure The pressure in the arteries when the heart contracts

T

tachypnea Rapid *(tachy)* breathing *(pnea);* respirations are more than 20 per minute

teamwork Staff members work together as a group; each person does his or her part to provide safe and effective care

terminal illness An illness or injury from which the person will not likely recover

tetraplegia See "quadriplegia"

tissue A group of cells with similar functions

transfer Moving the person from one place to another

transfer belt A device used to support a person who is unsteady or disabled; gait belt

Trendelenburg's position The head of the bed is lowered and the foot of the bed is raised

tumor A new growth of abnormal cells

U

ulcer A shallow or deep crater-like sore of the skin or a mucous membrane

urge incontinence The loss of urine in response to a sudden, urgent need to void; the person cannot get to a toilet in time

urinary frequency Voiding at frequent intervals

urinary incontinence The involuntary loss or leakage of urine

urinary urgency The need to void at once

urination The process of emptying urine from the bladder; voiding

V

vein A blood vessel that returns blood to the heart

verbal communication Communication that uses written or spoken words

vital signs Temperature, pulse, respirations, and blood pressure

voiding See "urination"

vomitus The food and fluids expelled from the stomach through the mouth; emesis

vulnerable adult A person 18 years old or older who has a disability or condition that makes him or her at risk to be wounded, attacked, or damaged

W

withdrawal syndrome The person's physical and mental response after stopping or severely reducing the use of a substance that was used regularly

work ethics Behavior in the workplace

workplace violence Violent acts (including assault and threat of assault) directed toward persons at work or while on duty

wound A break in the skin or mucous membrane

Y

young-old Persons between 65 and 74 years of age

KEY ABBREVIATIONS

A
AD Alzheimer's disease
ADL Activities of daily living
AED Automated external defibrillator
AHA American Heart Association
AIDS Acquired immunodeficiency syndrome
AIIR Airborne infection isolation room
ALR Assisted living residence
ALS Amyotrophic lateral sclerosis

B
BLS Basic Life Support
BM Bowel movement
BPH Benign prostatic hyperplasia

C
C Centigrade
CAD Coronary artery disease
CDC Centers for Disease Control and Prevention
CHF Congestive heart failure
CMS Centers for Medicare & Medicaid Services
CNA Certified nursing assistant; certified nurse aide
CO$_2$ Carbon dioxide
COPD Chronic obstructive pulmonary disease
CPR Cardiopulmonary resuscitation
CVA Cerebrovascular accident

D
DON Director of nursing
DNR Do not resuscitate

E
EMS Emergency Medical Services

F
F Fahrenheit
FBAO Foreign-body airway obstruction
FDA Food and Drug Administration

G
GI Gastro-intestinal

H
HAI Healthcare-associated infection
HBV Hepatitis B virus
Hg Mercury
HIPAA Health Insurance Portability and Accountability Act of 1996
HIV Human immunodeficiency virus
HMO Health maintenance organization

I
ID Identification
I&O Intake and output
IV Intravenous

L
L/min Liters per minute
LPN Licensed practical nurse
LVN Licensed vocational nurse

M
MDRO Multidrug-resistant organism
MDS Minimum Data Set
mg Milligram

MI Myocardial infarction
mL Milliliter
mm Millimeter
mm Hg Millimeters of mercury
MRSA Methicillin-resistant *Staphylococcus aureus*
MS Multiple sclerosis
MSD Musculoskeletal disorder
MS-DRG Medicare Severity-adjusted Diagnosis Related Group
MSDS Material safety data sheet

N
NANDA-I North American Nursing Diagnosis Association International
NATCEP Nursing assistant training and competency evaluation program
NCSBN National Council of State Boards of Nursing
NG Naso-gastric
NPO Non per os; nothing by mouth

O
O$_2$ Oxygen
OBRA Omnibus Budget Reconciliation Act of 1987
OPIM Other potentially infectious materials
OSHA Occupational Safety and Health Administration
oz Ounce

P
PDA Personal digital assistant
PHI Protected health information
PPE Personal protective equipment
PPO Preferred provider organization
PTSD Post-traumatic stress disorder

R
RA Rheumatoid arthritis
RAPs Resident Assessment Protocols
RBC Red blood cell
RN Registered nurse
ROM Range of motion
RRT Rapid Response Team
RUG Resource utilization group

S
SCA Sudden cardiac arrest
SNF Skilled nursing facility
SSE Soapsuds enema
STD Sexually transmitted disease

T
TB Tuberculosis
TBI Traumatic brain injury
TIA Transient ischemic attack
TJC The Joint Commission

U
UTI Urinary tract infection

V
VF Ventricular fibrillation
V-fib Ventricular fibrillation
VRE Vancomycin-resistant *Enterococcus*

W
WBC White blood cell

INDEX

Page numbers followed by f indicate figures,
t tables, and b boxes.